Handbook of

Pharmaceutical Manufacturing Formulations

Handbook of Pharmaceutical Manufacturing Formulations Second Edition

Volume Series

Sarfaraz K. Niazi

Volume 1
Handbook of Pharmaceutical Manufacturing Formulations: Compressed Solid Products

Volume 2
Handbook of Pharmaceutical Manufacturing Formulations: Uncompressed Solid Products

Volume 3
Handbook of Pharmaceutical Manufacturing Formulations: Liquid Products

Volume 4
Handbook of Pharmaceutical Manufacturing Formulations: Semisolid Products

Volume 5
Handbook of Pharmaceutical Manufacturing Formulations: Over-the-Counter Products

Volume 6
Handbook of Pharmaceutical Manufacturing Formulations: Sterile Products

VOLUME THREE

Second Edition

Handbook of Pharmaceutical Manufacturing Formulations

Liquid Products

SARFARAZ K. NIAZI

Pharmaceutical Scientist, Inc.
Deerfield, Illinois, USA

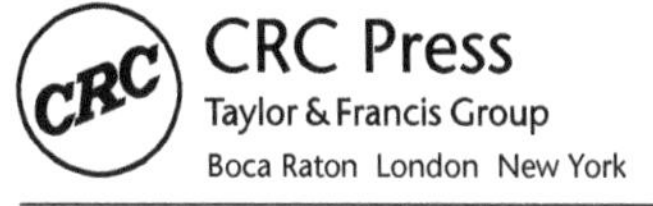

CRC Press is an imprint of the
Taylor & Francis Group, an **informa** business

CRC Press
Taylor & Francis Group
6000 Broken Sound Parkway NW, Suite 300
Boca Raton, FL 33487-2742

First issued in paperback 2017

ISBN 13: 978-1-138-11379-4 (pbk)
ISBN 13: 978-1-4200-8123-7 (hbk)

Library of Congress Cataloging-in-Publication Data

Niazi, Sarfaraz, 1949–
Handbook of pharmaceutical manufacturing formulations /
Sarfaraz K. Niazi. – 2nd ed.
p. ; cm.
Includes bibliographical references and index.
ISBN-13: 978-1-4200-8106-0 (set) (hardcover : alk. paper)
ISBN-10: 1-4200-8106-3 (set) (hardcover : alk. paper)
ISBN-13: 978-1-4200-8116-9 (v. 1) (hardcover : alk. paper)
ISBN-10: 1-4200-8116-0 (v. 1) (hardcover : alk. paper)
[etc.]
1. Drugs–Dosage forms–Handbooks, manuals, etc. I. Title.
[DNLM: 1. Drug Compounding–Handbooks. 2. Dosage Forms–Handbooks.
3. Formularies as Topic–Handbooks. 4. Technology, Pharmaceutical–Handbooks.
QV 735 N577h 2009]
RS200.N53 2009
615′.19–dc22

2009009979

Visit the Taylor & Francis Web site at
http://www.taylorandfrancis.com

and the CRC Press Web site at
http://www.crcpress.com

to August P. Lemberger

Preface to the Series—Second Edition

The science and the art of pharmaceutical formulation keeps evolving as new materials, methods, and machines become readily available to produce more reliable, stable, and release-controlled formulations. At the same time, globalization of sourcing of raw and finished pharmaceuticals brings challenges to regulatory authorities and results in more frequent revisions to the current good manufacturing practices, regulatory approval dossier requirements, and the growing need for cost optimization. Since the publication of the first edition of this book, a lot has changed in all of these areas of importance to pharmaceutical manufacturers. The second edition builds on the dynamic nature of the science and art of formulations and provides an evermore useful handbook that should be highly welcomed by the industry, the regulatory authorities, as well as the teaching institutions.

The first edition of this book was a great success as it brought under one umbrella the myriad of choices available to formulators. The readers were very responsive and communicated with me frequently pointing out to the weaknesses as well as the strengths of the book. The second edition totally revised attempts to achieve these by making major changes to the text, some of which include:

1. Complete, revised errors corrected and subject matter reorganized for easy reference. Whereas this series has six volumes differentiated on the basis of the type of dosage form and a separate inclusion of the U.S. OTC products, ideally the entire collection is needed to benefit from the myriad of topics relating to formulations, regulatory compliance, and dossier preparation.
2. Total number of pages is increased from 1684 to 2726.
3. Total number of formulations is expanded by about 30% with many newly approved formulations.
4. Novel formulations are now provided for a variety of drugs; these data are collected from the massive intellectual property data and suggest toward the future trend of formulations. While some of these formulations may not have been approved in the United States or Europe, these do provide additional choices, particularly for the NDA preparation. As always, it is the responsibility of the manufacturer to assure that the intellectual property rights are not violated.
5. A significant change in this edition is the inclusion of commercial products; while most of this information is culled out from the open source such as the FOIA (http://www.fda.gov/foi/default.htm), I have made attempts to reconstruct the critical portions of it based on what I call the generally acceptable standards. The drug companies are advised to assure that any intellectual property rights are not violated and this applies to all information contained in this book. The freedom of information act (FOIA) is an extremely useful conduit for reliable information and manufacturers are strongly urged to make use of this information. Whereas this information is provided free of charge, the process of obtaining the information may be cumbersome, in which case, commercial sources of these databases can prove useful, particularly for the non-U.S. companies.
6. Also included are the new Good Manufacturing Guidelines (2007) with amendments (2008) for the United States and similar updates for European Union and WHO; it is strongly urged that the companies discontinue using all old documents as there are significant changes in the revised form, and many of them are likely to reduce the cost of GMP compliance.
7. Details on design of clean rooms is a new entry that will be of great use to sterile product manufacturers; whereas the design and flow of personnel and material flow is of critical nature, regulatory agencies view these differently and the manufacturer is advised always to comply with most stringent requirements.
8. Addition of a self-auditing template in each volume of the series. While the cGMP compliance is a complex issue and the requirements diversified across the globe, the basic compliance remains universal. I have chosen the European Union guidelines (as these are more in tune with the ICH) to prepare a self-audit module that I recommend that every manufacturer adopt as a routine to assure GMP compliance. In most instances reading the template by those responsible for compliance with keep them sensitive to the needs of GMP.
9. OTC products cross-referenced in other volumes where appropriate. This was necessary since the regulatory authorities worldwide define this class of drug differently. It is important to iterate that regardless of the prescription or the OTC status of a product, the requirements for compliance with the cGMP apply equally.
10. OTC monograph status is a new section added to the OTC volume and this should allow manufacturers to chose appropriate formulations that may not require a filing with the regulatory agencies; it is important to iterate that an approved OTC monograph includes details of formulation including the types and quantities of active drug and excipients, labeling, and presentation. To qualify the exemption, the manufacturer must comply with the monograph in its entirety. However, subtle modifications that are merely cosmetic in nature and where there is an evidence that the modification will not affect the safety and efficacy of the products can be made but require prior approval of the regulatory agencies and generally these approvals are granted.
11. Expanded discussion on critical factors in the manufacturing of formulations provided; from basic shortcuts to smart modifications now extend to all dosage forms. Pharmaceutical compounding is one of the oldest professions and whereas the art of formulations has been

relegated to more objective parameters, the art nevertheless remains. An experienced formulator, like an artist, would know what goes with what and why; he avoids the pitfalls and stays with conservative choices. These sections of the book present advice that is time tested, although it may appear random at times; this is intended for experienced formulators.

12. Expanded details on critical steps in the manufacturing processes provided but to keep the size of the book manageable, and these are included for prototype formulations. The reader is advised to browse through similar formulations to gain more insight. Where multiple formulations are provided for the same drug, it intended to show the variety of possibilities in formulating a drug and whereas it pertains to a single drug, the basic formulation practices can be extended to many drugs of same class or even of diversified classes. Readers have often requested that more details be provided in the Manufacturing Direction sections. Whereas sufficient details are provided, this is restricted to prototype formulations to keep the size of the book manageable and to reduce redundancy.
13. Addition of a listing of approved excipients and the level allowed by regulatory authorities. This new section allows formulators a clear choice on which excipients to choose; the excipients are reported in each volume pertaining to the formulation type covered. The listing is drawn from the FDA-approved entities. For the developers of an ANDA, it is critical that the level of excipients be kept within the range generally approved to avoid large expense in justifying any unapproved level. The only category for which the listing is not provided separately is the OTC volume since it contains many dosage forms and the reader is referred to dosage form–specific title of the series. The choice of excipients forms keeps increasing with many new choices that can provide many special release characteristics to the dosage forms. Choosing correct excipients is thus a tedious exercise and requires sophisticated multivariate statistical analysis. Whereas the formulator may choose any number of novel or classical components, it is important to know the levels of excipients that are generally allowed in various formulations to reduce the cost of redundant exercises; I have therefore included, as an appendix to each volume, a list of all excipients that are currently approved by the U.S. FDA along their appropriate levels. I suggest that a formulator consult this table before deciding on which level of excipient to use; it does not mean that the excipient cannot be used outside this range but it obviates the need for a validation and lengthy justification studies in the submission of NDAs.
14. Expanded section on bioequivalence submission was required to highlight the recent changes in these requirements. New entries include a comprehensive listing of bioequivalence protocols in abbreviated form as approved by the U.S. FDA; these descriptions are provided in each volume where pertinent. To receive approval for an ANDA, an applicant must generally demonstrate, among other things, equivalence of the active ingredient, dosage form, strength, route of administration and conditions of use as the listed drug, and that the proposed drug product is bioequivalent to the reference listed drug [21 USC 355(j)(2)(A); 21 CFR 314.94(a)]. Bioequivalent drug products show no significant difference in the rate and extent of absorption of the therapeutic ingredient [21 U.S.C. 355(j)(8); 21 CFR 320.1(e)]. BE studies are undertaken in support of ANDA submissions with the goal of demonstrating BE between a proposed generic drug product and its reference listed drug. The regulations governing BE are provided at 21 CFR in part 320. The U.S. FDA has recently begun to promulgate individual bioequivalence requirements. To streamline the process for making guidance available to the public on how to design product-specific BE studies, the U.S. FDA will be issuing product-specific BE recommendations (www.fda.gov/cder/ogd/index.htm). To make this vital information available, an appendix to each volume includes a summary of all currently approved products by the U.S. FDA where a recommendation on conducting bioequivalence studies is made available by the U.S. FDA. When filing an NDA or an ANDA, the filer is faced with the choice of defending the methods used to justify the bioavailability or bioequivalence data. The U.S. FDA now allows application for waiver of bioequivalence requirement; a new chapter on this topic has been added along with details of the dissolution tests, where applicable, approved for various dosage forms.
15. Dissolution testing requirements are included for all dosage forms where this testing is required by the FDA. Surrogate testing to prove efficacy and compliance is getting more acceptance at regulatory agencies; in my experience, a well-designed dissolution test is the best measure of continuous compliance. Coupled with chapters on waivers of bioequivalence testing, this information on dissolution testing should be great value to all manufacturers; it is recommended that manufacturers develop their own in-house specifications, more stringent than those allowed in these listings and the USP.
16. Best-selling products (top 200 prescription products) are identified with an asterisk and a brand name where applicable; in all instances, composition of these products is provided and formulation of generic equivalents. Despite the vast expansion of pharmaceutical sales and shifting of categories of blockbuster drugs, basic drugs affecting gastrointestinal tract, vascular system, and brain remain most widely prescribed.
17. Updated list of approved coloring agents in the United States, Canada, European Union, and Japan is included to allow manufactures to design products for worldwide distribution.
18. Tablet-coating formulations that meet worldwide requirements of color selection are included in the Volume 1 (compressed solids) and Volume 5 (OTC) because these represent the products often coated.
19. Guidelines on preparing regulatory filings are now dispersed throughout the series depending on where these guidelines are more crucial. However, the reader would, as before, need access to all volumes to benefit from the advice and guidelines provided.

As always, comments and criticism from the readers are welcomed and these can be sent to me at Niazi@pharmsci.com or Niazi@niazi.com. I would try to respond to any inquiries requiring clarification of the information enclosed in these volumes.

I would like to express deep gratitude to Sherri R. Niziolek and Michelle Schmitt-DeBonis at Informa, the publisher of this work, for seeing an immediate value to the readers in publishing the second edition of this book and allowing me enough time to prepare this work. The diligent editing and composing staff at Informa, particularly Joseph Stubenrauch, Baljinder Kaur and others are highly appreciated. Regardless, all errors and omissions remain altogether mine.

In the first edition, I had dedicated each volume to one of my mentors; the second edition continues the dedication to these great teachers.

Sarfaraz K. Niazi, Ph.D.
Deerfield, Illinois, U.S.A.

Preface to the Series—First Edition

No industry in the world is more highly regulated than the pharmaceutical industry because of the potential threat to a patient's life from the use of pharmaceutical products. The cost of taking a new chemical entity to final regulatory approval is a staggering $800 million, making the pharmaceutical industry one of the most research-intensive industries in the world. It is anticipated that the industry will spend about $20 billion on research and development in 2004. Because patent protection on a number of drugs is expiring, the generic drug market is becoming one of the fastest growing segments of the pharmaceutical industry with every major multinational company having a significant presence in this field.

Many stages of new drug development are inherently constrained by time, but the formulation of drugs into desirable dosage forms remains an area where expediency can be practiced by those who have mastered the skills of pharmaceutical formulations. The *Handbook of Pharmaceutical Manufacturing Formulations* is the first major attempt to consolidate the available knowledge about formulations into a comprehensive and, by nature, rather voluminous presentation.

The book is divided into six volumes based strictly on the type of formulation science involved in the development of these dosage forms: sterile products, compressed solids, uncompressed solids, liquid products, semisolid products, and over-the-counter (OTC) products. Although they may easily fall into one of the other five categories, OTC products are considered separately to comply with the industry norms of separate research divisions for OTC products. Sterile products require skills related to sterilization of the product, and of less importance is the bioavailability issue, which is an inherent problem of compressed dosage forms. These types of considerations have led to the classification of pharmaceutical products into these six categories. Each volume includes a description of regulatory filing techniques for the formulations described. Also included are regulatory guidelines on complying with current good manufacturing practices (cGMPs) specific to the dosage form and advice is offered on how to scale up the production batches.

It is expected that formulation scientists will use this information to benchmark their internal development protocols and reduce the time required to file by adopting formulae that have survived the test of time. Many of us who have worked in the pharmaceutical industry suffer from a fixed paradigm when it comes to selecting formulations: "Not invented here" perhaps is kept in the back of the minds of many seasoned formulations scientists when they prefer certain platforms for development. It is expected that with a quick review of the formulation possibilities that are made available in this book such scientists would benefit from the experience of others. For teachers of formulation sciences, this series offers a wealth of information. Whether it is selection of a preservative system or the choice of a disintegrant, the series offers many choices to study and consider.

Sarfaraz K. Niazi, Ph.D.
Deerfield, Illinois, U.S.A.

Preface to the Volume—First Edition

Liquid products, for the purpose of inclusion in this volume, include nonsterile drugs administered by any route in the form of solutions (monomeric and multimeric), suspensions (powder and liquid), drops, extracts, elixirs, tinctures, paints, sprays, colloidons, emulsions, aerosols, and other fluid preparations. Sterile liquid products are presented in another volume. Whereas liquid drugs do not share the compression problems of solid dosage forms, the filling problems of powder dosage forms, and the consistency problems of semisolid dosage forms, they do have their own set of considerations in the formulation and manufacturing stages. The considerations of prime importance for liquid drugs include solubility of active drugs, preservation, taste masking, viscosity, flavoring, appearance, and stability (chemical, physical, and microbiological), raw materials, equipment, the compounding procedures (often the order of mixing), and finally the packaging (to allow a stable product to reach patients). Suspensions present a special situation in which even the powder for reconstitution needs to be formulated such that it can be stable after reconstitution; therefore, limited examples are included here.

Chapter 1 in section I (Regulatory and Manufacturing Guidance) describes the practical details in complying with the current good manufacturing practice (cGMP) requirements in liquid manufacturing. This chapter does not address the specific cGMP parameters but deals with the practical aspects as may arise during a U.S. Food and Drug Administration (FDA) inspection. This includes what an FDA inspector would be looking into when auditing a liquid manufacturing facility.

Chapter 2 describes the stability testing of new drugs and dosage forms. Drawn from the most current international conference on harmonization (ICH) guidelines, this chapter describes in detail the protocols used for stability testing not only for new drugs but also for new dosage forms. The chapter is placed in this volume because stability studies are of greater concern in liquid dosage forms; however, keeping in mind the overall perspective of the series of this title, this chapter would apply to all dosage forms. Again, emphasis is placed on the practical aspects, and the reader is referred to official guidelines for the development of complete testing protocols. It is noteworthy that the ICH guidelines divide the world into four zones; the discussion given in this chapter mainly refers to the U.S. and European regions, and again the formulator is referred to the original guideline for full guidance. Stability studies constitute one of the most expensive phases of product development because of their essential time investment. As a result, formulators often prepare a matrix of formulations to condense the development phase, particularly where there are known issues in compatibility, drug interactions, and packaging interactions. The FDA is always very helpful in this phase of study protocols, particularly where a generic drug is involved. It is also a good idea to benchmark the product against the innovator product. However, one should understand clearly that the FDA is not bound to accept stability data even though it might match that of the innovator product. The reason for this may lie in the improvements made since the innovator product was approved. For example, if a better packaging material that imparts greater safety and shelf life is available, the FDA would like this to be used (not for the purpose of shelf life, but for the safety factors). In recent years, the FDA has placed greater emphasis on the control of active pharmaceutical ingredient (API), particularly if it is sourced from a new manufacturer with a fresh DMF. Obviously, this is one way how the innovator controls the proliferation of generic equivalents. The original patents that pertain to synthesis or manufacturing of the active raw material may have been superseded by improved processes that are not likely to be a part of a later patent application (to protect the trade secret because of double-patenting issues). The innovator often goes on to revise the specifications of the active pharmaceutical ingredient to the detriment of the generic manufacturer. However, my experience tells me that such changes are not necessarily binding on the generic manufacturer, and as long as cGMP compliance in the API is demonstrated and the impurities do not exceed the reference standard (if one is available), there is no need to be concerned about this aspect. However, manufacturers are advised to seek a conference with the FDA should this be a serious concern. At times, the manufacturer changes the finished product specification as the patents expire or reformulates the product under a new patent. A good example of this practice was the reformulation of calcitriol injection by Abbott as its patent came to expiry. The new specifications include a tighter level of heavy metals, but a generic manufacturer should have no problem if the original specifications are met because the product was approvable with those specifications.

Chapter 3 describes the container closure systems; again, this discussion would apply to all dosage forms. It is noteworthy that the regulatory agencies consider containers and packaging systems, all those components that come in contact with the product, protect the product from environment, or are instrumental in the delivery of the product as part of the product definition. Whereas the industry is much attuned to studies of the effects of the API and dosage formulation components, the study of container or closure systems is often left to the end of the study trials. This is an imprudent practice, as it might result in loss of valuable time. The packaging industry generally undergoes faster changes than do the chemical or pharmaceutical industries. New materials, better tolerances, more environmentally friendly materials, and now, with the use of mechanical devices in many dosage forms, appropriate dosing systems emerge routinely. As a rule of thumb, the closure system for a product should be the first criterion selected before development of the dosage form. Switching between a glass and a plastic bottle at a later stage can be a very expensive exercise. Because many of these considerations are drawn by marketing teams, who may change their product positioning, the formulation team must be appropriately represented in marketing decision conferences. Once a decision has been made about the presentation of a product, the product development team should prepare several alternatives, based on the ease of formulation and the cost of the finished product involved. It should be emphasized at all stages of development that packaging scale-ups require just as much work as does a formulation scale-up or changes. As a result, the FDA provides the scale-up and postapproval change (SUPAC) guidelines for packaging components. Changes in the dimensions of a bottle may expose a large surface of liquid to the gaseous phase in the bottle and thus require a new stability testing exercise. This chapter forms an important reminder to formulators on the need to give consideration to every aspect of the container closure system as part of routine development.

Chapter 4 introduces the area of Preapproval Inspections, a process initiated by the FDA in the wake of the grand scandals in the generic pharmaceutical industry a few years ago. The FDA guidelines now allow "profiling" of companies and list the requirements of Preapproval Inspections when an application has been filed. Whereas the emphasis in this chapter is on "preapproval," the advice provided here applies to all regulatory inspections. A regulatory inspection can be an arduous exercise if the company has not prepared for it continuously. Preparedness for inspection is not something that can be achieved through a last-minute crash program. This chapter goes into considerable detail on how to create a cGMP culture, how to examine the documentary needs, assignment of responsibility, preparation of validation plan, and above all, the art of presenting the data to the FDA. Also discussed are the analyses of the outcome of inspection. Advice is provided on how to respond to Form 483 issued by the FDA, and the manufacturer is warned of the consequences of failing an inspection. Insight is also provided for foreign manufacturers, for whom a different set of rules may be applied because of the physical constraints of inspection. The inspection guidelines provided apply to both the manufacturers of API as well as to the finished products.

Chapter 5 includes highlights of topics of importance in the formulation of liquid products. However, this chapter is not an all-inclusive guide to formulation. Only highlights of points of concern are presented here, and the formulator is referred to several excellent treatises available on the subject.

Section II contains formulations of liquid products and lists a wide range of products that fall under this classification, as interpreted in the volume. There are three levels at which these formulations are described. First, the Bill of Materials is accompanied by detailed manufacturing directions; second, the manufacturing directions are abbreviated because they are already described in another product of similar nature; and third, only the composition is provided as supplied by the manufacturer. With the wide range of formulations included in this volume, it should be a simple matter for an experienced formulator to convert these formulations into quantitative Bills of Materials and then to benchmark it against similar formulations to come up with a working formula. The problems incumbent in the formulation of liquid products are highlighted in chapter 5, but these are generic problems, and the formulator should be aware of any specific situations or problems that may arise from time to time. I would like to hear from the formulators about these problems so that they could be included in future editions of this book. Again, the emphasis in this series is on a practical resolution of problems; the theoretical teachings are left to other, more comprehensive works on this topic. The key application of the data provided herein is to allow the formulator to select the ingredients that are reportedly compatible, avoiding need for long-term studies to establish compatibilities.

I am grateful to CRC Press for taking this lead in publishing what is possibility the largest such work in the field of pharmaceutical products. It has been a distinct privilege to know Mr. Stephen Zollo, senior editor at CRC Press. Stephen has done more than any editor can do to encourage an author into completing this work on a timely basis. The editorial assistance provided by CRC Press staff was indeed exemplary, particularly the help given by Erika Dery, Amy Rodriguez, and others. Although much care has gone into correcting errors, any errors remaining are altogether mine. I shall appreciate the readers bringing these to my attention for correction in future editions of this volume (niazi@pharmsci.com).

This volume is dedicated to one of the great educators and a leader in the pharmaceutical profession, August P. Lemberger, who is truly a Wisconsin man. At the University of Wisconsin in Madison, he was an undergraduate and graduate student. He was then a professor, and twice Dean of the School of Pharmacy (1943–44, 1946–52, 1953–69, 1980–91). During the period between 1969 and 1980, he assumed the responsibility of deanship at the University of Illinois, where I was a graduate student. In 1972, he offered me my first teaching job, as an instructor of pharmacy at the University of Illinois, while I was still in graduate school. I was one of the greatest beneficiaries of his kindness and attention. Gus has an unusual ability to put everyone at ease, respect everyone around him, and in the end, come out as a group leader. Whatever little I have accomplished in my life is mostly because of Gus. Many awards, recognitions, and salutations were offered to Gus during his celebrated career. His research contributions included stability studies, suspension, emulsion stabilization, and later in his career, the various aspects of pharmaceutical education. I wish him many years of happy retirement and shuttling back and forth between his homes in Arizona and Wisconsin. Thanks, Gus.

Sarfaraz K. Niazi, Ph.D.
Deerfield, Illinois, U.S.A.

About the Author

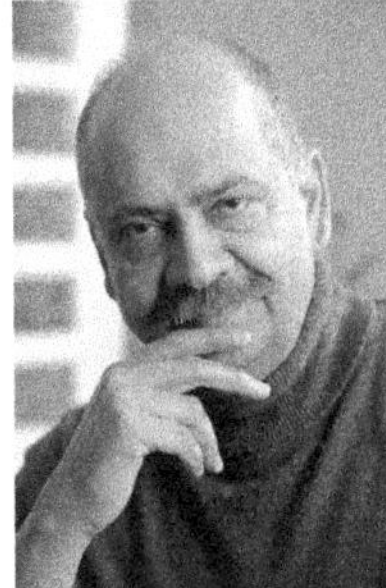

Sarfaraz K. Niazi has been teaching and conducting research in the pharmaceutical industry for over 35 years. He has authored hundreds of scientific papers, textbooks, and presentations on the topics of pharmaceutical formulation, biopharmaceutics, and pharmacokinetics of drugs. He is also an inventor with scores of patents in the field of drug and dosage form delivery systems; he is also licensed to practice law before the U.S. Patent and Trademark Office. Having formulated hundreds of products from the most popular consumer entries to complex biotechnology-derived products, he has accumulated a wealth of knowledge in the science and art of formulating and regulatory filings of investigational new drugs (INDs) and new drug applications (NDAs). Dr. Niazi advises the pharmaceutical industry internationally on issues related to formulations, cGMP compliance, pharmacokinetics and bioequivalence evaluation, and intellectual property issues (http://www.pharmsci.com). He can be contacted at Niazi@pharmsci.com.

Contents

Part I

Regulatory and Manufacturing Guidance

1

Manufacturing Practice Considerations in Liquid Formulations

I. INTRODUCTION

The manufacture and control of oral solutions and oral suspensions presents some unusual problems not common to other dosage forms. Although bioequivalency concerns are minimal (except for products in which dissolution is a rate-limiting or absorption-determining step, as in phenytoin suspension), other issues have frequently led to recalls of liquid products. These include microbiological, potency, and stability problems. In addition, because the population using these oral dosage forms includes newborns, pediatrics, and geriatrics, who may not be able to take oral solid dosage forms and who may have compromised drug metabolic or other clearance function, defective dosage forms can pose a greater risk if the absorption profiles are significantly altered from the profiles used in the development of drug safety profiles.

II. FACILITIES

The designs of the facilities are largely dependent on the type of products manufactured and the potential for cross-contamination and microbiological contamination. For example, the facilities used for the manufacture of over-the-counter oral products might not require the isolation that a steroid or sulfa product would require. However, the concern for contamination remains, and it is important to isolate processes that generate dust (such as those processes occurring before the addition of solvents). The HVAC (heating, ventilation, and air-conditioning) system should be validated just as required for processing of potent drugs. Should a manufacturer rely mainly on recirculation rather than filtration or fresh air intake, efficiency of air filtration must be validated by surface and air sampling. It is advisable not to take any shortcuts in the design of HVAC systems, as it is often very difficult to properly validate a system that is prone to breakdown; in such instances a fully validated protocol would need stress testing—something that may be more expensive than establishing proper HVAC systems in the first place. However, it is also unnecessary to overdo it in designing the facilities, as once the drug is present in a solution form, cross-contamination to other products becomes a lesser problem. It is, nevertheless, important to protect the drug from other powder sources (such as by maintaining appropriate pressure differentials in various cubicles).

III. EQUIPMENT

Equipment should be of sanitary design. This includes sanitary pumps, valves, flow meters, and other equipment that can be easily sanitized. Ball valves, the packing in pumps, and pockets in flow meters have been identified as sources of contamination. Contamination is an extremely important consideration, particularly for those sourcing manufacturing equipment from less developed countries; manufacturers of equipment often offer two grades of equipment: sanitary equipment, and equipment not qualified as sanitary and offered at substantial savings. All manufacturers intending to ship any product subject to U.S. Food and Drug Administration (FDA) inspection must insist on certification that the equipment is of sanitary design.

To facilitate cleaning and sanitization, manufacturing and filling lines should be identified and detailed in drawings and standard operating procedures. Long delivery lines between manufacturing areas and filling areas can be a source of contamination. Special attention should be paid to developing standard operating procedures that clearly establish validated limits for this purpose.

Equipment used for batching and mixing of oral solutions and suspensions is relatively basic. These products are generally formulated on a weight basis, with the batching tank on load cells so that a final volume can be made by weight; if you have not done so already, consider converting your systems to weight basis. Volumetric means, such as using a dipstick or a line on a tank, are not generally as accurate and should be avoided where possible. When volumetric means are chosen, make sure they are properly validated at different temperature conditions and other factors that might render this practice faulty. In most cases, manufacturers assay samples of the bulk solution or suspension before filling. A much greater variability is found with those batches that have been manufactured volumetrically rather than those that have been manufactured by weight. Again, the rule of thumb is to avoid any additional validation if possible.

The design of the batching tank with regard to the location of the bottom discharge valve often presents problems. Ideally, the bottom discharge valve is flush with the bottom of the tank. In some cases, valves—including undesirable ball valves—are several inches to a foot below the bottom of the tank. This is not acceptable. It is possible that in this situation the drug or preservative may not completely dissolve and may get trapped in the "dead leg" below the tank, with initial samples turning out subpotent. For the manufacture of suspensions, valves should be flush.

Transfer lines are generally hard piped and are easily cleaned and sanitized. In situations where manufacturers use flexible hoses to transfer product, it is not unusual to see these hoses lying on the floor, thus significantly increasing the potential for contamination. Such contamination can occur through operators picking up or handling hoses, and possibly even through operators placing them in transfer or batching tanks after the hoses had been lying on the floor. It is a good practice to store hoses in a way that allows them to drain, rather than coiling them, which may allow moisture to collect and be a potential source of microbial contamination.

Another common problem occurs when manifold or common connections are used, especially in water supply, premix, or raw material supply tanks. Such common connections can be a major source of contamination.

IV. RAW MATERIALS

The physical characteristics, particularly the particle size of the drug substance, are very important for suspensions. As with topical products in which the drug is suspended, particles are usually very fine to micronize (to <25 microns). For syrup, elixir, or solution dosage forms in which there is nothing suspended, particle size and physical characteristics of raw materials are not that important. However, they can affect the rate of dissolution of such raw materials in the manufacturing process. Raw materials of a finer particle size may dissolve faster than those of a larger particle size when the product is compounded.

Examples of a few oral suspensions in which a specific and well-defined particle-size specification for the drug substance is important include phenytoin suspension, carbamazepine suspension, trimethoprim and sulfamethoxazole suspension, and hydrocortisone suspension. It is therefore a good idea to indicate particle size in the raw material specification, even though it is meant for dissolving in the processing, to better validate the manufacturing process while avoiding scale-up problems.

V. COMPOUNDING

In addition to a determination of the final volume (on weight or volume basis) as previously discussed, there are microbiological concerns, and these are well covered in other chapters in this book.

For oral suspensions there is the additional concern of uniformity, particularly because of the potential for segregation during manufacture and storage of the bulk suspension, during transfer to the filling line, and during filling. It is necessary to establish procedures and time limits for such operations to address the potential for segregation or settling as well as other unexpected effects that may be caused by extended holding or stirring.

For oral solutions and suspensions, the amount and control of temperature is important from a microbiological as well as a potency aspect. For those products in which temperature is identified as a critical part of the operation, the batch records must demonstrate compliance using control charts. There are some processes in manufacturing in which heat is used during compounding to control the microbiological levels in the product. For such products, the addition of purified water to make up to final volume, the batch, and the temperatures during processing should be properly documented.

In addition to drug substances, some additives such as the most commonly used preservatives, parabens are difficult to dissolve, and require heat (often to 80°C). The control and verification of their dissolution during the compounding stage should be established in the method validation. From a potency aspect, the storage of product at high temperatures may increase the level of degradants. Storage limitations (time and temperature) should be justified.

There are also some oral liquids that are sensitive to oxygen and that have been known to undergo degradation. This is particularly true of the phenothiazine class of drugs, such as perphenazine and chlorpromazine. The manufacture of such products might require the removal of oxygen, as by nitrogen purging. In addition, such products might also require storage in sealed tanks, rather than in those with loose lids. Manufacturing directions provided in this book are particularly detailed about the purging steps, and these should be closely observed.

VI. MICROBIOLOGICAL QUALITY

Microbiological contamination can present significant health hazards in some oral liquids. For example, some oral liquids, such as nystatin suspension, are used in infants and immunocompromised patients, and microbiological contamination with organisms (such as Gram-negative organisms) is not acceptable. There are other oral liquid preparations such as antacids in which *Pseudomonas* sp. contamination is also objectionable. For other oral liquids such as cough preparations, contamination with *Pseudomonas* sp. might not present the same health hazard. However, the presence of a specific *Pseudomonas* sp. may also indicate other plant or raw material contamination and often points to defects in the water systems and environmental breaches; extensive investigations are often required to trace the source of contamination. Obviously, the contamination of any preparation with Gram-negative organisms is not desirable.

In addition to the specific contaminant being objectionable, such contamination would be indicative of a deficient process as well as an inadequate preservative system. For example, the presence of a *Pseudomonas putida* contaminant could also indicate that *P. aeruginosa*, a similar source organism, is also present.

Because FDA laboratories typically use more sensitive test methods than industry, samples of oral liquids in which manufacturers report microbiological counts well within limits may be found unacceptable by the federal laboratories. This result requires upgrading the sensitivity of testing procedures.

VII. ORAL SUSPENSIONS

Liquid products in which the drug is suspended (not in solution) present some unique manufacturing and control problems. Depending on the viscosity, many suspensions require continuous or periodic agitation during the filling process. If delivery lines are used between the bulk storage tank and the filling equipment, some segregation may occur, particularly if the product is not viscous. Procedures must therefore be established for filling and diagrams established for line setup prior to the filling equipment.

Good manufacturing practice would warrant testing bottles from the beginning, middle, and end of a batch to ensure that segregation has not occurred. Such samples should not be combined for the purpose of analysis. In-process testing for suspensions might also include an assay of a sample from the bulk tank. More important at this stage, however, may be testing for viscosity.

VIII. PRODUCT SPECIFICATIONS

Important specifications for the manufacture of all solutions include assay and microbial limits. Additional important specifications for suspensions include particle size of the suspended drug, viscosity, pH, and in some cases, dissolution. Viscosity can be important, from a processing aspect, to minimize segregation. In addition, viscosity has also been shown to be associated with bioequivalency. pH may also have some meaning regarding effectiveness of preservative systems and may even have an effect on the amount of drug in solution. With regard to dissolution, there are at least three products that have dissolution specifications. These products include phenytoin suspension, carbamazepine suspension, and sulfamethoxazole and trimethoprim suspension. Particle size is also important, and at this point it would seem that any suspension should have some type of particle-size specification. As with other dosage forms, the underlying data to support specifications should be established.

IX. PROCESS VALIDATION

As with other products, the amount of data needed to support the manufacturing process will vary from product to product. Development (data) should have identified critical phases of the operation, including the predetermined specifications that should be monitored during process validation.

For example, for solutions, the key aspects that should be addressed during validation include ensuring that the drug substance and preservatives are dissolved. Parameters such as heat and time should be measured. In-process assay of the bulk solution during or after compounding according to predetermined limits is also an important aspect of process validation. For solutions that are sensitive to oxygen or light, dissolved oxygen levels would also be an important test. Again, the development data and the protocol should provide limits.

As discussed, the manufacture of suspensions presents additional problems, particularly in the area of uniformity. The development data should address the key compounding and filling steps that ensure uniformity. The protocol should provide for the key in-process and finished product tests, along with their specifications. For oral solutions, bioequivalency studies may not always be needed. However, oral suspensions, with the possible exception of some of the over-the-counter antacids, usually require a bioequivalency or clinical study to demonstrate their effectiveness. Comparison of product batches with the biobatch is an important part of the validation process. Make sure there are properly written protocol and process validation reports and, if appropriate, data for comparing full-scale batches with biobatch available during FDA inspection.

X. STABILITY

One area that has presented a number of problems is ensuring the stability of oral liquid products throughout their expiry period. The presence of water or other solvents enhances all reaction rates: Because fluids can contain a certain amount of oxygen, the oxidation reactions are also enhanced, as in the case of vitamins and the phenothiazine class of drugs. Good practice for these classes of drug products should include quantitation of both the active and primary degradant. There should be well-established specifications for the primary degradant, including methods of quantitation of both the active drug and degradant.

Because interactions of products with closure systems are possible, liquids and suspensions undergoing stability studies should be stored on their side or inverted to determine whether contact of the drug product with the closure system affects product integrity.

Other problems associated with inadequate closure systems are moisture losses that can cause the remaining contents to become superpotent and microbiological contamination.

XI. PACKAGING

Problems in the packaging of oral liquids have included potency (fill) of unit dose products and accurate calibration of measuring devices such as droppers, which are often provided. For unit dose solution products the label claim quantity within the limits described should be delivered.

Another problem in the packaging of oral liquids is lack of cleanliness of the containers before filling. Fibers and even insects often appear as debris in containers, particularly in the plastic containers used for many of these products. Many manufacturers receive containers shrink wrapped in plastic to minimize contamination from fiberboard cartons, and many manufacturers use compressed air to clean the containers. Vapors, such as oil vapors, from the compressed air have occasionally been found to present problems, and it is a good practice to use compressed gas from oil-free compressors.

2

Oral Solutions and Suspensions

I. INTRODUCTION

The manufacture and control of oral solutions and oral suspensions present unique problems to the industry. While bioequivalency concerns are minimal (except for antibiotic suspensions, for example), other issues have led to recalls, including microbiological, potency, and stability problems. Additionally, because the population using these oral dosage forms includes newborn, pediatric, and geriatric patients who may not be able to take oral solid dosage forms and may be compromised, defective dosage forms can pose an even greater risk than for other patients.

II. FACILITIES

The design of production facilities is largely dependent on the type of products manufactured and the potential for cross-contamination and microbiological contamination. For example, facilities used for the manufacture of over-the-counter (OTC) oral products might not require the isolation that a steroid or sulfa product would require. The manufacturer must establish policies of isolation of processes to minimize contamination. It should be further established whether or not particular drug substances and powdered excipients generate dust, given the method of manufacture used. System design and efficiency of dust removal system must be considered. A firm's HVAC system requires particular attention, especially where potent or highly sensitizing drugs are processed. Some manufacturers recirculate air without adequate filtration. Where air is recirculated, a firm's data must demonstrate the efficiency of air filtration through surface and/or air sampling.

III. EQUIPMENT

Equipment should be of a sanitary design and should include sanitary pumps, valves, flow meters, and other equipment that can be easily sanitized. Ball valves, packing in pumps, and pockets in flow meters have been identified as sources of contamination. In order to facilitate cleaning and sanitization, manufacturing and filling lines should be identified and detailed in drawings and standard operating procedures. In some cases, long delivery lines between manufacturing areas and filling areas have been a source of contamination. The standard operating procedures of many manufacturers have been found to be deficient, particularly with regard to time limitations between batches and for cleaning. Equipment used for batching and mixing of oral solutions and suspensions is relatively basic. Generally, these products are formulated on a weight basis with the batching tank on load cells so that a final quantity sufficient (QS) can be made by weight. Volumetric means, such as using a dipstick or line on a tank, have been found to be inaccurate. In most cases, manufacturers will assay samples of the bulk solution or suspension prior to filling. A much greater variability has been found with batches that have been manufactured volumetrically rather than by weight.

The design of the batching tank with regard to the location of the bottom discharge valve also presents problems. Ideally, the bottom discharge valve should be flush with the bottom of the tank. In some cases, valves (including undesirable ball valves) are several inches below the bottom of the tank; in others, the drug or preservative is not completely dissolved and lies in the dead leg below the tank, with initial samples being found to be subpotent. For the manufacture of suspensions, valves should be flush.

With regard to transfer lines, they are generally hard piped and easily cleaned and sanitized. In some cases, manufacturers have used flexible hoses to transfer product, but it is not unusual to find flexible hoses on the floor, thus significantly increasing the potential for contamination. Such contamination can occur when operators pick up or handle the hoses, possibly even placing them in transfer or batching tanks after picking them up from the floor. It is also a good practice to store hoses in a way that allows them to drain rather than coiling them, which may allow moisture to collect and be a potential source of microbial contamination.

Another common problem occurs when a manifold or common connection is used, especially in water supply, premix, or raw material supply tanks. Such common connections have been shown to be a source of contamination.

IV. RAW MATERIALS

Physical characteristics, particularly the particle size of the drug substance, are very important for suspensions. As with topical products in which the drug is suspended, particles are usually very fine to micronize (less than 25 μm). For syrups, elixirs, or solution dosage forms in which nothing is suspended, the particle size and physical characteristics of the raw materials are not that important; however, they can affect the rate of dissolution of such raw materials during the manufacturing process. Raw materials of a finer particle size may dissolve faster than those of a larger particle size when the product is compounded.

V. COMPOUNDING

In addition to a determination of the final volume (QS) as previously discussed, microbiological concerns also exist. For oral suspensions, an additional concern is uniformity, particularly because of the potential for segregation during the manufacture and storage of the bulk suspension, during transfer to the filling line, and during filling. A manufacturer's data should support storage times and transfer operations. Procedures and time limits for such operations should be established to address the potential for segregation or settling, as well as other unexpected effects that may be caused by extended holding or stirring.

For oral solutions and suspensions, the amount and control of temperature are important from a microbiological as well as a potency aspect. For those products in which temperature is identified as a critical part of the operation, the manufacturer should maintain documentation of temperature, such as by control charts.

Some manufacturers rely on heat during compounding to control the microbiological levels in product. For such products, the addition of purified water to a final QS, the batch, and the temperatures during processing should be documented and available for review.

In addition to drug substances, some additives, such as paraben, are difficult to dissolve and require heat. The control and monitoring of their dissolution during the compounding stage should be documented. From a potency aspect, the storage of product at high temperatures may increase the level of degradants. Storage limitations (time and temperature) should be justified by manufacturers and are likely to be evaluated during an inspection.

Some oral liquids are sensitive to oxygen and have been known to undergo degradation. This is particularly true of the phenothiazine class of drugs, such as perphenazine and chlorpromazine. The manufacture of such products might require the removal of oxygen such as by nitrogen purging. Additionally, such products might also require storage in sealed tanks, rather than in tanks with loose lids. In the OTC category, the entire line of vitamins is subject to degradation if they are not properly protected against oxidation, particularly those products that contain minerals (which might contain highly active trace elements that catalyze degradation of vitamins).

VI. MICROBIOLOGICAL QUALITY

Microbiological contamination of some oral liquids can present significant health hazards. For example, some oral liquids, such as nystatin suspension, are used for infants and immunocompromised patients, and microbiological contamination with organisms such as Gram-negative organisms is objectionable. For other oral liquid preparations, such as antacids, *Pseudomonas* sp. contamination is also objectionable; however, for some oral liquids, such as cough preparations, contamination with *Pseudomonas* sp. might not present the same health hazard. Obviously, the contamination of any preparation with Gram-negative organisms is not desirable.

In addition to the specific contaminant being objectionable, such contamination would be indicative of a deficient process as well as an inadequate preservative system. The presence of a specific *Pseudomonas* sp. may also indicate that other plant or raw material contaminants could survive the process. For example, the fact that a *Pseudomonas putida* contaminant is present could also indicate that *Pseudomonas aeruginosa*, a similar source organism, could also be present.

VII. ORAL SUSPENSION UNIFORMITY

Liquid products in which the drug is suspended (and not in solution) present manufacturer control problems. Depending upon the viscosity, many suspensions require continuous or periodic agitation during the filling process. If delivery lines are used between the bulk storage tank and the filling equipment, some segregation may occur, particularly if the product is not viscous. Inspectors will review a manufacturer's procedures for filling and diagrams for line setup prior to the filling equipment. Good manufacturing practice would warrant testing bottles from the beginning, middle, and end to assure that segregation has not occurred. Such samples should not be composited or pooled. In-process testing for suspensions might also include an assay of a sample from the bulk tank. More important, however, may be testing for viscosity.

VIII. PRODUCT SPECIFICATIONS

Important specifications for the manufacture of all solutions include assay and microbial limits. Additional important specifications for suspensions include particle size of the suspended drug, viscosity, pH, and in some cases, dissolution. Maintaining an appropriate viscosity is important from a processing perspective to minimize segregation. Additionally, viscosity has also been shown to be associated with bioequivalency. The pH may also have some meaning regarding effectiveness of preservative systems and may even have an effect on the amount of drug in solution. With regard to dissolution, at least several products have dissolution specifications listed in their U.S. Pharmacopeia (USP) monographs. Particle size is also important, and at this point it would seem that any suspension should have some type of particle-size specification.

IX. PROCESS VALIDATION

As with other products, the amount of data required to support the manufacturing process will vary from product to product. Development (data) should identify critical phases of the operation, including the predetermined specifications that should be monitored during process validation. For example, for solutions the key aspects that should be addressed during validation include assurance that the drug substance and preservatives are dissolved. Parameters such as heat and time should be measured. In-process assay of the bulk solution during and/or after compounding according to predetermined limits is also an important aspect of process validation. For solutions that are sensitive to oxygen and/or light, dissolved oxygen levels would also be an important test. Again, the development data and the protocol should provide limits. The manufacture of suspensions presents additional problems, particularly in the area of uniformity. Again, development data should address the key compounding and filling steps that ensure uniformity. The protocol should provide for the key in-process and finished product tests, along with their specifications. For oral solutions, bioequivalency studies may not always be needed; however, oral suspensions, with the possible exception of some antacids and OTC products, usually require a bioequivalency or clinical study to demonstrate effectiveness. As with oral solid dosage forms, comparison to the biobatch is an important part of validating the process.

X. STABILITY

One area that has presented a number of problems includes maintaining the stability of oral liquid products throughout their expiry period. Vitamins with fluoride oral liquid products have had a number of recalls because of vitamin degradation. Drugs in the phenothiazine class, such as perphenazine, chlorpromazine, and promethazine, have also shown evidence of instability. Good practice for this class of drug products would include quantitation of both the active and primary degradant. Dosage form manufacturers should know and have specifications for the primary degradant. These manufacturers' data and validation data for methods used to quantitate both the active drug and degradant are likely to be reviewed during an inspection. Because interactions of products with closure systems are possible, liquids and suspensions undergoing stability studies should be stored on their side or inverted in order to determine whether contact of the drug product with the closure system affects product integrity. Moisture losses that can cause the remaining contents to become superpotent and microbiological contamination are other problems associated with inadequate closure systems.

XI. PACKAGING

Problems in the packaging of oral liquids have included potency (fill) of unit dose products and accurate calibration of measuring devices such as droppers that are often provided. The USP does not provide for dose uniformity testing for oral solutions. Thus, unit-dose solution products should deliver label claims within the limits described in the USP. Inspectors will review a manufacturer's data to ensure uniformity of fill and test procedures to ascertain that unit-dose samples are being tested. Another problem in the packaging of oral liquids is a lack of cleanliness of containers prior to filling. Fibers and even insects have been identified as debris in containers, particularly plastic containers used for these products. Many manufacturers receive containers shrink wrapped in plastic to minimize contamination from fiberboard cartons. Some manufacturers may utilize compressed air to clean containers, in which case vapors (such as oil vapors) from the compressed air have occasionally been found to present problems.

3

The FDA Drug Product Surveillance Program

I. BACKGROUND

A primary mission of the Food and Drug Administration (FDA) is to conduct comprehensive regulatory coverage of all aspects of production and distribution of drugs and drug products to assure that such products meet the 501(a)(2)(B) requirements of the Food, Drugs, and Cosmetics Act. The FDA has developed two basic strategies:

1. Evaluating through factory inspections, including the collection and analysis of associated samples, the conditions and practices under which drugs and drug products are manufactured, packed, tested, and held
2. Monitoring the quality of drugs and drug products through surveillance activities such as sampling and analyzing products in distribution

This compliance program is designed to provide guidance for implementing the first strategy. Products from production and distribution facilities covered under this program are consistently of acceptable quality if the firm is operating in a state of control. The Drug Product Surveillance Program (CP 7356.008) provides guidance for the latter strategy.

II. IMPLEMENTATION

A. Objectives

The goal of this program's activities is to minimize consumer's exposure to adulterated drug products. Under this program, inspections and investigations, sample collections and analyses, and regulatory or administrative follow-up are made:

- To determine whether inspected firms are operating in compliance with applicable current Good Manufacturing Practices (cGMPs) requirements and, if not, to provide the evidence for actions to prevent adulterated products from entering the market; and, as appropriate, to remove adulterated products from the market and to take action against persons responsible as appropriate
- To provide cGMP assessment, which may be used in efficient determination of acceptability of the firm in the preapproval review of a facility for new drug applications
- To provide input to firms during inspections to improve their compliance with regulations
- To continue the FDA's unique expertise in drug manufacturing in determining the adequacy of cGMP requirements, FDA cGMP regulatory policy, and guidance documents.

B. Strategy

1. Biennial Inspection of Manufacturing Sites

Drugs and drug products are manufactured using many physical operations to bring together components, containers, and closures into a product that is released for distribution. Activities found in drug firms can be organized into systems that are sets of operations and related activities. Control of all systems helps to ensure that the firm will produce drugs that are safe, have the identity and strength, and meet the quality and purity characteristics as intended.

Biennial inspections (every 2 years) of manufacturing sites, which include repackaging, contract labs, etc., help to

- reduce the risk that adulterated products are reaching the marketplace,
- increase communication between the industry and the Agency,
- provide for timely evaluation of new manufacturing operations in the firm, and
- provide for regular feedback from the Agency to individual firms on the continuing status of the firm's GMP compliance

This program applies to all drug manufacturing operations. Currently, not enough FDA resources are available to audit every aspect of cGMP in every manufacturing facility during every inspection visit. Profile classes generalize inspection coverage from a small number of specific products to all the products in that class. This program establishes a systems approach to further generalize inspection coverage from a small number of profile classes to an overall evaluation of the firm. Reporting coverage for every profile class as defined in Field Accomplishment and Compliance Tracking System (FACTS), in each biennial inspection, provides the most broadly resource-efficient approach. Biennial updating of all profile classes will allow for cGMP acceptability determinations to be made without delays resulting from revisiting the firm. This will speed the review process, in response to compressed time frames for application decisions and in response to provisions of the FDA Modernization Act of 1997 (FDAMA). This will allow for Preapproval Inspections/Investigations Program inspections and Postapproval Audit Inspections to focus on the specific issues related to a given application or the firm's ability to keep applications current.

The inspection is defined as audit coverage of two or more systems, with mandatory coverage of the Quality System (see the system definitions in section II.B.3.). Inspection options include different numbers of systems to be covered depending on the purpose of the inspection. Inspecting the minimum number of systems, or more systems as deemed necessary by the regional District of the FDA, will provide the basis for an overall cGMP decision.

2. Inspection of Systems

Inspections of drug manufacturers should be made and reported using the system definitions and organization in this compliance program. Focusing on systems instead of on profile classes will increase efficiency in conducting inspections because the systems are often applicable to multiple profile classes. One biennial inspection visit will result in a determination of acceptability/nonacceptability for all profile classes. Inspection coverage should be representative of all the profile classes manufactured by the firm. The efficiency will be realized, because multiple visits to a firm will not be needed to cover all profile classes; delays in approval decisions will be avoided because up-to-date profile class information will be available at all times.

Coverage of a system should be sufficiently detailed, with specific examples selected, so that the system inspection outcome reflects the state of control in that system for every profile class. If a particular system is adequate, it should be adequate for all profile classes manufactured by the firm. For example, the way a firm handles "materials" (i.e., receipt, sampling, testing, acceptance, etc.) should be the same for all profile classes. The investigator should not have to inspect the Material System for each profile class. Likewise, the Production System includes general requirements such as standard operating procedure (SOP) use, charge-in of components, equipment identification, and in-process sampling and testing, which can be evaluated through selection of example products in various profile classes. Under each system, there may be something unique for a particular profile class (e.g., under the Materials System, the production of Water for Injection USP (*US Pharmacopeia*) for use in manufacturing. Selecting unique functions within a system will be at the discretion of the lead investigator). Any given inspection need not cover every system (see section III).

Complete inspection of one system may necessitate further follow-up of some items within the activities of another/other system(s) to fully document the findings. However, this coverage neither constitute nor require complete coverage of these other systems.

3. A Scheme of Systems for the Manufacture of Drugs and Drug Products

A general scheme of systems for auditing the manufacture of drugs and drug products consists of the following:

1. *Quality System*—This system assures overall compliance with cGMPs and internal procedures and specifications. The system includes the quality control unit and all its review and approval duties (e.g., change control, reprocessing, batch release, annual record review, validation protocols, and reports). It includes all product defect evaluations and evaluation of returned and salvaged drug products. (See the cGMP regulation, 21 CFR 211 subparts B, E, F, G, I, J, and K.)
2. *Facilities and Equipment System*—This system includes the measures and activities that provide an appropriate physical environment and the resources used in the production of the drugs or drug products. It includes the following:
   a. Buildings and facilities along with maintenance
   b. Equipment qualifications (installation and operation); equipment calibration and preventative maintenance; and cleaning and validation of cleaning processes as appropriate process performance qualification will be evaluated as part of the inspection of the overall process validation that is done within the system where the process is employed
   c. Utilities not intended for incorporation into the product such as heating, ventilating, and air conditioning (HVAC), compressed gases, steam, and water systems. (See the cGMP regulation, 21 CFR 211 subparts B, C, D, and J.)
3. *Materials System*—This system includes measures and activities to control finished products, components, including water or gases that are incorporated into the product, containers, and closures. It includes validation of computerized inventory control processes, drug storage, distribution controls, and records. (See the cGMP regulation, 21 CFR 211 subparts B, E, H, and J.)
4. *Production System*—This system includes measures and activities to control the manufacture of drugs and drug products including batch compounding, dosage form production, in-process sampling and testing, and process validation. It also includes establishing, following, and documenting performance of approved manufacturing procedures. (See the cGMP regulation, 21 CFR 211 subparts B, F, and J.)
5. *Packaging and Labeling System*—This system includes measures and activities that control the packaging and labeling of drugs and drug products. It includes written procedures, label examination and usage, label storage and issuance, packaging and labeling operations controls, and validation of these operations. (See the cGMP regulation, 21 CFR 211 subparts B, G, and J.)
6. *Laboratory Control System*—This system includes measures and activities related to laboratory procedures, testing, analytical methods development and validation or verification, and the stability program. (See the cGMP regulation, 21 CFR 211 subparts B, I, J, and K.)

The overall theme in devising this scheme of systems was the subchapter structure of the cGMP regulation. Every effort was made to group whole subchapters together in a rational set of six systems that incorporates the general scheme of pharmaceutical manufacturing operations.

The organization and personnel, including appropriate qualifications and training, employed in any given system, is evaluated as part of that system's operation. Production, control, or distribution records required to be maintained by the cGMP regulation and selected for review should be included for inspection audit within the context of each of the previously described systems. Inspections of contract companies should be within the systems for which the products or services are contracted as well as their quality systems.

III. PROGRAM MANAGEMENT INSTRUCTIONS

A. Definitions

1. Surveillance Inspections

a. The Full Inspection Option

The Full Inspection Option is a surveillance or compliance inspection that is meant to provide a broad and deep evaluation of the firm's cGMP. This is done when little or no information is known about a firm's cGMP compliance (e.g., for new firms); or for firms where doubt exists about the cGMP compliance in the firm (e.g., a firm with a history of documented short-lived compliance and recidivism); or follow-up to previous regulatory actions. Based on findings of objectionable conditions (as listed in section V) in one or more systems—a minimum of two systems must be completed—a Full Inspection may revert to the Abbreviated Inspection Option, with District concurrence (see section III.B.1.). During the course of a Full Inspection, verification of Quality System activities may require limited coverage in other systems. The Full Inspection Option normally includes an inspection audit of at least four of the systems, one of which must be the Quality

System (the system that includes the responsibility for the annual product reviews).

b. The Abbreviated Inspection Option

The Abbreviated Inspection Option is a surveillance or compliance inspection that is meant to provide an efficient update evaluation of a firm's cGMP. The abbreviated inspection provides documentation for continuing a firm in a satisfactory cGMP compliance status. Generally, this is done when a firm has a record of satisfactory cGMP compliance, with no significant recall or product defect or alert incidents, or with little shift in the manufacturing profiles of the firm within the previous two years (see section III.B.2). A full inspection may revert to an abbreviated inspection based on findings of objectionable conditions as listed in section V in one or more systems. The Abbreviated Inspection Option normally includes an inspection audit of at least two of the systems, one of which must be the Quality System (the system which includes the responsibility for the annual product reviews). The District drug program managers should ensure that the optional systems are rotated in successive abbreviated inspections. During the course of an abbreviated inspection, verification of quality system activities may require limited coverage in other systems. Some firms participate in a limited part of the production of a drug or drug product (e.g., a contract laboratory). Such firms may employ only two of the systems defined. In these cases, the inspection of the two systems comprises inspection of the entire firm; this is considered as the Full Inspection Option.

c. Selecting Systems for Coverage

The selection of the system(s) for coverage will be made by the FDA's Regional District Office based on such factors as a given firm's specific operation, history of previous coverage, history of compliance, or other priorities determined by the District Office.

2. Compliance Inspections

Compliance inspections are inspections conducted to evaluate or verify compliance corrective actions after a regulatory action has been taken. First, the coverage given in compliance inspections must be related to the deficient areas and subjected to corrective actions.

In addition, coverage must be given to systems because a determination must be made on the overall compliance status of the firm after the corrective actions are taken. The firm is expected to address all its operations in its corrective action plan after a previously violative inspection, not just the deficiencies noted in the FDA-483 (inspectional observations). The Full Inspection Option should be used for a compliance inspection, especially if the Abbreviated Inspection Option was used during the violative inspection.

Compliance Inspections include "For Cause Inspections." For Cause Inspections are compliance inspections that are conducted to investigate a specific problem that has come to the attention of some level of the agency. The problems may be indicated in Field Alert Reports (FARs), industry complaints, recalls, indicators of defective products, etc. Coverage of these areas may be assigned under other compliance programs; however, expansion of the coverage to a GMP inspection must be reported under this program. For Cause Inspections may be assigned under this program as the need arises.

3. State of Control

A drug firm is considered to be operating in a "state of control" when it employs conditions and practices that assure compliance with the intent of sections 501(a)(2)(B) of the Act and portions of the cGMP regulations that pertain to their systems. A firm in a state of control produces finished drug products for which there is an adequate level of assurance of quality, strength, identity, and purity. A firm is "out of control" if any one system is out of control. A system is out of control if the quality, identity, strength, and purity of the products resulting from that (those) system(s) cannot be adequately assured. Documented cGMP deficiencies provide the evidence for concluding that a system is not operating in a state of control. See section V, "Regulatory/Administrative Strategy," for a discussion of compliance actions based on inspection findings demonstrating out of control systems/firm.

4. Drug Process

A drug process is a related series of operations that result in the preparation of a drug or drug product. Major operations or steps in a drug process may include mixing, granulation, encapsulation, tabletting, chemical synthesis, fermentation, aseptic filling, sterilization, packing, labeling, and testing.

5. Drug Manufacturing Inspection

A Drug Manufacturing Inspection is a factory inspection in which evaluation of two or more systems, including the Quality System, is done to determine if manufacturing is occurring in a state of control.

B. Inspection Planning

The Field Office will conduct drug manufacturing inspections and maintain profiles or other monitoring systems, which ensures that each drug firm receives biennial inspectional coverage, as provided for in the strategy.

The District Office is responsible for determining the depth of coverage given to each drug firm. cGMP inspectional coverage shall be sufficient to assess the state of compliance for each firm.

The frequency and depth of inspection should be determined by the statutory obligation, the firm's compliance history, the technology employed, and the characteristics of the products. When a system is inspected, the inspection of that system may be considered applicable to all products that use it. Investigators should select an adequate number and type of products to accomplish coverage of the system. Selection of products should be made so that coverage is representative of the firm's overall abilities to manufacture within cGMP requirements.

Review of new drug application/anticipated new drug application (NDA/ANDA) files may assist in selecting significant drug processes for coverage in the various systems. Significant drug processes are those that utilize all the systems in the firm very broadly and contain steps with unique or difficult manipulation in the performance of a step. Products posing special manufacturing features (e.g., low-dose products, narrow therapeutic range drugs, combination drugs, modified release products, etc.) and new products made under an approved drug application should be considered first in selecting products for coverage.

The health significance of certain cGMP deviations may be lower when the drug product involved has no major systemic effect or no dosage limitations, such as in products like calamine lotion or over-the-counter (OTC) medicated shampoos. Such products should be given inspection coverage with appropriate priority.

Inspections for this compliance program may be performed during visits to a firm when operations are being performed for other compliance programs or other investigations.

C. Profiles

The inspection findings will be used as the basis for updating all profile classes in the profile screen of the FACTS EIR coversheet that is used to record profile/class determinations. Normally, an inspection under this systems approach will result in the update of all profile classes.

IV. INSPECTIONAL OBSERVATIONS

A. Investigational Operations

1. General

Review and use the cGMPs for Finished Pharmaceuticals (21 CFR 210 and 211) to evaluate manufacturing processes. Use the Guides to Inspection published by the Office of Regional Operations for information on technical applications in various manufacturing systems.

The investigator should conduct inspections according to the "Strategy" section in part II of this compliance program. Recognizing that drug firms vary greatly in size and scope, and manufacturing systems are more or less sophisticated, the approach to inspecting each firm should be carefully planned. For example, it may be more appropriate to review the Quality System thoroughly before entering production areas in some firms; in others, the Quality System review should take place concurrently with inspection of another system or systems selected for coverage. The complexity and variability necessitate a flexible inspection approach—one that not only allows the investigator to choose the inspection focus and depth appropriate for a specific firm, but also directs the performance and reporting on the inspection within a framework that will provide for a uniform level of cGMP assessment. Furthermore, this inspection approach provides for fast communication and evaluation of findings.

Inspectional Observations noting cGMP deficiencies should be related to a requirement. Requirements for the manufacture of drug products (dosage forms) are in the cGMP regulation and are amplified by policy in the Compliance Policy Guides or case precedents. cGMP requirements apply to the manufacture of distributed prescription drug products, OTC drug products, approved products, and products not requiring approval, as well as drug products used in clinical trials. The cGMP regulations are not direct requirements for manufacture of active pharmaceutical ingredients (APIs); the regulations should not be referenced as the basis for a GMP deficiency in the manufacture of APIs, but they are guidance for cGMP in API manufacture.

Guidance documents do not establish requirements; they state examples of ways to meet requirements. Guidance documents are not to be referred to as the justification for an inspectional observation. The justification comes from the cGMPs. Current Guides to Inspection and Guidance to Industry documents provide interpretations of requirements, which may assist in the evaluation of the adequacy of cGMP systems.

Current inspectional observation policy as stated in the inspection operations manual (IOM) says that the FDA-483, when issued, should be specific and contain only significant items. For this program, inspection observations should be organized under separate captions by the systems defined in this program. List observations in order of importance within each system. Where repeated or similar observations are made, they should be consolidated under a unified observation. For those Districts utilizing Turbo EIR, a limited number of observations can be common to more than one system (e.g., organization and personnel including appropriate qualifications and training). In these instances, put the observation in the first system reported on the FDA-483 and in the text of the EIR, reference the applicability to other systems where appropriate. This should be done to accommodate the structure of Turbo EIR, which allows individual citation once per FDA-483. Refrain from using unsubstantiated conclusions. Do not use the term "inadequate" without explaining why and how. Refer to the policy in the IOM, chapter 5, section 512 and Field Management Directive 120 for further guidance on the content of Inspectional Observations.

Specific specialized inspectional guidance may be provided as attachments to this program, or in requests for inspection, assignments, etc.

2. Inspection Approaches

This program provides two surveillance inspectional options: Abbreviated Inspection Option and Full Inspection Option (see the definitions of the inspection options in part II of this compliance program).

1. *Selecting the Full Inspection Option*—The Full Inspection Option will include inspection of at least four of the systems as listed in part II "Strategy," one of which must be the Quality System.
   a. Select the Full Inspection Option for an initial FDA inspection of a facility. A full inspection may revert to the Abbreviated Inspection Option, *with District concurrence,* based on the finding of objectionable conditions as listed in part V in one or more systems (a minimum of two systems must be completed).
   b. Select the Full Inspection Option when the firm has a history of fluctuating into and out of compliance. To determine if the firm meets this criterion, the District should utilize all information at its disposal, such as, inspection results, results of sample analyses, complaints, drug quality reporting system (DQRS) reports, recalls, etc., and the compliance actions resulting from them or from past inspections. A Full Inspection may revert to the Abbreviated Inspection Option, *with District concurrence,* based on findings of objectionable conditions as listed in part V in one or more systems (a minimum of two systems must be completed).
   c. Evaluate if important changes have occurred by comparing current operations against the EIR for the previous full inspection. The following types of changes are typical of those that warrant the Full Inspection Option:
      - New potential for cross-contamination arising through change in process or product line
      - Use of new technology requiring new expertise, significant new equipment, or new facilities
   d. A Full Inspection may also be conducted on a surveillance basis at the District's discretion.
   e. The Full Inspection Option will satisfy the biennial inspection requirement.
   f. Follow-up to a Warning Letter or other significant regulatory actions should require a Full Inspection Option.

2. *Selecting the Abbreviated Inspection Option*—The Abbreviated Inspection Option normally will include inspection audit of at least two systems, one of which must be the Quality System. During the course of an abbreviated inspection, verification of quality system activities may require limited coverage in other systems.
   a. This option involves an inspection of the manufacturer to maintain surveillance over the firm's activities and to provide input to the firm on maintaining and improving the GMP level of assurance of quality of its products.
   b. A full inspection may revert to the Abbreviated Inspection Option, *with District concurrence,* based on findings of objectionable conditions as listed in part V in one or more systems (a minimum of two systems must be completed).
   c. An abbreviated inspection is adequate for routine coverage and will satisfy the biennial inspectional requirement.

a. Comprehensive Inspection Coverage
It is not anticipated that full inspections will be conducted every two years. They may be conducted at less frequent intervals, perhaps at every third or fourth inspection cycle. Districts should consider selecting different optional systems for inspection coverage as a cycle of Abbreviated inspections are carried out to build comprehensive information on the firm's total manufacturing activities.

3. System Inspection Coverage

a. Quality System
Assessment of the Quality System is two-phased:

1. The first phase evaluates whether the Quality Control Unit has fulfilled the responsibility to review and approve all procedures related to production, quality control, and quality assurance and assure the procedures are adequate for their intended use. This also includes the associated record-keeping systems.
2. The second phase assesses the data collected to identify quality problems and may link to other major systems for inspectional coverage.

For each of the following, the firm should have written and approved procedures and documentation resulting therefrom. The firm's adherence to written procedures should be verified through observation whenever possible. These areas are not limited to finished products, but may also incorporate components and in-process materials. These areas may indicate deficiencies not only in this system, but also in other major systems that would warrant expansion of coverage. All areas under this system should be covered; however, the depth of coverage may vary depending upon inspectional findings:

- *Product reviews*—at least annually; should include information from areas listed below as appropriate; batches reviewed for each product are representative of all batches manufactured; trends are identified [refer to 21 CFR 211.180(e)]
- *Complaint reviews (quality and medical)*—documented; evaluated; investigated in a timely manner; includes corrective action where appropriate
- *Discrepancy and failure investigations related to manufacturing and testing*—documented; evaluated; investigated in a timely manner; includes corrective action where appropriate
- *Change control*—documented; evaluated; approved; need for revalidation assessed
- *Product improvement projects*—for marketed products
- *Reprocess/rework*—evaluation, review, and approval; impact on validation and stability
- *Returns/salvages*—assessment; investigation expanded where warranted; disposition
- *Rejects*—investigation expanded where warranted; corrective action where appropriate
- *Stability failures*—investigation expanded where warranted; need for field alerts evaluated; disposition
- Quarantine products
- *Validation*—status of required validation/revalidation (e.g., computer, manufacturing process, laboratory methods)
- Training/qualification of employees in quality control unit functions

b. Facilities and Equipment System
For each of the following, the firm should have written and approved procedures and documentation resulting therefrom. The firm's adherence to written procedures should be verified through observation whenever possible. These areas may indicate deficiencies not only in this system but also in other systems that would warrant expansion of coverage. When this system is selected for coverage in addition to the Quality System, all areas listed next should be covered; however, the depth of coverage may vary depending upon inspectional findings:

1. *Facilities*
   - Cleaning and maintenance
   - Facility layout and air handling systems for prevention of cross-contamination (e.g., penicillin, beta-lactams, steroids, hormones, cytotoxics, etc.)
   - Specifically designed areas for the manufacturing operations performed by the firm to prevent contamination or mix-ups
   - General air handling systems
   - Control system for implementing changes in the building
   - Lighting, potable water, washing and toilet facilities, sewage and refuse disposal
   - Sanitation of the building, use of rodenticides, fungicides, insecticides, and cleaning and sanitizing agents
2. *Equipment*
   - Equipment installation and operational qualification where appropriate
   - Adequacy of equipment design, size, and location
   - Equipment surfaces should not be reactive, additive, or absorptive
   - Appropriate use of equipment operations substances (lubricants, coolants, refrigerants, etc.), contacting products, containers, etc.
   - Cleaning procedures and cleaning validation
   - Controls to prevent contamination, particularly with any pesticides or any other toxic materials, or other drug or nondrug chemicals
   - Qualification, calibration, and maintenance of storage equipment, such as refrigerators and freezers for ensuring that standards, raw materials, and reagents are stored at the proper temperatures

- Equipment qualification, calibration, and maintenance, including computer qualification/validation and security
- Control system for implementing changes in the equipment
- Equipment identification practices (where appropriate)
- Documented investigation into any unexpected discrepancy

c. Materials System

For each of the following, the firm should have written and approved procedures and documentation resulting therefrom. The firm's adherence to written procedures should be verified through observation whenever possible. These areas are not limited to finished products, but may also incorporate components and in-process materials. These areas may indicate deficiencies not only in this system, but also in other systems that would warrant expansion of coverage. When this system is selected for coverage in addition to the Quality System, all areas listed next should be covered; however, the depth of coverage may vary depending upon inspectional findings:

- Training/qualification of personnel
- Identification of components, containers, and closures
- Inventory of components, containers, and closures
- Storage conditions
- Storage under quarantine until tested or examined and released
- Representative samples collected, tested, or examined using appropriate means
- At least one specific identity test is conducted on each lot of each component
- A visual identification is conducted on each lot of containers and closures
- Testing or validation of supplier's test results for components, containers, and closures
- Rejection of any component, container, or closure not meeting acceptance requirements
- Investigate fully the firm's procedures for verification of the source of components
- Appropriate retesting/reexamination of components, containers, and closures
- First in–first out use of components, containers, and closures
- Quarantine of rejected materials
- Water and process gas supply, design, maintenance, validation, and operation
- Containers and closures should not be additive, reactive, or absorptive to the drug product
- Control system for implementing changes in the materials handling operations
- Qualification/validation and security of computerized or automated processes
- Finished product distribution records by lot
- Documented investigation into any unexpected discrepancy

d. Production System

For each of the following, the firm should have written and approved procedures and documentation resulting therefrom. The firm's adherence to written procedures should be verified through observation whenever possible. These areas are not limited to finished products, but may also incorporate components and in-process materials. These areas may indicate deficiencies not only in this system, but also in other systems that would warrant expansion of coverage. When this system is selected for coverage in addition to the Quality System, all areas listed next should be covered; however, the depth of coverage may vary depending upon inspectional findings:

- Training/qualification of personnel
- Control system for implementing changes in processes
- Adequate procedure and practice for charge-in of components
- Formulation/manufacturing at not less than 100%
- Identification of equipment with contents, and, where appropriate, phase of manufacturing or status
- Validation and verification of cleaning/sterilization/depyrogenation of containers and closures
- Calculation and documentation of actual yields and percentage of theoretical yields
- Contemporaneous and complete batch production documentation
- Establishing time limits for completion of phases of production
- Implementation and documentation of in-process controls, tests, and examinations (e.g., pH, adequacy of mix, weight variation, clarity)
- Justification and consistency of in-process specifications and drug product final specifications
- Prevention of objectionable microorganisms in unsterile drug products
- Adherence to preprocessing procedures (e.g., setup, line clearance, etc.)
- Equipment cleaning and use logs
- Master production and control records
- Batch production and control records
- Process validation, including validation and security of computerized or automated processes
- Change control; the need for revalidation evaluated
- Documented investigation into any unexpected discrepancy

e. Packaging and Labeling System

For each of the following, the firm should have written and approved procedures and documentation resulting therefrom. The firm's adherence to written procedures should be verified through observation whenever possible. These areas are not limited only to finished products, but may also incorporate components and in-process materials. These areas may indicate deficiencies not only in this system, but also in other systems that would warrant expansion of coverage. When this system is selected for coverage in addition to the Quality System, all areas listed next should be covered; however, the depth of coverage may vary depending upon inspectional findings:

- Training/qualification of personnel
- Acceptance operations for packaging and labeling materials
- Control system for implementing changes in packaging and labeling operations
- Adequate storage for labels and labeling, both approved and returned after issued
- Control of labels that are similar in size, shape, and color for different products

- Finished product cut labels for immediate containers that are similar in appearance without some type of 100% electronic or visual verification system or the use of dedicated lines
- Labels are not gang printed unless they are differentiated by size, shape, or color
- Control of filled unlabeled containers that are later labeled under multiple private labels
- Adequate packaging records that will include specimens of all labels used
- Control of issuance of labeling, examination of issued labels, and reconciliation of used labels
- Examination of the labeled finished product
- Adequate inspection (proofing) of incoming labeling
- Use of lot numbers and the destruction of excess labeling bearing lot/control numbers
- Physical/spatial separation between different labeling and packaging lines
- Monitoring of printing devices associated with manufacturing lines
- Line clearance, inspection, and documentation
- Adequate expiration dates on the label
- Conformance to tamper-evident packaging (TEP) requirements (see 21CFR 211.132 and Compliance Policy Guide, 7132a.17)
- Validation of packaging and labeling operations, including validation and security of computerized processes
- Documented investigation into any unexpected discrepancy

f. Laboratory Control System

For each of the following, the firm should have written and approved procedures and documentation resulting therefrom. The firm's adherence to written procedures should be verified through observation whenever possible. These areas are not limited only to finished products, but may also incorporate components and in-process materials. These areas may indicate deficiencies not only in this system, but also in other systems that would warrant expansion of coverage. When this system is selected for coverage in addition to the Quality System, all areas listed next should be covered; however, the depth of coverage may vary depending upon inspectional findings:

- Training/qualification of personnel
- Adequacy of staffing for laboratory operations
- Adequacy of equipment and facility for intended use
- Calibration and maintenance programs for analytical instruments and equipment
- Validation and security of computerized or automated processes
- Reference standards: source, purity and assay, and tests to establish equivalency to current official reference standards as appropriate
- System suitability checks on chromatographic systems [e.g., gas chromatography (GC) or high pressure liquid chromatography (HPLC)]
- Specifications, standards, and representative sampling plans
- Adherence to the written methods of analysis
- Validation/verification of analytical methods
- Control system for implementing changes in laboratory operations
- Required testing is performed on the correct samples
- Documented investigation into any unexpected discrepancy
- Complete analytical records from all tests and summaries of results
- Quality and retention of raw data (e.g., chromatograms and spectra)
- Correlation of result summaries to raw data; presence of unused data
- Adherence to an adequate Out of Specification (OOS) procedure that includes timely completion of the investigation
- Adequate reserve samples; documentation of reserve sample examination
- Stability testing program, including demonstration of stability indicating capability of the test methods

4. Sampling

Samples of defective product constitute persuasive evidence that significant cGMP problems exist. Physical samples may be an integral part of a cGMP inspection where control deficiencies are observed. Physical samples should be correlated with observed control deficiencies. Consider consulting your servicing laboratory for guidance on quantity and type of samples (in-process or finished) to be collected. Documentary samples may be submitted when the documentation illustrates the deficiencies better than a physical sample. Districts may elect to collect, but not analyze, physical samples or to collect documentary samples to document cGMP deficiencies. Physical sample analysis is not necessary to document cGMP deficiencies.

When a large number of products have been produced under deficient controls, collect physical or documentary samples of products that have the greatest therapeutic significance, narrow range of toxicity, or low dosage strength. Include samples of products of minimal therapeutic significance only when they illustrate highly significant cGMP deficiencies.

5. Inspection Teams

An inspection team (see IOM 502.4) composed of experts from within the District, other Districts, or Headquarters is encouraged when it provides needed expertise and experience. Contact the ORO/Division of Field Investigations if technical assistance is needed (see also FMD 142). Participation of an analyst (chemist or microbiologist) on an inspection team is also encouraged, especially where laboratory issues are extensive or complex. Contact your Drug Servicing Laboratory or ORO/Division of Field Science.

6. Reporting

The investigator utilizes Subchapter 590 of the IOM for guidance in reporting of inspectional findings. The Summary of Findings should identify systems covered. The body of the report should identify and explain the rationale for inspecting the profile classes covered. Any adverse findings by systems under separate captions should be reported and discussed in full. Additional information should be provided as needed or desired, for example, a description of any significant changes that have occurred since previous inspections.

Reports with specific, specialized information required should be prepared as instructed within the individual assignment/attachment.

V. ANALYTICAL OBSERVATIONS

A. Analyzing Laboratories

1. Routine chemical analyses—all Servicing Laboratories except WEAC.
2. Sterility testing:
   Region Examining Laboratory
3. Other microbiological examinations—NRL (for the CE Region), SRL, SAN, and DEN; *Salmonella* Serotyping Lab—ARL.
4. Chemical cross-contamination analyses by mass spectrometry (MS)—NRL, SRL, DEN, PRL/NW, and PHI. Non–mass-spectrometry laboratories should call one of their own regional MS-capable laboratories or Division of Field Science (HFC-140) to determine the most appropriate lab for the determinations to be performed.
5. Chemical cross-contamination analyses by nuclear magnetic resonance (NMR) spectroscopy—NRL. Non-NMR laboratories should call one of their own regional labs equipped with NMR or Division of Field Science (HFC-140) to determine the most appropriate lab for the determinations to be performed.
6. Dissolution testing—NRL, KAN, SRL, SJN, DET, PHI, DEN, PRL/SW, and PRL-NW. Districts without dissolution testing capability should use one of their own regional labs for dissolution testing. Otherwise, call DFS.
7. Antibiotic analyses: ORA Examining Laboratory,
   Denver District Lab (HFR-SW260): Tetracyclines, erythromycins
   Northeast Regional Lab (HFR-NE500): Penicillins, cephalosporins
   CDER Examining Laboratory, Office of Testing and Research, Division of Pharmaceutical Analysis (HFD-473): All other antibiotics
8. Bioassays—Division of Testing and Applied Analytical Research, Drug Bioanalysis Branch(HFN-471).
9. Particulate Matter in Injectables—NRL, SRL.
10. Pyrogen/LAL Testing— SRL

B. Analysis

1. Samples must be examined for compliance with applicable specifications as they relate to deficiencies noted during the inspection. The official method should be used for check analyses or, when no official method exists, by other validated procedures.
2. The presence of cross-contamination must be confirmed by a second method. Spectroscopic methods, such as MS, NMR, ultraviolet (UV)-Visible, or infrared (IR) are preferred. A second confirmatory method should be employed by different mechanisms than the initial analysis (i.e., ion-pairing vs. conventional reverse phase HPLC).
3. Check Analysis for dissolution rate must be performed by a second dissolution-testing laboratory.
4. Sterility testing methods should be based on current editions of USP and the *Sterility Analytical Manual*. Other microbiological examinations should be based on appropriate sections of USP and BAM.

VI. REGULATORY/ADMINISTRATIVE STRATEGY

Inspection findings that demonstrate that a firm is not operating in a state of control may be used as evidence for taking appropriate advisory, administrative, or judicial actions.

When the management of the firm is unwilling or unable to provide adequate corrective actions in an appropriate time frame, formal agency regulatory actions will be recommended that are designed to meet the situation encountered.

When deciding the type of action to recommend, the initial decision should be based on the seriousness of the problem and the most effective way to protect consumers. Outstanding instructions in the *Regulatory Procedures Manual* (*RPM*) should be followed.

The endorsement to the inspection report should point out the actions that have been taken or will be taken and when. All deficiencies noted in inspections/audits under this program must be addressed by stating the firm's corrective actions, accomplished or projected, for each as established in the discussion with management at the close of the inspection.

All corrective action approaches in domestic firms are monitored and managed by the District Offices. The approaches may range from shutdown of operations, recall of products, conducting testing programs, development of new procedures, modifications of plants and equipment, to simple immediate corrections of conditions. CDER/DMPQ/CMGB/HFD-325 will assist District Offices as requested.

An inspection report that documents that one or more systems is/are out of control should be classified as OAI. District Offices may issue Warning Letters per RPM to warn firms of violations, to solicit voluntary corrections, and to provide for the initial phase of formal agency regulatory actions.

Issuance of a Warning Letter or taking other regulatory actions pursuant to a surveillance inspection (other than a For Cause Inspection) should result in the classification of all profile classes as unacceptable. Also, the inspection findings will be used as the basis for updating profile classes in FACTS.

The FDA laboratory tests that demonstrate the effects of absent or inadequate cGMPs are strong evidence for supporting regulatory actions. Such evidence development should be considered as an inspection progresses and deficiencies are found; however, the lack of violative physical samples is *not* a barrier to pursuing regulatory or administrative action, provided that cGMP deficiencies have been well documented. Likewise, physical samples found to be in compliance are *not* a barrier to pursuing action under cGMP charges.

Evidence to support significant deficiencies or a trend of deficiencies within a system covered could demonstrate the failure of a system and should result in consideration of the issuance of a Warning Letter or other regulatory action by the District. When deciding the type of action to recommend, the initial decision should be based on the seriousness or the frequency of the problem. Examples include the following:

Quality System

1. Pattern of failure to review/approve procedures
2. Pattern of failure to document execution of operations as required
3. Pattern of failure to review documentation
4. Pattern of failure to conduct investigations and resolve discrepancies/failures/deviations/complaints
5. Pattern of failure to assess other systems to assure compliance with GMP and SOPs

Facilities and Equipment

1. Contamination with filth, objectionable microorganisms, toxic chemicals or other drug chemicals, or a reasonable potential for contamination, with demonstrated

avenues of contamination, such as airborne or through unclean equipment
2. Pattern of failure to validate cleaning procedures for nondedicated equipment; lack of demonstration of effectiveness of cleaning for dedicated equipment
3. Pattern of failure to document investigation of discrepancies
4. Pattern of failure to establish/follow a control system for implementing changes in the equipment
5. Pattern of failure to qualify equipment, including computers

Materials System
1. Release of materials for use or distribution that do not conform to established specifications
2. Pattern of failure to conduct one specific identity test for components
3. Pattern of failure to document investigation of discrepancies
4. Pattern of failure to establish/follow a control system for implementing changes in the materials handling operations
5. Lack of validation of water systems as required depending upon the intended use of the water
6. Lack of validation of computerized processes

Production System
1. Pattern of failure to establish/follow a control system for implementing changes in the production system operations
2. Pattern of failure to document investigation of discrepancies
3. Lack of process validation
4. Lack of validation of computerized processes
5. Pattern of incomplete or missing batch production records
6. Pattern of nonconformance to established in-process controls, tests, and specifications

Packaging and Labeling
1. Pattern of failure to establish/follow a control system for implementing changes in the packaging or labeling operations
2. Pattern of failure to document investigation of discrepancies
3. Lack of validation of computerized processes
4. Lack of control of packaging and labeling operations that may introduce a potential for mislabeling
5. Lack of packaging validation

Laboratory Control System
1. Pattern of failure to establish/follow a control system for implementing changes in the laboratory operations
2. Pattern of failure to document investigation of discrepancies
3. Lack of validation of computerized and/or automated processes
4. Pattern of inadequate sampling practices
5. Lack of validated analytical methods
6. Pattern of failure to follow approved analytical procedures
7. Pattern of failure to follow an adequate OOS procedure
8. Pattern of failure to retain raw data
9. Lack of stability indicating methods
10. Pattern of failure to follow stability programs

Follow-up to a Warning Letter or other significant regulatory action because of an abbreviated inspection should warrant full inspection coverage as defined in this program.

GLOSSARY

Acceptance Criteria—Numerical limits, ranges, or other suitable measures for acceptance of test results.

Active Pharmaceutical Ingredient (API) ***(or Drug Substance)***—Any substance or mixture of substances intended to be used in the manufacture of a drug (medicinal) product and that, when used in the production of a drug, becomes an active ingredient of the drug product. Such substances are intended to furnish pharmacological activity or other direct effect in the diagnosis, cure, mitigation, treatment, or prevention of disease or to affect the structure and function of the body.

Airlock—An enclosed space with two or more doors, which is interposed between two or more rooms, for example, of differing classes of cleanliness, for the purpose of controlling the airflow between those rooms when they need to be entered. An airlock is designed for use either by people or for goods and/or equipment.

API Starting Material—A raw material, intermediate, or an API that is used in the production of an API and that is incorporated as a significant structural fragment into the structure of the API. An API Starting Material can be an article of commerce, a material purchased from one or more suppliers under contract or commercial agreement, or produced in-house. API Starting Materials are normally of defined chemical properties and structure.

Authorized person—The person recognized by the national regulatory authority as having the responsibility for ensuring that each batch of finished product has been manufactured, tested, and approved for release in compliance with the laws and regulations in force in that country.

Batch (or Lot)—A specific quantity of material produced in a process or series of processes so that it is expected to be homogeneous within specified limits. In the case of continuous production, a batch may correspond to a defined fraction of the production. The batch size can be defined either by a fixed quantity or by the amount produced in a fixed time interval. A defined quantity of starting material, packaging material, or product processed in a single process or series of processes so that it is expected to be homogeneous. It may sometimes be necessary to divide a batch into a number of sub-batches, which are later brought together to form a final homogeneous batch. In the case of terminal sterilization, the batch size is determined by the capacity of the autoclave. In continuous manufacture, the batch must correspond to a defined fraction of the production, characterized by its intended homogeneity. The batch size can be defined either as a fixed quantity or as the amount produced in a fixed time interval.

Batch Number (or Lot Number)—A unique combination of numbers, letters, and/or symbols that identifies a batch (or lot) and from which the production and distribution history can be determined. A distinctive combination of numbers and/or letters which uniquely identifies a batch on the labels, its batch records and corresponding certificates of analysis, etc.

Batch Records—All documents associated with the manufacture of a batch of bulk product or finished product. They provide a history of each batch of product and of all circumstances pertinent to the quality of the final product.

Bioburden—The level and type (e.g., objectionable or not) of micro-organisms that can be present in raw materials, API starting materials, intermediates or APIs. Bioburden should not be considered contamination unless the levels have been exceeded or defined objectionable organisms have been detected.

Bulk Product—Any product that has completed all processing stages up to, but not including, final packaging.

Calibration—The demonstration that a particular instrument or device produces results within specified limits by comparison with those produced by a reference or traceable standard over an appropriate range of measurements. The set of operations that establish, under specified conditions, the relationship between values indicated by an instrument or system for measuring (especially weighing), recording, and controlling, or the values represented by a material measure, and the corresponding known values of a reference standard. Limits for acceptance of the results of measuring should be established.

Clean Area—An area with defined environmental control of particulate and microbial contamination, constructed and used in such a way as to reduce the introduction, generation, and retention of contaminants within the area.

Computer System—A group of hardware components and associated software, designed and assembled to perform a specific function or group of functions. A process or operation integrated with a computer system.

Consignment (or Delivery)—The quantity of a pharmaceutical(s), made by one manufacturer and supplied at one time in response to a particular request or order. A consignment may comprise one or more packages or containers and may include material belonging to more than one batch.

Contamination—The undesired introduction of impurities of a chemical or microbiological nature, or of foreign matter, into or onto a raw material, intermediate, or API during production, sampling, packaging or repackaging, storage, or transport.

Contract Manufacturer—A manufacturer performing some aspect of manufacturing on behalf of the original manufacturer.

Critical—Describes a process step, process condition, test requirement, or other relevant parameter or item that must be controlled within predetermined criteria to ensure that the API meets its specification.

Critical Operation—An operation in the manufacturing process that may cause variation in the quality of the pharmaceutical product.

Cross-Contamination—Contamination of a material or product with another material or product. Contamination of a starting material, intermediate product, or finished product with another starting material or product during production.

Deviation—Departure from an approved instruction or established standard.

Drug (Medicinal) Product—The dosage form in the final immediate packaging intended for marketing. (Reference Q1A)

Drug Substance—See Active Pharmaceutical Ingredient

Expiry Date (or Expiration Date)—The date placed on the container/labels of an API designating the time during which the API is expected to remain within established shelf life specifications if stored under defined conditions, and after which it should not be used.

Fnished Product—A finished dosage form that has undergone all stages of manufacture, including packaging in its final container and labeling.

Impurity—Any component present in the intermediate or API that is not the desired entity.

Impurity Profile—A description of the identified and unidentified impurities present in an API.

In-Process Control—Checks performed during production in order to monitor and, if necessary, to adjust the process to ensure that the product conforms to its specifications. The control of the environment or equipment may also be regarded as a part of in-process control.

Intermediate—A material produced during steps of the processing of an API that undergoes further molecular change or purification before it becomes an API. Intermediates may or may not be isolated. Partly processed product that must undergo further manufacturing steps before it becomes a bulk product.

Large-Volume Parenterals—Sterile solutions intended for parenteral application with a volume of 100 mL or more in one container of the finished dosage form.

Lot—See Batch

Lot Number—see Batch Number

Manufacture—All operations of receipt of materials, production, packaging, repackaging, labeling, relabeling, quality control, release, storage, and distribution of APIs and related controls.

Manufacturer—A company that carries out operations such as production, packaging, repackaging, labeling, and relabeling of pharmaceuticals.

Marketing Authorization (Product License, Registration Certificate)—A legal document issued by the competent drug regulatory authority that establishes the detailed composition and formulation of the product and the pharmacopoeial or other recognized specifications of its ingredients and of the final product itself, and includes details of packaging, labeling, and shelf-life.

Master Formula—A document or set of documents specifying the starting materials with their quantities and the packaging materials, together with a description of the procedures and precautions required to produce a specified quantity of a finished product as well as the processing instructions, including the in-process controls.

Master Record—A document or set of documents that serve as a basis for the batch documentation (blank batch record).

Material—A general term used to denote raw materials (starting materials, reagents, solvents), process aids, intermediates, APIs and packaging and labeling materials.

Mother Liquor—The residual liquid which remains after the crystallization or isolation processes. A mother liquor may contain unreacted materials, intermediates, levels of the API, and/or impurities. It may be used for further processing.

Packaging—All operations, including filling and labeling, that a bulk product has to undergo in order to become a finished product. Filling of a sterile product under aseptic conditions or a product intended to be terminally sterilized, would not normally be regarded as part of packaging.

Packaging Material—Any material intended to protect an intermediate or API during storage and transport. Any material, including printed material, employed in the packaging of a pharmaceutical, but excluding any outer packaging used for transportation or shipment. Packaging materials are referred to as primary or secondary according to whether or not they are intended to be in direct contact with the product.

Pharmaceutical Product—Any material or product intended for human or veterinary use presented in its finished dosage form or as a starting material for use in such a dosage form, that is subject to control by pharmaceutical legislation in the exporting state and/or the importing state.

Procedure—A documented description of the operations to be performed, the precautions to be taken, and measures to be applied directly or indirectly related to the manufacture of an intermediate or API.

Process Aids—Materials, excluding solvents, used as an aid in the manufacture of an intermediate or API that do not themselves participate in a chemical or biological reaction (e.g., filter aid, activated carbon, etc).

Process Control—See In-Process Control

Production—All operations involved in the preparation of a pharmaceutical product, from receipt of materials, through processing, packaging and repackaging, labeling and relabeling, to completion of the finished product.

Qualification—Action of proving and documenting that equipment or ancillary systems are properly installed, work correctly, and actually lead to the expected results. Qualification is part of validation, but the individual qualification steps alone do not constitute process validation.

Quality Assurance (QA)—The sum total of the organized arrangements made with the object of ensuring that all APIs are of the quality required for their intended use and that quality systems are maintained.

Quality Control (QC)—Checking or testing that specifications are met.

Quality Unit(s)—An organizational unit independent of production which fulfills both Quality Assurance and Quality Control responsibilities. This can be in the form of separate QA and QC units or a single individual or group, depending upon the size and structure of the organization.

Quarantine—The status of starting or packaging materials, intermediates, or bulk or finished products isolated physically or by other effective means while a decision is awaited on their release, rejection, or reprocessing.

Raw Material—A general term used to denote starting materials, reagents, and solvents intended for use in the production of intermediates or APIs.

Reconciliation—A comparison between the theoretical quantity and the actual quantity.

Recovery—The introduction of all or part of previous batches (or of redistilled solvents and similar products) of the required quality into another batch at a defined stage of manufacture. It includes the removal of impurities from waste to obtain a pure substance or the recovery of used materials for a separate use.

Reference Standard, Primary—A substance that has been shown by an extensive set of analytical tests to be authentic material that should be of high purity.

Reference Standard, Secondary—A substance of established quality and purity, as shown by comparison to a primary reference standard, used as a reference standard for routine laboratory analysis.

Reprocessing—Subjecting all or part of a batch or lot of an in-process drug, bulk process intermediate (final biological bulk intermediate) or bulk product of a single batch/ lot to a previous step in the validated manufacturing process due to failure to meet predetermined specifications. Reprocessing procedures are foreseen as occasionally necessary for biological drugs and, in such cases, are validated and preapproved as part of the marketing authorization.

Retest Date—The date when a material should be reexamined to ensure that it is still suitable for use.

Reworking—Subjecting an in-process or bulk process intermediate (final biological bulk intermediate) or final product of a single batch to an alternate manufacturing process due to a failure to meet predetermined specifications. Reworking is an unexpected occurrence and is not pre-approved as part of the marketing authorization.

Self-Contained Area—Premises which provide complete and total separation of all aspects of an operation, including personnel and equipment movement, with well-established procedures, controls, and monitoring. This includes physical barriers as well as separate air-handling systems, but does not necessarily imply two distinct and separate buildings.

Signature (Signed)—See definition for signed

Signed (Signature)—The record of the individual who performed a particular action or review. This record can be initials, full handwritten signature, personal seal, or authenticated and secure electronic signature.

Solvent—An inorganic or organic liquid used as a vehicle for the preparation of solutions or suspensions in the manufacture of an intermediate or API.

Specification—A list of detailed requirements with which the products or materials used or obtained during manufacture have to conform. They serve as a basis for quality evaluation.

Standard Operating Procedure (SOP)—An authorized written procedure giving instructions for performing operations not necessarily specific to a given product or material (e.g., equipment operation, maintenance and cleaning; validation; cleaning of premises and environmental control; sampling and inspection). Certain SOPs may be used to supplement product-specific master and batch production documentation.

Starting Material—Any substance of a defined quality used in the production of a pharmaceutical product, but excluding packaging materials.

Validation—A documented program that provides a high degree of assurance that a specific process, method, or system will consistently produce a result meeting predetermined acceptance criteria. Action of proving, in accordance with the principles of GMP, that any procedure, process, equipment, material, activity, or system actually leads to the expected results (see also Qualification).

Validation Protocol—A written plan stating how validation will be conducted and defining acceptance criteria. For example, the protocol for a manufacturing process identifies processing equipment, critical process parameters/operating ranges, product characteristics, sampling, test data to be collected, number of validation runs, and acceptable test results.

Yield, Expected—The quantity of material or the percentage of theoretical yield anticipated at any appropriate phase of production based on previous laboratory, pilot scale, or manufacturing data.

Yield, Theoretical—The quantity that would be produced at any appropriate phase of production, based upon the quantity of material to be used, in the absence of any loss or error in actual production.

4

Changes to Approved NDAs and ANDAs

I. INTRODUCTION

The holders of new drug applications (NDAs) and abbreviated new drug applications (ANDAs) can make postapproval changes in accordance with added section 506A of the FDA Modernization Act. There are specific reporting requirements for postapproval changes in components and composition, manufacturing sites, manufacturing process, specifications, package labeling, miscellaneous changes, and multiple related changes. Reporting categories for changes relating to specified biotechnology and specified synthetic biological products regulated by the Center for Drug Evaluation and Research (CDER) are found in the guidance for industry entitled *Changes to an Approved Application for Specified Biotechnology and Specified Synthetic Biological Products* (July 1997). Information specific to products is developed by an applicant to assess the effect of the change on the identity, strength (e.g., assay, content uniformity), quality (e.g., physical, chemical, and biological properties), purity (e.g., impurities and degradation products), or potency (e.g., biological activity, bioavailability, bioequivalence) of a product as they may relate to the safety or effectiveness of the product. CDER has published guidances, including the SUPAC (scale-up and postapproval changes) guidances that provide recommendations on reporting categories.

II. REPORTING CATEGORIES

Section 506A of the act provides for four reporting categories that are distinguished in the following paragraphs. A "major change" is a change that has a substantial potential to have an adverse effect on the identity, strength, quality, purity, or potency of a product as these factors may relate to the safety or effectiveness of the product [506A(c)(2)]. A major change requires the submission of a supplement and approval by the FDA before distribution of the product made using the change [506A(c)(1)]. This type of supplement is called, and should be clearly labeled as, a Prior Approval Supplement. An applicant may ask the FDA to expedite its review of a Prior Approval Supplement for public health reasons (e.g., drug shortage) or if a delay in making the change described in the supplement would impose an extraordinary hardship on the applicant. This type of supplement is called, and should be clearly labeled as, a Prior Approval Supplement—Expedited Review Requested. Requests for expedited review based on extraordinary hardship should be reserved for manufacturing changes made necessary by catastrophic events (e.g., fire) or by events that could not be reasonably foreseen and for which the applicant could not plan.

A "moderate change" is a change that has a moderate potential to have an adverse effect on the identity, strength, quality, purity, or potency of the product as these factors may relate to the safety or effectiveness of the product. There are two types of moderate change. One type of moderate change requires the submission of a supplement to the FDA at least 30 days before the distribution of the product made using the change [506A(d)(3)(B)(i)]. This type of supplement is called, and should be clearly labeled as, a Supplement—Changes Being Effected in 30 Days. The product made using a moderate change cannot be distributed if the FDA informs the applicant within 30 days of receipt of the supplement that a Prior Approval Supplement is required [506A(d)(3)(B)(i)]. For each change, the supplement must contain information determined by the FDA to be appropriate and must include the information developed by the applicant in assessing the effects of the change [506A(b)]. If the FDA informs the applicant within 30 days of receipt of the supplement that information is missing, distribution must be delayed until the supplement has been amended with the missing information. The FDA may identify certain moderate changes for which distribution can occur when the FDA receives the supplement [506A(d)(3)(B)(ii)]. This type of supplement is called, and should be clearly labeled as, a Supplement—Changes Being Effected. If, after review, the FDA disapproves a Changes Being Effected in 30 Days Supplement or a Changes Being Effected Supplement, the FDA may order the manufacturer to cease distribution of the drugs that have been made using the disapproved change [506A(d)(3)(B)(iii)].

A "minor change" is a change that has minimal potential to have an adverse effect on the identity, strength, quality, purity, or potency of the product as these factors may relate to the safety or effectiveness of the product. The applicant must describe minor changes in its next annual report [506A(d)(1)(A) and (d)(2)].

An applicant can submit one or more protocols (i.e., comparability protocols) describing tests, validation studies, and acceptable limits to be achieved to demonstrate the absence of an adverse effect from specified types of changes. A comparability protocol can be used to reduce the reporting category for specified changes. A proposed comparability protocol should be submitted as a Prior Approval Supplement if not approved as part of the original application.

III. GENERAL REQUIREMENTS

Other than for editorial changes in previously submitted information (e.g., correction of spelling or typographical errors, reformatting of batch records), an applicant must notify the FDA about each change in each condition established in an approved application beyond the variations already provided for in the application [506A(a)].

An applicant making a change to an approved application under section 506A of the Act must also conform to other applicable laws and regulations, including current good manufacturing practice (cGMP) requirements of the Act [21 USC 351(a)(2)(B)] and applicable regulations in Title 21 of the Code of Federal Regulations (e.g., 21 CFR parts 210, 211, 314). For example, manufacturers must comply with relevant cGMP validation and record-keeping requirements and must ensure that relevant records are readily available for examination by authorized FDA personnel during an inspection. A Changes Being Effected Supplement for labeling changes must include 12 copies of the final printed labeling [21 CFR 314.50(e)(2)(ii)].

Except for a supplemental application providing for a change in labeling, an applicant should include a statement in a supplemental application or amendment certifying that the required field copy (21 CFR 314.50) of the supplement or amendment has been provided.

IV. ASSESSING THE EFFECT OF MANUFACTURING CHANGES

A. Assessment of the Effects of the Change

A drug made with a manufacturing change, whether a major manufacturing change or otherwise, may be distributed only after the holder validates (i.e., assesses) the effects of the change on the identity, strength, quality, purity, and potency of the product as these factors may relate to the safety or effectiveness of the product [506A(b)]. For each change, the supplement or annual report must contain information determined by the FDA to be appropriate and must include the information developed by the applicant in assessing the effects of the change [506A(b), (c)(1), (d)(2)(A), and (d)(3)(A)]. Recommendations on the type of information that should be included in a supplemental application or annual report are available in guidance documents. If no guidance is available on the type of information that should be submitted to support a change, the applicant is encouraged to contact the appropriate chemistry or microbiology review staff.

1. Conformance to Specifications

An assessment of the effect of a change on the identity, strength, quality, purity, or potency of the drug product should include a determination that the drug substance intermediates, drug substance, in-process materials, or drug product affected by the change conforms to the approved specifications. A "specification" is a quality standard (i.e., tests, analytical procedures, and acceptance criteria) provided in an approved application to confirm the quality of drug substances, drug products, intermediates, raw materials, reagents, and other components, including container closure systems and their components and in-process materials. For the purpose of defining specifications, "acceptance criteria" are numerical limits, ranges, or other criteria for the tests described. Conformance to a specification means that the material, when tested according to the analytical procedures listed in the specification, will meet the listed acceptance criteria.

2. Additional Testing

In addition to confirmation that the material affected by manufacturing changes continues to meet its specification, the applicant should perform additional testing, when appropriate, to assess whether the identity, strength, quality, purity, or potency of the product as these factors may relate to the safety or effectiveness of the product have been or will be affected. The assessment should include, as appropriate, evaluation of any changes in the chemical, physical, microbiological, biological, bioavailability, or stability profiles. This additional assessment could involve testing of the postchange drug product itself or, if appropriate, the component directly affected by the change. The type of additional testing that an applicant should perform would depend on the type of manufacturing change, the type of drug substance or drug product, and the effect of the change on the quality of the product. For example:

- Evaluation of changes in the impurity or degradation product profile could first involve profiling using appropriate chromatographic techniques and then, depending on the observed changes in the impurity profile, toxicology tests to qualify a new impurity or degradant or to qualify an impurity that is above a previously qualified level.
- Evaluation of the hardness or friability of a tablet after changes in formulation or manufacturing procedure.
- Assessment of the effect of a change on bioequivalence when required under 21 CFR part 320 could include, for example, multipoint or multimedia dissolution profiling or an in vivo bioequivalence study.
- Evaluation of extractables from new packaging components or moisture permeability of a new container closure system.

B. Equivalence

When testing is performed, the applicant should usually assess the extent to which the manufacturing change has affected the identity, strength, quality, purity, or potency of the drug product. Typically, this is accomplished by comparing test results from prechange and postchange material and determining whether the test results are equivalent or not. Simply stated: Is the product made after the change equivalent to the product made before the change? An exception to this general approach is that when bioequivalence should be redocumented for certain ANDA postapproval changes, the comparator should be the reference-listed drug. Equivalence comparisons frequently require a criterion for comparison with calculation of confidence intervals relative to a predetermined equivalence interval. For this reason, as well as for other reasons, "equivalent" does not necessarily mean "identical." Equivalence may also relate to maintenance of a quality characteristic (e.g., stability) rather than a single performance of a test.

C. Adverse Effect

Sometimes manufacturing changes have an adverse effect on the identity, strength, quality, purity, or potency of the drug product. In many cases, the applicant chooses not to implement these suboptimal manufacturing changes, but sometimes the applicant wishes to put them into practice. If an assessment concludes that a change has adversely affected the identity, strength, quality, purity, or potency of the drug product, the change should be filed in a Prior Approval Supplement, regardless of the recommended reporting category for the change. For example, a type of process change with a recommended filing category of a Supplement—Changes Being Effected in 30 Days could cause a new degradant to be formed that requires qualification or identification. However, the applicant's degradation qualification procedures may indicate that there are no safety concerns relating to the new degradant. The applicant should submit this change in a Prior Approval Supplement with appropriate information to support the continued safety and effectiveness of the product. During the review of the Prior Approval Supplement, the FDA will assess the impact of any adverse effect on the product as it may relate to the safety or effectiveness of the product.

V. COMPONENTS AND COMPOSITION

Changes in the qualitative or quantitative formulation, including inactive ingredients, as provided in the approved application, are considered major changes and should be filed in a Prior Approval Supplement, unless exempted by regulation or guidance [506A(c)(2)(A)]. The deletion or reduction of an ingredient intended to affect only the color of a product may be reported in an annual report. Guidance on changes in components and composition that may be filed in a Changes Being Effected Supplement or annual report is not included in this document because of the complexity of these recommendations, but it may be covered in one or more guidance documents describing postapproval changes (e.g., SUPAC documents).

VI. MANUFACTURING SITES

A. General Considerations

CDER should be notified about a change to a different manufacturing site used by an applicant to manufacture or process drug products, in-process materials, drug substances, or drug substance intermediates; package drug products; label drug products; or test components, drug product containers, closures, packaging materials, in-process materials, or drug products. Sites include those owned by the applicant or contract sites used by an applicant. Testing sites include those performing physical, chemical, biological, and microbiological testing to monitor, accept, or reject materials, as well as those performing stability testing. Sites used to label drug products are considered to be those that perform labeling of the drug product's primary or secondary packaging components. Sites performing operations that place identifying information on the dosage form itself (e.g., ink imprint on a filled capsule) are considered to be facilities that manufacture or process the drug product. The supplement or annual report should identify whether the proposed manufacturing site is an alternative or replacement to those provided for in the approved application.

A move to a different manufacturing site, when it is a type of site routinely subject to FDA inspection, should be filed as a Prior Approval Supplement if the site does not have a satisfactory cGMP inspection for the type of operation being moved. For labeling, secondary packaging, and testing site changes, the potential for adverse effect on the identity, strength, quality, purity, or potency of a product as these factors may relate to the safety or effectiveness of the product is considered to be independent of the type of drug product dosage form or specific type of operation being performed. Therefore, the recommended reporting category for any one of these manufacturing site changes will be the same for all types of drug products and operations. For manufacturing sites used to manufacture or process drug products, in-process materials, drug substances, or drug substance intermediates or perform primary packaging operations, the potential for adverse effect and, consequently, the recommended reporting category depend on various factors such as the type of product and operation being performed. For this reason, recommended reporting categories may differ depending on the type of drug product and operations.

Except for those situations described in sections VI.B.4, VI.C.1.b, and VI.D.5, moving production operations between buildings at the same manufacturing site or within a building, or having construction activities occur at a manufacturing site, do not have to be reported to CDER. A move to a different manufacturing site that involves other changes (e.g., process, equipment) should be evaluated as a multiple related change (see section XII) to determine the appropriate reporting category.

B. Major Changes (Prior Approval Supplement)

The following are examples of changes that are considered to have substantial potential to have an adverse effect on the identity, strength, quality, purity, or potency of a product, as these factors may relate to the safety or effectiveness of the product:

1. A move to a different manufacturing site, except one used to manufacture or process a drug substance intermediate, when the new manufacturing site has never been inspected by the FDA for the type of operation that is being moved, or the move results in a restart at the new manufacturing site of a type of operation that has been discontinued for more than 2 years.
2. A move to a different manufacturing site, except one used to manufacture or process a drug; substance intermediate, when the new manufacturing site has not had a satisfactory cGMP inspection for the type of operation being moved.
3. A move to a different manufacturing site for (1) the manufacture, processing, or primary packaging of drug products when the primary packaging components control the dose delivered to the patient or when the formulation modifies the rate or extent of availability of the drug; or for (2) the manufacture or processing of in-process materials with modified-release characteristics; examples of these types of drug products include modified-release solid oral dosage forms, transdermal systems, liposomal products, depot products, oral and nasal metered-dose inhalers, dry powder inhalers, and nasal spray pumps.
4. Transfer of manufacturing of an aseptically processed sterile drug substance or aseptically processed sterile drug product to a newly constructed or refurbished aseptic processing facility or area or to an existing aseptic processing facility or area that does not manufacture similar (including container types and sizes) approved products; for example, transferring the manufacture of a lyophilized product to an existing aseptic process area where no approved lyophilized products are manufactured or where the approved lyophilized products being manufactured have dissimilar container types or sizes to the product being transferred.
5. Transfer of the manufacture of a finished product sterilized by terminal processes to a newly constructed facility at a different manufacturing site: Once this change has been approved, subsequent site changes to the facility for similar product types and processes may be filed as a Supplement—Changes Being Effected in 30 Days.

C. Moderate Changes (Supplement—Changes Being Effected)

The following are examples of changes that are considered to have a moderate potential to have an adverse effect on the identity, strength, quality, purity, or potency of a product as these factors may relate to the safety or effectiveness of the product.

The following manufacturing site changes (excluding changes relating to drug substance intermediate manufacturing sites) should be filed in a Prior Approval Supplement if the new site does not have a satisfactory cGMP inspection for the type of operation being moved (see sections VI.B.1 and 2):

1. Supplement—Changes Being Effected in 30 Days
   a. A move to a different manufacturing site for the manufacture or processing of any drug product, in-process material, or drug substance that is not otherwise provided for in this guidance
   b. For aseptically processed sterile drug substance or aseptically processed sterile drug product, a move to an aseptic processing facility or area at the same or different manufacturing site, except as provided for in section VI.B.4
   c. A move to a different manufacturing site for the primary packaging of (1) any drug product that is not otherwise listed as a major change and of (2) modified-release solid oral dosage–form products
   d. A move to a different manufacturing site for testing whether (1) the test procedures approved in the application or procedures that have been implemented via an annual report are used, (2) all postapproval commitments made by the applicant relating to the test procedures have been fulfilled (e.g., providing methods validation samples), and (3) the new testing facility has the capability to perform the intended testing
2. Supplement—Changes Being Effected
   a. A move to a different manufacturing site for the manufacture or processing of the final intermediate

D. Minor Changes (Annual Report)

The following are examples of changes that are considered to have a minimal potential to have an adverse effect on the identity, strength, quality, purity, or potency of a product as these factors may relate to the safety or effectiveness of the product.

The following manufacturing site changes (excluding changes relating to drug substance intermediate manufacturing sites) should be filed in a Prior Approval Supplement if the new site does not have a satisfactory cGMP inspection for the type of operation being moved (see sections VI.B.1 and 2):

1. A move to a different manufacturing site for secondary packaging.
2. A move to a different manufacturing site for labeling.
3. A move to a different manufacturing site for the manufacture or processing of drug substance intermediates, other than the final intermediate.
4. A change in the contract sterilization site for packaging components when the process is not materially different from that provided for in the approved application, and the facility has a satisfactory cGMP inspection for the type of operation being performed.
5. A transfer of the manufacture of a finished product sterilized by terminal processes to a newly constructed building or existing building at the same manufacturing site.
6. A move to a different manufacturing site for the ink imprinting of solid oral dosage–form products.

VII. MANUFACTURING PROCESS

A. General Considerations

The potential for adverse effects on the identity, strength, quality, purity, or potency of a drug product as these factors may relate to the safety or effectiveness of the product depends on the type of manufacturing process and the changes being instituted for the drug substance or drug product. In some cases, there may be a substantial potential for adverse effect, regardless of direct testing of the drug substance or drug product for conformance with the approved specification. When there is a substantial potential for adverse effects, a change should be filed in a Prior Approval Supplement.

B. Major Changes (Prior Approval Supplement)

The following are examples of changes that are considered to have a substantial potential to have an adverse effect on the identity, strength, quality, purity, or potency of a product as these factors may relate to the safety or effectiveness of the product:

1. Changes that may affect the controlled (or modified) release, metering, or other characteristics (e.g., particle size) of the dose delivered to the patient, including the addition or deletion of a code imprint by embossing, debossing, or engraving on a modified-release solid oral dosage form.
2. Changes that may affect product sterility assurance including, where appropriate, process changes for sterile drug substances and sterile packaging components, including
   Changes in the sterilization method (e.g., gas, dry heat, irradiation); these include changes from sterile filtered or aseptic processing to terminal sterilization, or vice versa
   Addition, deletion, or substitution of sterilization steps or procedures for handling sterile materials in an aseptic processing operation
   Replacing sterilizers that operate by one set of principles with sterilizers that operate by another principle (e.g., substituting a gravity-displacement steam process with a process using superheated water spray)
   Addition to an aseptic processing line of new equipment made of different materials (e.g., stainless steel vs. glass, changes between plastics) that will come in contact with sterilized bulk solution or sterile drug components, or deletion of equipment from an aseptic processing line
   Replacing a class 100 aseptic fill area with a barrier system or isolator for aseptic filling: Once this change has been approved, subsequent process changes for similar product types in the same barrier system or isolator may be filed as a Supplement—Changes Being Effected in 30 Days
   Replacement or addition of lyophilization equipment of a different size that uses different operating parameters or lengthens the overall process time
   Changes from bioburden-based terminal sterilization to the use of an overkill process, and vice versa
   Changes to aseptic processing methods, including scale, that extend the total processing, including bulk storage time, by more than 50% beyond the validated limits in the approved application
   Changes in sterilizer load configurations that are outside the range of previously validated loads
   Changes in materials or pore size rating of filters used in aseptic processing
3. The following changes for a natural product: Changes in the virus or adventitious agent removal or inactivation methods; this is applicable to any material for which such procedures are necessary, including drug substance, drug product, reagents, and excipients.
4. The following changes for drug substance and drug product: Changes in the source material (e.g., microorganism, plant) or cell line.

5. The following changes for drug substance and drug product: Establishment of a new master cell bank or seed.
6. Any fundamental change in the manufacturing process or technology from that currently used by the applicant, for example:
   a. Drug product
      Dry to wet granulation, or vice versa change from one type of drying process to another (e.g., oven tray, fluid bed, microwave)
   b. Drug substance
      Filtration to centrifugation, or vice versa change in the route of synthesis of a drug substance
7. The following changes for drug substance: Any process change made after the final intermediate processing step in drug substance manufacture.
8. Changes in the synthesis or manufacture of the drug substance that may affect its impurity profile or the physical, chemical, or biological properties.
9. Addition of an ink code imprint or change to or in the ink used for an existing imprint code for a solid oral dosage–form drug product when the ink as changed is not currently used on CDER-approved products.
10. Establishing a new procedure for reprocessing a batch of drug substance or drug product that fails to meet the approved specification.

C. Moderate Changes (Supplement—Changes Being Effected)

The following are examples of changes that are considered to have a moderate potential to have an adverse effect on the identity, strength, quality, purity, or potency of a product as these factors may relate to the safety or effectiveness of the product:

1. Supplement—Changes Being Effected in 30 Days
   a. For drug products, any change in the process, process parameters, or equipment, except as otherwise provided for in this guidance
   b. For drug substances, any change in process or process parameters, except as otherwise provided for in this guidance
   c. For natural protein drug substances and drug products:
      Any change in the process, process parameters, or equipment, except as otherwise provided for in this guidance
      An increase or decrease in production scale during finishing steps that involves new or different equipment
      Replacement of equipment with that of similar, but not identical, design and operating principle that does not affect the process methodology or process operating parameters
   d. For sterile products, drug substances, and components, as appropriate:
      Changes in dry heat depyrogenation processes for glass container systems for products that are produced by terminal sterilization processes or aseptic processing
      Changes to filtration parameters for aseptic processing (including flow rate, pressure, time, or volume but not filter materials or pore size rating) that require additional validation studies for the new parameters
      Filtration process changes that provide for a change from single to dual product sterilizing filters in series, or for repeated filtration of a bulk
      Changes from one qualified sterilization chamber to another for in-process or terminal sterilization that results in changes to validated operating parameters (time, temperature, F_0, and others)
      Changes in scale of manufacturing for terminally sterilized products that increase the bulk solution storage time by more than 50% beyond the validated limits in the approved application when bioburden limits are unchanged
   e. For drug substances, redefinition of an intermediate, excluding the final intermediate, as a starting material
2. Supplement—Changes Being Effected
   a. A change in methods or controls that provides increased assurance that the drug substance or drug product will have the characteristics of identity, strength, purity, or potency that it purports to or is represented to possess
   b. For sterile drug products, elimination of in-process filtration performed as part of the manufacture of a terminally sterilized product

D. Minor Changes (Annual Report)

The following are examples of changes that are considered to have a minimal potential to have an adverse effect on the identity, strength, quality, purity, or potency of a product as these factors may relate to the safety or effectiveness of the product:

1. For drug products and protein drug substances, changes to equipment of the same design and operating principle or changes in scale, except as otherwise provided for in this guidance [e.g., section VII.C.1.c; see FDA guidance for industry on the *Submission of Documentation for Sterilization Process Validation in Applications for Human and Veterinary Drug Products* (November 1994)].
2. A minor change in an existing code imprint for a dosage form; for example, changing from a numeric to alphanumeric code.
3. Addition of an ink code imprint or a change in the ink used in an existing code imprint for a solid oral dosage–form drug product when the ink is currently used on CDER-approved products.
4. Addition or deletion of a code imprint by embossing, debossing, or engraving on a solid dosage–form drug product other than a modified-release dosage form.
5. A change in the order of addition of ingredients for solution dosage forms or solutions used in unit operations (e.g., granulation solutions).
6. Changes in scale of manufacturing for terminally sterilized products that increase the bulk solution storage time by no more than 50% beyond the validated limits in the approved application when bioburden limits are unchanged.

VIII. SPECIFICATIONS

A. General Considerations

All changes in specifications from those in the approved application must be submitted in a Prior Approval Supplement unless otherwise exempted by regulation or guidance [506A(c)(2)(A)].

Specifications (i.e., tests, analytical procedures, and acceptance criteria) are the quality standards provided in an approved application to confirm the quality of drug substances, drug products, intermediates, raw materials, reagents, and other components, including container and closure systems and in-process materials. For the purpose of defining specifications, acceptance criteria are numerical limits, ranges, or other criteria for the tests described. Examples of a test, an analytical procedure, and acceptance criteria are an assay, a specific fully described high-pressure liquid chromatography procedure, and 98.0% to 102.0%. The recommendations in this section also apply to specifications associated with sterility assurance that are included in NDA and ANDA submissions. A regulatory analytical procedure is the analytical procedure used to evaluate a defined characteristic of the drug substance or drug product. The analytical procedures in the U.S. Pharmacopeia/National Formulary (USP/NF) are those legally recognized under section 501(b) of the Act as the regulatory analytical procedures for compendial items. The applicant may include in its application alternative analytical procedures to the approved regulatory procedure for testing the drug substance and drug product. However, for purposes of determining compliance with the Act, the regulatory analytical procedure is used. In sections B to D below, the use of the term "analytical procedure" without a qualifier such as "regulatory" or "alternative" refers to analytical procedures used to test materials other than the drug substance or drug product.

B. Major Changes (Prior Approval Supplement)

The following are examples of changes in specifications that are considered to have a substantial potential to have an adverse effect on the identity, strength, quality, purity, or potency of a product as these factors may relate to the safety or effectiveness of the product:

1. Relaxing an acceptance criterion, except as otherwise provided for in this guidance (e.g., section VIII.C.1.b).
2. Deleting any part of a specification, except as otherwise provided for in this guidance (e.g., section VIII.D.2).
3. Establishing a new regulatory analytical procedure.
4. A change in a regulatory analytical procedure that does not provide the same or increased assurance of the identity, strength, quality, purity, or potency of the material being tested as the regulatory analytical procedure described in the approved application.
5. A change in an analytical procedure used for testing components, packaging components, the final intermediate, in-process materials after the final intermediate, or starting materials introduced after the final intermediate that does not provide the same or increased assurance of the identity, strength, quality, purity, or potency of the material being tested as the analytical procedure described in the approved application, except as otherwise noted; for example, a change from a high-pressure liquid chromatography procedure that distinguishes impurities to one that does not, to another type of analytical procedure (e.g., titrimetric) that does not, or to one that distinguishes impurities but for which the limit of detection or limit of quantitation is higher.
6. Relating to testing of raw materials for viruses or adventitious agents (1) relaxing an acceptance criteria, (2) deleting a test, or (3) a change in the analytical procedure that does not provide the same or increased assurance of the identity, strength, quality, purity, or potency of the material being tested as the analytical procedure described in the approved application.

C. Moderate Changes (Supplement—Changes Being Effected)

The following are examples of changes in specifications that are considered to have a moderate potential to have an adverse effect on the identity, strength, quality, purity, or potency of a product as these factors may relate to the safety or effectiveness of the product:

1. Supplement—Changes Being Effected in 30 Days
   a. Any change in a regulatory analytical procedure other than editorial or those identified as major changes
   b. Relaxing an acceptance criterion or deleting a test for raw materials used in drug substance manufacturing, in-process materials before the final intermediate, starting materials introduced before the final drug substance intermediate, or drug substance intermediates (excluding final intermediate), except as provided for in section VIII.B.6.
   c. A change in an analytical procedure used for testing raw materials used in drug substance manufacturing, in-process materials before the intermediate, starting materials introduced before the final drug substance intermediate, or drug substance intermediates (excluding final intermediate) that does not provide the same or increased assurance of the identity, strength, quality, purity, or potency of the material being tested as the analytical procedure described in the approved application, except as provided for in section VIII.B.6.
   d. Relaxing an in-process acceptance criterion associated with microbiological monitoring of the production environment, materials, and components that are included in NDA and ANDA submissions; for example, increasing the microbiological alert or action limits for critical processing environments in an aseptic fill facility or increasing the acceptance limit for bioburden in bulk solution intended for filtration and aseptic filling.
2. Supplement—Changes Being Effected
   a. An addition to a specification that provides increased assurance that the drug substance or drug product will have the characteristics of identity, strength, purity, or potency that it purports to or is represented to possess; for example, adding a new test and associated analytical procedure and acceptance criterion
   b. A change in an analytical procedure used for testing components, packaging components, the final intermediate, in-process materials after the final intermediate, or starting materials introduced after the final intermediate that provides the same or increased assurance of the identity, strength, quality, purity, or potency of the material being tested as the analytical procedure described in the approved application

D. Minor Changes (Annual Report)

The following are examples of changes in specifications that are considered to have a minimal potential to have an adverse effect on the identity, strength, quality, purity, or potency of a product as these factors may relate to the safety or effectiveness of the product:

1. Any change in a specification made to comply with an official compendium.
2. For drug substance and drug product, the addition, deletion, or revision of an alternative analytical procedure that provides the same or greater level of assurance of the identity, strength, quality, purity, or potency of the material being tested as the analytical procedure described in the approved application.
3. Tightening of acceptance criteria.
4. A change in an analytical procedure used for testing raw materials used in drug substance synthesis, starting materials introduced before the final drug substance intermediate, in-process materials before the final intermediate, or

drug substance intermediates (excluding final intermediate) that provides the same or increased assurance of the identity, strength, quality, purity, or potency of the material being tested as the analytical procedure described in the approved application.

IX. PACKAGE

A. General Considerations

The potential for adverse effect on the identity, strength, quality, purity, or potency of a product, as these factors may relate to the safety or effectiveness of the product when making a change to or in the container closure system is generally dependent on the route of administration of the drug product, performance of the container closure system, and likelihood of interaction between the packaging component and the dosage form. In some cases, there may be a substantial potential for adverse effect, regardless of direct product testing for conformance with the approved specification.

A change to or in a packaging component will often result in a new or revised specification for the packaging component. This situation does not have to be considered a multiple related change. Only the reporting category for the packaging change needs to be considered.

B. Major Changes (Prior Approval Supplement)

The following are examples of changes that are considered to have a substantial potential to have an adverse effect on the identity, strength, quality, purity, or potency of a product as these factors may relate to the safety or effectiveness of the product:

1. For liquid (e.g., solution, suspension, elixir) and semisolid (e.g., creams, ointments) dosage forms, a change to or in polymeric materials (e.g., plastic, rubber) of primary packaging components, when the composition of the component as changed has never been used in a CDER-approved product of the same dosage form and same route of administration; for example, a polymeric material that has been used in a CDER-approved topical ointment would not be considered CDER-approved for use with an ophthalmic ointment.
2. For liquid (e.g., solution, suspension, elixir) and semisolid (e.g., creams, ointments) dosage forms in permeable or semipermeable container closure systems, a change to an ink or an adhesive used on the permeable or semipermeable packaging component to one that has never been used in a CDER-approved product of the same dosage form, same route of administration, and same type of permeable or semipermeable packaging component (e.g., low-density polyethylene, polyvinyl chloride).
3. A change in the primary packaging components for any product when the primary packaging components control the dose delivered to the patient (e.g., the valve or actuator of a metered-dose inhaler).
4. For sterile products, any other change that may affect product sterility assurance, such as:
   A change from a glass ampule to a glass vial with an elastomeric closure
   A change to a flexible container system (bag) from another container system
   A change to a prefilled syringe dosage form from another container system
   A change from a single-unit-dose container to a multiple-dose container system
   Changes that add or delete silicone treatments to container closure systems (such as elastomeric closures or syringe barrels)
   Changes in the size or shape of a container for a sterile drug product
5. Deletion of a secondary packaging component intended to provide additional protection to the drug product (e.g., carton to protect from light, overwrap to limit transmission of moisture or gases).
6. A change to a new container closure system if the new container closure system does not provide the same or better protective properties than the approved container closure system.

C. Moderate Changes (Supplement—Changes Being Effected)

The following are examples of changes that are considered to have a moderate potential to have an adverse effect on the identity, strength, quality, purity, or potency of a product as these factors may relate to the safety or effectiveness of the product:

1. Supplement—Changes Being Effected in 30 Days
   a. A change to or in a container closure system, except as otherwise provided for in this guidance
   b. Changes in the size or shape of a container for a sterile drug substance
2. Supplement—Changes Being Effected
   a. A change in the size or shape of a container for a nonsterile drug product, except for solid dosage forms (see section IX.D.2 regarding solid dosage forms)
   b. A change in or addition or deletion of a desiccant

D. Minor Changes (Annual Report)

The following are examples of changes that are considered to have a minimal potential to have an adverse effect on the identity, strength, quality, purity, or potency of a product as these factors may relate to the safety or effectiveness of the product:

1. A change in the container closure system for a nonsterile drug product, based on a showing of equivalency to the approved system under a protocol approved in the application or published in an official compendium.
2. A change in the size or shape of a container containing the same number of dose units, for a nonsterile solid dosage form.
3. The following changes in the container closure system of solid oral dosage–form products as long as the new package provides the same or better protective properties (e.g., light, moisture) and any new primary packaging component materials have been used in and been in contact with CDER-approved solid oral dosage–form products:
   Adding or changing a child-resistant closure, changing from a metal to plastic screw cap, or changing from a plastic to metal screw cap
   Changing from one plastic container to another of the same type of plastic (e.g., high-density polyethylene container to another high-density polyethylene container)
   Changes in packaging materials used to control odor (e.g., charcoal packets)
   Changes in bottle filler (e.g., change in weight of cotton or amount used) without changes in the type of filler (e.g., cotton to rayon)
   Increasing the wall thickness of the container
   A change in or addition of a cap liner
   A change in or addition of a seal (e.g., heat induction seal)

A change in an antioxidant, colorant, stabilizer, or mold-releasing agent for production of the container or closure to one that is used at similar levels in the packaging of CDER-approved solid oral dosage–form products
A change to a new container closure system when the container closure system is already approved in the NDA or ANDA for other strengths of the product

4. The following changes in the container closure system of nonsterile liquid products, as long as the new package provides the same or better protective properties and any new primary packaging component materials have been used in and been in contact with CDER-approved liquid products with the same route of administration (i.e., the material in contact with a liquid topical should already have been used with other CDER-approved liquid topical products):
   Adding or changing a child-resistant closure
   Changing from a metal to plastic screw cap
   Changing from a plastic to metal screw cap
   Increasing the wall thickness of the container
   A change in or addition of a cap liner
   A change in or addition of a seal (e.g., heat induction seal)
5. A change in the container closure system of unit-dose packaging (e.g., blister packs) for nonsterile solid dosage form–products, as long as the new package provides the same or better protective properties and any new primary packaging component materials have been used in and been in contact with CDER-approved products of the same type (e.g., solid oral dosage form, rectal suppository).
6. The following changes in the container closure system of nonsterile semisolid products, as long as the new package provides the same or better protective properties and any new primary packaging component materials have been used in and been in contact with CDER-approved semisolid products:
   Changes in the closure or cap
   Increasing the wall thickness of the container
   A change in or addition of a cap liner
   A change in or addition of a seal
   A change in the crimp sealant
7. A change in the flip seal cap color, as long as the cap color is consistent with any established color-coding system for that class of drug products.

X. LABELING

A. General Considerations

A drug product labeling change includes changes in the package insert, package labeling, or container label. An applicant should promptly revise all promotional labeling and drug advertising to make it consistent with any labeling change implemented in accordance with the regulations. All labeling changes for ANDA products must be consistent with section 505(j) of the Act.

B. Major Changes (Prior Approval Supplement)

Any proposed change in the labeling, except those that are designated as moderate or minor changes by regulation or guidance, should be submitted as a Prior Approval Supplement. The following list contains some examples of changes that are currently considered by CDER to fall into this reporting category:

1. Changes based on postmarketing study results, including, but not limited to, labeling changes associated with new indications and usage.
2. Change in, or addition of, pharmacoeconomic claims based on clinical studies.
3. Changes to the clinical pharmacology or the clinical study section reflecting new or modified data.
4. Changes based on data from preclinical studies.
5. Revision (expansion or contraction) of population based on data.
6. Claims of superiority to another product.
7. Change in the labeled storage conditions, unless exempted by regulation or guidance.

C. Moderate Changes (Supplement—Changes Being Effected)

A Changes Being Effected Supplement should be submitted for any labeling change that adds or strengthens a contraindication, warning, precaution, or adverse reaction; adds or strengthens a statement about drug abuse, dependence, psychological effect, or overdosage; adds or strengthens an instruction about dosage and administration that is intended to increase the safe use of the product; deletes false, misleading, or unsupported indications for use or claims for effectiveness; or is specifically requested by the FDA. The submission should include 12 copies of final printed labeling. The following list includes some examples of changes that are currently considered by CDER to fall into this reporting category:

1. Addition of an adverse event because of information reported to the applicant or agency.
2. Addition of a precaution arising out of a postmarketing study.
3. Clarification of the administration statement to ensure proper administration of the product.
4. Labeling changes, normally classified as major changes, that the FDA specifically requests be implemented using a Changes Being Effected Supplement.

D. Minor Changes (Annual Report)

Labeling with editorial or similar minor changes or with a change in the information concerning the description of the drug product or information about how the drug is supplied that does not involve a change in the dosage strength or dosage form should be described in an annual report. The following list includes some examples that are currently considered by CDER to fall into this reporting category:

1. Changes in the layout of the package or container label that are consistent with FDA regulations (e.g., 21 CFR part 201) without a change in the content of the labeling.
2. Editorial changes, such as adding a distributor's name.
3. Foreign language versions of the labeling, if no change is made to the content of the approved labeling and a certified translation is included.
4. Labeling changes made to comply with an official compendium.

XI. MISCELLANEOUS CHANGES

A. Major Changes (Prior Approval Supplement)

The following are examples of changes that are considered to have a substantial potential to have an adverse effect on the identity, strength, quality, purity, or potency of a product as these factors may relate to the safety or effectiveness of the product:

1. Changes requiring completion of studies in accordance with 21 CFR part 320 to demonstrate equivalence of the drug to the drug as manufactured without the change or to a reference-listed drug [506A(c)(2)(B)].

2. Addition of a stability protocol or comparability protocol.
3. Changes to an approved stability protocol or comparability protocol unless otherwise provided for in this guidance (e.g., VIII.C, VIII.D, XI.C.2).
4. An extension of an expiration dating period based on data obtained under a new or revised stability testing protocol that has not been approved in the application or on full shelf-life data on pilot-scale batches using an approved protocol.

B. Moderate Changes (Supplement—Changes Being Effected)

The following are examples of changes that are considered to have a moderate potential to have an adverse effect on the identity, strength, quality, purity, or potency of a product as these factors may relate to the safety or effectiveness of the product:

1. Supplement—Changes Being Effected in 30 Days
   a. Reduction of an expiration dating period to provide increased assurance of the identity, strength, quality, purity, or potency of the drug product; extension of an expiration date that has previously been reduced under this provision should be filed in a Supplement—Changes Being Effected in 30 Days even if it is based on data obtained under a protocol approved in the application
2. Supplement—Changes Being Effected
   a. No changes have been identified

C. Minor Changes (Annual Report)

The following are examples of changes that are considered to have a minimal potential to have an adverse effect on the identity, strength, quality, purity, or potency of a product as these factors may relate to the safety or effectiveness of the product:

1. An extension of an expiration dating period based on full shelf life data on full production batches obtained under a protocol approved in the application.
2. Addition of time points to the stability protocol or deletion of time points beyond the approved expiration dating period.
3. A change from previously approved stability storage conditions to storage conditions recommended in ICH guidances.
4. Non-USP reference standards:
   Replacement of an in-house reference standard or reference panel (or panel member) according to procedures in an approved application
   Tightening of acceptance criteria for existing reference standards to provide greater assurance of product purity and potency

XII. MULTIPLE RELATED CHANGES

Multiple related changes involve various combinations of individual changes. For example, a site change may also involve equipment and manufacturing process changes, or a component and composition change may necessitate a change in a specification. For multiple related changes for which the recommended reporting categories for the individual changes differ, CDER recommends that the filing be in accordance with the most restrictive of those reporting categories recommended for the individual changes. When the multiple related changes all have the same recommended reporting category, CDER recommends that the filing be in accordance with the reporting category for the individual changes. For the purposes of determining the reporting category for moves between buildings, the terms "different manufacturing site" and "same manufacturing site" are defined as follows. Same manufacturing site: The new and old buildings are included under the same drug establishment registration number, and the same FDA district office is responsible for inspecting the operations in both the new and old buildings. Different manufacturing site: The new and old buildings have different drug establishment registration numbers, or different FDA district offices are responsible for inspecting operations in the new and old building.

The change to a different manufacturing site should be filed in a Prior Approval Supplement when the new manufacturing site has never been inspected by the FDA for the type of operation being moved, the move results in a restart at the new manufacturing site of a type of operation that has been discontinued for more than 2 years, or the new manufacturing site does not have a satisfactory cGMP inspection for the type of operation being moved.

Examples of postapproval manufacturing site changes and filing consequences include

- An applicant wants to move the manufacture of an immediate-release tablet to a different manufacturing site that currently manufactures, and has satisfactory cGMP status for, capsules and powders for oral solution. This manufacturing site change should be filed in a Prior Approval Supplement because the new manufacturing site does not have a satisfactory cGMP inspection for immediate-release tablets.
- An applicant wants to contract out his or her packaging operations for immediate-release tablets and capsules and modified-release capsules. The potential contract packager has a satisfactory cGMP status for immediate-release and modified-release capsules but has never packaged immediate-release tablets. The packaging site change for the immediate-release tablet products should be filed in a Prior Approval Supplement. The packaging site change for the capsule products should be filed as recommended in section VI of this guidance for packaging sites with a satisfactory cGMP inspection.
- An applicant wishes to consolidate his or her product testing to a single analytical laboratory at a manufacturing site. This manufacturing site produces various solid oral dosage–form products, has an operational analytical laboratory currently at the site, and has satisfactory cGMP inspections for the manufacturing occurring at the facility. Some of the products that will be tested at the analytical laboratory when the consolidation occurs are not solid oral dosage form products. Unlike most other production operations, testing laboratories are not inspected on a dosage form/type of drug substance-specific basis. The satisfactory cGMP inspection of the analytical laboratory, which was performed as part of the cGMP inspection for manufacture of the solid oral dosage form products, is considered to apply to all dosage forms, including those not actually produced at the site.

Different reporting categories are proposed for changes to or the addition of certain components based on whether the component/material has been used in and has been in contact with CDER-approved products. Different reporting categories are recommended once CDER has reviewed certain components/materials in association with a product approval because similar subsequent changes then have a reduced potential to have an adverse effect on the identity, strength, quality, purity, or potency of a product as they may relate to the safety or effectiveness of the product. For example, certain changes in the container closure systems of solid oral dosage form products may be included in the annual report, as long as the new package provides the same or better protective properties and any new primary packaging component materials have been used in and been in contact with CDER-approved solid oral dosage–form products (see section IX.D.3). If the primary packaging component material has not been used in or has not been in contact with CDER-approved solid oral dosage–form products, then submission of the change in an annual report is not recommended. CDER-approved products are considered those subject to an approved NDA or ANDA. When information is not available, an applicant should use reliable sources of information to determine that the component or material has been used in and has been in contact with a CDER-approved product of the same dosage form and route of administration, as appropriate. The applicant should identify in the supplement or annual report the basis for the conclusion that the component or material is used in a CDER-approved product.

If an applicant cannot confirm that a component or material has been used in and has been in contact with a CDER-approved product of the same dosage form and route of administration, the applicant has the option of filing the change for a single NDA or ANDA, using the higher recommended reporting category and, after approval, filing similar subsequent changes for other NDAs and ANDAs, using the lower recommended reporting category.

GLOSSARY

Acceptance Criteria—Numerical limits, ranges, or other criteria for the tests described

Active Ingredient/Drug Substance—Any component that is intended to furnish pharmacological activity or other direct effect in the diagnosis, cure, mitigation, treatment, or prevention of a disease, or to affect the structure or any function of the human body, but does not include intermediates used in the synthesis of such ingredient, including those components that may undergo chemical change in the manufacture of the drug product and are present in the drug product in a modified form intended to furnish the specified activity or effect [21 CFR 210.3(b)(7) and 314.3]

Component—Any ingredient intended for use in the manufacture of a drug product, including those that may not appear in such drug product [21 CFR 210.3(b)(3)]

Container Closure System—The sum of packaging components that together contain and protect the dosage form; this includes primary packaging components and secondary packaging components, if the latter are intended to provide additional protection to the drug product

Drug Product—A finished dosage form, for example, tablet, capsule, or solution, that contains an active ingredient, generally, but not necessarily, in association with inactive ingredients [21 CFR 210.3(b)(4)]

Final Intermediate—The last compound synthesized before the reaction that produces the drug substance. The final step forming the drug substance must involve covalent bond formation or breakage; ionic bond formation (i.e., making the salt of a compound) does not qualify. As a consequence, when the drug substance is a salt, the precursors to the organic acid or base, rather than the acid or base itself, should be considered the final intermediate

Inactive Ingredients—Any intended component of the drug product other than an active ingredient

In-Process Material—Any material fabricated, compounded, blended, or derived by chemical reaction that is produced for, and used in, the preparation of the drug product [21 CFR 210.3(b)(9)]. For drug substance, in-process materials are considered those materials that are undergoing change (e.g., molecular, physical)

Intermediate—A material produced during steps of the synthesis of a drug substance that must undergo further molecular change before it becomes a drug substance

Package—The container closure system and labeling, associated components (e.g., dosing cups, droppers, spoons), and external packaging (e.g., cartons, shrink wrap)

Packaging Component—Any single part of a container closure system

Primary Packaging Component—A packaging component that is or may be in direct contact with the dosage form

Reference-Listed Drug—The listed drug identified by the FDA as the drug product on which an applicant relies in seeking approval of its abbreviated application (21 CFR 314.3)

Satisfactory cGMP Inspection—A satisfactory cGMP inspection is an FDA inspection during which no objectionable conditions or practices were found during (no action indicated), or an inspection during which objectionable conditions were found, but corrective action is left to the firm to take voluntarily, and the objectionable conditions will not be the subject of further administrative or regulatory actions (voluntary action indicated). Information about the cGMP status of a firm may be obtained by requesting a copy of the Quality Assurance Profile (QAP) from the FDAs Freedom of Information (FOI) Office. The QAP reports information on the cGMP compliance status of firms that manufacture, package, assemble, repack, relabel, or test human drugs, devices, biologics, and veterinary drugs. All FOI requests must be in writing and should follow the instructions found in the reference entitled *A Handbook for Requesting Information and Records from FDA*. An electronic version of this reference is available at the Web site http://www.fda.gov/opacom/backgrounders/foiahand.html

Secondary Packaging Component—A packaging component that is not and will not be in direct contact with the dosage form

Specifications—The quality standards (i.e., tests, analytical procedures, and acceptance criteria) provided in an approved application to confirm the quality of drug substances, drug products, intermediates, raw materials, reagents, and other components including container closure systems and in-process materials

Validate the Effects of the Change—To assess the effect of a manufacturing change on the identity, strength, quality, purity, or potency of a drug as these factors relate to the safety or effectiveness of the drug

5

Formulation Considerations of Liquid Products

Liquid formulations offer many advantages, from ease in dosing to ease in administration (easy to swallow), and myriad possibilities of innovative drug delivery systems. One of the most desirable features of liquid formulations, particularly the solution forms, is the relatively lower importance of bioavailability considerations, as the drug molecules are already in the dispersed phase, removing many rate-limiting steps in the absorption of drugs. For the purpose of this volume, liquid formulations include formulations that have liquid characteristics, meaning they can flow and thus include clear liquids, suspensions, and extemporaneous powder suspensions (which could easily be classified as uncompressed solids but for the stability considerations postreconstitution, which are common to liquid preparations). However, all of the advantages of liquid dosage forms are balanced by the many problems in their formulation. These include stability problems, taste masking needs, phase separations, and so forth, all of which require highly specialized formulation techniques.

I. SOLUBILITY

The amount of active drug dissolved per unit of a solvent or liquid base is a critical parameter subject to many factors including temperature, presence of electrolytes (salting-out effect), complexation with other components, state of crystallinity (such as amorphous), nature of crystals (inclusion or imperfections), hydration, or salvation, and so forth. One of the most important studies conducted on new chemical entities is the solubility characteristics, phase conversion studies, and saturation limits under different conditions. Where the amount of drug is above saturation solubility, an equilibrium between the solution (monomolecular dispersion) is established with undissolved particles (often multimolecular dispersions), the direction and extent of which are governed by many physicochemical factors. Because the absorption of drugs takes place only from a monomolecular dispersion (except those instances of pinocytosis, etc.), the equilibrium of the two states is critical to drug absorption. A large number of pH-adjusting buffers are used in the liquid products to modify the solubility of drugs as well as to provide the most optimal pH for drug absorption and drug stability. The dielectric constant of the solvent (or composite dispersion phase) is important in determining the solubility. With available values of dielectric constant, for both pure systems and binary systems, it is easy to project the solubility characteristics of many new drugs. Another factor determining the solubility of drugs is the degree of solubilization in the dispersion phase.

Solubilization is defined as spontaneous passage of poorly water-soluble drugs into an aqueous solution of a detergent, the mechanism being entrapment of drug molecules in the micelles of surface-active agent. As a result, many liquid preparations contain surfactants, not only to solubilize but also to "wet" the powders to allow better mixing with liquid phase. Because the critical micelle concentration of surfactants is highly dependent on the presence of other polar or dielectric molecules, the use of surfactants to solubilized drugs requires extensive compatability studies. The most common solubilizers used include polyoxyethylene sorbital, fatty acid esters, polyoxyethylene monoalklyl ethers, sucrose monoesters, lanolin esters and ethers, and so forth.

Complexation with other components of formulation can give rise to enhanced or reduced solubility. Organic compounds in solution generally tend to associate with each other to some extent, but these are weak bonds, and the complex readily disassociates. Where the drug forms a stronger complex, such as with caffeine or other binders, solubility can be extensively altered. Some polyols are known to disrupt complexes, reducing the solubility. Often complexation results in loss of active drug or a preservative used in the system, leading to serious stability problems. Examples of complexation include when xanthines, polyvinyl pyrrolidone, and so on bind to drugs.

Hydrotrophy is defined as an increase in solubility in water caused by presence of large amounts of additives. It is another type of "solubilization," except the solubilizing agent is not necessarily a surfactant. The phenomenon is closer to complexation, but the change in solvent characteristics play a significant role as well. In general, the quantity of other components must be in the range of 20% to 50% to induce hydrotrophy.

II. CHEMICAL MODIFICATION

Many poorly soluble drugs can be made more water soluble by modifying their chemistry, such as introducing by a hydrophilic group on the molecule. Salts and derivates of poorly soluble drugs are widely used, and modification requires a careful selection because different salts and forms may not have the same chemical stability, and also because the biologic activity may be modified.

III. PRESERVATION

Preservatives are almost always a part of liquid formulations unless there is sufficient preservative efficacy in the formulation itself, such as due to high sugar content, presence of antimicrobial drugs, or solvents that inhibit growth such as alcohol. In all instances a preservative efficacy challenge is needed to prove adequate protection against the growth of microorganisms during the shelf life and use of the product (such as in the case of reconstituted powder suspensions). A large number of approved preservatives are available, including such universal preservatives as parabens, to protect liquid preparations. Among the acidic group, the most prominent preservatives are phenol, chlorocresol, O-pheyl phenol, alkyl esters of parahydroxybenzoic acid, benzoic acid and its salts, boric acid and its salts, and sorbic acid and its salts; neutral preservatives include chlorbutanol, benzyl alcohol, and β-phenylethyl alcohol; mercurial preservatives include thiomersal, phenylmercuric acetate, and nitrate; and nitromersol and quarternary compounds include benzalkonium chloride and cetylpyridinium chloride. The admissible levels of preservatives are defined in the pharmacopoeia. It should be noted that although preservatives provide an essential function, they often cause an unpleasant taste and allergic reactions in some individuals, requiring proper labeling of all products containing preservatives.

IV. SWEETENING AGENTS

Because taste is of prime importance in the administration of liquid products, sweetening agents ranging from sugar to potassium acesulfame are widely used; appropriate warnings are required when using artificial sweetening agents. Often a combination of sweetening agents is used, in combination with various flavors (which are often included to make the product more palatable), to impart the best taste. When formulating granules for dispersion, solid flavors are preferred.

V. FLAVORS

There are four basic sensations: salty, bitter, sweet, and sour. A combination of efforts is required to mask these tastes. For example, menthol and chloroform act as desensitizing agents; a large number of natural and artificial flavors and their combinations are available to mask the bitterness most often found in organic compounds. Most formulators refer the selection of compatible flavors to companies manufacturing these flavors, as they may allow use of their drug master file for the purpose of filing regulatory applications. The formulator is referred to Givaudan (http://www.givaudan.com/), International Flavors and Fragrances (http://www.iff.com), and Flavors of North America (http://www.fonaflavors.com). Detailed information about other companies can be obtained from the National Association of Flavor and Fragrances (http://www.naffs.org/naffs/public/members.htm). It is noteworthy that as of the end of 2003, all foreign manufacturers of flavors are required to file a registration with the U.S. Food and Drug Administration under the Public Health Security and Bioterrorism Preparedness and Response Act of 2002.

VI. VISCOSITY

Because the flow of liquid for dispensing and dosing is important, an appropriate control of viscosity is required to prevent the liquid from running and, at the same time, to allow good dosing control; many thickening agents are available including carboxymethyl cellulose, methyl cellulose, polyvinylpyrrolidone, and sugar. Because of the significant opportunities available for interacting with salts and other formulation ingredients, the viscosity control should be studied in the final formulation and over the shelf life of the product.

VII. APPEARANCE

The appearance or color of liquid products is often synchronized with the flavors used, for example, green or blue for mint, red for berry, and so forth. Because the amount of dyestuffs allowed in pharmaceutical products is strongly regulated, this presents problems—especially where there is a need to mask features of a preparation. In some instances, solutions are made to "sparkle" by passing them through a filtration process. Often, adsorbents are used in the liquid preparations to remove fine particles, imparting a greater clarity to solutions. Filtration often presents problems, but with the help now available from major filter manufacturers, most problems can be readily solved. The formulators are urged to consult these commercial suppliers.

VIII. CHEMICAL STABILITY

Drugs are more unstable in solution or liquid dispersion than they are in solid state because the molecular interactions are more plausible in liquid surroundings.

IX. PHYSICAL STABILITY

Physically stable liquid products are supposed to retain their color, viscosity, clarity, taste, and odor throughout the shelf life; however, the limits of the specifications for physical attributes are often kept flexible to allow for subjective evaluation criteria often involved and for inevitable, inconsequential, changes in the physical characteristics of these products. Ideally, a freshly prepared product is used as the reference standard; alternately, many companies develop more objective evaluation criteria using instrumental evaluation instead of subjective evaluation. Similar to chemical stability, physical stability can be significantly altered by the packaging type and design; as a result, the New Drug Application for every product requires a package interaction description; obviously, final stability data are to be developed in the final package form. Although glass bottles are fairly resistant to many products, caps and liners are often not. Even the integrity of the caps needs to be evaluated, applying exact torque in closing the bottles intended for stability evaluation; this is important to prevent any cap breakage that might adversely affect stability.

X. RAW MATERIAL

Raw material specifications are more important in liquid products, as the contaminants can adversely affect the formulation more than in solid dosage form. Also, the many features of a liquid product are controlled by including several raw materials such as sweeteners, thickening agents, and so forth, further complicating the matrixing of formulation at the development stage. The microbial quality of raw materials (both solid and liquid) needs to be critically evaluated. It is noteworthy that several raw materials used in liquid products may fall into the "food" category, and even though one is purchasing pharmaceutical-grade material, newly enacted laws in the United States require all foreign manufacturers to make a complete declaration of the composition of materials. Companies are encouraged to revise their specifications based on this additional information, to control the quality of raw materials more tightly.

Water is the most common raw material used, and it is recommended that the manufacturer fully comply with the standards of at least purified water for inclusion in the formulation, although there is no requirement. Efforts should be made to provide as much microbial-free water as possible; this can be readily achieved by installing a loop system in which the incoming water is first subjected to ultraviolet sterilizer, carbon filter, demineralizer, and a 5-μm filter, and then sent to a heated tank, from which it is passed again through an ultraviolet sterilizer and then a 0.22-μm filter before bringing it into the product; water coming out of the 5-μm filter can be circulated. When using a loop, it is important to establish methods for draining the dead water in the tap and the loop before using it. Also make sure that the flow rate of water does not exceed the sterilizing capacity of the ultraviolet systems installed.

XI. MANUFACTURING EQUIPMENT

Fully sanitizable stainless steel 314 or better quality is recommended. Equipment must be cleaned or sterilized; appropriate disinfectants include dilute solutions of hydrogen peroxide, phenol derivatives, and peracetic acid. Equipment lines can be sterilized by using alcohol, boiling water, autoclaving, steam, or dry heat. Where lids are used, be cautious of the condensate, which may be a source of microbial contamination. Operators must conform to all sanitary presentation requirements, including head covering, gloves, and face masks. Use of portable laminar flow hoods to expose ingredients before addition is often desirable.

XII. MANUFACTURING DIRECTIONS

Provided in this volume are hundreds of formulations with manufacturing directions; in some instances, for the sake of brevity, general details are left out that pertain to basic compounding techniques. For example, the order of addition and techniques of adding solutes to a liquid tank can be very important. Flavors are generally added after first mixing them in a smaller volume of the solvent or liquid base and rinsing them with a portion of liquid as well. This also holds for all other additions, particularly those of smaller quantities of ingredients. Proper mixing is validated; however, unlike solid mixing, where overmixing may result in segregation, the problems in liquid mixing pertain to air entrapment. Appropriate temperature of the liquid phase is often important to ensure that there is no precipitation of the solute added. Classic examples include use of syrup base, which must be heated to bring it to proper viscosity and to allow proper mixing. Parabens, when used as preservatives, must be dissolved in hot water because the quantity used is small and can be readily lost if complete dissolution is not ensured. In most instances, small quantities of solutes should be predissolved in a smaller quantity of solvent before adding it to the main tank. It is customary to bring the batch to the final volume of weight. The gravimetric adjustments are preferred, as they can be done while taring the vessel. Problems arise when solvents like alcohol are used wherein volume contraction and density are subject to temperature changes. Also, formulations are often presented in a volumetric format and require careful conversion calculation, especially where one or two components are used to compensate for the amount of active used (e.g., based on potency factors).

XIII. PACKAGING

Filling of liquid products is determined by their viscosity, surface tension, foam producing, and compatibility with filling machine components. Liquids are often filled at a higher temperature to allow better flow. In most instances, some type of piston filling and delivery is used to fill bottles, for which proper control of volume is required. The filling can be done on the basis of fixed volume or on the level of fill in the container. The filling can be accomplished through positive pressure or through a vacuum created in the container. If the latter is used, care should be taken not to lose any volatile components through the vacuum process; proper validation is required. Liquid product exposed to environment should be protected and filled under a laminar flow hood where possible. All points of contact of product to the environment should be similarly protected; however, once the product has been filled and capped, the bottles can be safely taken to an uncontrolled environment. In most instances, either plastic or aluminum caps are applied to bottles. The liners used in the caps should demonstrate full compatibility with the product, including any adhesive used. Proper torque should be applied to ensure a tight seal. Pilfer-evident packaging where used must comply with the regulatory requirements. It is not uncommon for syrups to crystallize out at the edge of the bottles, which the consumer might think a defect. Efforts should be made to formulate products to avoid this type of crystallization; use of sugar-free formulations is becoming more acceptable and offers a good alternate. However, taste masking without using sugar or liquid glucose remains a challenge. Stability testing in final packaged containers should include trial shipment runs as well to ensure that the caps do not come off or leak during the shipment.

XIV. PARTICLE SIZE AND SHAPE

When suspensions are formulated to provide a stable system, the particle size becomes critical. Flocculated suspensions also require careful particle-size control either in the process of manufacturing or in the starting material. Equally important is the crystal habit—the outward appearance of an agglomeration of crystals. Crystal structure can be altered during the manufacturing process, particularly if the product is subject to temperature cycling, and this can alter the stability of suspensions.

XV. SUSPENSIONS

Suspensions are manufactured either by a precipitation or by dispersed methods requiring use of suspending agents whose characteristic can significantly change because of the presence of other components such as electrolytes.

XVI. EMULSIONS

Heterogeneous systems comprising emulsions offer greater difficulties in manufacturing, where not only a careful calculation of formulation additives such as surfactants is required but also the manufacturing techniques such as mixing times, intensity of mixing, and temperature become critical in the formation of proper emulsion of the stable type. Microemulsion manufacturing requires special equipment, and recently the use of nanoparticles has created a need for highly specialized handling systems. Homogenizers are used to emulsify liquids along with ultrasonifiers and colloid mills. In some instances, spontaneous emulsification is obtained by a careful order of mixing. The choice of emulsifying agent depends on the type of emulsion desired and determined by the use of hydrophilic–lipophilic balance evaluation. The temperature at which an emulsion is formed can often affect the particle size and, thus, later, the tendency to coalesce or break. Auxiliary emulsification aids include use of fine solids. Hydrophilic colloids are commonly used to impart proper viscosity that enhances stability of emulsions. However, there is a tendency to build up viscosity with time in freshly prepared emulsions. The flow characteristics of emulsions are important and are determined by the emulsion's yield value. Consistency in the density character of emulsion is therefore important. Clear emulsions have a lower proportion of internal phase and require solubilization techniques more frequently than do opaque emulsions. The antimicrobial preservatives used in emulsions are selected on the basis of the type of emulsion manufactured (oil-in-water or water-in-oil). Because water is one of the phases often encountered in emulsions, these must be properly preserved. Classical preservatives are used, but care must be exercised in not selecting preservatives that might interact with surfactants; get adsorbed onto the packaging material such as plastic bottles, caps, or cap liners; and be lost to a point at which they are rendered inactive. Parabens remain a good choice. The presence of oil phase also requires inclusion of antioxidants where necessary, and these may include such examples as gallic acid, propyl gallate, butylated hydroxy-anisole, butylated hydroxytoluene (BHT), ascorbic acid, sulfites, l-tocopherol, butyl phenol, and so forth. Scaling up of emulsion formulations from laboratory scale to manufacturing scales often presents significant problems related to temperature distribution studies; often the two phases are mixed at a specific temperature that may change during the mixing process and thus require a certain mixing rate. Stability testing of emulsions is subject to different protocols than those used for other liquid products, for example, higher-temperature studies may cause an emulsion to break but may not be reflective of the log-linear effect of temperature but, rather, of phase change or inversion. Centrifugation is a common technique to study emulsion stability, and so is the agitation test, which may cause suspended phases to coalesce. Of prime importance in the stability evaluation of emulsions are the phase separation, viscosity changes, changes in light reflection, viscosity, particle size, electrical conductivity, and chemical composition.

XVII. POWDER FOR RECONSTITUTION

Whereas, classically, powder forms would fall under solids, they are included in liquids because of the requirements of formulation after the powder is reconstituted. In some instances, preservatives are required to protect the product during use by the patient. It is important to note that the FDA considers this phase of use of product a part of the product development strategy. The manufacturer must ensure label compliance through the use period, as indicated on the package and under the conditions prescribed, such as keeping it in a refrigerator. Whereas the instructions require the product to be stored in a refrigerator, product development should evaluate a wider range of temperatures, as the temperature inside the consumer's refrigerator may not correspond to the official definition of refrigeration. The method of granulation for the powders intended for resuspension before use is a traditional one, as is used in the preparation of uncompressed or even compressed solids; the difference here is obviously the consideration of the effects of stability on reconstitution, which may require addition of stabilizers. In general, the method of granulation requires wet massing, screening, drying, and screening again; fluid bed dryers may be used as well.

XVIII. NASAL SPRAY PRODUCTS

Nasal spray drug products contain therapeutically active ingredients (drug substances) that are dissolved or suspended in solutions or mixtures of excipients (e.g., preservatives, viscosity modifiers, emulsifiers, and buffering agents) in nonpressurized dispensers that deliver a spray containing a metered dose of the active ingredient. The dose can be metered by the spray pump or can be premetered during manufacture. A nasal spray unit can be designed for unit dosing or can discharge up to several hundred metered sprays of formulation containing the drug substance. Nasal sprays are applied to the nasal cavity for local or systemic effects. Although similar in many features to other drug products, some aspects of nasal sprays may be unique (e.g., formulation, container closure system, manufacturing, stability, controls of critical steps, intermediates, and drug product). These aspects should be considered carefully during the development program because changes can affect the ability of the product to deliver reproducible doses to patients throughout the product's shelf life. Some of the unique features of nasal sprays are listed below:

- Metering and spray producing (e.g., orifice, nozzle, jet) pump mechanisms and components are used for reproducible delivery of drug formulation, and these can be constructed of many parts of different design that are precisely controlled in terms of dimensions and composition.
- Energy is required for dispersion of the formulation as a spray. This is typically accomplished by forcing the formulation through the nasal actuator and its orifice.
- The formulation and the container closure system (container, closure, pump, and any protective packaging) collectively constitute the drug product. The design of the container closure system affects the dosing performance of the drug product.
- The concept of classical bioequivalence and bioavailability may not be applicable for all nasal sprays, depending on the intended site of action. The doses administered are typically so small that blood or serum concentrations are generally undetectable by routine analytical procedures.

A. Inhalation Solutions and Suspensions

Inhalation solution and suspension drug products are typically aqueous-based formulations that contain therapeutically active ingredients and can also contain additional excipients. Aqueous-based oral inhalation solutions and suspension must be sterile (21 CFR 200.51). Inhalation solutions and suspensions are intended for delivery to the lungs by oral inhalation for local or systemic effects and are used with a specified nebulizer. Unit-dose presentation is recommended for these drug products to prevent microbial contamination during use. The container closure system for these drug products consists of the container and closure and can include protective packaging such as foil overwrap.

B. Inhalation Sprays

An inhalation spray drug product consists of the formulation and the container closure system. The formulations are typically aqueous based and, by definition, do not contain any propellant. Aqueous-based oral inhalation sprays must be sterile (21 CFR 200.51). Inhalation sprays are intended for delivery to the lungs by oral inhalation for local or systemic effects. The products contain therapeutically active ingredients and can also contain additional excipients. The formulation can be in unit-dose or multidose presentations. The use of preservatives or stabilizing agents in inhalation spray formulations is discouraged. If these excipients are included in a formulation, their use should be justified by assessment in a clinical setting to ensure the safety and tolerability of the drug product. The dose is delivered by the integral pump components of the container closure system to the lungs by oral inhalation for local or systemic effects. The container closure system of these drug products consists of the container, closure, and pump, and it can also include protective packaging. Current container closure system designs for inhalation spray drug products include both premetered and device-metered presentations using mechanical or power assistance or energy from patient inspiration for production of the spray plume. Premetered presentations contain previously measured doses or a dose fraction in some type of units (e.g., single or multiple blisters or other cavities) that are subsequently inserted into the device during manufacture or by the patient before use. Typical device-metered units have a reservoir containing formulation sufficient for multiple doses that are delivered as metered sprays by the device itself when activated by the patient. Inhalation spray and nasal spray drug products have many similarities. Many of the characteristics for nasal sprays are also characteristic of inhalation spray drug products. Moreover, the potential wide array of inhalation spray drug product designs with unique characteristics will present a variety of development challenges. Regardless of the design, the most crucial attributes are the reproducibility of the dose, the spray plume, and the particle-/droplet-size distribution, as these parameters can affect the delivery of the drug substance to the intended biological target. Maintaining the reproducibility of these parameters through the expiration dating period and ensuring the sterility of the content and the functionality of the device (e.g., spray mechanism, electronic features, and sensors) through its lifetime under patient-use conditions will probably present the most formidable challenges. Therefore, changes in components of the drug product or changes in the manufacturer or manufacturing process that can affect these parameters should be carefully evaluated for their effect on the safety, clinical effectiveness, and stability of the product. If such changes are made subsequent to the preparation of the batches used in critical clinical, bioequivalence, or primary stability studies, adequate supportive comparative data should be provided to demonstrate equivalency in terms of safety, clinical effectiveness, and stability of the product.

C. Pump Delivery of Nasal Products

A test to assess pump-to-pump reproducibility in terms of drug product performance and to evaluate the delivery from the pump should be performed. The proper performance of the pump should be ensured primarily by the pump manufacturer, who should assemble the pump with parts of precise dimensions. Pump spray weight delivery should be verified by the applicant for the drug product. In general, pump spray weight delivery acceptance criteria should control the weight of individual sprays to within "15% of the target weight" and their USP mean weight to within "10% of the target weight." However, for small-dosage pumps (e.g., 20 mL), other acceptance criteria may be justified. Acceptance testing for pump delivery on incoming pump lots can substitute for the release testing of pump delivery for the drug product, if justified. However, the acceptance criteria for pump delivery should be included in the drug product specification.

D. Spray Content Uniformity for Nasal Products

The spray discharged from the nasal actuator should be thoroughly analyzed for the drug substance content of multiple sprays from beginning to the end of an individual container, among containers, and among batches of drug product. This test should provide an overall performance evaluation of a batch, assessing the formulation, the manufacturing process, and the pump. At most, two sprays per determination should be used except when the number of sprays per minimum dose specified in the product labeling is one. Then the number of sprays per determination should be one spray. To ensure reproducible in vitro dose collection, the procedure should have controls for actuation parameters (e.g., stroke length, actuation force). The test can be performed with units primed following the instructions in the labeling. The amount of drug substance delivered from the nasal actuator should be expressed both as the actual amount and as a percentage of label claim. This test is designed to demonstrate the uniformity of medication per spray (or minimum dose) consistent with the label claim, discharged from the nasal actuator, of an appropriate number ($n = 10$ from beginning and $n = 10$ from end) of containers from a batch. The primary purpose is to ensure spray content uniformity within the same container and among multiple containers of a batch. The following acceptance criteria are recommended, but alternative approaches (e.g., statistical) can be proposed and used if they are demonstrated to provide equal or greater assurance of spray content uniformity. For acceptance of a batch:

- The amount of active ingredient per determination is not outside 80% to 120% of label claim for more than 2 of 20 determinations (10 from beginning and 10 from end) from 10 containers.
- None of the determinations is outside 75% to 125% of the label claim.
- The mean for each of the beginning and end determinations is not outside 85% to 115% of label claim.

If the above acceptance criteria are not met because 3 to 6 of the 20 determinations are outside 80% to 120% of the label claim, 14 units but none are outside 75% to 125% of label claim, and the means for each of the beginning and end determinations are not outside 85% to 115% of label claim, an additional 20 containers should be sampled for second-tier testing.

For the second-tier testing of a batch, the acceptance criteria are met if

- the amount of active ingredient per determination is not outside 80% to 120% of the label claim for more than 6 of all 60 determinations;
- none of the 60 determinations is outside 75% to 125% of label claim; and
- the mean for each of the beginning and end determinations is not outside 85% to 115% of label claim.

E. Spray Pattern and Plume Geometry of Nasal Products

Characterization of spray pattern and plume geometry is important for evaluating the performance of the pump. Various factors can affect the spray pattern and plume geometry, including the size and shape of the nozzle, the design of the pump, the size of the metering chamber, and the characteristics of the formulation. Spray-pattern testing should be performed on a routine basis as a quality control for release of the drug product. However, the characterization of plume geometry typically should be established during the characterization of the product and is not necessarily tested routinely thereafter. The proposed test procedure for spray pattern should be provided in detail to allow duplication by FDA laboratories. For example, in the evaluation of the spray pattern, the spray distance between the nozzle and the collection surface, number of sprays per spray pattern, position and orientation of the collection surface relative to the nozzle, and visualization procedure should be specified. The acceptance criteria for spray pattern should include the shape (e.g., ellipsoid of relative uniform density) as well as the size of the pattern (e.g., no axis is greater than x millimeters and the ratio of the longest to the shortest axes should lie in a specified range). Data should be provided to demonstrate that the collection distance selected for the spray pattern test will provide the optimal discriminatory capability. Variability in the test can be reduced by the development of a sensitive detection procedure and by providing procedure-specific training to the analyst. Acceptance testing for spray pattern on incoming pump lots can substitute for the release testing of spray pattern for the drug product, if justified (e.g., spray patterns from pumps with drug product formulation and with the proposed simulating media are the same).

However, the 15 acceptance criteria for spray pattern should be included in the drug product specification.

F. Droplet-Size Distribution in Nasal Products

For both suspension and solution nasal sprays, the specifications should include an appropriate control for the droplet-size distribution (e.g., three to four cutoff values) of the delivered plume subsequent to spraying under specified experimental and instrumental conditions. If a laser diffraction method is used, droplet-size distribution can be controlled in terms of ranges for the D_{10}, D_{50}, D_{90}, span $[(D_{90} - D_{10})/D_{50}]$, and percentage of droplets less than 10 mm. Appropriate and validated or calibrated droplet-size analytical procedures should be described in sufficient detail to allow accurate assessment by agency laboratories (e.g., apparatus and accessories, calculation theory, correction principles, software version, sample placement, laser trigger condition, measurement range, and beam width). For solution nasal sprays, acceptance testing for droplet-size distribution on incoming pump lots with placebo formulation can substitute for the release testing of droplet-size distribution for the drug product, if justified (i.e., droplet-size distributions from pumps with drug product formulation and those with the placebo are the same). However, the acceptance criteria for droplet-size distribution should be included in the drug product specification.

G. Particle-Size Distribution for Nasal Suspensions

For suspension nasal sprays, the specification should include tests and acceptance criteria for the particle-size distribution of the drug substance particles in the formulation. The quantitative procedure should be appropriately validated, if feasible, in terms of its sensitivity and ability to detect shifts that may occur in the distribution. When examining formulations containing suspending agents in the presence of suspended drug substance, when it is demonstrated that the currently available technology cannot be acceptably validated, a qualitative and semiquantitative method for examination of drug and aggregated drug particle-size distribution can be used. Supportive data, along with available validation information, should be submitted. For example, microscopic evaluation can be used, and such an examination can provide information and data on the presence of large particles, changes in morphology of the drug substance particles, extent of agglomerates, and crystal growth.

XIX. EMULSIFICATION AND SOLUBILIZATION

To solubilize insoluble lypophilic or hydrophobic active substances in an aqueous medium, BASF pharmaceutical excipients offer several possibilities and mechanisms. For microemulsions, Cremophor RH 40, Cremophor EL, and Solutol HS 15 act as surface-active solubilizers in water and form the structures of micelles. The micelle that envelops the active substance is so small that it is invisible, or perhaps visible in the form of opalescence. Typical fields of application are oil-soluble vitamins, antimycotics of the miconazole type, mouth disinfectants (e.g., hexiditin), and etherian oils or fragrances. Solutol HS 15 is recommended for parenteral use of this solubilizing system and has been specially developed for this purpose.

XX. COMPLEXING

The soluble Kollidon products form reversible complexes with many hydrophobic active substances, and clear solutions in water are thus obtained. This may be affected by the molecular weight. The longer the chains or the higher the K-value of the Kollidon type are, the stronger the solubility effect is, and thus the greater the solubility that can be obtained by the active substance. In practice, this effect was mostly exploited for the solubilization of antibiotics in human and veterinary medicine. There are also restrictions on the use of this substance in human parenterals. In many countries the K-value must not exceed 18, and there is also a restriction on the amount to be used for each dose administered in intramuscular application.

XXI. HYDROPHILIZATION

Active substances can also be solubilized by Lutrol F 68 in addition to the Cremophor and Kollidon products. The mechanism is probably based, for the most part, on the principle of hydrophilization. Micelle formation is certainly of minor significance, if it exists at all.

XXII. STABILIZING SUSPENSIONS

Various BASF pharmaceutical excipients with different functions can be used for stabilizing suspensions. The following groups of products can be offered for stabilizing oral and topical suspensions. Soluble Kollidon products can be used at low concentrations, that is, at 2% to 5%, Kollidon

90°F suffices to stabilize aqueous suspensions. A combination consisting of 2% Kollidon 90°F and 5% to 9% Kollidon CL-M has proved to be an effective system for stabilizing suspensions. Kollidon 30 is also used for this purpose. It can be combined with all conventional suspension stabilizers (thickeners, surfactants, etc.). The use of Kollidon CL-M as a suspension stabilizer has nothing whatever to do with the principle of increasing the viscosity. The addition of 5% to 9% Kollidon CL-M has practically no effect in changing the viscosity, but it strongly reduces the rate of sedimentation and facilitates the redispersability, in particular—an effect that is consistent with the low viscosity. One of the reasons for this Kollidon CL-M effect is its low (bulk) density, which is only half of that of conventional crospovidone (e.g., Kollidon CL). The polyoxamers, Lutrol F 68, and Lutrol F 127, in concentrations of 2% to 5%, expressed in terms of the final weight of the suspension, offer a further opportunity of stabilizing suspensions. They also do not increase viscosity when used in these amounts and can be combined with all other conventional suspension stabilizers.

6

Container Closure Systems

I. INTRODUCTION

According to the Federal Food, Drug, and Cosmetic Act (the act), section 501(a)(3), a drug is deemed to be adulterated "if its container is composed, in whole or in part, of any poisonous or deleterious substance which may render the contents injurious to health." In addition, section 502 of the act states that a drug is considered misbranded if there are packaging omissions. Also, section 505 of the act requires a full description of the methods used in, and the facilities and controls used for, the packaging of drugs. Section 505(b)(1)(D) of the act states that an application shall include a full description of the methods used in the manufacturing, processing, and packing of such drug. This includes facilities and controls used in the packaging of a drug product.

A. Definitions

Materials of construction are the substances [e.g., glass, high-density polyethylene (HDPE) resin, metal] used to manufacture a packaging component. A packaging component is any single part of a container closure system. Typical components are containers (e.g., ampoules, vials, bottles), container liners (e.g., tube liners), closures (e.g., screw caps, stoppers), closure liners, stopper overseals, container inner seals, administration ports (e.g., on large-volume parenterals), overwraps, administration accessories, and container labels. A primary packaging component is a packaging component that is or may be in direct contact with the dosage form. A secondary packaging component is a packaging component that is not and will not be in direct contact with the dosage form.

A container closure system is the sum of packaging components that together contain and protect the dosage form. This includes primary packaging components and secondary packaging components, if the latter is intended to provide additional protection to the drug product. A packaging system is equivalent to a container closure system.

A package, or market package, is the container closure system and labeling, associated components (e.g., dosing cups, droppers, spoons), and external packaging (e.g., cartons or shrink-wrap). A market package is the article provided to a pharmacist or retail customer on purchase and does not include packaging used solely for the purpose of shipping such articles.

The term "quality" refers to the physical, chemical, microbiological, biological, bioavailability, and stability attributes that a drug product should maintain if it is to be deemed suitable for therapeutic or diagnostic use. In this guidance, the term is also understood to convey the properties of safety, identity, strength, quality, and purity [see Title 21 Code of Federal Register (CFR) 211.94(a)].

An extraction profile is the analysis (usually by chromatographic means) of extracts obtained from a packaging component. A quantitative extraction profile is one in which the amount of each detected substance is determined.

B. Current Good Manufacturing Practice, the Consumer Product Safety Commission, and Requirements on Containers and Closures

Current good manufacturing practice requirements for the control of drug product containers and closures are included in 21 CFR Parts 210 and 211. The U.S. Food and Drug Administration (FDA) requirement for tamper-resistant closures is included in 21 CFR 211.132 and the Consumer Product Safety Commission requirements for child-resistant closures are included in 16 CFR 1700.

The United States Pharmacopeial Convention has established requirements for containers that are described in many of the drug product monographs in *The United States Pharmacopeia/National Formulary*. For capsules and tablets, these requirements generally relate to the design characteristics of the container (e.g., tight, well closed, or light resistant). For injectable products, materials of construction are also addressed (e.g., "Preserve in single-dose or in multiple-dose containers, preferably of type I glass, protected from light"). These requirements are defined in the "General Notices and Requirements" (Preservation, Packaging, Storage, and Labeling) section of the USP. The requirements for materials of construction are defined in the "General Chapters" of the USP.

C. Additional Considerations

The packaging information in the chemistry, manufacturing, and controls (CMC) section of an investigational new drug application (IND) usually includes a brief description of the components, the assembled packaging system, and any precautions needed to ensure the protection and preservation of the drug substance and drug product during their use in the clinical trials.

A contract packager is a firm retained by the applicant to package a drug product. The applicant remains responsible for the quality of the drug product during shipping, storage, and packaging. The information regarding the container closure system used by a contract packager that should be submitted in the CMC section of an application [new drug application (NDA), abbreviated new drug application (ANDA), or biological license application (BLA)], or in a drug master file (DMF) that is referenced in the application, is no different from that which would be submitted if the applicant performed its own packaging operations. If the information is provided in a DMF, then a copy of the letter of authorization for the DMF should be provided in the application.

II. QUALIFICATION AND QUALITY CONTROL OF PACKAGING COMPONENTS

A packaging system found acceptable for one drug product is not automatically assumed to be appropriate for another. Each application should contain enough information to show that each proposed container closure system and its components are suitable for its intended use.

The type and extent of information that should be provided in an application will depend on the dosage form and the route of administration. For example, the kind of information that should be provided about a packaging system for an injectable dosage form or a drug product for inhalation is often more detailed than that which should be provided about a packaging system for a solid oral dosage form. More detailed information usually should be provided for a liquid-based dosage form than for a powder or a solid, as a liquid-based dosage form is more likely to interact with the packaging components. There is a correlation between the degree of concern regarding the route of administration and the likelihood of packaging component–dosage form interactions for different classes of drug products:

Highest: inhalation, aerosols, sterile powders, and solutions; powders for injections and injection; and inhalation, injectable, powders, and suspensions
High: ophthalmic solutions and suspensions, transdermal ointments and patches, and nasal aerosols and sprays
Low: topical solutions and topical powders; oral tablets and oral suspensions; and topical oral powders (hard and soft and lingual aerosols; gelatin), capsules, oral solutions, and suspensions

"Suitability" refers to the tests and studies used and accepted for the initial qualification of a component, or a container closure system, for its intended use. "Quality control" refers to the tests typically used and accepted to establish that, after the application is approved, the components and the container closure system continue to possess the characteristics established in the suitability studies. The subsections on associated components and secondary components describe the tests and studies for establishing suitability and quality control for these types of components. However, the ultimate proof of the suitability of the container closure system and the packaging process is established by full shelf-life stability studies.

Every proposed packaging system should be shown to be suitable for its intended use: It should adequately protect the dosage form, it should be compatible with the dosage form, and it should be composed of materials that are considered safe for use with the dosage form and the route of administration. If the packaging system has a performance feature in addition to containing the product, the assembled container closure system should be shown to function properly. Information intended to establish suitability may be generated by the applicant, by the supplier of the material of construction or the component, or by a laboratory under contract to either the applicant or the firm. An adequately detailed description of the tests, methods, acceptance criteria, reference standards, and validation information for the studies should be provided. The information may be submitted directly in the application or indirectly by reference to a DMF. If a DMF is used, a letter authorizing reference (i.e., letter of authorization) to the DMF must be included in the application.

A container closure system should provide the dosage form with adequate protection from factors (e.g., temperature, light) that can cause a degradation in the quality of that dosage form over its shelf life. Common causes of such degradation are exposure to light, loss of solvent, exposure to reactive gases (e.g., oxygen), absorption of water vapor, and microbial contamination. A drug product can also suffer an unacceptable loss in quality if it is contaminated by filth.

Not every drug product is susceptible to degradation by all of these factors: not all drug products are light sensitive. Not all tablets are subject to loss of quality caused by absorption of moisture. Sensitivity to oxygen is most commonly found with liquid-based dosage forms. Laboratory studies can be used to determine which of these factors actually have an influence on a particular drug product.

Light protection is typically provided by an opaque or amber-colored container or by an opaque secondary packaging component (e.g., cartons or overwrap). The test for light transmission (USP <661>) is an accepted standard for evaluating the light transmission properties of a container. Situations exist in which solid- and liquid-based oral drug products have been exposed to light during storage because the opaque secondary packaging component was removed, contrary to the approved labeling and the monograph recommendation. A firm, therefore, may want to consider using additional or alternate measures to provide light protection for these drug products when necessary.

Loss of solvent can occur through a permeable barrier (e.g., a polyethylene container wall), through an inadequate seal, or through leakage. Leaks can develop through rough handling or from inadequate contact between the container and the closure (e.g., because of the buildup of pressure during storage). Leaks can also occur in tubes as a result of failure of the crimp seal. Water vapor or reactive gases (e.g., oxygen) may penetrate a container closure system either by passing through a permeable container surface [e.g., the wall of a low-density polyethylene (LDPE) bottle] or by diffusing past a seal. Plastic containers are susceptible to both routes. Although glass containers would seem to offer better protection, because glass is relatively impermeable, glass containers are more effective only if there is a good seal between the container and the closure.

Protection from microbial contamination is provided by maintaining adequate container integrity after the packaging system has been sealed. An adequate and validated procedure should be used for drug product manufacture and packaging.

Packaging components that are compatible with a dosage form will not interact sufficiently to cause unacceptable changes in the quality of either the dosage form or the packaging component. Examples of interactions include loss of potency, caused by absorption or adsorption of the active drug substance, or degradation of the active drug substance, induced by a chemical entity leached from a packaging component; reduction in the concentration of an excipient caused by absorption, adsorption, or leachable-induced degradation; precipitation; changes in drug product pH; discoloration of either the dosage form or the packaging component; or increase in brittleness of the packaging component.

Some interactions between a packaging component and dosage form will be detected during qualification studies on the container closure system and its components. Others may not show up except in the stability studies. Therefore, any change noted during a stability study that may be attributable to interaction between the dosage form and a packaging component should be investigated, and appropriate action should be taken, regardless of whether the stability study is being conducted for an original application, a supplemental application, or as fulfillment of a commitment to conduct postapproval stability studies.

Packaging components should be constructed of materials that will not leach harmful or undesirable amounts of substances to which a patient will be exposed when being treated with the drug product. This consideration is especially important for those packaging components that may be in direct contact with the dosage form, but it is also applicable to any component from which substances may migrate into the dosage form (e.g., an ink or adhesive). Making the determination that a material of construction used in the manufacture of a packaging component is safe for its intended use is not a simple process, and a standardized approach has not been established. There is, however, a body of experience that supports the use of certain approaches that depend on the route of administration and the likelihood of interactions between the component and the dosage form. For a drug product such as an injection, inhalation, ophthalmic, or transdermal product, a comprehensive study is appropriate. This involves two parts: first, an extraction study on the packaging component to determine which chemical species may migrate into the dosage form (and at what concentration), and second, a toxicological evaluation of those substances that are extracted to determine the safe level of exposure via the label-specified route of administration. This technique is used by the Center for Food Safety and Applied Nutrition to evaluate the safety of substances that are proposed as indirect food additives (e.g., polymers or additives that may be used in for packaging foods).

The approach for toxicological evaluation of the safety of extractables should be based on good scientific principles and should take into account the specific container closure system, drug product formulation, dosage form, route of administration, and dose regimen (chronic or short-term dosing). For many injectable and ophthalmic drug products, data from the Biological Reactivity tests and Elastomeric Closures for Injections tests will typically be considered sufficient evidence of material safety.

For many solid and liquid oral drug products, an appropriate reference to the indirect food additive regulations (21 CFR 174–186) promulgated by Center for Food Safety and Applied Nutrition for the materials of construction used in the packaging component will typically be considered sufficient. Although these regulations do not specifically apply to materials for packaging drug products, they include purity criteria and limitations pertaining to the use of specific materials for packaging foods that may be acceptable for the evaluation of drug product packaging components. Applicants are cautioned that this approach may not be acceptable for liquid oral dosage forms intended for chronic use.

For drug products that undergo clinical trials, the absence of adverse reactions traceable to the packaging components is considered supporting evidence of material safety. Performance of the container closure system refers to its ability to function in the manner for which it was designed. A container closure system is often called on to do more than simply contain the dosage form. When evaluating performance, two major considerations are container closure system functionality and drug delivery.

First, consider container closure system functionality: the container closure system may be designed to improve patient compliance (e.g., a cap that contains a counter), minimize waste (e.g., a two-chamber vial or IV bag), improve ease of use (e.g., a prefilled syringe), or have other functions.

The second consideration is drug delivery: Drug delivery refers to the ability of the packaging system to deliver the dosage form in the amount or at the rate described in the package insert. Some examples of a packaging system for which drug delivery aspects are relevant are a prefilled syringe, a transdermal patch, a metered tube, a dropper or spray bottle, a dry powder inhaler, and a metered dose inhaler.

Container closure system functionality or drug delivery are compromised when the packaging system fails to operate as designed. Failure can result from misuse, faulty design, manufacturing defect, improper assembly, or wear and tear during use. Tests and acceptance criteria regarding dosage form delivery and container closure system functionality should be appropriate to the particular dosage form, route of administration, and design features. If there is a special performance function built into the drug product (e.g., a counter cap), it is of importance for any dosage form or route of administration to show that the container closure system performs that function properly.

In addition to providing data to show that a proposed container closure system is suitable for its intended use, an application should also describe the quality control measures that will be used to ensure consistency in the packaging components. These controls are intended to limit unintended postapproval variations in the manufacturing procedures or the materials of construction for a packaging component and to prevent adverse effects on the quality of a dosage form.

Principal consideration is usually given to consistency in physical characteristics and chemical composition. The physical characteristics of interest include dimensional criteria (e.g., shape, neck finish, wall thickness, design tolerances), physical parameters critical to the consistent manufacture of a packaging component (e.g., unit weight), and performance characteristics (e.g., metering valve delivery volume or the ease of movement of syringe plungers). Unintended variations in dimensional parameters, if undetected, may affect package permeability, drug delivery performance, or the adequacy of the seal between the container and the closure. Variation in any physical parameter is considered important if it can affect the quality of a dosage form.

The chemical composition of the materials of construction may affect the safety of a packaging component. New materials may result in new substances being extracted into the dosage form or in a change in the amount of known extractables. Chemical composition may also affect the compatibility, functional characteristics, or protective properties of packaging components by changing rheological or other physical properties (e.g., elasticity, resistance to solvents, or gas permeability). A composition change may occur as a result of a change in formulation or a change in a processing aid (e.g., using a different mold release agent) or through the use of a new supplier of a raw material. A change in the supplier of a polymeric material or a substance of biological origin is more likely to bring with it an unexpected composition change than is a change in the supplier of a pure chemical compound because polymeric and natural materials are often complex mixtures. A composition change may also occur with a change in the manufacturing process, such as the use of different operating conditions (e.g., a significantly different curing temperature), different equipment, or both. A change in formulation is considered a change in the specifications for the packaging component. Changes in the formulation of a packaging component by its manufacturer should be reported to the firm that purchases that component and to any appropriate DMF. The firm that purchases the component should, in turn, report the change to its application as required under 21 CFR 314.70(a) or 601.12. Manufacturers who supply a raw material or an intermediate packaging component should inform their customers of any intended changes to formulations or manufacturing procedures and should update the DMF in advance of implementing such a change. Changes that seem innocuous may have unintended consequences on the dosage form marketed in the affected packaging system.

The use of stability studies for monitoring the consistency of a container closure system in terms of compatibility with the dosage form and the degree of protection provided to the dosage form is accepted. At present, there is no general policy concerning the monitoring of a packaging system and components with regard to safety. One exception involves inhalation drug products, for which batch-to-batch monitoring of the extraction profile for the polymeric and elastomeric components is routine.

"Associated components" are packaging components that are typically intended to deliver the dosage form to the patient but that are not stored in contact with the dosage form for its entire shelf life. These components are packaged separately in the market package and are either attached to the container on opening or used only when a dose is to be administered. Measuring spoons, dosing cups, measuring syringes, and vaginal delivery tubes are examples of associated components that typically contact the dosage form only during administration. A hand pump or dropper combined into a closure are examples of an associated component that would contact the dosage form from the time the packaging system is opened until the dosing regimen is completed.

The complete and assembled component and its parts should meet suitability criteria appropriate for the drug product and the actual use of the component. Safety and functionality are the most common factors to be established for suitability. The length of time that the associated component and the dosage form are in direct contact should also be taken into consideration when assessing the suitability of an associated component.

Unlike primary and associated packaging components, secondary packaging components are not intended to make contact with the dosage form. Examples are cartons, which are generally constructed of paper or plastic, and overwraps, which may be fabricated from a single layer of plastic or from a laminate made of metal foil, plastic, or paper. A secondary packaging component generally provides one or more of the following additional services:

- Protection from excessive transmission of moisture or solvents into or out of the packaging system
- Protection from excessive transmission of reactive gases (atmospheric oxygen, inert head-space filler gas, or other organic vapors) into or out of the packaging system
- Light protection for the packaging system
- Protection for a packaging system that is flexible or that needs extra protection from rough handling
- Additional measure of microbiological protection (i.e., by maintaining sterility or by protecting the packaging system from microbial intrusion)

When information on a container closure system is submitted in an application, the emphasis would normally be on the primary packaging components. For a secondary packaging component, a brief description will usually suffice unless the component is intended to provide some additional measure of protection to the drug product. In this case, more complete information should be provided, along with data showing that the secondary packaging component actually provides the additional protection.

Because secondary packaging components are not intended to make contact with the dosage form, there is usually less concern regarding the materials from which they are constructed. However, if the packaging system is relatively permeable, the possibility increases that the dosage form could be contaminated by the migration of an ink or adhesive component or from a volatile substance present in the secondary packaging component. (For example, a solution packaged in an LDPE container was found to be contaminated by a volatile constituent of the secondary packaging components that enclosed it.) In such a case, the secondary packaging component should be considered a potential source of contamination, and the safety of its materials of construction should be taken into consideration.

A. Description

A general description of the entire container closure system should be provided in the CMC section of the application. In addition, the following information should be provided by the applicant for each individual component of the packaging system:

- Identification by product name, product code (if available), name and address of the manufacturer, and a physical description of the packaging component (e.g., type, size, shape, and color)
- Identification of the materials of construction (i.e., plastics, paper, metal, glass, elastomers, coatings, adhesives, and other such materials) should be identified by a specific product designation (code name and/or code number) and the source (name of the manufacturer); alternate materials of construction should be indicated; postconsumer recycled plastic should not be used in the manufacture of a primary packaging component, and if it is used for a secondary or associated component, then the safety and compatibility of the material for its intended use should be addressed appropriately
- Description of any operations or preparations that are performed on a packaging component by the applicant (such as washing, coating, sterilization, or depyrogenation)

B. Information about Suitability

To establish safety and to ensure consistency, the complete chemical composition should be provided for every material used in the manufacture of a packaging component. Test results from appropriate qualification and characterization tests should be provided. Adequate information regarding the tests, methods, acceptance criteria, reference standards, and validation information should also be provided.

To address protection, use of tests for light transmission, moisture permeation, microbial limits, and sterility are generally considered sufficient. Testing for properties other than those described above (e.g., gas transmission, solvent leakage container integrity) may also be necessary.

To address safety and compatibility, the results of extraction/toxicological evaluation studies should be provided for drug products that are likely to interact with the packaging components and to introduce extracted substances into the patient. For drug products less likely to interact, other tests (e.g., Biological Reactivity test) or information (e.g., appropriate reference to the indirect food additive regulations at 21 CFR 174–186) could be used to address the issue of safety and compatibility. For example, an appropriate reference to an indirect food additive regulation is generally sufficient for a solid oral dosage form product.

To address performance, the results of nonfunctionality tests are considered sufficient if the test and acceptance criteria are appropriate for the intended purpose. Tests described there are typically considered sufficient standards for establishing specified properties and characteristics of specified materials of construction or packaging components. For nonfunctionality tests, an applicant should provide justification for the use of the test, a complete and detailed description of how the test was performed, and an explanation of what the test is intended to establish. If a related test is available, comparative data should be provided using both methods. Supporting data should include a demonstration of the suitability of the test for its intended use and its validation.

Testing on an assembled container closure system is usually performed by the applicant (or a testing laboratory commissioned by the applicant), and the test results are provided in the application. Such tests may include vacuum-leak testing, moisture permeation, and weight loss or media fill. Testing on an individual packaging component is typically performed by the manufacturer of the component and is reported via a DMF (see section V).

The fabricator/manufacturer of a packaging component and the drug product manufacturer who uses this firm share the responsibility for ensuring the quality of packaging components. These firms should have a quality control program in place so that consistent components are produced. The drug product manufacturer must have an inspection program for incoming packaging components and materials (21 CFR 211.22, 211.84, and 211.122). For most drug products, a drug product manufacturer may accept a packaging component lot based on receiving a certificate of analysis (COA) or certificate of certification (COC) from the component supplier and on the performance of an appropriate identification test, provided the supplier's test data are periodically validated [21 CFR 211.84(d)(3)]. Acceptance of a packaging component lot based on a supplier's COA or COC may not be appropriate in all cases (e.g., some packaging components for certain inhalation drug products).

The tests and methods used by the applicant for acceptance of each batch of a packaging component that they receive should be described. If a batch is to be accepted based on a supplier's COA or COC, then the procedure for supplier validation should be described. The data from the supplier's COA or COC should clearly indicate that the lot meets the applicant's acceptance criteria. Acceptance criteria for extractables should also be included, if appropriate.

Dimensional and performance criteria should be provided. Dimensional information is frequently provided via a detailed schematic drawing, complete with target dimensions and tolerances, and it may be provided via the packaging component manufacturer's DMF. A separate drawing may not be necessary if the packaging component is part of a larger unit for which a drawing is provided or if the component is uncomplicated in design (e.g., a cap liner).

Each manufacturer of a packaging component consistency is the physical and chemical characteristics of the component. These measures generally include release criteria (and test methods, if appropriate) and a description of the manufacturing procedure. If the release of the packaging component is based on statistical process control, a complete description of the process (including control criteria) and its validation should be provided.

The description of the manufacturing process is generally brief and should include any operations performed on the packaging component after manufacture but before shipping (e.g., washing, coating, or sterilization). In some cases, it may be desirable for the description to be more detailed and to include in-process controls. This information may be provided via a DMF.

The quality control procedures of the manufacturer of a packaging component may sometimes rely in whole or in part on the quality control procedures of a manufacturer who makes an intermediate packaging component that is used to create the component. If so, each contributor to the final packaging system should provide a description of the quality control measures used to maintain consistency in the physical and chemical characteristics of the separate components and of the assembled packaging system that they provide.

The manufacturer of each material of construction should be prepared to describe the quality control measures used to maintain consistency in the chemical characteristics of their product. This information may be provided via a DMF.

C. Stability Data (Packaging Concerns)

Stability testing of the drug product should be conducted using the container closure systems proposed in the application. The packaging system used in each stability study should be clearly identified, and the container closure system should be monitored for signs of instability. When appropriate, an evaluation of the packaging system should be included in the stability protocol. Even when a formal test for quality of the packaging system is not performed, the applicant should investigate any observed change in the packaging system used in the stability studies. The observations, results of the investigation, and corrective actions should be included in the stability report. If the corrective action requires a change in an approved container closure system, a supplemental application should be submitted.

D. Inhalation Drug Products

Inhalation drug products include inhalation aerosols (metered dose inhalers); inhalation solutions, suspensions, and sprays (administered via nebulizers); inhalation powders (dry powder inhalers); and nasal sprays. The CMC and preclinical considerations for inhalation drug products are unique in that these drug products are intended for respiratory tract-compromised patients. This is reflected in the level of concern given to the nature of the packaging components that may come in contact with the dosage form or the patient.

E. Injection and Ophthalmic Drug Products

These dosage forms share the common attributes that they are generally solutions, emulsions, or suspensions, and that all are required to be sterile. Injectable dosage forms represent one of the highest-risk drug products. Any contaminants present (as a result of contact with a packaging component or caused by the packaging system's failure to provide adequate protection) can be rapidly and completely introduced into the patient's general circulation. Although the risk factors associated with ophthalmics are generally considered to be lower than for injectables, any potential for causing harm to the eyes demands caution.

Injectable drug products may be liquids in the form of solutions, emulsions, suspensions, or dry solids that are to be combined with an appropriate vehicle to yield a solution or suspension. Injections are classified as small-volume parenterals if they have a solution volume of 100 mL or less, or as large-volume parenterals if the solution volume exceeds 100 mL. For solids that must be dissolved or dispersed in an appropriate diluent before being injected, the diluent may be in the same container closure system (e.g., a two-part vial) or be part of the same market package (e.g., a kit containing a vial of diluent). A small-volume parenteral may be packaged in a disposable cartridge, a disposable syringe, a vial, an ampoule, or a flexible bag. A large-volume parenteral may be packaged in a vial, a flexible bag, a glass bottle, or in some cases, as a disposable syringe.

Cartridges, syringes, vials, and ampoules are usually composed of type I or II glass or of polypropylene. Flexible bags are typically constructed with multilayered plastic. Stoppers and septa in cartridges, syringes, and vials are typically composed of elastomeric materials. The input (medication) and output (administration) ports for flexible bags may be plastic or elastomeric materials. An overwrap may be used with flexible bags to retard solvent loss and to protect the flexible packaging system from rough handling.

The potential effects of packaging component/dosage form interactions are numerous. Hemolytic effects may result from a decrease in tonicity, and pyrogenic effects may result from the presence of impurities. The potency of the drug product or the concentration of the antimicrobial preservatives may decrease because of adsorption or absorption. A cosolvent system essential to the solubilization of a poorly soluble drug can also serve as a potent extractant of plastic additives. A disposable syringe may be made of plastic, glass, rubber, and metal components, and such multicomponent construction provides a potential for interaction that is greater than when a container consists of a single material.

Injectable drug products require protection from microbial contamination (loss of sterility or added bioburden) and may also need to be protected from light or from exposure to gases (e.g., oxygen). Liquid-based injectables may need to be protected from solvent loss, whereas sterile powders or powders for injection may need to be protected from exposure to water vapor. For elastomeric components, data showing that a component meets the requirements of elastomeric closures for injections will typically be considered sufficient evidence of safety. For plastic components, data from Biological Reactivity tests will typically be considered sufficient evidence of safety. Whenever possible, the extraction studies should be performed using the drug product. If the extraction properties of the drug product vehicle may reasonably be expected to differ from that of water (e.g., because of high or low pH or a solubilizing excipient), then drug product should be used as the extracting medium. If the drug substance significantly affects extraction characteristics, it may be necessary to perform the extractions using the drug product vehicle. If the total of the extracts significantly exceeds the amount obtained from water extraction, then an extraction profile should be obtained. It may be advisable to obtain a quantitative extraction profile of an elastomeric or plastic packaging component and to compare this periodically to the profile from a new batch of the packaging component. Extractables should be identified whenever possible. For a glass packaging component, data from *Containers: Chemical Resistance—Glass Containers* will typically be considered sufficient evidence of safety and compatibility. In some cases (e.g., for some chelating agents), a glass packaging component may need to meet additional criteria to ensure the absence of significant interactions between the packaging component and the dosage form.

Performance of a syringe is usually addressed by establishing the force to initiate and maintain plunger movement down the barrel and the capability of the syringe to deliver the labeled amount of the drug product.

These drug products are usually solutions marketed in an LDPE bottle with a dropper built into the neck (sometimes referred to as droptainer) or ointments marketed in a metal tube with an ophthalmic tip. A few solution products use a glass container because of stability concerns regarding plastic packaging components. Ophthalmic ointments that are reactive toward metal may be packaged in a tube lined with an epoxy or vinyl plastic coating. A large-volume intraocular solution (for irrigation) may be packaged in a glass or polyolefin (polyethylene or polypropylene) container. The American Academy of Ophthalmology recommended to the FDA that a uniform color coding system be established for the caps and labels of all topical ocular medications. An applicant should either follow this system or provide an adequate justification for any deviations from the system.

Although ophthalmic drug products can be considered topical products, they have been grouped here with injectables because they are required to be sterile [21 CFR 200.50(a)(2)] and the descriptive, suitability, and quality control information is typically the same as that for an injectable drug product. Because ophthalmic drug products are applied to the eye, compatibility and safety should also address the container closure system's potential to form substances which irritate the eye or introduce particulate matter into the product (see USP <771> Ophthalmic Ointments).

F. Liquid-Based Oral and Topical Drug Products and Topical Delivery Systems

A wide variety of drug products falls into this category. The presence of a liquid phase implies a significant potential for the transfer of materials from a packaging component into the dosage form. The higher viscosity of semisolid dosage forms and transdermal systems may cause the rate of migration of leachable substances into these dosage forms to be slower than for aqueous solutions. Because of extended contact, the amount of leachables in these drug products may depend more on a leachable material's affinity for the liquid/semisolid phase than on the rate of migration.

Typical liquid-based oral dosage forms are elixirs, emulsions, extracts, fluid extracts, solutions, gels, syrups, spirits, tinctures, aromatic waters, and suspensions. These products are usually nonsterile but may be monitored for changes in bioburden or for the presence of specific microbes. These dosage forms are generally marketed in multiple-unit bottles or in unit-dose or single-use pouches or cups. The dosage form may be used as is or admixed first with a compatible diluent or dispersant. A bottle is usually glass or plastic, often with a screw cap with a liner, and possibly with a tamper-resistant seal or an overcap that is welded to the bottle. The same cap liners and inner seals are sometimes used with solid oral dosage forms. A pouch may be a single-layer plastic or a laminated material. Both bottles and pouches may use an overwrap, which is usually a laminated material. A single-dose cup may be metal or plastic with a heat-sealed lid made of a laminated material.

A liquid-based oral drug product typically needs to be protected from solvent loss, microbial contamination, and sometimes, from exposure to light or reactive gases (e.g., oxygen). For glass components, data showing that a component meets the requirements of *Containers: Glass Containers* are accepted as sufficient evidence of safety and compatibility. For LDPE components, data from Containers tests are typically considered sufficient evidence of compatibility. The General Chapters do not specifically address safety for polyethylene (HDPE or LDPE), polypropylene, or laminate components. A patient's exposure to substances extracted from a plastic packaging component (e.g., HDPE, LDPE, polypropylene, laminated components) into a liquid-based oral dosage form is expected to be comparable to a patient's exposure to the same substances through the use of the same material when it is used to package food. On the basis of this assumption, an appropriate reference to the indirect food additive regulations (21 CFR 174–186) is typically considered sufficient to establish safety of the material of construction, provided any limitations specified in the regulations are taken into consideration. This assumption is considered valid for liquid-based oral dosage forms that the patient will take only for a relatively short time (acute dosing regimen). For liquid-based oral drug products that the patient will continue to take for an extended period (i.e., months or years [chronic drug regimen]), a material of construction that meets the requirements for indirect food additives will be considered safe—on that basis alone—only if the patient's exposure to extractables can be expected to be no greater than the exposure through foods or if the length of exposure is supported by toxicological information. For example, if the dosage form is aqueous-based and contains little or no cosolvent (or other substance, including the active drug substance, liable to cause greater extraction of substances from plastic packaging components than would be extracted by water), meeting the requirements of the indirect food additive regulations will usually satisfy the issue of safety.

If the dosage form contains cosolvents (or if, for any reason, it may be expected to extract greater amounts of substances from plastic packaging components than water), then additional extractable information may be needed to address safety issues. Performance is typically not a factor for liquid-based oral drug products.

Topical dosage forms include aerosols, creams, emulsions, gels, lotions, ointments, pastes, powders, solutions, and suspensions. These dosage forms are generally intended for local (not systemic) effect and are generally applied to the skin or oral mucosal surfaces. Topical products also include some nasal and otic preparations as well as some ophthalmic drug products. Vaginal and rectal drug products may be considered to be topical if they are intended to have a local effect. Some topical drug products are sterile or may be subject to microbial limits. In these cases, additional evaluation may be necessary when determining the appropriate packaging.

A liquid-based topical product typically has a fluid or semisolid consistency and is marketed in a single- or multiple-unit container (e.g., a rigid bottle or jar, a collapsible tube, or a flexible pouch). A powder product may be marketed in a sifter-top container. An antibacterial product may be marketed as part of a sterile dressing; there are also a number of products marketed as a pressurized aerosol or a hand-pumped spray. A rigid bottle or jar is usually made of glass or polypropylene with a screw cap. The same cap liners and inner seals are sometimes used as with solid oral dosage forms. A collapsible tube is usually constructed from metal—or is metal-lined, from LDPE, or from a laminated material. Tubes are identified as either blind end or open end. In the former, there is no product contact with the cap on storage. Usually, the size of the tube is controlled by trimming it to an appropriate length for the target fill volume. Fill volume is commonly determined as an in-process measurement, using bulk density. Usually there is no cap liner, although the tube may have a liner. Aluminum tubes usually include a liner. A tube liner is frequently a lacquer or shellac whose composition should be stated. A tube is closed by folding or crimping the open end. The type of fold (roll or saddle) should be described, as well as the type and composition of any sealant. If the tube material is self-sealing through the application of heat alone, this should be stated. If the market package includes a separate applicator device, this should be described. Product contact is possible if the applicator is part of the closure, and therefore, an applicator's compatibility with the drug product should be established as appropriate. Dressings consist of dosage form on a bandage material (e.g., absorbent gauze or gauze bandage) within a flexible pouch. The pouch should maintain the sterility and physical stability of the dressing.

Topical aerosols are not intended to be inhaled; therefore, the droplet size of the spray does not need to be carefully controlled, nor is the dose usually metered. The spray may be used to apply dosage form to the skin (topical aerosol) or mouth (lingual aerosol), and functionality of the sprayer should be addressed. A topical aerosol may be sterile or may conform to acceptance criteria for microbial limits. The packaging system for a liquid-based topical product should deter solvent loss and should provide protection from light when appropriate. Because these dosage forms may be placed in contact with mucosal membranes or with skin that has been broken or otherwise compromised, the safety of the materials of construction for the packaging components should be evaluated. For solid dosage forms, an appropriate reference to the indirect food additive regulations is typically considered sufficient to establish safety.

Topical delivery systems are self-contained, discrete dosage forms that are designed to deliver drug via intact skin or body surface. There are three types of topical delivery systems: transdermal, ocular, and intrauterine.

Transdermal systems are usually applied to the skin with an adhesive and may be in place for an extended period. Ocular systems are inserted under the lower eyelid, typically for 7 days. Intrauterine systems are held in place without adhesive and may stay in place for a year. A transdermal system usually comprises an outer barrier, a drug reservoir (with or without a rate-controlling membrane), a contact adhesive, and a protective liner. An ocular system usually consists of the drug formulation contained in a rate-controlling membrane. An intrauterine system may be constructed of a plastic material impregnated with active ingredients or a coated metal. It is shaped to remain in place after being inserted in the uterus. Each of these systems is generally marketed in a single-unit soft blister pack or a preformed tray with a preformed cover or overwrap.

Compatibility and safety for topical delivery systems are addressed in the same manner as for topical drug products. Performance and quality control should be addressed for the rate-controlling membrane. Appropriate microbial limits should be established and justified for each delivery system. Microbiological standards are under development; therefore, the review division for a specific application should be consulted.

G. Solid Oral Dosage Forms and Powders for Reconstitution

The most common solid oral dosage forms are capsules and tablets. For the purpose of this guidance, oral powders and granules for reconstitution are also included in this group.

The risk of interaction between packaging components and a solid oral dosage form is generally recognized to be small. Powders that are reconstituted in their market container, however, have an additional possibility of an interaction between the packaging components and the reconstituting fluid. Although the contact time will be relatively short when compared with the component/dosage form contact time for liquid-based oral dosage forms, it should still be taken into consideration when the compatibility and safety of the container closure system are being evaluated.

A typical container closure system is a plastic (usually HDPE) bottle with a screw-on or snap-off closure and a flexible packaging system, such as a pouch or a blister package. A typical closure consists of a cap—often with a liner—frequently with an inner seal. If used, fillers, desiccants, and other absorbent materials are considered primary packaging components.

The most common forms of flexible packaging are the blister package and the pouch. A blister package usually consists of a lid material and a forming film. The lid material is usually a laminate, which includes a barrier layer (e.g., aluminum foil) with a print primer on one side and a sealing agent (e.g., a heat-sealing lacquer) on the other side.

The sealing agent contacts the dosage form and the forming film. The forming film may be a single film, a coated film, or a laminate. A pouch typically consists of film or laminate that is sealed at the edges by heat or adhesive. Leak testing is usually performed on flexible packages as part of the in-process controls.

Solid oral dosage forms generally need to be protected from the potential adverse effects of water vapor. Protection from light and reactive gases may also be needed. For example, the presence of moisture may affect the decomposition rate of the active drug substance or the dissolution rate of the dosage form. The container should have an intrinsically low rate of water vapor permeation, and the container closure system should establish a seal to protect the drug product. Three standard tests for water vapor permeation have been established by the USP for use with solid oral dosage forms.

1. Polyethylene Containers (USP <661>)

This test is conducted on containers heat sealed with foil laminate; therefore, only the properties of the container are evaluated. The level of protection from water vapor permeation provided by a packaging system marketed with a heat-sealed foil laminate inner seal (up to the time the inner seal is removed) is expected to be approximately the same as that determined by this test. The acceptance criteria are those established in USP <671>.

2. Single-Unit Containers and Unit-Dose Containers for Capsules and Tablets (USP <671>)

This test measures the water vapor permeation of a single-unit or unit-dose container closure system and establishes acceptance criteria for five standards (Class A–E containers).

3. Multiple-Unit Containers for Capsules and Tablets (USP <671>)

This test is intended for drugs being dispensed on prescription, but it has also been applied to the drug product manufacturer's container closure system. If the container closure system has an inner seal, it should be removed before testing. The results from this study reflect the contributions to water vapor permeation through the container and through the seal between the container and the closure.

Acceptance criteria have been established for two standards (tight containers and well-closed containers).

For solid oral dosage forms, a reference to the appropriate indirect food additive regulation for each material of construction is typically considered sufficient evidence of safety. However, for a powder for reconstitution dosage form, reference only to the indirect food additive regulations as evidence of safety for the materials of construction is not recommended. Compatibility for solid oral dosage forms and for powders for reconstitution is typically addressed for plastics and glass by meeting the requirements of the Containers test.

The monographs for Purified Cotton and Purified Rayon USP will typically be considered sufficient standards to establish the safety of these materials as fillers in the packaging of tablets or capsules, with the following caveats: cotton need not meet the monograph requirements for sterility, fiber length, or absorbency; and rayon need not meet the monograph requirements for fiber length or absorbency. Appropriate tests and acceptance criteria for identification and for moisture content should be provided for both cotton and rayon filler. Rayon has been found to be a potential source of dissolution problems for gelatin capsules and gelatin-coated tablets, and this characteristic should be considered when choosing filler. The use of other fillers may be considered with appropriate tests and acceptance criteria. If a desiccant or other absorbent material is used, the composition should be provided (or an appropriate DMF referenced). The component should differ in shape or size from the tablets or capsules with which it is packaged. This will help distinguish between the component and the dosage form. Because these are considered primary packaging components, appropriate tests and acceptance criteria to establish suitability should be provided.

H. Other Dosage Forms

The current good manufacturing practice requirements for container closure systems for compressed medical gases are described in 21 CFR 210 and 211. The containers are regulated by the U.S. Department of Transportation. When submitting information for a drug product or dosage form not specifically covered by the sections above, a firm should take into consideration the compatibility and safety concerns raised by the route of administration of the drug product and the nature of the dosage form (e.g., solid or liquid based); the kinds of protection the container closure system should provide to the dosage form; and the potential effect of any treatment or handling that may be unique to the drug product in the packaging system. Quality control procedures for each packaging component should ensure the maintenance of the safety and quality of future production batches of the drug product.

III. POSTAPPROVAL PACKAGING CHANGES

For an approved application (NDA, ANDA, or BLA), a change to a container closure system, to a component of the container closure system, to a material of construction for a component, or to a process involving one of the above must be reported to the application. The filing requirements are specified under 21 CFR 314.70 (supplements and other changes to an approved application) for an NDA or ANDA and under 21 CFR 601.12 (changes to an approved application) for a BLA.

IV. TYPE III DRUG MASTER FILES

The responsibility for providing information about packaging components rests foremost with the applicant of an NDA, ANDA, or BLA, or with the sponsor of an IND. This information may be provided to the applicant by the manufacturer of a packaging component or material of construction and may be included directly in the application. Any information that a manufacturer does not wish to share with the applicant or sponsor (i.e., because it is considered proprietary) may be placed in a type III DMF and incorporated into the application by a letter from the manufacturer to the applicant that authorizes reference to the DMF. The letter of authorization should specify the firm to whom authorization is granted, the component or material of construction being described, and where the information or data is located in the file by page number or date of submission. This last item is especially important for files that contain information on multiple components or have several volumes. Information in a type III DMF is not restricted to data of a proprietary nature. DMF holders may include in their files as much or as little information as they choose. In addition, a manufacturer of a packaging component is not required to maintain a type III DMF. Without a DMF, there is no procedure for the FDA to review proprietary information except by submission to the application.

The FDA ordinarily reviews a DMF only in connection with an application (IND, NDA, ANDA, or BLA). If the combined information from the application and the DMF is not adequate to support approval of the application or safety for the IND, then the agency may request additional information from the applicant or the DMF holder, as appropriate.

In the event of a change in the DMF, the holder of a DMF must notify the holder of each application supported by the DMF [21 CFR 314.420(c)]. Notice should be provided well before the change is implemented to allow the applicant or sponsor enough time to file a supplement or an amendment to the affected application.

V. BULK CONTAINERS

Drug substances are generally solids, but some are liquids or gases. The container closure system for storage or shipment of a bulk solid drug substance is typically a drum with double LDPE liners that are usually heat sealed or closed with a twist tie. A desiccant may be placed between the bags.

The drum provides protection from light and mechanical strength to protect the liner during shipment and handling. The majority of the protection from air and moisture is provided by the liner. Because LDPE is not a particularly good moisture barrier, a drug substance that is moisture sensitive may need additional protection. An alternative to an LDPE bag is a heat-sealable laminate bag with a comparatively low rate of water vapor transmission.

Qualification of the packaging system is usually based on establishing compatibility and safety of the liner but may also include characterization for solvent or gas transmission. The container closure system for the storage or shipment of a bulk liquid drug substance is typically plastic, stainless steel, a glass-lined metal container, or an epoxy-lined metal container with a rugged, tamper-resistant closure. Qualification of the container closure system may include characterization for solvent and gas permeation, light transmittance, closure integrity, ruggedness in shipment, protection against microbial contamination through the closure, and compatibility and safety of the packaging components as appropriate.

The application (or type II DMF) should include a detailed description of the complete container closure system for the bulk drug substance as well as a description of the specific container, closure, all liners, inner seal, and desiccant (if any), and a description of the composition of each component. A reference to the appropriate indirect food additive regulation is typically considered sufficient to establish the safety of the materials of construction. The tests, methods, and criteria for the acceptance and release of each packaging component should be provided. Stability studies to establish a retest period for bulk drug substance in the proposed container closure system should be conducted with fillers or desiccant packs in place (if used). Smaller versions that simulate the actual container closure system may be used.

A container closure system for bulk drug products may be used for storage before packaging or for shipment to repackagers or contract packagers. In all cases, the container closure system should adequately protect the dosage form and should be constructed of materials that are compatible and safe. Container closure systems for on-site storage have generally been considered a current good manufacturing practice issue under 21 CFR 211.65. However, if a firm plans to hold bulk drug products in storage, then the container closure system and the maximum storage time should be described and justified in the application. In addition, stability data should be provided to demonstrate that extended storage in the described containers does not adversely affect the dosage form. Even when the storage time before packaging will be short, a firm should use a container closure system that provides adequate protection and that is manufactured from materials that are compatible and safe for the intended use.

A container closure system for the transportation of bulk drug products to contract packagers should be described in the application. The container closure system should be adequate to protect the dosage form, be constructed with materials that are compatible with product being stored, and be safe for the intended use. The protective properties of the shipping container are verified by the practice of including annual batches of the packaged product in postapproval stability studies.

A container closure system specifically intended for the transportation of a large volume of drug product to a repackager, whether for a solid or liquid dosage form, is considered a market package. The package should meet the same requirements for protection, compatibility, and safety as a smaller market package; should be included in the stability studies for application approval and in the long-term stability protocol; and should be fully described in the application. The length of time that the dosage form will spend in the bulk container may be a factor in determining the level of detail of the supporting information. Two examples of a large-volume shipping package are a 10,000-tablet HDPE pail with tamper-evident closure and a 10-L polyethylene terephthalate container with a screw-cap closure with dispenser attachment for a liquid drug product. Both are intended for sale to a mass distribution pharmacy.

REFERENCES

FDA guidelines are available at http://www.fda.gov/guidance. Compressed Medical Gases Guideline (February 1989).

FDA Guideline for Drug Master Files (September 1989). http://www.fda.gov/CDER/GUIDANCE/dmf.htm.

FDA Guidance for Industry on the Submission of Documentation for the Sterilization Process Validation in Applications for Human and Veterinary Drug Products (November 1994).

FDA Guidance for Industry on the Content and Format on Investigational New Drug Applications (INDs) for Phase 1 Studies of Drugs, Including Well Characterized, Therapeutic, Biotechnology-Derived Products (November 1995).

FDA Guidance for Industry on the Submission of Chemistry, Manufacturing, and Controls Information for a Therapeutic Recombinant DNA-Derived Product or a Monoclonal Antibody Product for *In Vivo* Use (August 1996).

FDA Guidance for Industry on the Submission of Chemistry, Manufacturing, and Controls Information and Establishment Description for Autologous Somatic Cell Therapy Products (January 1997).

FDA Guidance for the Photostability Testing of New Drug Substance and Products (May 1997).

FDA Guidance for Industry on the Submission of Chemistry, Manufacturing, and Controls Information for Synthetic Peptide Substances (January 1998).

FDA Guidance for Industry on the Content and Format of Chemistry, Manufacturing, and Controls and Establishment Description Information for a Vaccine or Related Product (January 1999).

FDA Guidance for Industry for the Submission of Chemistry, Manufacturing, and Controls and Establishment Description Information for Human Plasma-Derived Biological Product or Animal Plasma or Serum-Derived Products (February 1999).

FDA Guidance for Industry on the Content and Format of Chemistry, Manufacturing, and Controls and Establishment Description Information for a Biological *In Vitro* Diagnostic Product (March 1999).

FDA Guidance for Industry on the Content and Format of Chemistry, Manufacturing, and Controls and Establishment Description Information for Allergenic Extract or Allergen Patch Test (April 1999).

FDA Guidance for Industry for the Submission of Chemistry, Manufacturing, and Controls and Establishment Description Information for Human Blood and Blood Components Intended for Transfusion or for Further Manufacture and for the Completion of the FDA Form 356 h, Application to Market a New Drug, Biologic, or an Antibiotic Drug for Human Use (May 1999).

7

Material for Containers

A container for pharmaceutical use is an article that contains or is intended to contain a product and is, or may be, in direct contact with it. The closure is a part of the container.

The container is so designed that the contents may be removed in a manner appropriate to the intended use of the preparation. It provides a varying degree of protection depending on the nature of the product and the hazards of the environment and minimizes the loss of constituents. The container does not interact physically or chemically with the contents in a way that alters their quality beyond the limits tolerated by official requirements.

Single-dose container. A single-dose container holds a quantity of the preparation intended for total or partial use on one occasion only.

Multidose container. A multidose container holds a quantity of the preparation suitable for two or more doses.

Well-closed container. A well-closed container protects the contents from contamination with extraneous solids and liquids and from loss of contents under ordinary conditions of handling, storage, and transport.

Airtight container. An airtight container is impermeable to solids, liquids, and gases under ordinary conditions of handling, storage, and transport. If the container is intended to be opened on more than one occasion, it must be so designed that it remains airtight after reclosure.

Sealed container. A sealed container is a container closed by fusion of the material of the container.

Tamper-proof container. A tamper-proof container is a closed container fitted with a device that reveals irreversibly whether the container has been opened.

Childproof container. A container that is fitted with a closure that prevents opening by children.

I. GLASS CONTAINERS

Glass containers for pharmaceutical use are glass articles intended to come into direct contact with pharmaceutical preparations. Colorless glass is highly transparent in the visible spectrum. Colored glass is obtained by the addition of small amounts of metal oxides, chosen according to the desired spectral absorbance. *Neutral glass* is a borosilicate glass containing significant amounts of boric oxide, aluminum oxide alkali, and/or alkaline earth oxides. Because of its composition, neutral glass has a high hydrolytic resistance and a high thermal shock resistance. *Soda-lime-silica glass* is a silica glass containing alkali metal oxides, mainly sodium oxide and alkaline earth oxides, mainly calcium oxide. Because of its composition, soda-lime-silica glass has only a moderate hydrolytic resistance. The hydrolytic stability of glass containers for pharmaceutical use is expressed by the resistance to the release of soluble mineral substances into water under the prescribed conditions of contact between the inner surface of the container or glass grains and water. The hydrolytic resistance is evaluated by titrating released alkali. According to their hydrolytic resistance, glass containers are classified as follows:

1. Type I glass containers: Neutral glass, with a high hydrolytic resistance due to the chemical composition of the glass itself.
2. Type II glass containers: Usually of soda-lime-silica glass with a high hydrolytic resistance resulting from suitable treatment of the surface.
3. Type III glass containers: Usually of soda-lime-silica glass with only moderate hydrolytic resistance. The following italicized statements constitute general recommendations concerning the type of glass container that may be used for different types of pharmaceutical preparations. The manufacturer of a pharmaceutical product is responsible for ensuring the suitability of the chosen container.

Type I glass containers are suitable for most preparations whether or not for parenteral use. Type II glass containers are suitable for most acidic and neutral, aqueous preparations whether or not for parenteral use. Type III glass containers are in general suitable for nonaqueous preparations for parenteral use, for powders for parenteral use (except for freeze-dried preparations), and for preparations not for parenteral use. Glass containers with a hydrolytic resistance higher than that recommended earlier for a particular type of preparation may generally also be used. The container chosen for a given preparation shall be such that the glass material does not release substances in quantities sufficient to affect the stability of the preparation or to present a risk of toxicity. In justified cases, it may be necessary to have detailed information on the glass composition, so that the potential hazards can be assessed. Preparations for parenteral use are normally presented in colorless glass, but colored glass may be used for substances known to be light sensitive. Colorless or colored glass is used for the other pharmaceutical preparations. It is recommended that all glass containers for liquid preparations and for powders for parenteral use permit the visual inspection of the contents. The inner surface of glass containers may be specially treated to improve hydrolytic resistance, to confer water repellency. The outer surface may also be treated, for example, to reduce friction and to improve resistance to abrasion. The outer treatment is such that it does not contaminate the inner surface of the container. Except for type I glass containers, glass containers for pharmaceutical preparations are not to be reused. Containers for human blood and blood components must not be reused. Glass containers for pharmaceutical use comply with the relevant test or tests for hydrolytic resistance. When glass containers have nonglass components, the tests apply only to the glass part of the container.

II. NONPLASTICIZED POLY(VINYL CHLORIDE) FOR CONTAINERS FOR NONINJECTABLE AQUEOUS SOLUTIONS

Materials based on nonplasticized poly(vinyl chloride) that comply with the following specifications are suitable for the manufacture of containers for noninjectable aqueous solutions. They may also be used for solid forms for oral administration and, in some cases, subject to special studies on the compatibility of the container with its contents; these materials may be suitable for the preparation of containers for suppositories. They consist of one or more poly(vinyl chloride/vinyl acetate) or of a mixture of poly(vinyl chloride) and poly(vinyl acetate) or of poly(vinyl chloride). They contain not more than 1 ppm of vinyl chloride. The chlorine content expressed in poly(vinyl chloride) is not less than 80%. They may contain not more than 15% of copolymers based on acrylic and/or methacrylic acids and/or their esters, and/or on styrene and/or butadiene. Materials based on nonplasticized poly(vinyl chloride) are produced by polymerization methods, which guarantee a residual vinyl chloride content of less than 1 ppm.

III. POLYETHYLENE TEREPHTHALATE FOR CONTAINERS FOR PREPARATIONS NOT FOR PARENTERAL USE

Polyethylene terephthalate is obtained from the polymerization of terephthalic acid or dimethyl terephthalate with ethylene glycol. Isophthalic acid, dimethyl isophthalate, 1,4-bis(hydroxymethyl)cyclohexane (cyclohexane-1,4-dimethanol), or diethylene glycol may be used in the polymerization. It may contain not more than 0.5% of silica or silicates and coloring matter approved by the competent authority. The manufacturing process is validated to demonstrate that the residual acetaldehyde content is not greater than 10 ppm in the granules.

IV. NONPLASTICIZED POLY(VINYL CHLORIDE) FOR CONTAINERS FOR DRY DOSAGE FORMS FOR ORAL ADMINISTRATION

Materials based on nonplasticized poly(vinyl chloride) for containers for dry dosage forms for oral administration are suitable for the manufacture of sheets or containers. They consist of one or more poly(vinyl chloride/vinyl acetate) or of a mixture of poly(vinyl chloride) and poly(vinyl acetate) or of poly(vinyl chloride). They contain not more than 1 ppm of vinyl chloride. The chlorine content expressed in poly(vinyl chloride) is not less than 80%. They may contain not more than 15% of copolymers based on acrylic and/or methacrylic acids and/or their esters and/or on styrene and/or butadiene. Materials based on nonplasticized poly(vinyl chloride) are produced by polymerization methods, which guarantee a residual vinyl chloride content of less than 1 ppm.

V. PLASTICIZED POLY(VINYL CHLORIDE) FOR CONTAINERS FOR AQUEOUS SOLUTIONS FOR INTRAVENOUS INFUSION

Materials based on plasticized poly(vinyl chloride) contain not less than 55% of poly(vinyl chloride) and contain various additives, in addition to the high-molecular-mass polymer obtained by polymerization of vinyl chloride. Materials based on plasticized poly(vinyl chloride) for containers for aqueous solutions for intravenous infusion are defined by the nature and the proportions of the substances used in their manufacture. Materials based on plasticized poly(vinyl chloride) are produced by polymerization methods, which guarantee a residual vinyl chloride content of less than 1 ppm.

VI. POLYETHYLENE TEREPHTHALATE FOR CONTAINERS FOR PREPARATIONS NOT FOR PARENTERAL USE

Polyethylene terephthalate is obtained from the polymerization of terephthalic acid or dimethyl terephthalate with ethylene glycol. Isophthalic acid, dimethyl isophthalate, 1,4-bis(hydroxymethyl)cyclohexane (cyclohexane-1,4-dimethanol), or diethylene glycol may be used in the polymerization. It may contain not more than 0.5% of silica or silicates and coloring matter approved by the competent authority. The manufacturing process is validated to demonstrate that the residual acetaldehyde content is not more than 10 ppm in the granules.

VII. POLYOLEFINES

Polyolefines are obtained by polymerization of ethylene or propylene or by copolymerization of these substances with not more than 25% of higher homologues (C_4–C_{10}) or of carboxylic acids or of esters. Certain materials may be mixtures of polyolefines. A certain number of additives are added to the polymer to optimize their chemical, physical, and mechanical properties to adapt them for the intended use. All of these additives are chosen from the appended list, which specifies for each product the maximum allowable content. They may contain at most three antioxidants, one or several lubricants or antiblocking agents, as well as titanium dioxide as an opacifying agent when the material must provide protection from light.

1. Butyl hydroxytoluene (plastic additive 07) (not more than 0.125%)
2. Pentaerythrityl tetrakis[3-(3,5-di-*tert*-butyl-4-hydroxyphenyl)propionate] (plastic additive 09) (not more than 0.3%)
3. 1,3,5-tris(3,5-di-*tert*-butyl-4-hydroxybenzyl)-*s*-triazine-2,4,6(1*H*, 3*H*, 5*H*)-trione, (plastic additive 13) (not more than 0.3%)
4. Octadecyl 3-(3,5-di-*tert*-butyl-4-hydroxyphenyl)propionate (plastic additive 11) (not more than 0.3%), ethylene bis[3,3-bis[3-(1,1-dimethylethyl)-4-hydroxyphenyl] butanoate] (plastic additive 08) (not more than 0.3%)
5. Dioctadecyl disulphide (plastic additive 15) (not more than 0.3%)
6. 4,4′,4″-(2,4,6-trimethylbenzene-1,3,5-triyltrismethylene) trio[2,6-bis(1,1-dimethylethyl)phenol] (plastic additive 10) (not more than 0.3%)
7. 2,2′-bis(octadecyloxy)-5,5′-spirobi(1,3,2-dioxaphosphinane) (plastic additive 14) (not more than 0.3%)
8. Didodecyl 3,3′-thiodipropionate (plastic additive 16) (not more than 0.3%),
9. Dioctadecyl 3,3′-thiodipropionate (plastic additive 17) (not more than 0.3%)
10. Tris[2,4-bis(1,1-dimethylethyl)phenyl] phosphite (plastic additive 12) (not more than 0.3%)
11. Plastic additive 18 (not more than 0.1%)

12. Copolymer of dimethyl succinate and (4-hydroxy-2,2,6,6-tetramethylpiperidin-1-yl)ethanol (plastic additive 22) (not more than 0.3%%)
    The total of antioxidant additives listed above does not exceed 0.3%—hydrotalcite (not more than 0.5%).
13. Alkanamides (not more than 0.5%)
14. Alkenamides (not more than 0.5%)
15. Sodium silicoaluminate (not more than 0.5%)
16. Silica (not more than 0.5%)
17. Sodium benzoate (not more than 0.5%)
18. Fatty acid esters or salts (not more than 0.5%)
19. Trisodium phosphate (not more than 0.5%)
20. Liquid paraffin (not more than 0.5%)
21. Zinc oxide (not more than 0.5%)
22. Talc (not more than 0.5%)
23. Magnesium oxide (not more than 0.2%)
24. Calcium stearate or zinc stearate or a mixture of both (not more than 0.5%)
25. Titanium dioxide (not more than 4%)

VIII. POLYETHYLENE WITH ADDITIVES FOR CONTAINERS FOR PARENTERAL PREPARATIONS AND FOR OPHTHALMIC PREPARATIONS

Polyethylene with additives is obtained by the polymerization of ethylene under pressure in the presence of a catalyst or by copolymerization of ethylene with not more than 25% of higher alkene homologues (C_3–C_{10}). A certain number of additives are added to the polymer to optimize their chemical, physical, and mechanical properties to adapt them for the intended use. All these additives are chosen from the appended list, which specifies for each product the maximum allowable content. They may contain at most three antioxidants, one or several lubricants or antiblocking agents, as well as titanium dioxide as an opacifying agent when the material must provide protection from light.

1. Butyl hydroxytoluene (plastic additive 07) (not more than 0.125%).
2. Pentaerythrityl tetrakis[3-(3,5-di-*tert*-butyl-4-hydroxyphenyl)propionate] (plastic additive 09) (not more than 0.3%).
3. 1,3,5-tris(3,5-di-*tert*-butyl-4-hydroxybenzyl)-*s*-triazine-2,4,6(1*H*, 3*H*, 5*H*)-trione (plastic additive 13) (not more than 0.3%).
4. Octadecyl 3-(3,5-di-*tert*-butyl-4-hydroxyphenyl) propionate, (plastic additive 11) (not more than 0.3%).
5. Ethylene bis[3,3-bis(3-[1,1-dimethylethyl]-4-hydroxyphenyl)butanoate] (plastic additive 08) (not more than 0.3%).
6. Dioctadecyl disulphide (plastic additive 15) (not more than 0.3%).
7. 4,4′,4″-(2,4,6-trimethylbenzene-1,3,5-triyltrismethylene) tris[2,6-bis(1,1-dimethylethyl)phenol] (plastic additive 10) (not more than 0.3%).
8. 2,2′-bis(octadecyloxy)-5,5′-spirobi(1,3,2-dioxaphosphinane) (plastic additive 14) (not more than 0.3%).
9. Didodecyl 3,3′-thiodipropionate (plastic additive 16) (not more than 0.3%).
10. Dioctadecyl 3,3′-thiodipropionate (plastic additive 17) (not more than 0.3%).
11. Tris [2,4-bis(1,1-dimethylethyl)phenyl] phosphite (plastic additive 12) (not more than 0.3%).

    The total of antioxidant additives listed above does not exceed 0.3%.
12. Hydrotalcite (not more than 0.5%).
13. Alkanamides (not more than 0.5%).
14. Alkenamides (not more than 0.5%).
15. Sodium silicoaluminate (not more than 0.5%).
16. Silica (not more than 0.5%).
17. Sodium benzoate (not more than 0.5%).
18. Fatty acid esters or salts (not more than 0.5%).
19. Trisodium phosphate (not more than 0.5%).
20. Liquid paraffin (not more than 0.5%).
21. Zinc oxide (not more than 0.5%).
22. Magnesium oxide (not more than 0.2%).
23. Calcium stearate or zinc stearate or a mixture of both (not more than 0.5%).
24. Titanium dioxide (not more than 4%) only for materials for containers for ophthalmic use. The supplier of the material must be able to demonstrate that the qualitative and quantitative composition of the type sample is satisfactory for each production batch.

IX. POLYPROPYLENE FOR CONTAINERS AND CLOSURES FOR PARENTERAL PREPARATIONS AND OPHTHALMIC PREPARATIONS

Polypropylene consists of the homopolymer of propylene or of a copolymer of propylene with not more than 25% of ethylene or of a mixture (alloy) of polypropylene with not more than 25% of polyethylene. It may contain additives. A certain number of additives are added to the polymer to optimize their chemical, physical, and mechanical properties to adapt them for the intended use. All these additives are chosen from the appended list, which specifies for each product the maximum allowable content. They may contain at most three antioxidants, one or several lubricants or antiblocking agents, as well as titanium dioxide as opacifying agent when the material must provide protection from light.

1. Butyl hydroxytoluene (plastic additive 07) (not more than 0.125%).
2. Pentaerythrityl tetrakis[3-(3,5-di-*tert*-butyl-4-hydroxyphenyl)propionate] (plastic additive 09) (not more than 0.3%).
3. 1,3,5-tris(3,5-di-*tert*-butyl-4-hydroxybenzyl)-*s*-triazine-2,4,6(1*H*,3*H*,5*H*)-trione (plastic additive 13) (not more than 0.3%).
4. Octadecyl 3-(3,5-di-*tert*-butyl-4-hydroxyphenyl)propionate, (plastic additive 11) (not more than 0.3%).
5. Ethylene bis[3,3-bis(3-[1,1-dimethylethyl]-4-hydroxyphenyl)butanoate] (plastic additive 08) (not more than 0.3%).
6. Dioctadecyl disulphide (plastic additive 15) (not more than 0.3%).
7. 2,2′,2″,6,6′,6″-hexa-*tert*-butyl-4,4′,4″-[(2,4,6-trimethyl-1,3,5-benzenetriyl)trismethylene]triphenol (plastic additive 10) (not more than 0.3%).
8. 2,2′-bis(octadecyloxy)-5,5′-spirobi[1,3,2-dioxaphosphinane] (plastic additive 14) (not more than 0.3%).
9. Didodecyl 3,3′-thiodipropionate (plastic additive 16) (not more than 0.3%).
10. Dioctadecyl 3,3′-thiodipropionate (plastic additive 17) (not more than 0.3%).
11. Tris(2,4-di-*tert*-butylphenyl) phosphite (plastic additive 12) (not more than 0.3%).

The total of antioxidant additives listed above does not exceed 0.3%.

12. Hydrotalcite (not more than 0.5%).
13. Alkanamides (not more than 0.5%).
14. Alkenamides (not more than 0.5%).
15. Sodium silicoaluminate (not more than 0.5%).
16. Silica (not more than 0.5%), sodium benzoate (not more than 0.5%), fatty acid esters or salts (not more than 0.5%).
17. Trisodium phosphate (not more than 0.5%).
18. Liquid paraffin (not more than 0.5%).
19. Zinc oxide (not more than 0.5%), talc (not more than 0.5%).
20. Magnesium oxide (not more than 0.2%).
21. Calcium stearate or zinc stearate or a mixture of both (not more than 0.5%).
22. Titanium dioxide (not more than 4%) only for materials for containers for ophthalmic use. The supplier of the material must be able to demonstrate that the qualitative and quantitative composition of the type sample is satisfactory for each production batch.

X. POLY(ETHYLENE/VINYL ACETATE) FOR CONTAINERS AND TUBING FOR TOTAL PARENTERAL NUTRITION PREPARATIONS

Poly(ethylene/vinyl acetate), complying with the following requirements, is suitable for the manufacture of containers and tubing for total parenteral nutrition preparations. Poly(ethylene/vinyl acetate) is obtained by copolymerization of mixtures of ethylene and vinyl acetate. This copolymer contains a defined quantity of not more than 25% of vinyl acetate for material to be used for containers and not more than 30% for material to be used for tubing. A certain number of additives are added to the polymer to optimize their chemical, physical, and mechanical properties to adapt them for the intended use. All these additives are chosen from the appended list, which specifies for each product the maximum allowable content. Poly(ethylene/vinyl acetate) may contain not more than three of the following antioxidants:

1. Butyl hydroxytoluene (plastic additive 07) (not more than 0.125%)
2. Pentaerythrityl tetrakis[3-(3,5-di-*tert*-butyl-4-hydroxyphenyl)propionate] (plastic additive 09) (not more than 0.2%)
3. Octadecyl 3-(3,5-di-*tert*-butyl-4-hydroxyphenyl)propionate (plastic additive 11) (not more than 0.2%),
4. Tris(2,4-di-*tert*-butylphenyl) phosphite (plastic additive 12) (not more than 0.2%)
5. 2,2′,2″,6,6′,6″-hexa-*tert*-butyl-4,4′,4″-[(2,4,6-trimethyl-1,3,5-benzenetriyl)trismethylene]triphenol (plastic additive 10) (not more than 0.2%). It may also contain
   a. oleamide (plastic additive 20) (not more than 0.5%),
   b. erucamide (plastic additive 21) (not more than 0.5%),
   c. calcium stearate or zinc stearate or a mixture of both (not more than 0.5%),
   d. calcium carbonate or potassium hydroxide (not more than 0.5% of each),
   e. colloidal silica (not more than 0.2%). The supplier of the material must be able to demonstrate that the qualitative and quantitative composition of the type sample is satisfactory for each production batch.

XI. PLASTIC CONTAINERS FOR AQUEOUS SOLUTIONS FOR INFUSION

Plastic containers for aqueous solutions for infusion are manufactured from one or more polymers, if necessary with additives. The containers described in this section are not necessarily suitable for emulsions. The polymers most commonly used are polyethylene, polypropylene, and poly(vinyl chloride). The containers may be bags or bottles. They have a site suitable for the attachment of an infusion set designed to ensure a secure connection. They may have a site that allows an injection to be made at the time of use. They usually have a part that allows them to be suspended and which will withstand the tension occurring during use. The containers must withstand the sterilization conditions to which they will be submitted. The design of the container and the method of sterilization chosen are such that all parts of the containers that may be in contact with the infusion are sterilized. The containers are impermeable to microorganisms after closure. The containers are such that after filling they are resistant to damage from accidental freezing which may occur during transport of the final preparation. The containers are and remain sufficiently transparent to allow the appearance of the contents to be examined at any time, unless otherwise justified and authorized. The empty containers display no defects that may lead to leakage and the filled and closed containers show no leakage. For satisfactory storage of some preparations, the container has to be enclosed in a protective envelope. The initial evaluation of storage has then to be carried out using the container enclosed in the envelope.

A plastic container for pharmaceutical use is a plastic article, which contains or is intended to contain a pharmaceutical product and is, or may be, in direct contact with it. The closure is a part of the container. Plastic containers and closures for pharmaceutical use are made of materials in which may be included certain additives; these materials do not include in their composition any substance that can be extracted by the contents in such quantities as to alter the efficacy or the stability of the product or to present a risk of toxicity. The most commonly used polymers are polyethylene (with and without additives), polypropylene, poly(vinyl chloride), poly(ethylene terephthalate), and poly(ethylene/vinyl acetate). The nature and amount of the additives are determined by the type of the polymer, the process used to convert the polymer into the container, and the intended purpose of the container. Additives may consist of antioxidants, stabilizers, plasticizes, lubricants, coloring matter, and impact modifiers. Antistatic agents and mould-release agents may be used only for containers for preparations for oral use or for external use for which they are authorized Acceptable additives are indicated in the type specification for each material described in the *Pharmacopoeia*. Other additives may be used provided they are approved in each case by the competent authority responsible for the licensing for sale of the preparation. For selection of a suitable plastic container, it is necessary to know the full manufacturing formula of the plastic, including all materials added during formation of the container so that the potential hazards can be assessed. The plastic container chosen for any particular preparation should be such that

1. the ingredients of the preparation in contact with the plastic material are not significantly adsorbed on its surface and do not significantly migrate into or through the plastic,
2. the plastic material does not release substances in quantities sufficient to affect the stability of the preparation or

to present a risk of toxicity. Using material (or materials) selected to satisfy these criteria, a number of identical type samples of the container are made by a well-defined procedure and submitted to practical testing in conditions that reproduce those of the intended use, including, where appropriate, sterilization. To confirm the compatibility of the container and the contents and to ensure that there are no changes detrimental to the quality of the preparation, various tests are carried out, such as verification of the absence of changes in physical characteristics, assessment of any loss or gain through permeation, detection of pH changes, assessment of changes caused by light, chemical tests, and, where appropriate, biological tests. The method of manufacture is such as to ensure reproducibility for subsequent bulk manufacture and the conditions of manufacture are chosen so as to preclude the possibility of contamination with other plastic materials or their ingredients. The manufacturer of the product must ensure that containers made in production are similar in every respect to the type samples.

For the results of the testing on type samples to remain valid, it is important that

1. there is no change in the composition of the material as defined for the type samples,
2. there is no change in the manufacturing process as defined for the type samples, especially as regards the temperatures to which the plastic material is exposed during conversion or subsequent procedures such as sterilization,
3. scrap material is not used. Recycling of excess material of well-defined nature and proportions may be permitted after appropriate validation. Subject to satisfactory testing for compatibility of each different combination of container and contents, the materials described in the *Pharmacopoeia* are recognized as being suitable for the specific purposes indicated, as defined above.

XII. STERILE SINGLE-USE PLASTIC SYRINGES

Sterile single-use plastic syringes are medical devices intended for immediate use for the administration of injectable preparations. They are supplied sterile and pyrogen-free and are not to be resterilized or reused. They consist of a syringe barrel and a piston which may have an elastomer sealing ring; they may be fitted with a needle which may be nondetachable. Each syringe is presented with individual protection for maintaining sterility. The barrel of the syringe is sufficiently transparent to permit dosages to be read without difficulty and allow air bubbles and foreign particles to be discerned. The plastics and elastomer materials of which the barrel and piston are made comply with the appropriate specification or with the requirements of the competent authority. The most commonly used materials are polypropylene and polyethylene. The syringes comply with current standards regarding dimensions and performance. Silicone oil may be applied to the internal wall of the barrel to assist in the smooth operation of the syringe but there remains no excess capable of contaminating the contents at the time of use. The inks, glues, and adhesives for the marking on the syringe or on the package and, where necessary, the assembly of the syringe and its package do not migrate across the walls.

XIII. RUBBER CLOSURES FOR CONTAINERS FOR AQUEOUS PARENTERAL PREPARATIONS, FOR POWDERS, AND FOR FREEZE-DRIED POWDERS

Rubber closures for containers for aqueous parenteral preparations for powders and for freeze-dried powders are made of materials obtained by vulcanization (cross-linking) of macromolecular organic substances (elastomers) with appropriate additives. The specification also applies to closures for containers for powders and freeze-dried products to be dissolved in water immediately before use. The elastomers are produced from natural or synthetic substances by polymerization, polyaddition, or polycondensation. The nature of the principal components and of the various additives (e.g., vulcanizers, accelerators, stabilizers, pigments) depends on the properties required for the finished article. Rubber closures may be classified in two types: type I closures are those which meet the strictest requirements and which are to be preferred; type II closures are those which, having mechanical properties suitable for special uses (e.g., multiple piercing), cannot meet requirements as severe as those for the first category because of their chemical composition. The closures chosen for use with a particular preparation are such that

1. the components of the preparation in contact with the closure are not adsorbed onto the surface of the closure and do not migrate into or through the closure to an extent sufficient to affect the preparation adversely,
2. the closure does not yield to the preparation substances in quantities sufficient to affect its stability or to present a risk of toxicity. The closures are compatible with the preparation for which they are used throughout its period of validity. The manufacturer of the preparation must obtain from the supplier an assurance that the composition of the closure does not vary and that it is identical to that of the closure used during compatibility testing. When the supplier informs the manufacturer of the preparation of changes in the composition, compatibility testing must be repeated, totally or partly, depending on the nature of the changes. The closures are washed and may be sterilized before use.

XIV. SILICONE OIL USED AS A LUBRICANT

Silicone oil used as a lubricant is a poly(dimethylsiloxane) obtained by hydrolysis and polycondensation of dichlorodimethylsilane and chlorotrimethylsilane. Different grades exist which are characterized by a number indicating the nominal viscosity placed after the name. Silicone oil used as lubricants have a degree of polymerization (n = 400–1200) such that their kinematic viscosities are nominally between 1000 $mm^2{\cdot}s^{-1}$ and 30,000 $mm^2{\cdot}s^{-1}$.

XV. SILICONE ELASTOMER FOR CLOSURES AND TUBING

Silicone elastomer complying with the following requirements is suitable for the manufacture of closures and tubing. Silicone elastomer is obtained by cross-linking a linear polysiloxane constructed mainly of dimethylsiloxy units with small quantities of methylvinylsiloxy groups; the chain ends are blocked by trimethylsiloxy or dimethylvinylsiloxy groups. In all cases, appropriate additives are used, such as silica, and sometimes small quantities of organosilicon additives (α,ω-dihydroxypolydimethylsiloxane).

8

Stability Testing of New Drug Substances and Products

I. INTRODUCTION

A. Objectives of the Guideline

The following guideline is a revised version of the ICH Q1A guideline and defines the stability data package for a new drug substance or drug product that is sufficient for a registration application within the three regions of the European Commission, Japan, and the United States. It does not seek necessarily to cover the testing for registration in or export to other areas of the world.

The guideline seeks to exemplify the core stability data package for new drug substances and products, but leaves sufficient flexibility to encompass the variety of different practical situations that may be encountered due to specific scientific considerations and characteristics of the materials being evaluated. Alternative approaches can be used when there are scientifically justifiable reasons.

B. Scope of the Guideline

The guideline addresses the information to be submitted in registration applications for new molecular entities and associated drug products. This guideline does not currently seek to cover the information to be submitted for abbreviated or abridged applications, variations, clinical trial applications, etc.

Specific details of the sampling and testing for particular dosage forms in their proposed container closures are not covered in this guideline.

C. General Principles

The purpose of stability testing is to provide evidence on how the quality of a drug substance or drug product varies with time under the influence of a variety of environmental factors such as temperature, humidity, and light, and to establish a retest period for the drug substance or a shelf life for the drug product and recommended storage conditions.

The choice of test conditions defined in this guideline is based on an analysis of the effects of climatic conditions in the three regions of the European Commission, Japan, and the United States. The mean kinetic temperature in any part of the world can be derived from climatic data, and the world can be divided into four climatic zones, I to IV. This guideline addresses climatic zones I and II. The principle has been established that stability information generated in any one of the three regions of the European Commission, Japan, and the United States would be mutually acceptable to the other two regions, provided the information is consistent with this guideline and the labeling is in accordance with national/regional requirements.

II. GUIDELINES

A. Drug Substance

1. General

Information on the stability of the drug substance is an integral part of the systematic approach to stability evaluation.

2. Stress Testing

Stress testing of the drug substance can help identify the likely degradation products, which can in turn help establish the degradation pathways and the intrinsic stability of the molecule and validate the stability indicating power of the analytical procedures used. The nature of the stress testing will depend on the individual drug substance and the type of drug product involved.

Stress testing is likely to be carried out on a single batch of the drug substance. It should include the effect of temperatures [in 10°C increments (e.g., 50°C, 60°C) above that for accelerated testing], humidity (e.g., 75% RH or greater) where appropriate, oxidation, and photolysis on the drug substance. The testing should also evaluate the susceptibility of the drug substance to hydrolysis across a wide range of pH values when in solution or suspension. Photostability testing should be an integral part of stress testing.

Examining degradation products under stress conditions is useful in establishing degradation pathways and developing and validating suitable analytical procedures. However, it may not be necessary to examine specifically for certain degradation products if it has been demonstrated that they are not formed under accelerated or long-term storage conditions.

Results from these studies will form an integral part of the information provided to regulatory authorities.

3. Selection of Batches

Data from formal stability studies should be provided on at least three primary batches of the drug substance. The batches should be manufactured to a minimum of pilot scale by the same synthetic route as, and using a method of manufacture and procedure that simulates the final process to be used for, production batches. The overall quality of the batches of drug substance placed on formal stability studies should be representative of the quality of the material to be made on a production scale.

Other supporting data can be provided.

4. Container Closure System

The stability studies should be conducted on the drug substance packaged in a container closure system that is the same as or simulates the packaging proposed for storage and distribution.

5. Specification

Specification, which is a list of tests, reference to analytical procedures, and proposed acceptance criteria, is addressed in ICH Q6A and Q6B. In addition, specification for degradation products in a drug substance is discussed in Q3A.

Stability studies should include testing of those attributes of the drug substance that are susceptible to change during storage and are likely to influence quality, safety, and/or efficacy. The testing should cover, as appropriate, the physical, chemical, biological, and microbiological attributes.

Validated stability indicating analytical procedures should be applied. Whether and to what extent replication should be performed will depend on the results from validation studies.

6. Testing Frequency

For long-term studies, frequency of testing should be sufficient to establish the stability profile of the drug substance. For drug substances with a proposed retest period of at least 12 months, the frequency of testing at the long-term storage condition should normally be every 3 months over the first year, every 6 months over the second year, and annually thereafter through the proposed retest period.

At the accelerated storage condition, a minimum of three time points, including the initial and final time points (e.g., 0, 3, and 6 months), a 6-month study is recommended. Where an expectation (based on development experience) exists that results from accelerated studies that are likely to approach significant change criteria, increased testing should be conducted either by adding samples at the final time point or by including a fourth time point in the study design.

When testing at the intermediate storage condition is called for as a result of significant change at the accelerated storage condition, a minimum of four time points, including the initial and final time points (e.g., 0, 6, 9, 12 months), from a 12-month study is recommended.

7. Storage Conditions

In general, a drug substance should be evaluated under storage conditions (with appropriate tolerances) that test its thermal stability and, if applicable, its sensitivity to moisture. The storage conditions and the lengths of studies chosen should be sufficient to cover storage, shipment, and subsequent use.

The long-term testing should cover a minimum of 12 months duration on at least three primary batches at the time of submission and should be continued for a period of time sufficient to cover the proposed retest period. Additional data accumulated during the assessment period of the registration application should be submitted to the authorities if requested. Data from the accelerated storage condition and, if appropriate, from the intermediate storage condition can be used to evaluate the effect of short-term excursions outside the label storage conditions (such as might occur during shipping).

Long-term, accelerated, and, where appropriate, intermediate storage conditions for drug substances are detailed in the sections below. The general case applies if the drug substance is not specifically covered by a subsequent section. Alternative storage conditions can be used if justified.

a. General Case

Study	Storage condition	Minimum time period covered by data at submission
Long term[a]	25°C ± 2°C/60% RH ± 5% RH or 30°C ± 2°C/65% RH ± 5% RH	12 mo
Intermediate[b]	30°C ± 2°C/65% RH ± 5% RH	6 mo
Accelerated	40°C ± 2°C/75% RH ± 5% RH	6 mo

[a]It is up to the applicant to decide whether long-term stability studies are performed at 25 ± 2°C/60% RH ± 5% RH or 30°C ± 2°C/65% RH ± 5% RH.

[b]If 30°C ± 2°C/65% RH ± 5% RH is the long-term condition, there is no intermediate condition.

If long-term studies are conducted at 25°C ± 2°C/60% RH ± 5% RH and "significant change" occurs at any time during 6 months' testing at the accelerated storage condition, additional testing at the intermediate storage condition should be conducted and evaluated against significant change criteria. Testing at the intermediate storage condition should include all tests, unless otherwise justified. The initial application should include a minimum of 6 months' data from a 12-month study at the intermediate storage condition.

"Significant change" for a drug substance is defined as failure to meet its specification.

b. Drug Substances Intended for Storage in a Refrigerator

Study	Storage condition	Minimum time period covered by data at submission
Long term	5°C ± 3°C	12 mo
Accelerated	25°C ± 2°C/60% RH ± 5% RH	6 mo

Data from refrigerated storage should be assessed according to the evaluation section of this guideline, except where explicitly noted below.

If significant change occurs between 3 and 6 months' testing at the accelerated storage condition, the proposed retest period should be based on the real-time data available at the long-term storage condition.

If significant change occurs within the first 3 months' testing at the accelerated storage condition, a discussion should be provided to address the effect of short-term excursions outside the label storage condition, for example, during shipping or handling. This discussion can be supported, if appropriate, by further testing on a single batch of the drug substance for a period shorter than 3 months but with more frequent testing than usual. It is considered unnecessary to continue to test a drug substance through 6 months when a significant change has occurred within the first 3 months.

c. Drug Substances Intended for Storage in a Freezer

Study	Storage condition	Minimum time period covered by data at submission
Long term	−20°C ± 5°C	12 mo

For drug substances intended for storage in a freezer, the retest period should be based on the real-time data obtained at the long term storage condition. In the absence of an accelerated storage condition for drug substances intended to be stored in a freezer, testing on a single batch at an elevated temperature (e.g., 5°C ± 3°C or 25°C ± 2°C) for an appropriate time period should be conducted to address the effect of short term excursions outside the proposed label storage condition, for example, during shipping or handling.

d. Drug Substances Intended for Storage Below −20°C

Drug substances intended for storage below −20°C should be treated on a case-by-case basis.

8. Stability Commitment

When available, long-term stability data on primary batches do not cover the proposed retest period granted at the time of approval; a commitment should be made to continue the stability studies post approval to firmly establish the retest period.

Where the submission includes long-term stability data on three production batches covering the proposed retest period, a postapproval commitment is considered unnecessary. Otherwise, one of the following commitments should be made.

1. If the submission includes data from stability studies on at least three production batches, a commitment should be made to continue these studies through the proposed retest period.
2. If the submission includes data from stability studies on fewer than three production batches, a commitment should be made to continue these studies through the proposed retest period and to place additional production batches, to a total of at least three, on long-term stability studies through the proposed retest period.
3. If the submission does not include stability data on production batches, a commitment should be made to place the first three production batches on long-term stability studies through the proposed retest period.

The stability protocol used for long-term studies for the stability commitment should be the same as that for the primary batches, unless otherwise scientifically justified.

9. Evaluation

The purpose of the stability study is to establish, based on testing a minimum of three batches of the drug substance and evaluating the stability information (including, as appropriate, results of the physical, chemical, biological, and microbiological tests), a retest period applicable to all future batches of the drug substance manufactured under similar circumstances. The degree of variability of individual batches affects the confidence that a future production batch will remain within specification throughout the assigned retest period.

The data may show so little degradation and so little variability that it is apparent from looking at the data that the requested retest period will be granted. Under these circumstances, it is normally unnecessary to go through the formal statistical analysis. Providing a justification for the omission should be sufficient.

An approach for analyzing the data on a quantitative attribute that is expected to change with time is to determine the time at which the 95% one-sided confidence limit for the mean curve intersects the acceptance criterion. If analysis shows that the batch-to-batch variability is small, it is advantageous to combine the data into one overall estimate. This can be done by first applying appropriate statistical tests (e.g., p values for level of significance of rejection of more than 0.25) to the slopes of the regression lines and zero time intercepts for the individual batches. If it is inappropriate to combine data from several batches, the overall retest period should be based on the minimum time a batch can be expected to remain within acceptance criteria.

The nature of any degradation relationship will determine whether the data should be transformed for linear regression analysis. Usually the relationship can be represented by a linear, quadratic, or cubic function on an arithmetic or logarithmic scale. Statistical methods should be employed to test the goodness of fit of the data on all batches and combined batches (where appropriate) to the assumed degradation line or curve.

Limited extrapolation of the real-time data from the long-term storage condition beyond the observed range to extend the retest period can be undertaken at approval time, if justified. This justification should be based on what is known about the mechanism of degradation, the results of testing under accelerated conditions, the goodness of fit of any mathematical model, batch size, existence of supporting stability data, etc. However, this extrapolation assumes that the same degradation relationship will continue to apply beyond the observed data.

Any evaluation should cover not only the assay, but also the levels of degradation products and other appropriate attributes.

10. Statements/Labeling

A storage statement should be established for the labeling in accordance with relevant national/regional requirements. The statement should be based on the stability evaluation of the drug substance. Where applicable, specific instructions should be provided, particularly for drug substances that cannot tolerate freezing. Terms such as "ambient conditions" or "room temperature" should be avoided.

A retest period should be derived from the stability information, and a retest date should be displayed on the container label if appropriate.

B. Drug Product

1. General

The design of the formal stability studies for the drug product should be based on knowledge of the behavior and properties of the drug substance and from stability studies on the drug substance and on experience gained from clinical formulation studies. The likely changes on storage and the rationale for the selection of attributes to be tested in the formal stability studies should be stated.

2. Photostability Testing

Photostability testing should be conducted on at least one primary batch of the drug product if appropriate. The standard conditions for photostability testing are described in ICH Q1B.

3. Selection of Batches

Data from stability studies should be provided on at least three primary batches of the drug product. The primary batches should be of the same formulation and packaged in the same container closure system as proposed for marketing. The manufacturing process used for primary batches should simulate as that to be applied to production batches and should provide product of the same quality and meeting the same specification as that intended for marketing. Two of the three batches should be at least pilot scale batches and the third one can be smaller, if justified. Where possible, batches of the drug product should be manufactured by using different batches of the drug substance.

Stability studies should be performed on each individual strength and container size of the drug product unless bracketing or matrixing is applied.

Other supporting data can be provided.

4. Container Closure System

Stability testing should be conducted on the dosage form packaged in the container closure system proposed for marketing (including, as appropriate, any secondary packaging and container label). Any available studies carried out on the drug product outside its immediate container or in other packaging materials can form a useful part of the stress testing of the dosage form or can be considered as supporting information respectively.

5. Specification

Specification, which is a list of tests, reference to analytical procedures, and proposed acceptance criteria, including the concept of different acceptance criteria for release and shelf life specifications, is addressed in ICH Q6A and Q6B. In addition, specification for degradation products in a drug product is addressed in Q3B.

Stability studies should include testing of those attributes of the drug product that are susceptible to change during storage and are likely to influence quality, safety, and/or efficacy. The testing should cover, as appropriate, the physical, chemical, biological, and microbiological attributes, preservative content (e.g., antioxidant, antimicrobial preservative), and functionality tests (e.g., for a dose delivery system). Analytical procedures should be fully validated and stability indicating. Whether and to what extent replication should be performed will depend on the results of validation studies.

Shelf life acceptance criteria should be derived from consideration of all available stability information. It may be appropriate to have justifiable differences between the shelf life and release acceptance criteria based on the stability evaluation and the changes observed on storage. Any differences between the release and shelf life acceptance criteria for antimicrobial preservative content should be supported by a validated correlation of chemical content and preservative effectiveness demonstrated during drug development on the product in its final formulation (except for preservative concentration) intended for marketing.A single primary stability batch of the drug product should be tested for antimicrobial preservative effectiveness (in addition to preservative content) at the proposed shelf life for verification purposes, regardless of whether there is a difference between the release and shelf life acceptance criteria for preservative content.

6. Testing Frequency

For long-term studies, frequency of testing should be sufficient to establish the stability profile of the drug product. For products with a proposed shelf life of at least 12 months, the frequency of testing at the long-term storage condition should normally be every 3 months over the first year, every 6 months over the second year, and annually thereafter through the proposed shelf life.

At the accelerated storage condition, a minimum of three time points, including the initial and final time points (e.g., 0, 3, and 6 months), from a 6-month study is recommended. Where an expectation (based on development experience) exists that results from accelerated testing are likely to approach significant change criteria, increased testing should be conducted either by adding samples at the final time point or by including a fourth time point in the study design.

When testing at the intermediate storage condition is called for as a result of significant change at the accelerated storage condition, a minimum of four time points, including the initial and final time points (e.g., 0, 6, 9, 12 months), from a 12-month study is recommended.

Reduced designs, that is, matrixing or bracketing, where the testing frequency is reduced or certain factor combinations are not tested at all, can be applied if justified.

7. Storage Conditions

In general, a drug product should be evaluated under storage conditions (with appropriate tolerances) that test its thermal stability and, if applicable, its sensitivity to moisture or potential for solvent loss. The storage conditions and the lengths of studies chosen should be sufficient to cover storage, shipment, and subsequent use.

Stability testing of the drug product after constitution or dilution, if applicable, should be conducted to provide information for the labeling on the preparation, storage condition, and in-use period of the constituted or diluted product. This testing should be performed on the constituted or diluted product through the proposed in-use period on primary batches as part of the formal stability studies at initial and final time points and, if full shelf life long-term data will not be available before submission, at 12 months or the last time point for which data will be available. In general, this testing need not be repeated on commitment batches.

The long-term testing should cover a minimum of 12 months' duration on at least three primary batches at the time of submission and should be continued for a period of time sufficient to cover the proposed shelf life. Additional data accumulated during the assessment period of the registration application should be submitted to the authorities if requested. Data from the accelerated storage condition and, if appropriate, from the intermediate storage condition can be used to evaluate the effect of short-term excursions outside the label storage conditions (such as might occur during shipping).

Long-term, accelerated, and, where appropriate, intermediate storage conditions for drug products are detailed in the sections below. The general case applies if the drug product is not specifically covered by a subsequent section. Alternative storage conditions can be used, if justified.

a. General Case

Study	Storage condition	Minimum time period covered by data at submission
Long term[a]	25°C ± 2°C/60% RH ± 5% RH or 30°C ± 2°C/65% RH ± 5% RH	12 mo
Intermediate[b]	30°C ± 2°C/65% RH ± 5% RH	6 mo
Accelerated	40°C ± 2°C/75% RH ± 5% RH	6 mo

[a]It is up to the applicant to decide whether long term stability studies are performed at 25 ± 2°C/60% RH ± 5% RH or 30°C ± 2°C/65% RH ± 5% RH.

[b]If 30°C ± 2°C/65% RH ± 5% RH is the long-term condition, there is no intermediate condition.

If long-term studies are conducted at 25°C ± 2°C/60% RH ± 5% RH and "significant change" occurs at any time during 6 months' testing at the accelerated storage condition, additional testing at the intermediate storage condition should be conducted and evaluated against significant change criteria. The initial application should include a minimum of 6 months' data from a 12-month study at the intermediate storage condition.

In general, "significant change" for a drug product is defined as

1. a 5% change in assay from its initial value, or failure to meet the acceptance criteria for potency when using biological or immunological procedures;

2. any degradation product's exceeding its acceptance criterion;
3. failure to meet the acceptance criteria for appearance, physical attributes, and functionality test (e.g., color, phase separation, resuspendibility, caking, hardness, dose delivery per actuation); however, some changes in physical attributes (e.g., softening of suppositories, melting of creams) may be expected under accelerated conditions; and, as appropriate for the dosage form;
4. failure to meet the acceptance criterion for pH; or
5. Failure to meet the acceptance criteria for dissolution for twelve dosage units.

b. Drug Products Packaged in Impermeable Containers

Sensitivity to moisture or potential for solvent loss is not a concern for drug products packaged in impermeable containers that provide a permanent barrier to passage of moisture or solvent. Thus, stability studies for products stored in impermeable containers can be conducted under any controlled or ambient humidity condition.

c. Drug Products Packaged in Semipermeable Containers

Aqueous-based products packaged in semipermeable containers should be evaluated for potential water loss in addition to physical, chemical, biological, and microbiological stability. This evaluation can be carried out under conditions of low relative humidity, as discussed below. Ultimately, it should be demonstrated that aqueous-based drug products stored in semipermeable containers can withstand low relative humidity environments.

Other comparable approaches can be developed and reported for nonaqueous, solvent-based products.

Study	Storage condition	Minimum time period covered by data at submission
Long term[a]	25°C ± 2°C/40% RH ± 5% RH or 30°C ± 2°C/35% RH ± 5% RH	12 mo
Intermediate[b]	30°C ± 2°C/65% RH ± 5% RH	6 mo
Accelerated	40°C ± 2°C/not more than (NMT) 25% RH	6 mo

[a]It is up to the applicant to decide whether long-term stability studies are performed at 25 ± 2°C/40% RH ± 5% RH or 30°C ± 2°C/35% RH ± 5% RH.
[b]If 30°C ± 2°C/35% RH ± 5% RH is the long-term condition, there is no intermediate condition.

For long-term studies conducted at 25°C ± 2°C/40% RH ± 5% RH, additional testing at the intermediate storage condition should be performed as described under the general case to evaluate the temperature effect at 30°C if significant change other than water loss occurs during the 6 months' testing at the accelerated storage condition.A significant change in water loss alone at the accelerated storage condition does not necessitate testing at the intermediate storage condition. However, data should be provided to demonstrate that the drug product will not have significant water loss throughout the proposed shelf life if stored at 25°C and the reference relative humidity of 40% RH.

A 5% loss in water from its initial value is considered a significant change for a product packaged in a semipermeable container after an equivalent of 3 months' storage at 40°C/NMT 25% RH. However, for small containers (1mL or less) or unit-dose products, a water loss of 5% or more after an equivalent of 3 months' storage at 40°C/NMT 25% RH may be appropriate, if justified.

An alternative approach to studying at the reference relative humidity as recommended in the table above (for either long-term or accelerated testing) is performing the stability studies under higher relative humidity and deriving the water loss at the reference relative humidity through calculation. This can be achieved by experimentally determining the permeation coefficient for the container closure system or, as shown in the example below, using the calculated ratio of water loss rates between the two humidity conditions at the same temperature. The permeation coefficient for a container closure system can be experimentally determined by using the worst-case scenario (e.g., the most diluted of a series of concentrations) for the proposed drug product.

Example of an approach for determining water loss: For a product in a given container closure system, container size, and fill, an appropriate approach for deriving the water loss rate at the reference relative humidity is to multiply the water loss rate measured at an alternative relative humidity at the same temperature by a water loss rate ratio shown in the table below.A linear water loss rate at the alternative relative humidity over the storage period should be demonstrated.

For example, at a given temperature, for example, 40°C, the calculated water loss rate during storage at NMT 25% RH is the water loss rate measured at 75% RH multiplied by 3, the corresponding water loss rate ratio.

Alternative relative humidity	Reference relative humidity	Ratio of water loss rates at a given temperature
60% RH	25% RH	1.9
60% RH	40% RH	1.5
65% RH	35% RH	1.9
75% RH	25% RH	3.0

Valid water loss rate ratios at relative humidity conditions other than those shown in the table above can also be used.

d. Drug Products Intended for Storage in a Refrigerator

Study	Storage condition	Minimum time period covered by data at submission
Long term	5°C ± 3°C	12 mo
Accelerated	25°C ± 2°C/60% RH ± 5% RH	6 mo

If the drug product is packaged in a semipermeable container, appropriate information should be provided to assess the extent of water loss.

Data from refrigerated storage should be assessed according to the evaluation section of this guideline, except where explicitly noted below.

If significant change occurs between 3 and 6 months' testing at the accelerated storage condition, the proposed shelf life should be based on the real-time data available from the long-term storage condition.

If significant change occurs within the first 3 months' testing at the accelerated storage condition, a discussion should be provided to address the effect of short-term excursions outside the label storage condition, for example, during shipment and handling. This discussion can be supported, if appropriate, by further testing on a single batch of the drug product for a period less than 3 months but with more frequent testing than usual. It is considered unnecessary to continue to test a product through 6 months when a significant change has occurred within the first 3 months.

e. Drug Products Intended for Storage in a Freezer

Study	Storage condition	Minimum time period covered by data at submission
Long term	−20°C ± 5°C	12 mo

For drug products intended for storage in a freezer, the shelf life should be based on the real-time data obtained at the long-term storage condition. In the absence of an accelerated storage condition for drug products intended to be stored in a freezer, testing on a single batch at an elevated temperature (e.g., 5°C ± 3°C or 25°C ± 2°C) for an appropriate time period should be conducted to address the effect of short-term excursions outside the proposed label storage condition.

f. Drug Products Intended for Storage Below −20°C

Drug products intended for storage below −20°C should be treated on a case-by-case basis.

8. Stability Commitment

When available, long-term stability data on primary batches do not cover the proposed shelf life granted at the time of approval; a commitment should be made to continue the stability studies post approval to firmly establish the shelf life.

Where the submission includes long-term stability data from three production batches covering the proposed shelf life, a postapproval commitment is considered unnecessary. Otherwise, one of the following commitments should be made.

1. If the submission includes data from stability studies on at least three production batches, a commitment should be made to continue the long-term studies through the proposed shelf life and the accelerated studies for 6 months.
2. If the submission includes data from stability studies on fewer than three production batches, a commitment should be made to continue the long-term studies through the proposed shelf life and the accelerated studies for 6 months, and to place additional production batches, to a total of at least three, on long-term stability studies through the proposed shelf life and on accelerated studies for 6 months.
3. If the submission does not include stability data on production batches, a commitment should be made to place the first three production batches on long-term stability studies through the proposed shelf life and on accelerated studies for 6 months.

The stability protocol used for studies on commitment batches should be the same as that for the primary batches, unless otherwise scientifically justified.

Where intermediate testing is called for by a significant change at the accelerated storage condition for the primary batches, testing on the commitment batches can be conducted at either the intermediate or the accelerated storage condition. However, if significant change occurs at the accelerated storage condition on the commitment batches, testing at the intermediate storage condition should also be conducted.

9. Evaluation

A systematic approach should be adopted in the presentation and evaluation of the stability information, which should include, as appropriate, results from the physical, chemical, biological, and microbiological tests, including particular attributes of the dosage form (e.g., dissolution rate for solid oral dosage forms).

The purpose of the stability study is to establish, based on testing a minimum of three batches of the drug product, shelf life and label storage instructions applicable to all future batches of the drug product manufactured and packaged under similar circumstances. The degree of variability of individual batches affects the confidence that a future production batch will remain within specification throughout its shelf life.

Where the data show so little degradation and so little variability that it is apparent from looking at the data that the requested shelf life will be granted, it is normally unnecessary to go through the formal statistical analysis; providing a justification for the omission should be sufficient.

An approach for analyzing data of a quantitative attribute that is expected to change with time is to determine the time at which the 95% one-sided confidence limit for the mean curve intersects the acceptance criterion. If analysis shows that the batch-to-batch variability is small, it is advantageous to combine the data into one overall estimate. This can be done by first applying appropriate statistical tests (e.g., p values for level of significance of rejection of more than 0.25) to the slopes of the regression lines and zero time intercepts for the individual batches. If it is inappropriate to combine data from several batches, the overall shelf life should be based on the minimum time a batch can be expected to remain within acceptance criteria.

The nature of the degradation relationship will determine whether the data should be transformed for linear regression analysis. Usually the relationship can be represented by a linear, quadratic, or cubic function on an arithmetic or logarithmic scale. Statistical methods should be employed to test the goodness of fit on all batches and combined batches (where appropriate) to the assumed degradation line or curve.

Limited extrapolation of the real-time data from the long-term storage condition beyond the observed range to extend the shelf life can be undertaken at approval time, if justified. This justification should be based on what is known about the mechanisms of degradation, the results of testing under accelerated conditions, the goodness of fit of any mathematical model, batch size, existence of supporting stability data, etc. However, this extrapolation assumes that the same degradation relationship will continue to apply beyond the observed data.

Any evaluation should consider not only the assay but also the degradation products and other appropriate attributes. Where appropriate, attention should be paid to reviewing the adequacy of the mass balance and different stability and degradation performance.

10. Statements/Labeling

A storage statement should be established for the labeling in accordance with relevant national/regional requirements. The statement should be based on the stability evaluation of the drug product. Where applicable, specific instruction should be provided, particularly for drug products that cannot tolerate freezing. Terms such as "ambient conditions" or "room temperature" should be avoided.

There should be a direct link between the label storage statement and the demonstrated stability of the drug product. An expiration date should be displayed on the container label.

GLOSSARY

The following definitions are provided to facilitate interpretation of the guideline.

Accelerated testing—Studies designed to increase the rate of chemical degradation or physical change of a drug substance or drug product by using exaggerated storage conditions as part of the formal stability studies. Data from these studies, in addition to long-term stability studies, can be used to assess longer-term chemical effects at nonaccelerated conditions and to evaluate the effect of short-term excursions outside the label storage conditions such as might occur during shipping. Results from accelerated testing studies are not always predictive of physical changes.

Bracketing—The design of a stability schedule such that only samples on the extremes of certain design factors, for example, strength, package size, are tested at all time points as in a full design. The design assumes that the stability of any intermediate level is represented by the stability of the extremes tested. Where a range of strengths is to be tested, bracketing is applicable if the strengths are identical or closely related in composition (e.g., for a tablet range made with different compression weights of a similar basic granulation, or a capsule range made by filling different plug fill weights of the same basic composition into different size capsule shells). Bracketing can be applied to different container sizes or different fills in the same container closure system.

Climatic zones—The four zones in the world that are distinguished by their characteristic prevalent annual climatic conditions. This is based on the concept described by W. Grimm (*Drugs Made in Germany*, 28:196–202, 1985 and 29:39–47, 1986).

Commitment batches—Production batches of a drug substance or drug product for which the stability studies are initiated or completed post approval through a commitment made in the registration application.

Container closure system—The sum of packaging components that together contain and protect the dosage form. This includes primary packaging components and secondary packaging components, if the latter are intended to provide additional protection to the drug product.A packaging system is equivalent to a container closure system.

Dosage form—A pharmaceutical product type (e.g., tablet, capsule, solution, cream) that contains a drug substance generally, but not necessarily, in association with excipients.

Drug product—The dosage form in the final immediate packaging intended for marketing.

Drug substance—The unformulated drug substance that may subsequently be formulated with excipients to produce the dosage form.

Excipient—Anything other than the drug substance in the dosage form.

Expiration date—The date placed on the container label of a drug product designating the time prior to which a batch of the product is expected to remain within the approved shelf life specification if stored under defined conditions, and after which it must not be used.

Formal stability studies—Long-term and accelerated (and intermediate) studies undertaken on primary and/or commitment batches according to a prescribed stability protocol to establish or confirm the retest period of a drug substance or the shelf life of a drug product.

Impermeable containers—Containers that provide a permanent barrier to the passage of gases or solvents, for example, sealed aluminum tubes for semisolids, sealed glass ampoules for solutions.

Intermediate testing—Studies conducted at 30°C/65% RH and designed to moderately increase the rate of chemical degradation or physical changes for a drug substance or drug product intended to be stored long term at 25°C.

Long-term testing—Stability studies under the recommended storage condition for the retest period or shelf life proposed (or approved) for labeling.

Mass balance—The process of adding together the assay value and levels of degradation products to see how closely these add up to 100% of the initial value, with due consideration of the margin of analytical error.

Matrixing—The design of a stability schedule such that a selected subset of the total number of possible samples for all factor combinations is tested at a specified time point. At a subsequent time point, another subset of samples for all factor combinations is tested. The design assumes that the stability of each subset of samples tested represents the stability of all samples at a given time point. The differences in the samples for the same drug product should be identified as, for example, covering different batches, different strengths, different sizes of the same container closure system, and, possibly in some cases, different container closure systems.

Mean kinetic temperature—A single derived temperature that, if maintained over a defined period of time, affords the same thermal challenge to a drug substance or drug product as would be experienced over a range of both higher and lower temperatures for an equivalent defined period. The mean kinetic temperature is higher than the arithmetic mean temperature and takes into account the Arrhenius equation.

When establishing the mean kinetic temperature for a defined period, the formula of J. D. Haynes (*J. Pharm. Sci.*, 60:927–929, 1971) can be used.

New molecular entity—An active pharmaceutical substance not previously contained in any drug product registered with the national or regional authority concerned.A new salt, ester, or non–covalent-bond derivative of an approved drug substance is considered a new molecular entity for the purpose of stability testing under this guidance.

Pilot scale batch—A batch of a drug substance or drug product manufactured by a procedure fully representative of and simulating that to be applied to a full production scale batch. For solid oral dosage forms, a pilot scale is generally, at a minimum, one-tenth that of a full production scale or 100000 tablets or capsules, whichever is the larger.

Primary batch—A batch of a drug substance or drug product used in a formal stability study, from which stability data are submitted in a registration application for the purpose of establishing a retest period or shelf life respectively.A primary batch of a drug substance should be at least a pilot scale batch. For a drug product, two of the three batches should be at least pilot scale batch, and the third batch can be smaller if it is representative with regard to the critical manufacturing steps. However, a primary batch may be a production batch.

Production batch—A batch of a drug substance or drug product manufactured at production scale by using production equipment in a production facility as specified in the application.

Retest date—The date after which samples of the drug substance should be examined to ensure that the material is still in compliance with the specification and thus suitable for use in the manufacture of a given drug product.

Retest period—The period of time during which the drug substance is expected to remain within its specification and, therefore, can be used in the manufacture of a given drug product, provided that the drug substance has been stored under the defined conditions. After this period, a batch of drug substance destined for use in the manufacture of a drug product should be retested for compliance with the specification and then used immediately.A batch of drug substance can be retested multiple times and a different portion of the batch used after each retest, as long as it continues to comply with the specification. For most biotechnological/biological substances known to be labile, it is more appropriate to establish a shelf life than a retest period. The same may be true for certain antibiotics.

Semipermeable containers—Containers that allow the passage of solvent, usually water, while preventing solute loss. The mechanism for solvent transport occurs by absorption into one container surface, diffusion through the bulk of the container material, and desorption from the other surface. Transport is driven by a partial-pressure gradient. Examples of semipermeable containers include plastic bags and semirigid, low-density polyethylene (LDPE) pouches for large-volume parenterals (LVPs), and LDPE ampoules, bottles, and vials.

Shelf life (also referred to as expiration dating period)—The time period during which a drug product is expected to remain within the approved shelf life specification, provided that it is stored under the conditions defined on the container label.

Specification—See Q6A and Q6B.

Specification Release—The combination of physical, chemical, biological, and microbiological tests and acceptance criteria that determine the suitability of a drug product at the time of its release.

Specification—Shelf life—The combination of physical, chemical, biological, and microbiological tests and acceptance criteria that determine the suitability of a drug substance throughout its retest period, or that a drug product should meet throughout its shelf life.

Storage condition tolerances—The acceptable variations in temperature and relative humidity of storage facilities for formal stability studies. The equipment should be capable of controlling the storage condition within the ranges defined in this guideline. The actual temperature and humidity (when controlled) should be monitored during stability storage. Short-term spikes caused by opening of doors of the storage facility are accepted as unavoidable. The effect of excursions owing to equipment failure should be addressed, and reported if judged to affect stability results. Excursions that exceed the defined tolerances for more than 24 hours should be described in the study report and their effect assessed.

Stress testing (drug substance)—Studies undertaken to elucidate the intrinsic stability of the drug substance. Such testing is part of the development strategy and is normally carried out under more severe conditions than those used for accelerated testing.

Stress testing (drug product)—Studies undertaken to assess the effect of severe conditions on the drug product. Such studies include photostability testing (see ICH Q1B) and specific testing on certain products, (e.g., metered dose inhalers, creams, emulsions, refrigerated aqueous liquid products).

Supporting data—Data, other than those from formal stability studies, that support the analytical procedures, the proposed retest period or shelf life, and the label storage statements. Such data include (1) stability data on early synthetic route batches of drug substance, small-scale batches of materials, investigational formulations not proposed for marketing, related formulations, and product presented in containers and closures other than those proposed for marketing, (2) information regarding test results on containers, and (3) other scientific rationales.

REFERENCES

Grimm W (1985). Storage Conditions for stability testing—long term testing and stress tests. Drugs Made Germany 28: 196–202; (Part I) and 29: 39–47, 1986 (Part II).

Haynes JD (1971). Worldwide virtual temperature for product stability testing. Pharm Sci 60: 927–929.

ICH Q1B: *Stability Testing: Photostability Testing of New Drug Substances and Products*

ICH Q1C: *Stability Testing of New Dosage Forms*

ICH Q3A: *Impurities in New Drug Substances*

ICH Q3B: *Impurities in New Drug Products*

ICH Q5C: *Quality of Biotechnological Products: Stability Testing of Biotechnological/Biological Products*

ICH Q6A: *Specifications: Test Procedures and Acceptance Criteria for New Drug Substances and New Drug Products: Chemical Substances (Including Decision Trees)*

ICH Q6B: *Specifications: Test Procedures and Acceptance Criteria for Biotechnological/Biological Products*

9

Stability Testing: Photostability Testing of New Drug Substances and Products

I. GENERAL

The ICH Harmonized Tripartite Guideline covering the Stability Testing of New Drug Substances and Products notes that light testing should be an integral part of stress testing.

A. Preamble

The intrinsic photostability characteristics of new drug substances and products should be evaluated to demonstrate that, as appropriate, light exposure does not result in unacceptable change. Normally, photostability testing is carried out on a single batch of material selected as described under Selection of Batches in the Parent Guideline. Under some circumstances these studies should be repeated if certain variations and changes are made to the product (e.g., formulation, packaging). Whether these studies should be repeated depends on the photostability characteristics determined at the time of initial filing and the type of variation and/or change made.

The guideline primarily addresses the generation of photostability information for submission in Registration Applications for new molecular entities and associated drug products. The guideline does not cover the photostability of drugs after administration (i.e., under conditions of use) and those applications not covered by the Parent Guideline. Alternative approaches may be used if they are scientifically sound and justification is provided.

A systematic approach to photostability testing is recommended covering, as appropriate, studies such as:

i. Tests on the drug substance;
ii. Tests on the exposed drug product outside of the immediate pack; and if necessary;
iii. Tests on the drug product in the immediate pack; and if necessary;
iv. Tests on the drug product in the marketing pack.

B. Light Sources

The light sources described below may be used for photostability testing. The applicant should either maintain an appropriate control of temperature to minimize the effect of localized temperature changes or include a dark control in the same environment unless otherwise justified. For both options 1 and 2, a pharmaceutical manufacturer/applicant may rely on the spectral distribution specification of the light source manufacturer.

Option 1

Any light source that is designed to produce an output similar to the D65/ID65 emission standard such as an artificial daylight fluorescent lamp combining visible and ultraviolet (UV) outputs, xenon, or metal halide lamp. D65 is the internationally recognized standard for outdoor daylight as defined in ISO 10977 (1993). ID65 is the equivalent indoor indirect daylight standard. For a light source emitting significant radiation below 320 nm, an appropriate filter(s) may be fitted to eliminate such radiation.

Option 2

For option 2 the same sample should be exposed to both the cool white fluorescent and near UV lamp.

1. A cool white fluorescent lamp designed to produce an output similar to that specified in ISO 10977(1993); and
2. A near UV fluorescent lamp having a spectral distribution from 320 nm to 400 nm with a maximum energy emission between 350 nm and 370 nm; a significant proportion of UV should be in both bands of 320 to 360 nm and 360 to 400 nm.

C. Procedure

For confirmatory studies, samples should be exposed to light providing an overall illumination of not less than 1.2 million lux hours and an integrated near UV energy of not less than 200 W hr/m^2 to allow direct comparisons to be made between the drug substance and drug product.

Samples may be exposed side-by-side with a validated chemical actinometric system to ensure the specified light exposure is obtained, or for the appropriate duration of time when conditions have been monitored using calibrated radiometers/lux meters. An example of an actinometric procedure is provided in the Annex.

If protected samples (e.g., wrapped in aluminum foil) are used as dark controls to evaluate the contribution of thermally induced change to the total observed change, these should be placed alongside the authentic sample.

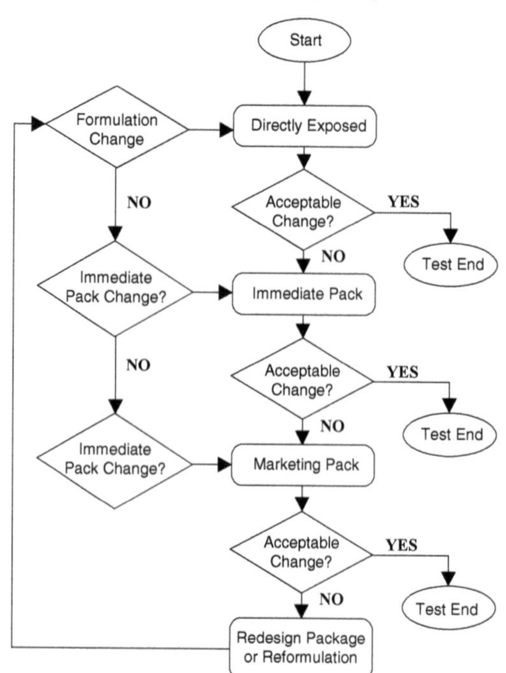

II. DRUG SUBSTANCE

For drug substances, photostability testing should consist of two parts: forced degradation testing and confirmatory testing.

The purpose of forced degradation testing studies is to evaluate the overall photosensitivity of the material for method development purposes and/or degradation pathway elucidation. This testing may involve the drug substance alone and/or in simple solutions/suspensions to validate the analytical procedures. In these studies, the samples should be in chemically inert and transparent containers. In these forced degradation studies, a variety of exposure conditions may be used, depending on the photosensitivity of the drug substance involved and the intensity of the light sources used. For development and validation purposes, it is appropriate to limit exposure and end the studies if extensive decomposition occurs. For photostable materials, studies may be terminated after an appropriate exposure level has been used. The design of these experiments is left to the applicant's discretion although the exposure levels used should be justified.

Under forcing conditions, decomposition products may be observed that are unlikely to be formed under the conditions used for confirmatory studies. This information may be useful in developing and validating suitable analytical methods. If in practice it has been demonstrated that they are not formed in the confirmatory studies, these degradation products need not be further examined.

Confirmatory studies should then be undertaken to provide the information necessary for handling, packaging, and labeling (see section I.C., Procedure, and II. A., Presentation, for information on the design of these studies).

Normally, only one batch of drug substance is tested during the development phase, and then the photostability characteristics should be confirmed on a single batch selected as described in the Parent Guideline if the drug is clearly photostable or photolabile. If the results of the confirmatory study are equivocal, testing of up to two additional batches should be conducted. Samples should be selected as described in the Parent Guideline.

A. Presentation of Samples

Care should be taken to ensure that the physical characteristics of the samples under test are taken into account and efforts should be made, such as cooling and/or placing the samples in sealed containers, to ensure that the effects of the changes in physical states such as sublimation, evaporation or melting are minimized. All such precautions should be chosen to provide minimal interference with the exposure of samples under test. Possible interactions between the samples and any material used for containers or for general protection of the sample should also be considered and eliminated wherever not relevant to the test being carried out.

As a direct challenge for samples of solid drug substances, an appropriate amount of sample should be taken and placed in a suitable glass or plastic dish and protected with a suitable transparent cover if considered necessary. Solid drug substances should be spread across the container to give a thickness of typically not more than 3 mL. Drug substances that are liquids should be exposed in chemically inert and transparent containers.

B. Analysis of Samples

At the end of the exposure period, the samples should be examined for any changes in physical properties (e.g., appearance, clarity, or color of solution) and for assay and degradants by a method suitably validated for products likely to arise from photochemical degradation processes.

Where solid drug substance samples are involved, sampling should ensure that a representative portion is used in individual tests. Similar sampling considerations, such as homogenization of the entire sample, apply to other materials that may not be homogeneous after exposure. The analysis of the exposed sample should be performed concomitantly with that of any protected samples used as dark controls if these are used in the test.

C. Judgement of Results

The forced degradation studies should be designed to provide suitable information to develop and validate test methods for the confirmatory studies. These test methods should be capable of resolving and detecting photolytic degradants that appear during the confirmatory studies. When evaluating the results of these studies, it is important to recognize that they form part of the stress testing and are not therefore designed to establish qualitative or quantitative limits for change.

The confirmatory studies should identify precautionary measures needed in manufacturing or in formulation of the drug product, and if light resistant packaging is needed. When evaluating the results of confirmatory studies to determine whether change due to exposure to light is acceptable, it is important to consider the results from other formal stability studies in order to assure that the drug will be within justified limits at time of use (see the relevant ICH Stability and Impurity Guidelines).

III. DRUG PRODUCT

Normally, the studies on drug products should be carried out in a sequential manner starting with testing the fully exposed product then progressing as necessary to the product in the immediate pack and then in the marketing pack. Testing should progress until the results demonstrate that the drug product is adequately protected from exposure to light. The drug product should be exposed to the light conditions described under the procedure in section I.C.

Normally, only one batch of drug product is tested during the development phase, and then the photostability characteristics should be confirmed on a single batch selected as described in the Parent Guideline if the product is clearly photostable or photolabile. If the results of the confirmatory study are equivocal, testing of up to two additional batches should be conducted.

For some products where it has been demonstrated that the immediate pack is completely impenetrable to light, such as aluminum tubes or cans, testing should normally only be conducted on directly exposed drug product.

It may be appropriate to test certain products such as infusion liquids, dermal creams, etc., to support their photostability in-use. The extent of this testing should depend on and relate to the directions for use, and is left to the applicant's discretion.

The analytical procedures used should be suitably validated.

A. Presentation of Samples

Care should be taken to ensure that the physical characteristics of the samples under test are taken into account and efforts, such as cooling and/or placing the samples in sealed containers, should be made to ensure that the effects of the changes in physical states are minimized, such as sublimation, evaporation, or melting. All such precautions should be chosen to provide a minimal interference with the irradiation of samples under test. Possible interactions between the samples and any material used for containers or for general protection of the sample should also be considered and eliminated wherever not relevant to the test being carried out.

Where practicable when testing samples of the drug product outside of the primary pack, these should be presented in a way similar to the conditions mentioned for the drug substance. The samples should be positioned to provide maximum area of exposure to the light source. For example, tablets, capsules, etc., should be spread in a single layer.

If direct exposure is not practical (e.g., due to oxidation of a product), the sample should be placed in a suitable protective inert transparent container (e.g., quartz).

If testing of the drug product in the immediate container or as marketed is needed, the samples should be placed horizontally or transversely with respect to the light source, whichever provides for the most uniform exposure of the samples. Some adjustment of testing conditions may have to be made when testing large volume containers (e.g., dispensing packs).

B. Analysis of Samples

At the end of the exposure period, the samples should be examined for any changes in physical properties (e.g., appearance, clarity or color of solution, dissolution/disintegration for dosage forms such as capsules, etc.) and for assay and degradants by a method suitably validated for products likely to arise from photochemical degradation processes.

When powder samples are involved, sampling should ensure that a representative portion is used in individual tests. For solid oral dosage form products, testing should be conducted on an appropriately sized composite of, for example, 20 tablets or capsules. Similar sampling considerations, such as homogenization or solubilization of the entire sample, apply to other materials that may not be homogeneous after exposure (e.g., creams, ointments, suspensions, etc.). The analysis of the exposed sample should be performed concomitantly with that of any protected samples used as dark controls if these are used in the test.

C. Judgement of Results

Depending on the extent of change special labeling or packaging may be needed to mitigate exposure to light. When evaluating the results of photostability studies to determine whether change due to exposure to light is acceptable, it is important to consider the results obtained from other formal stability studies in order to assure that the product will be within proposed specifications during the shelf life (see the relevant ICH Stability and Impurity Guidelines).

IV. ANNEX

A. Quinine Chemical Actinometry

The following provides details of an actinometric procedure for monitoring exposure to a near UV fluorescent lamp (based on FDA/National Institute of Standards and Technology study). For other light sources/actinometric systems, the same approach may be used, but each actinometric system should be calibrated for the light source used.

Prepare a sufficient quantity of a 2% weight/volume aqueous solution of quinine monohydrochloride dihydrate (if necessary, dissolve by heating).

Option 1

Put 10 mL of the solution into a 20 mL colorless ampoule seal it hermetically, and use this as the sample. Separately, put 10 mL of the solution into a 20 mL colorless ampoule (see note 1), seal it hermetically, wrap in aluminum foil to protect completely from light, and use this as the control. Expose the sample and control to the light source for an appropriate number of hours. After exposure determine the absorbances of the sample (AT) and the control (Ao) at 400 nm using a 1 cm path length. Calculate the change in absorbance, $\Delta A = AT - Ao$. The length of exposure should be sufficient to ensure a change in absorbance of at least 0.9.

Option 2

Fill a 1 cm quartz cell and use this as the sample. Separately fill a 1 cm quartz cell, wrap in aluminum foil to protect completely from light, and use this as the control. Expose the sample and control to the light source for an appropriate number of hours. After exposure determine the absorbances of the sample (AT) and the control (Ao) at 400 nm. Calculate the change in absorbance, $\Delta A = AT - Ao$. The length of exposure should be sufficient to ensure a change in absorbance of at least 0.5.

Alternative packaging configurations may be used if appropriately validated. Alternative validated chemical actinometers may be used.

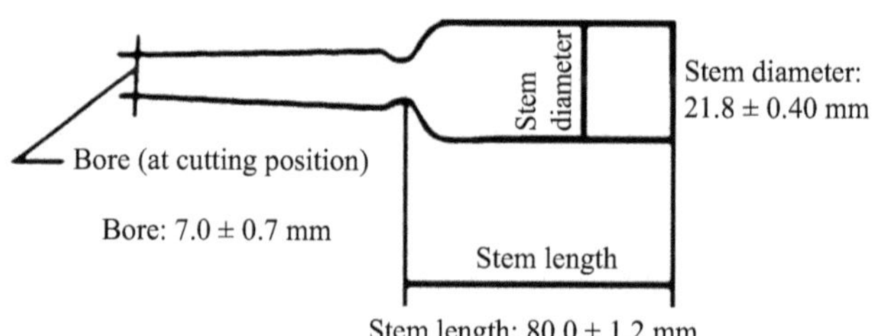

Note 1: Shape and Dimensions (See Japanese Industry Standard (JIS) R3512 (1974) for ampoule specifications).

10

Stability Testing for New Dosage Forms

I. GENERAL

This document discusses stability guideline and addresses the recommendations on what should be submitted regarding stability of new dosage forms by the owner of the original application, after the original submission for new drug substances and products.

II. NEW DOSAGE FORMS

A new dosage form is defined as a drug product, which is a different pharmaceutical product type, but contains the same active substance as included in the existing drug product approved by the pertinent regulatory authority.

Such pharmaceutical product types include products of different administration route (e.g., oral to parenteral), new specific functionality/delivery systems (e.g., immediate-release tablet to modified-release tablet), and different dosage forms of the same administration route (e.g., capsule to tablet, solution to suspension).

Stability protocols for new dosage forms should follow the guidance in the parent stability guideline in principle. However, a reduced stability database at submission time (e.g., 6 months accelerated and 6 months long-term data from ongoing studies) may be acceptable in certain justified cases.

GLOSSARY

Immediate (primary) pack is that constituent of the packaging that is in direct contact with the drug substance or drug product, and includes any appropriate label.

Marketing pack is the combination of immediate pack and other secondary packaging such as a carton.

Forced degradation testing studies are those undertaken to degrade the sample deliberately. These studies, which may be undertaken in the development phase normally on the drug substances, are used to evaluate the overall photosensitivity of the material for method development purposes and/or degradation pathway elucidation.

Confirmatory studies are those undertaken to establish photostability characteristics under standardized conditions. These studies are used to identify precautionary measures needed in manufacturing or formulation and whether light resistant packaging and/or special labeling is needed to mitigate exposure to light. For the confirmatory studies, the batches should be selected according to batch selection for long-term and accelerated testings, which is described in the Parent Guideline.

BIBLIOGRAPHY

Yoshioka S, Ishihara Y, Terazono T, et al. (1994). Quinine actinometry as a method for calibrating ultraviolet radiation intensity in light-stability testing of pharmaceuticals. Drug Dev Ind Pharm 20(13):2049–2062.

11

Bracketing and Matrixing Designs for Stability Testing of New Drug Substances and Products

I. INTRODUCTION

A. Objectives of the Guideline

This guideline is intended to address recommendations on the application of bracketing and matrixing to stability studies conducted in accordance with principles outlined in the ICH Q1A(R) Harmonised Tripartite guideline on Stability Testing of New Drug Substances and Products (hereafter referred to as the parent guideline).

B. Background

The parent guideline notes that the use of matrixing and bracketing can be applied, if justified, to the testing of new drug substances and products, but provides no further guidance on the subject.

C. Scope of the Guideline

This document provides guidance on bracketing and matrixing study designs. Specific principles are defined in this guideline for situations in which bracketing or matrixing can be applied. Sample designs are provided for illustrative purposes, and should not be considered the only, or the most appropriate, designs in all cases.

II. GUIDELINES

A. General

A full study design is one in which samples for every combination of all design factors are tested at all time points. A reduced design is one in which samples for every factor combination are not all tested at all time points. A reduced design can be a suitable alternative to a full design when multiple design factors are involved. Any reduced design should have the ability to adequately predict the retest period or shelf life. Before a reduced design is considered, certain assumptions should be assessed and justified. The potential risk should be considered of establishing a shorter retest period or shelf life than could be derived from a full design due to the reduced amount of data collected.

During the course of a reduced design study, a change to full testing or to a less reduced design can be considered if a justification is provided and the principles of full designs and reduced designs are followed. However, proper adjustments should be made to the statistical analysis, where applicable, to account for the increase in sample size as a result of the change. Once the design is changed, full testing or less reduced testing should be carried out through the remaining time points of the stability study.

B. Applicability of Reduced Designs

Reduced designs can be applied to the formal stability study of most types of drug products, although additional justification should be provided for certain complex drug delivery systems where there are a large number of potential drug-device interactions. For the study of drug substances, matrixing is of limited utility and bracketing is generally not applicable.

Whether bracketing or matrixing can be applied depends on the circumstances, as discussed in detail below. The use of any reduced design should be justified. In certain cases, the condition described in this guideline is sufficient justification for use, while in other cases, additional justification should be provided. The type and level of justification in each of these cases will depend on the available supporting data. Data variability and product stability, as shown by supporting data, should be considered when a matrixing design is applied.

Bracketing and matrixing are reduced designs based on different principles. Therefore, careful consideration and scientific justification should precede the use of bracketing and matrixing together in one design.

C. Bracketing

As defined in the glossary to the parent guideline, bracketing is the design of a stability schedule such that only samples on the extremes of certain design factors (e.g., strength, container size, and/or fill) are tested at all time points as in a full design. The design assumes that the stability of any intermediate levels is represented by the stability of the extremes tested.

The use of a bracketing design would not be considered appropriate if it cannot be demonstrated that the strengths or container sizes and/or fills selected for testing are indeed the extremes.

1. Design Factors

Design factors are variables (e.g., strength, container size, and/or fill) to be evaluated in a study design for their effect on product stability.

a. Strength

Bracketing can be applied to studies with multiple strengths of identical or closely related formulations. Examples include but are not limited to (1) capsules of different strengths made with different fill plug sizes from the same powder blend, (2) tablets of different strengths manufactured by compressing varying amounts of the same granulation, and (3) oral solutions of different strengths with formulations that differ only in minor excipients (e.g., colorants, flavorings).

With justification, bracketing can be applied to studies with multiple strengths where the relative amounts of drug substance and excipients change in a formulation. Such justification can include a demonstration of comparable stability profiles among the different strengths of clinical or development batches.

In cases where different excipients are used among strengths, bracketing generally should not be applied.

Table 11.1 Example of a Bracketing Design

Strength		50 mg			75 mg			100 mg		
Batch		1	2	3	1	2	3	1	2	3
Container size	15 mL	T	T	T				T	T	T
	100 mL									
	500 mL	T	T	T				T	T	T

Key: T = Sample tested.

b. Container Closure Sizes and/or Fills

Bracketing can be applied to studies of the same container closure system where either container size or fill varies while the other remains constant. However, if a bracketing design is considered where both container size and fill vary, it should not be assumed that the largest and smallest containers represent the extremes of all packaging configurations. Care should be taken to select the extremes by comparing the various characteristics of the container closure system that may affect product stability. These characteristics include container wall thickness, closure geometry, surface area to volume ratio, headspace to volume ratio, water vapor permeation rate or oxygen permeation rate per dosage unit or unit fill volume, as appropriate.

With justification, bracketing can be applied to studies for the same container when the closure varies. Justification could include a discussion of the relative permeation rates of the bracketed container closure systems.

2. Design Considerations and Potential Risks

If, after starting the studies, one of the extremes is no longer expected to be marketed, the study design can be maintained to support the bracketed intermediates. A commitment should be provided to carry out stability studies on the marketed extremes postapproval.

Before a bracketing design is applied, its effect on the retest period or shelf life estimation should be assessed. If the stability of the extremes is shown to be different, the intermediates should be considered no more stable than the least stable extreme (i.e., the shelf life for the intermediates should not exceed that for the least stable extreme).

3. Design Example

An example of a bracketing design is given in Table 11.1. This example is based on a product available in three strengths and three container sizes. In this example, it should be demonstrated that the 15 and 500 mL high-density polyethylene container sizes truly represent the extremes. The batches for each selected combination should be tested at each time point as in a full design.

D. Matrixing

As defined in the glossary of the parent guideline, matrixing is the design of a stability schedule such that a selected subset of the total number of possible samples for all factor combinations would be tested at a specified time point. At a subsequent time point, another subset of samples for all factor combinations would be tested. The design assumes that the stability of each subset of samples tested represents the stability of all samples at a given time point. The differences in the samples for the same drug product should be identified as, for example, covering different batches, different strengths, different sizes of the same container closure system, and possibly, in some cases, different container closure systems.

When a secondary packaging system contributes to the stability of the drug product, matrixing can be performed across the packaging systems.

Each storage condition should be treated separately under its own matrixing design. Matrixing should not be performed across test attributes. However, alternative matrixing designs for different test attributes can be applied if justified.

1. Design Factors

Matrixing designs can be applied to strengths with identical or closely related formulations. Examples include but are not limited to (1) capsules of different strengths made with different fill plug sizes from the same powder blend, (2) tablets of different strengths manufactured by compressing varying amounts of the same granulation, and (3) oral solutions of different strengths with formulations that differ only in minor excipients (e.g., colorants or flavorings).

Other examples of design factors that can be matrixed include batches made by using the same process and equipment, and container sizes and/or fills in the same container closure system.

With justification, matrixing designs can be applied, for example, to different strengths where the relative amounts of drug substance and excipients change or where different excipients are used or to different container closure systems. Justification should generally be based on supporting data. For example, to matrix across two different closures or container closure systems, supporting data could be supplied showing relative moisture vapor transmission rates or similar protection against light. Alternatively, supporting data could be supplied to show that the drug product is not affected by oxygen, moisture, or light.

2. Design Considerations

A matrixing design should be balanced as far as possible so that each combination of factors is tested to the same extent over the intended duration of the study and through the last time point prior to submission. However, due to the recommended full testing at certain time points, as discussed below, it may be difficult to achieve a complete balance in a design where time points are matrixed.

In a design where time points are matrixed, all selected factor combinations should be tested at the initial and final time points, while only certain fractions of the designated combinations should be tested at each intermediate time point. If full long-term data for the proposed shelf life will not be available for review before approval, all selected combinations of batch, strength, container size, and fill, among other things, should also be tested at 12 months or at the last time point prior to submission. In addition, data from at least three time points, including initial, should be available for each selected combination through the first 12 months of the study. For matrixing at an accelerated or intermediate storage condition, care should be taken to ensure testing occurs at a minimum of three time points, including initial and final, for each selected combination of factors.

When a matrix on design factors is applied, if one strength or container size and/or fill is no longer intended for marketing, stability testing of that strength or container size and/or fill can be continued to support the other strengths or container sizes and/or fills in the design.

3. Design Examples

Examples of matrixing designs on time points for a product in two strengths (S1 and S2) are shown in Table 11.2. The terms "one-half reduction" and "one-third reduction" refer to the

Table 11.2 Examples of Matrixing Designs on Time Points for a Product with Two Strengths

Time Point (Months)			0	3	6	9	12	18	24	36
One-half reduction										
	S1	Batch 1	T	T		T	T		T	T
		Batch 2	T	T		T	T	T		T
		Batch 3	T		T		T	T		T
Strength	S2	Batch 1	T		T		T		T	T
		Batch 2	T	T		T	T	T		T
		Batch 3	T		T		T		T	T
One-third reduction										
	S1	Batch 1	T	T		T	T		T	T
		Batch 2	T	T	T		T	T		T
		Batch 3	T		T	T	T	T	T	T
Strength	S2	Batch 1	T		T	T	T	T	T	T
		Batch 2	T	T		T	T		T	T
		Batch 3	T	T	T		T	T		T

Key: T = Sample tested.

reduction strategy initially applied to the full study design. For example, a "one-half reduction" initially eliminates one in every two time points from the full study design and a "one-third reduction" initially removes one in every three. In the examples shown in Table 11.2, the reductions are less than one-half and one-third due to the inclusion of full testing of all factor combinations at some time points as discussed in section 2.4.2. These examples include full testing at the initial, final, and 12-month time points. The ultimate reduction is therefore less than one-half (24/48) or one-third (16/48), and is actually 15/48 or 10/48, respectively.

Additional examples of matrixing designs for a product with three strengths and three container sizes are given in Table 11.3. Table 11.3(A) shows a design with matrixing on time points only and Table 11.3(B) depicts a design with matrixing on time points and factors. In Table 11.3(A), all combinations of batch, strength, and container size are tested, while in Table 11.3(B), certain combinations of batch, strength, and container size are not tested.

4. Applicability and Degree of Reduction

The following, although not an exhaustive list, should be considered when a matrixing design is contemplated:

- Knowledge of data variability
- Expected stability of the product
- Availability of supporting data
- Stability differences in the product within a factor or among factors

and/or

- Number of factor combinations in the study

In general, a matrixing design is applicable if the supporting data indicate predictable product stability. Matrixing is appropriate when the supporting data exhibit only small variability. However, where the supporting data exhibit moderate variability, a matrixing design should be statistically justified. If the supportive data show large variability, a matrixing design should not be applied.

Table 11.3 Examples of Matrixing Designs for a Product with Three Strengths and Three Container Sizes

Strength		S1			S2			S3	
A. Matrixing on time points									
Container size	A	B	C	A	B	C	A	B	C
Batch 1	T1	T2	T3	T2	T3	T1	T3	T1	T2
Batch 2	T2	T3	T1	T3	T1	T2	T1	T2	T3
Batch 3	T3	T1	T2	T1	T2	T3	T2	T3	T1
B. Matrixing on time points and factors									
Container size	A	B	C	A	B	C	A	B	C
Batch 1	T1	T2		T2		T1		T1	T2
Batch 2		T3	T1	T3	T1		T1		T3
Batch 3	T3		T2		T2	T3	T2	T3	
Time-point (months)	0	3	6	9	12	18	24	36	
T1	T		T	T	T	T	T	T	
T2	T	T		T	T		T	T	
T3	T	T	T		T	T		T	

S1, S2, and S3 are different strengths. A, B, and C are different container sizes.
Key: T = Sample tested.

A statistical justification could be based on an evaluation of the proposed matrixing design with respect to its power to detect differences among factors in the degradation rates or its precision in shelf life estimation.

If a matrixing design is considered applicable, the degree of reduction that can be made from a full design depends on the number of factor combinations being evaluated. The more factors associated with a product and the more levels in each factor, the larger the degree of reduction that can be considered. However, any reduced design should have the ability to adequately predict the product shelf life.

5. Potential Risk

Because of the reduced amount of data collected, a matrixing design on factors other than time points generally has less precision in shelf life estimation and yields a shorter shelf life than the corresponding full design. In addition, such a matrixing design may have insufficient power to detect certain main or interaction effects, thus leading to incorrect pooling of data from different design factors during shelf life estimation. If there is an excessive reduction in the number of factor combinations tested and data from the tested factor combinations cannot be pooled to establish a single shelf life, it may be impossible to estimate the shelf lives for the missing factor combinations.

A study design that matrixes on time points only would often have similar ability to that of a full design to detect differences in rates of change among factors and to establish a reliable shelf life. This feature exists because linearity is assumed and because full testing of all factor combinations would still be performed at both the initial time point and the last time point prior to submission.

E. Data Evaluation

Stability data from studies in a reduced design should be treated in the same manner as data from full design studies.

12

Evaluation of Stability Data

I. INTRODUCTION

A. Objectives of the Guideline

This guideline is intended to provide recommendations on how to use stability data generated in accordance with the principles detailed in the ICH guideline "Q1A(R) Stability Testing of New Drug Substances and Products" (hereafter referred to as the parent guideline) to propose a retest period or shelf life in a registration application. This guideline describes when and how extrapolation can be considered when proposing a retest period for a drug substance or a shelf life for a drug product that extends beyond the period covered by "available data from the stability study under the long-term storage condition" (hereafter referred to as long-term data).

B. Background

The guidance on the evaluation and statistical analysis of stability data provided in the parent guideline is brief in nature and limited in scope. The parent guideline states that regression analysis is an appropriate approach to analyzing quantitative stability data for retest period or shelf-life estimation and recommends that a statistical test for batch poolability be performed using a level of significance of 0.25. However, the parent guideline includes few details and does not cover situations where multiple factors are involved in a full- or reduced-design study.

This guideline is an expansion of the guidance presented in the Evaluation sections of the parent guideline.

C. Scope of the Guideline

This guideline addresses the evaluation of stability data that should be submitted in registration applications for new molecular entities and associated drug products. The guideline provides recommendations on establishing retest periods and shelf lives for drug substances and drug products intended for storage at or below "room temperature"*. It covers stability studies using single- or multifactor designs and full or reduced designs.

ICH Q6A and Q6B should be consulted for recommendations on the setting and justification of acceptance criteria, and ICH Q1D should be referenced for recommendations on the use of full- versus reduced-design studies.

II. GUIDELINES

A. General Principles

The design and execution of formal stability studies should follow the principles outlined in the parent guideline. The purpose of a stability study is to establish, based on testing a minimum of three batches of the drug substance or product, a retest period or shelf life and label storage instructions applicable to all future batches manufactured and packaged under similar circumstances. The degree of variability of individual batches affects the confidence that a future production batch will remain within acceptance criteria throughout its retest period or shelf life.

Although normal manufacturing and analytical variations are to be expected, it is important that the drug product be formulated with the intent to provide 100% of the labeled amount of the drug substance at the time of batch release. If the assay values of the batches used to support the registration application are higher than 100% of label claim at the time of batch release, after taking into account manufacturing and analytical variations, the shelf life proposed in the application can be overestimated. On the other hand, if the assay value of a batch is lower than 100% of label claim at the time of batch release, it might fall below the lower acceptance criterion before the end of the proposed shelf life.

A systematic approach should be adopted in the presentation and evaluation of the stability information. The stability information should include, as appropriate, results from the physical, chemical, biological, and microbiological tests, including those related to particular attributes of the dosage form (e.g., dissolution rate for solid oral dosage forms). The adequacy of the mass balance should be assessed. Factors that can cause an apparent lack of mass balance should be considered, including, for example, the mechanisms of degradation and the stability-indicating capability and inherent variability of the analytical procedures.

The basic concepts of stability data evaluation are the same for single- versus multifactor studies and for full- versus reduced-design studies. Data from formal stability studies and, as appropriate, supporting data should be evaluated to determine the critical quality attributes likely to influence the quality and performance of the drug substance or product. Each attribute should be assessed separately, and an overall assessment should be made of the findings for the purpose of proposing a retest period or shelf life. The retest period or shelf life proposed should not exceed that predicted for any single attribute.

The decision tree in Appendix A outlines a stepwise approach to stability data evaluation and when and how much extrapolation can be considered for a proposed retest period or shelf life. Appendix B provides (1) information on how to analyze long-term data for appropriate quantitative test attributes from a study with a multifactor, full, or reduced design; (2) information on how to use regression analysis for retest period or shelf life estimation; and (3) examples of statistical procedures to determine poolability of data from different batches or other factors. Additional guidance can be found in the references listed; however, the examples and references do not cover all applicable statistical approaches.

In general, certain quantitative chemical attributes (e.g., assay, degradation products, preservative content) for a drug

**Note*: The term "room temperature" refers to the general customary environment and should not be inferred to be the storage statement for labeling.

substance or product can be assumed to follow zero-order kinetics during long-term storage (Carstensen, 1977). Data for these attributes are therefore amenable to the type of statistical analysis described in Appendix B, including linear regression and poolability testing. Although the kinetics of other quantitative attributes (e.g., pH, dissolution) is generally not known, the same statistical analysis can be applied, if appropriate. Qualitative attributes and microbiological attributes are not amenable to this kind of statistical analysis.

The recommendations on statistical approaches in this guideline are not intended to imply that use of statistical evaluation is preferred when it can be justified to be unnecessary. However, statistical analysis can be useful in supporting the extrapolation of retest periods or shelf lives in certain situations and can be called for to verify the proposed retest periods or shelf lives in other cases.

B. Data Presentation

Data for all attributes should be presented in an appropriate format (e.g., tabular, graphical, narrative) and an evaluation of such data should be included in the application. The values of quantitative attributes at all time points should be reported as measured (e.g., assay as percent of label claim). If a statistical analysis is performed, the procedure used and the assumptions underlying the model should be stated and justified. A tabulated summary of the outcome of statistical analysis and/or graphical presentation of the long-term data should be included.

C. Extrapolation

Extrapolation is the practice of using a known data set to infer information about future data. Extrapolation to extend the retest period or shelf life beyond the period covered by long-term data can be proposed in the application, particularly if no significant change is observed at the accelerated condition. Whether extrapolation of stability data is appropriate depends on the extent of knowledge about the change pattern, the goodness of fit of any mathematical model, and the existence of relevant supporting data. Any extrapolation should be performed such that the extended retest period or shelf life will be valid for a future batch released with test results close to the release acceptance criteria.

An extrapolation of stability data assumes that the same change pattern will continue to apply beyond the period covered by long-term data. The correctness of the assumed change pattern is critical when extrapolation is considered. When estimating a regression line or curve to fit the long-term data, the data themselves provide a check on the correctness of the assumed change pattern, and statistical methods can be applied to test the goodness of fit of the data to the assumed line or curve. No such internal check is possible beyond the period covered by long-term data. Thus, a retest period or shelf life granted on the basis of extrapolation should always be verified by additional long-term stability data as soon as these data become available. Care should be taken to include in the protocol for commitment batches a time point that corresponds to the end of the extrapolated retest period or shelf life.

D. Data Evaluation for Retest Period or Shelf-Life Estimation for Drug Substances or Products Intended for Room Temperature Storage

A systematic evaluation of the data from formal stability studies should be performed as illustrated in this section. Stability data for each attribute should be assessed sequentially. For drug substances or products intended for storage at room temperature, the assessment should begin with any significant change at the accelerated condition and, if appropriate, at the intermediate condition, and progress through the trends and variability of the long-term data. The circumstances are delineated under which extrapolation of retest period or shelf life beyond the period covered by long-term data can be appropriate. A decision tree is provided in Appendix A as an aid.

1. No Significant Change at Accelerated Condition

Where no significant change occurs at the accelerated condition, the retest period or shelf life would depend on the nature of the long-term and accelerated data.

a. Long-Term and Accelerated Data Showing Little or No Change Over Time and Little or No Variability

Where the long-term data and accelerated data for an attribute show little or no change over time and little or no variability, it might be apparent that the drug substance or product will remain well within the acceptance criteria for that attribute during the proposed retest period or shelf life. In these circumstances, a statistical analysis is normally considered unnecessary but justification for the omission should be provided. Justification can include a discussion of the change pattern or lack of change, relevance of the accelerated data, mass balance, and/or other supporting data as described in the parent guideline. Extrapolation of the retest period or shelf life beyond the period covered by long-term data can be proposed. The proposed retest period or shelf life can be up to twice, but should not be more than 12 months beyond, the period covered by long-term data.

b. Long-Term or Accelerated Data Showing Change Over Time and/or Variability

If the long-term or accelerated data for an attribute show change over time and/or variability within a factor or among factors, statistical analysis of the long-term data can be useful in establishing a retest period or shelf life. Where there are differences in stability observed among batches or among other factors (e.g., strength, container size, and/or fill) or factor combinations (e.g., strength-by-container size and/or fill) that preclude the combining of data, the proposed retest period or shelf life should not exceed the shortest period supported by any batch, other factor, or factor combination. Alternatively, where the differences are readily attributed to a particular factor (e.g., strength), different shelf lives can be assigned to different levels within the factor (e.g., different strengths). A discussion should be provided to address the cause for the differences and the overall significance of such differences on the product. Extrapolation beyond the period covered by long-term data can be proposed; however, the extent of extrapolation would depend on whether long-term data for the attribute are amenable to statistical analysis.

- *Data not amenable to statistical analysis:* Where long-term data are not amenable to statistical analysis, but relevant supporting data are provided, the proposed retest period or shelf life can be up to one-and-a-half times, but should not be more than 6 months beyond, the period covered by long-term data. Relevant supporting data include satisfactory long-term data from development batches that are (1) made with a closely related formulation to, (2)

manufactured on a smaller scale than, or (3) packaged in a container closure system similar to, that of the primary stability batches.
- *Data amenable to statistical analysis:* If long-term data are amenable to statistical analysis but no analysis is performed, the extent of extrapolation should be the same as when data are not amenable to statistical analysis. However, if a statistical analysis is performed, it can be appropriate to propose a retest period or shelf life of up to twice, but not more than 12 months beyond, the period covered by long-term data, when the proposal is backed by the result of the analysis and relevant supporting data.

2. Significant Change at Accelerated Condition

Where significant change* occurs at the accelerated condition, the retest period or shelf life would depend on the outcome of stability testing at the intermediate condition, as well as at the long-term condition.

However, if phase separation of a semisolid dosage form occurs at the accelerated condition, testing at the intermediate condition should be performed. Potential interaction effects should also be considered in establishing that there is no other significant change.

a. No Significant Change at Intermediate Condition

If there is no significant change at the intermediate condition, extrapolation beyond the period covered by long-term data can be proposed; however, the extent of extrapolation would depend on whether long-term data for the attribute are amenable to statistical analysis.

- *Data not amenable to statistical analysis:* When the long-term data for an attribute are not amenable to statistical analysis, the proposed retest period or shelf life can be up to 3 months beyond the period covered by long-term data, if backed by relevant supporting data.
- *Data amenable to statistical analysis:* When the long-term data for an attribute are amenable to statistical analysis but no analysis is performed, the extent of extrapolation should be the same as when data are not amenable to statistical analysis. However, if a statistical analysis is performed, the proposed retest period or shelf life can be up to one-and-half times, but should not be more than 6 months beyond, the period covered by long-term data, when backed by statistical analysis and relevant supporting data.

b. Significant Change at Intermediate Condition

Where significant change occurs at the intermediate condition, the proposed retest period or shelf life should not exceed the period covered by long-term data. In addition, a retest period or shelf life shorter than the period covered by long-term data could be called for.

**Note:* The following physical changes can be expected to occur at the accelerated condition and would not be considered significant change that calls for intermediate testing if there is no other significant change:

- softening of a suppository that is designed to melt at 37°C, if the melting point is clearly demonstrated and
- failure to meet acceptance criteria for dissolution for 12 units of a gelatin capsule or gel-coated tablet if the failure can be unequivocally attributed to cross-linking.

E. Data Evaluation for Retest Period or Shelf-Life Estimation for Drug Substances or Products Intended for Storage Below Room Temperature

1. Drug Substances or Products Intended for Storage in a Refrigerator

Data from drug substances or products intended to be stored in a refrigerator should be assessed according to the same principles as described in section D for drug substances or products intended for room temperature storage, except where explicitly noted in the section below. The decision tree in Appendix A can be used as an aid.

a. No Significant Change at Accelerated Condition

Where no significant change occurs at the accelerated condition, extrapolation of retest period or shelf life beyond the period covered by long-term data can be proposed based on the principles outlined in subsection 1 of section D, except that the extent of extrapolation should be more limited.

If the long-term and accelerated data show little change over time and little variability, the proposed retest period or shelf life can be up to one-and-a-half times, but should not be more than 6 months beyond, the period covered by long-term data normally without the support of statistical analysis.

Where the long-term or accelerated data show change over time and/or variability, the proposed retest period or shelf life can be up to 3 months beyond the period covered by long-term data if (1) the long-term data are amenable to statistical analysis but a statistical analysis is not performed, or (2) the long-term data are not amenable to statistical analysis but relevant supporting data are provided.

Where the long-term or accelerated data show change over time and/or variability, the proposed retest period or shelf life can be up to one-and-a-half times, but should not be more than 6 months beyond, the period covered by long-term data if (1) the long-term data are amenable to statistical analysis and a statistical analysis is performed, and (2) the proposal is backed by the result of the analysis and relevant supporting data.

b. Significant Change at Accelerated Condition

If significant change occurs between 3 and 6 months' testing at the accelerated storage condition, the proposed retest period or shelf life should be based on the long-term data. Extrapolation is not considered appropriate. In addition, a retest period or shelf life shorter than the period covered by long-term data could be called for. If the long-term data show variability, verification of the proposed retest period or shelf life by statistical analysis can be appropriate.

If significant change occurs within the first 3 months' testing at the accelerated storage condition, the proposed retest period or shelf life should be based on long-term data. Extrapolation is not considered appropriate. A retest period or shelf life shorter than the period covered by long-term data could be called for. If the long-term data show variability, verification of the proposed retest period or shelf life by statistical analysis can be appropriate. In addition, a discussion should be provided to address the effect of short-term excursions outside the label storage condition (e.g., during shipping or handling). This discussion can be supported, if appropriate, by further testing on a single batch of the drug substance or product at the accelerated condition for a period shorter than 3 months.

2. Drug Substances or Products Intended for Storage in a Freezer

For drug substances or products intended for storage in a freezer, the retest period or shelf life should be based on long-term data. In the absence of an accelerated storage condition for drug substances or products intended to be stored in a freezer, testing on a single batch at an elevated temperature (e.g., 5°C ± 3°C or 25°C ± 2°C) for an appropriate time period should be conducted to address the effect of short-term excursions outside the proposed label storage condition (e.g., during shipping or handling).

3. Drug Substances or Products Intended for Storage Below −20°C

For drug substances or products intended for storage below −20°C, the retest period or shelf life should be based on long-term data and should be assessed on a case-by-case basis.

F. General Statistical Approaches

Where applicable, an appropriate statistical method should be employed to analyze the long-term primary stability data in an original application. The purpose of this analysis is to establish, with a high degree of confidence, a retest period or shelf life during which a quantitative attribute will remain within acceptance criteria for all future batches manufactured, packaged, and stored under similar circumstances.

In cases where a statistical analysis was employed to evaluate long-term data due to a change over time and/or variability, the same statistical method should also be used to analyze data from commitment batches to verify or extend the originally approved retest period or shelf life.

Regression analysis is considered an appropriate approach to evaluating the stability data for a quantitative attribute and establishing a retest period or shelf life. The nature of the relationship between an attribute and time will determine whether data should be transformed for linear regression analysis. The relationship can be represented by a linear or nonlinear function on an arithmetic or logarithmic scale. In some cases, a nonlinear regression can better reflect the true relationship.

An appropriate approach to retest period or shelf-life estimation is to analyze a quantitative attribute (e.g., assay, degradation products) by determining the earliest time at which the 95% confidence limit for the mean intersects the proposed acceptance criterion.

For an attribute known to decrease with time, the lower one-sided 95% confidence limit should be compared to the acceptance criterion. For an attribute known to increase with time, the upper one-sided 95% confidence limit should be compared to the acceptance criterion. For an attribute that can either increase or decrease, or whose direction of change is not known, two-sided 95% confidence limits should be calculated and compared to the upper and lower acceptance criteria.

The statistical method used for data analysis should take into account the stability study design to provide a valid statistical inference for the estimated retest period or shelf life. The approach described above can be used to estimate the retest period or shelf life for a single batch or for multiple batches when the data are combined after an appropriate statistical test. Examples of statistical approaches to the analysis of stability data from single or multifactor, full- or reduced-design studies are included in Appendix B. References to current literature sources can be found in Appendix B.6.

III. APPENDICES

Appendix A: Decision Tree for Data Evaluation for Retest Period or Shelf-Life Estimation for Drug Substances or Products (Excluding Frozen Products)

(See chart on page 72.)

Appendix B: Examples of Statistical Approaches to Stability Data Analysis

Linear regression, poolability tests, and statistical modeling, described below, are examples of statistical methods and procedures that can be used in the analysis of stability data that are amenable to statistical analysis for a quantitative attribute for which there is a proposed acceptance criterion.

B.1. DATA ANALYSIS FOR A SINGLE BATCH

In general, the relationship between certain quantitative attributes and time is assumed to be linear (Carstensen, 1977). Figure 12.1 shows the regression line for assay of a drug product with upper and lower acceptance criteria of 105% and 95% of label claim, respectively, with 12 months of long-term data and a proposed shelf life of 24 months. In this example, two-sided 95% confidence limits for the mean are applied because it is not known ahead of time whether the assay would increase or decrease with time (e.g., in the case of an aqueous-based product packaged in a semipermeable container). The lower confidence limit intersects the lower acceptance criterion at 30 months, while the upper confidence limit does not intersect with the upper acceptance criterion until later. Therefore, the proposed shelf life of 24 months can be supported by the statistical analysis of the assay, provided the recommendations in sections D and E are followed.

When data for an attribute with only an upper or a lower acceptance criterion are analyzed, the corresponding one-sided 95% confidence limit for the mean is recommended. Figure 12.2 shows the regression line for a degradation product in a drug product with 12 months of long-term data and a proposed shelf life of 24 months, where the acceptance criterion is not more than 1.4%. The upper one-sided 95% confidence limit for the mean intersects the acceptance criterion at 31 months. Therefore, the proposed shelf life of 24 months can be supported by statistical analysis of the degradation product data, provided the recommendations in sections D and E are followed.

If the above approach is used, the mean value of the quantitative attribute (e.g., assay, degradation products) can be expected to remain within the acceptance criteria through the end of the retest period or shelf life at a confidence level of 95%.

The approach described above can be used to estimate the retest period or shelf life for a single batch, individual batches, or multiple batches when combined after appropriate statistical tests described in sections B.2 through B.5.

B.2. DATA ANALYSIS FOR ONE-FACTOR, FULL-DESIGN STUDIES

For a drug substance or for a drug product available in a single strength and a single container size and/or fill, the retest period or shelf life is generally estimated based on the stability data from a minimum of three batches. When

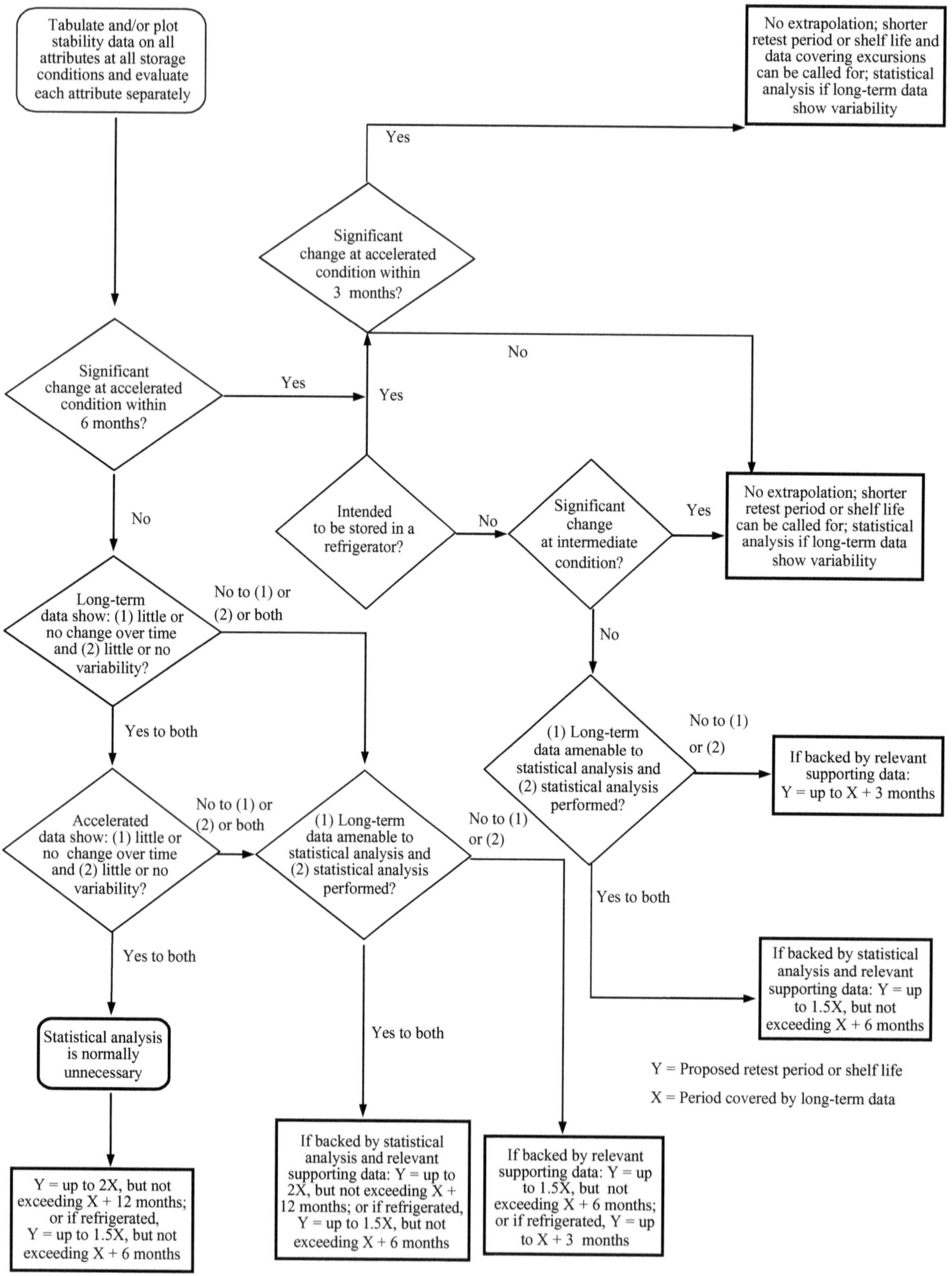
Tabulate and/or plot stability data on all attributes at all storage conditions and evaluate each attribute separately
Significant change at accelerated condition within 6 months?
Yes
No
Long-term data show: (1) little or no change over time and (2) little or no variability?
No to (1) or (2) or both
Yes to both
Accelerated data show: (1) little or no change over time and (2) little or no variability?
No to (1) or (2) or both
Yes to both
Statistical analysis is normally unnecessary
Y = up to 2X, but not exceeding X + 12 months; or if refrigerated, Y = up to 1.5X, but not exceeding X + 6 months
(1) Long-term data amenable to statistical analysis and (2) statistical analysis performed?
Yes to both
No to (1) or (2)
If backed by statistical analysis and relevant supporting data: Y = up to 2X, but not exceeding X + 12 months; or if refrigerated, Y = up to 1.5X, but not exceeding X + 6 months
If backed by relevant supporting data: Y = up to 1.5X, but not exceeding X + 6 months; or if refrigerated, Y = up to X + 3 months
Significant change at accelerated condition within 3 months?
Yes
No extrapolation; shorter retest period or shelf life and data covering excursions can be called for; statistical analysis if long-term data show variability
No
Yes
Intended to be stored in a refrigerator?
No
Significant change at intermediate condition?
Yes
No extrapolation; shorter retest period or shelf life can be called for; statistical analysis if long-term data show variability
No
(1) Long-term data amenable to statistical analysis and (2) statistical analysis performed?
No to (1) or (2)
If backed by relevant supporting data: Y = up to X + 3 months
Yes to both
If backed by statistical analysis and relevant supporting data: Y = up to 1.5X, but not exceeding X + 6 months
Y = Proposed retest period or shelf life
X = Period covered by long-term data

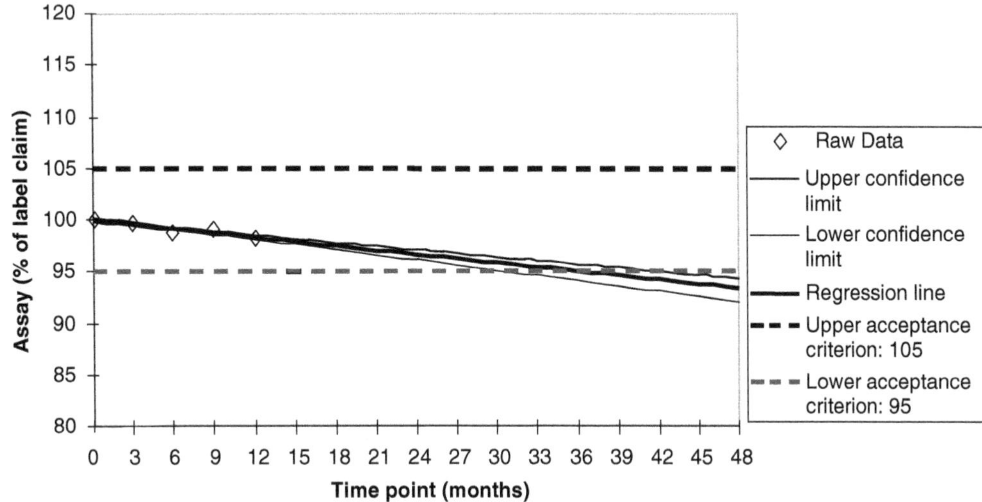

Figure 12.1 Shelf-life estimation with upper and lower acceptance criteria based on assay at 25°C/60% RH.

analyzing data from such one-factor, batch-only, full-design studies, two statistical approaches can be considered:

- The objective of the first approach is to determine whether the data from all batches support the proposed retest period or shelf life.
- The objective of the second approach, testing for poolability, is to determine whether the data from different batches can be combined for an overall estimate of a single retest period or shelf life.

B.2.1. Evaluating whether all batches support the proposed retest period or shelf life

The objective of this approach is to evaluate whether the estimated retest periods or shelf lives from all batches are longer than the one proposed. Retest periods or shelf lives for individual batches should first be estimated using the procedure described in section B.1 with individual intercepts, individual slopes, and the pooled mean square error calculated from all batches. If each batch has an estimated retest period or shelf life longer than that proposed, the proposed retest period or shelf life will generally be considered appropriate, as long as the guidance for extrapolation in sections D and E is followed. There is generally no need to perform poolability tests or identify the most reduced model. If, however, one or more of the estimated retest periods or shelf lives are shorter than that proposed, poolability tests can be performed to determine whether the batches can be combined to estimate a longer retest period or shelf life.

Alternatively, the above approach can be taken during the pooling process described in section B.2.2. If the regression lines for the batches are found to have a common slope and the estimated retest periods or shelf lives based on the common slope and individual intercepts are all longer than the proposed retest period or shelf life, there is generally no need to continue to test the intercepts for poolability.

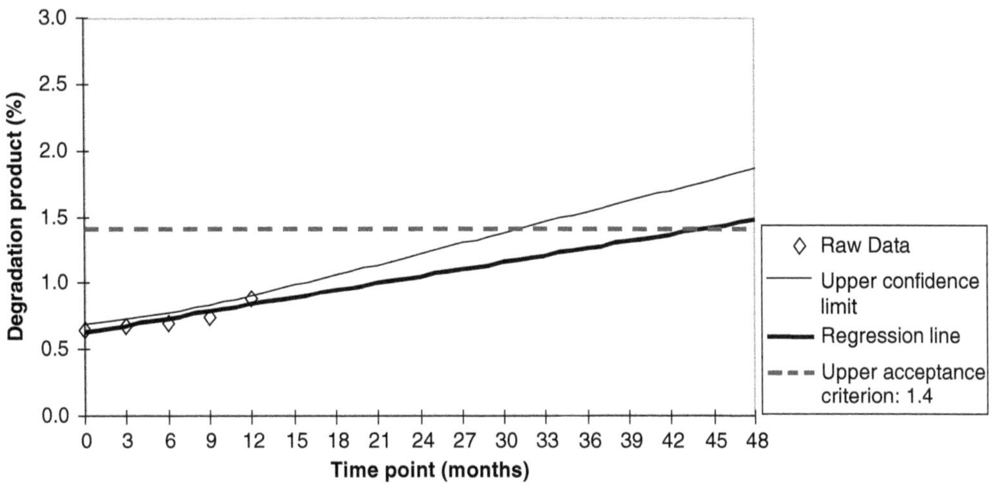

Figure 12.2 Shelf-life estimation with upper acceptance criterion based on a degradation product at 25°C/60% RH.

B.2.2. Testing for poolability of batches

B.2.2.1. Analysis of covariance

Before pooling the data from several batches to estimate a retest period or shelf life, a preliminary statistical test should be performed to determine whether the regression lines from different batches have a common slope and a common time-zero intercept. Analysis of covariance (ANCOVA) can be employed, where time is considered the covariate, to test the differences in slopes and intercepts of the regression lines among batches. Each of these tests should be conducted using a significance level of 0.25 to compensate for the expected low power of the design due to the relatively limited sample size in a typical formal stability study.

If the test rejects the hypothesis of equality of slopes (i.e., if there is a significant difference in slopes among batches), it is not considered appropriate to combine the data from all batches. The retest periods or shelf lives for individual batches in the stability study can be estimated by applying the approach described in section B.1 using individual intercepts and individual slopes and the pooled mean square error calculated from all batches. The shortest estimate among the batches should be chosen as the retest period or shelf life for all batches.

If the test rejects the hypothesis of equality of intercepts but fails to reject that the slopes are equal (i.e., if there is a significant difference in intercepts but no significant difference in slopes among the batches), the data can be combined for the purpose of estimating the common slope. The retest periods or shelf lives for individual batches in the stability study should be estimated by applying the approach described in section B.1, using the common slope and individual intercepts. The shortest estimate among the batches should be chosen as the retest period or shelf life for all batches.

If the tests for equality of slopes and equality of intercepts do not result in rejection at a level of significance of 0.25 (i.e., if there is no significant difference in slope and intercepts among the batches), the data from all batches can be combined. A single retest period or shelf life can be estimated from the combined data by using the approach described in section B.1 and applied to all batches. The estimated retest period or shelf life from the combined data is usually longer than that from individual batches because the width of the confidence limit(s) for the mean will become narrower as the amount of data increases when batches are combined.

The pooling tests described above should be performed in a proper order such that the slope terms are tested before the intercept terms. The most reduced model (i.e., individual slopes, common slope with individual intercepts, or common slope with common intercept, as appropriate) can be selected for retest period or shelf-life estimation.

B.2.2.2. Other methods

Statistical procedures other than those described above can be used in retest period or shelf-life estimation (Murphy and Weisman, 1990; Ruberg and Stegeman, 1991; Ruberg and Hsu, 1992; Shao and Chow, 1994; Yoshioka et al., 1997). For example, if it is possible to decide in advance the acceptable difference in slope or in mean retest period or shelf life among batches, an appropriate procedure for assessing the equivalence in slope or in mean retest period or shelf life can be used to determine the data poolability. However, such a procedure should be prospectively defined, evaluated, and justified and, where appropriate, discussed with the regulatory authority. A simulation study can be useful, if applicable, to demonstrate that the statistical properties of the alternative procedure selected are appropriate (Chen et al., 1997).

B.3. DATA ANALYSIS FOR MULTIFACTOR, FULL-DESIGN STUDIES

The stability of the drug product could differ to a certain degree among different factor combinations in a multifactor, full-design study. Two approaches can be considered when analyzing such data.

- The objective of the first approach is to determine whether the data from all factor combinations support the proposed shelf life.
- The objective of the second approach, testing for poolability, is to determine whether the data from different factor combinations can be combined for an overall estimate of a single shelf life.

B.3.1. Evaluating whether all factor combinations support the proposed shelf life

The objective of this approach is to evaluate whether the estimated shelf lives from all factor combinations are longer than the one proposed. A statistical model that includes all appropriate factors and factor combinations should be constructed as described in section B.3.2.2.1, and the shelf life should be estimated for each level of each factor and factor combination.

If all shelf lives estimated by the original model are longer than the proposed shelf life, further model building is considered unnecessary and the proposed shelf life will generally be appropriate as long as the guidance in sections D and E is followed. If one or more of the estimated shelf lives fall short of the proposed shelf life, model building as described in section B.3.2.2.1 can be employed. However, it is considered unnecessary to identify the final model before evaluating whether the data support the proposed shelf life. Shelf lives can be estimated at each stage of the model building process, and if all shelf lives at any stage are longer than the one proposed, further attempts to reduce the model are considered unnecessary.

This approach can simplify the data analysis of a complicated multifactor stability study compared to the data analysis described in section B.3.2.2.1.

B.3.2. Testing for poolability

The stability data from different combinations of factors should not be combined unless supported by statistical tests for poolability.

B.3.2.1. Testing for poolability of batch factor only

If each factor combination is considered separately, the stability data can be tested for poolability of batches only, and the shelf life for each nonbatch factor combination can be estimated separately by applying the procedure described in section B.2. For example, for a drug product available in two strengths and four container sizes, eight sets of data from the 2×4 strength-size combinations can be analyzed and eight separate shelf lives should be estimated accordingly. If a single shelf life is desired, the shortest estimated shelf life among all factor combinations should become the shelf life for the product. However, this approach does not take advantage of the available data from all factor combinations, thus generally resulting in shorter shelf lives than does the approach in section B.3.2.2.

B.3.2.2. Testing for poolability of all factors and factor combinations

If the stability data are tested for poolability of all factors and factor combinations and the results show that the data can be combined, a single shelf life longer than that estimated based on individual factor combinations is generally obtainable. The shelf life is longer because the width of the confidence limit(s) for the mean will become narrower as the amount of data increases when batches, strengths, container sizes and/or fills, and so forth are combined.

B.3.2.2.1. Analysis of covariance

Analysis of covariance can be employed to test the difference in slopes and intercepts of the regression lines among factors and factor combinations (Chen et al., 1997; Fairweather et al., 1995). The purpose of the procedure is to determine whether data from multiple factor combinations can be combined for the estimation of a single shelf life.

The full statistical model should include the intercept and slope terms of all main effects and interaction effects and a term reflecting the random error of measurement. If it can be justified that the higher-order interactions are very small, there is generally no need to include these terms in the model. In cases where the analytical results at the initial time point are obtained from the finished dosage form prior to its packaging, the container intercept term can be excluded from the full model because the results are common among the different container sizes and/or fills.

The tests for poolability should be specified to determine whether there are statistically significant differences among factors and factor combinations. Generally, the pooling tests should be performed in a proper order such that the slope terms are tested before the intercept terms and the interaction effects are tested before the main effects. For example, the tests can start with the slope and then the intercept terms of the highest-order interaction, and proceed to the slope and then the intercept terms of the simple main effects. The most reduced model, obtained when all remaining terms are found to be statistically significant, can be used to estimate the shelf lives.

All tests should be conducted using appropriate levels of significance. It is recommended that a significance level of 0.25 be used for batch-related terms, and a significance level of 0.05 be used for non-batch-related terms. If the tests for poolability show that the data from different factor combinations can be combined, the shelf life can be estimated according to the procedure described in section B.1 using the combined data.

If the tests for poolability show that the data from certain factors or factor combinations should not be combined, either of two alternatives can be applied: (1) a separate shelf life can be estimated for each level of the factors and of the factor combinations remaining in the model; or (2) a single shelf life can be estimated based on the shortest estimated shelf life among all levels of factors and factor combinations remaining in the model.

B.3.2.2.2. Other methods

Alternative statistical procedures to those described above can be applied (Murphy and Weisman, 1990; Ruberg and Stegeman, 1991; Ruberg and Hsu, 1992; Shao and Chow, 1994; Yoshioka et al., 1997). For example, an appropriate procedure for assessing the equivalence in slope or in mean shelf life can be used to determine the data poolability. However, such a procedure should be prospectively defined, evaluated, properly justified, and, where appropriate, discussed with the regulatory authority. A simulation study can be useful, if applicable, to demonstrate that the statistical properties of the alternative procedure selected are appropriate (Chen et al., 1997).

B.4. DATA ANALYSIS FOR BRACKETING DESIGN STUDIES

The statistical procedures described in section B.3 can be applied to the analysis of stability data obtained from a bracketing design study. For example, for a drug product available in three strengths (S1, S2, and S3) and three container sizes (P1, P2, and P3) and studied according to a bracketing design where only the two extremes of the container sizes (P1 and P3) are tested, six sets of data from the 3 × 2 strength-size combinations will be obtained. The data can be analyzed separately for each of the six combinations for shelf-life estimation according to section B.3.2.1, or tested for poolability prior to shelf-life estimation according to section B.3.2.2.

The bracketing design assumes that the stability of the intermediate strengths or sizes is represented by the stability at the extremes. If the statistical analysis indicates that the stability of the extreme strengths or sizes is different, the intermediate strengths or sizes should be considered no more stable than the least stable extreme. For example, if P1 from the above bracketing design is found to be less stable than P3, the shelf life for P2 should not exceed that for P1. No interpolation between P1 and P3 should be considered.

B.5. DATA ANALYSIS FOR MATRIXING DESIGN STUDIES

A matrixing design has only a fraction of the total number of samples tested at any specified time point. Therefore, it is important to ascertain that all factors and factor combinations that can have an impact on shelf-life estimation have been appropriately tested. For a meaningful interpretation of the study results and shelf-life estimation, certain assumptions should be made and justified. For instance, the assumption that the stability of the samples tested represents the stability of all samples should be valid. In addition, if the design is not balanced, some factors or factor interactions might not be estimable. Furthermore, for different levels of factor combinations to be poolable, it might have to be assumed that the higher-order factor interactions are negligible. Because it is usually impossible to statistically test the assumption that the higher-order terms are negligible, a matrixing design should be used only when it is reasonable to assume that these interactions are indeed very small, based on supporting data.

The statistical procedure described in section B.3 can be applied to the analysis of stability data obtained from a matrixing design study. The statistical analysis should clearly identify the procedure and assumptions used. For instance, the assumptions underlying the model in which interaction terms are negligible should be stated. If a preliminary test is performed for the purpose of eliminating factor interactions from the model, the procedure used should be provided and justified. The final model on which the estimation of shelf life will be based should be stated. The estimation of shelf life should be performed for each of the terms remaining in the model. The use of a matrixing design can result in an estimated shelf life shorter than that resulting from a full design.

Where bracketing and matrixing are combined in one design, the statistical procedure described in section B.3 can be applied.

REFERENCES

Carstensen JT (1977). Stability and dating of solid dosage forms. In: Pharmaceutics of Solids and Solid Dosage Forms. Wiley-Interscience, 182–185.

Ruberg SJ, Stegeman JW (1991). Pooling Data for stability studies: Testing the equality of batch degradation slopes. Biometrics 47:1059–1069.

Ruberg SJ, Hsu JC (1992). Multiple comparison procedures for pooling batches in stability studies. Technometrics 34:465–472.

Shao J, Chow SC (1994). Statistical inference in stability analysis. Biometrics 50:753–763.

Murphy JR, Weisman D (1990). Using random slopes for estimating shelf-life. In: Proceedings of American Statistical Association of the Biopharmaceutical Section 196–200.

Yoshioka S, Aso Y, Kojima S (1997). Assessment of shelf-life equivalence of pharmaceutical products. Chem Pharm Bull 45:1482–1484.

Chen JJ, Ahn H, Tsong Y (1997). Shelf-life estimation for multifactor stability studies. Drug Inf J 31:573–587.

Fairweather W, Lin TD, Kelly R (1995). Regulatory, design, and analysis aspects of complex stability studies. J Pharm Sci 84:1322–1326.

13

Stability Data Package for Registration Applications in Climatic Zones III and IV

I. INTRODUCTION

A. Objectives of the Guideline

This guideline describes an approach to broader use of the ICH guideline "Q1A(R) Stability Testing of New Drug Substances and Products" (hereafter referred to as the parent guideline) and outlines the stability data package for a new drug substance or drug product that is considered sufficient for a registration application in territories in Climatic Zones III and IV (Schumacher, 1974; Grimm, 1985).

B. Background

The parent guideline describes the stability data package for the ICH tripartite regions (EC, Japan, and the United States), which are in Climatic Zones I and II. The parent guideline can be followed to generate stability data packages for registration applications in other countries or regions in Zones I and II. For territories in Climatic Zones III and IV, the data package as described in the parent guideline can be considered applicable except for certain storage conditions. An approach for classification of countries according to Climatic Zones I, II, III, and IV can be found in the literature (Dietz et al., 1993; Grimm, 1998).

The World Health Organization (WHO) has published a guideline "Stability testing of pharmaceutical products containing well-established drug substances in conventional dosage forms" (WHO Technical Report Series, No 863, Annex 5), updated in the Report of the thirty-seventh meeting of the WHO Expert Committee on Specifications for Pharmaceutical Preparations, Geneva, 22–26 October 2001. The WHO guideline describes stability testing recommendations, including storage conditions for all four climatic zones.

The stability testing recommendations in this guideline are based on the parent guideline and the WHO guideline. To harmonize with the long-term storage condition for Zones III and IV, the intermediate storage condition in the General Case for Zones I and II in the parent guideline is changed to 30°C ± 2°C/65% RH ± 5% RH. This condition of 30°C ± 2°C/65% RH ± 5% RH can also be a suitable alternative to 25°C ± 2°C/60% RH ± 5% RH as the long-term storage condition for Zones I and II.

C. Scope of the Guideline

This document is an annex to the parent guideline and recommends the long-term storage condition for stability testing of a new drug substance or drug product for a registration application in territories in Climatic Zones III and IV.

II. GUIDELINES

A. Continuity with the Parent Guideline

This guideline should be used in conjunction with the parent guideline and subsequently published annexes (Q1B, Q1C, Q1D, Q1E, Q5C). The recommendations in the parent guideline and annexes should be followed unless specific alternatives are described within this guideline. The following sections of the parent guideline can be considered common to any territory in the world and are not reproduced here.

- Stress testing
- Selection of batches
- Container closure system
- Specification
- Testing frequency
- Storage conditions for drug substance or product in a refrigerator
- Storage conditions for drug substance or product in a freezer
- Stability commitment
- Evaluation
- Statements/labelling

B. Storage Conditions

1. General Case

For the "General case" (as described in the parent guideline), the recommended long-term and accelerated storage conditions for Climatic Zones III and IV are shown below:

Study	Storage Condition	Minimum Time Period Covered by Data at Submission
Long-term	30°C ± 2°C/65% RH ± 5% RH	12 mo
Accelerated	40°C ± 2°C/75% RH ± 5% RH	6 mo

No intermediate storage condition for stability studies is recommended for Climatic Zones III and IV. Therefore, the intermediate storage condition is not relevant when the principles of retest period or shelf life extrapolation described in Q1E are applied.

2. Aqueous-Based Drug Products Packaged in Semipermeable Containers

For aqueous-based drug products packaged in semipermeable containers (as described in the parent guideline), the recommended long-term and accelerated storage conditions for Climatic Zones III and IV are shown below:

Study	Storage Condition	Minimum Time Period Covered by Data at Submission
Long-term	30°C ± 2°C/35% RH ± 5% RH	12 mo
Accelerated	40°C ± 2°C/not more than 25% RH ± 5% RH	6 mo

As described in the parent guideline, an appropriate approach for deriving the water loss rate at the reference relative humidity is to multiply the water loss rate measured at an alternative relative humidity at the same temperature by a water loss rate ratio (see table below for examples).

The ratio of water loss rates at a given temperature is calculated by the general formula (100 – reference% RH)/(100 – alternative% RH).

Alternative Relative Humidity	Reference Relative Humidity	Ratio of Water Loss Rates at a Given Temperature
65% RH	35% RH	1.9
75% RH	25% RH	3.0

Valid water loss rate ratios at relative humidity conditions other than those shown in the table above can be used. A linear water loss rate at the alternative relative humidity over the storage period should be demonstrated.

3. Tests at Elevated Temperature and/or Extremes of Humidity

Special transportation and climatic conditions outside the storage conditions recommended in this guideline should be supported by additional data. For example, these data can be obtained from studies on one batch of drug product conducted for up to 3 months at 50°C/ambient humidity to cover extremely hot and dry conditions and at 25°C/80% RH to cover extremely high humidity conditions (Grimm, 1985).

Stability testing at a high humidity condition, for example, 25°C/80% RH, is recommended for solid dosage forms in water-vapor permeable packaging, for example, tablets in PVC/aluminum blisters, intended to be marketed in territories with extremely high humidity conditions in Zone IV. However, for solid dosage forms in primary containers designed to provide a barrier to water vapor, for example, aluminum/aluminum blisters, stability testing at a storage condition of extremely high humidity is not considered necessary.

C. Additional Considerations

If it cannot be demonstrated that the drug substance or drug product will remain within its acceptance criteria when stored at 30°C ± 2°C/65% RH ± 5% RH for the duration of the proposed retest period or shelf life, the following options should be considered: (1) a reduced retest period or shelf life, (2) a more protective container closure system, or (3) additional cautionary statements in the labeling.

REFERENCES

Schumacher P (1974). Aktuelle Fragen zur Haltbarkeit von Arzneimitteln [Current questions on drug stability]. Pharm Ztg 119:321–324.

Grimm W (1985). Storage conditions for stability testing – long term testing and stress tests. Drugs Made Ger 28;196–202; (Part I) and 29: 39–47, 1986 (Part II).

Dietz R, Feilner K, Gerst F, et al. (1993). Drug stability testing – classification of countries according to climatic zone. Drugs Made Ger 36:99–103.

Grimm W (1998). Extension of the international conference on harmonization tripartite guideline for stability testing of new drug substances and products to countries of climatic zones III and IV. Drug Dev Ind Pharm 24:313–325.

14

EU Guidelines to Good Manufacturing Practice Medicinal Products for Human and Veterinary Use

I. INTRODUCTION

The pharmaceutical industry of the European Union maintains high standards of quality assurance in the development, manufacture, and control of medicinal products. A system of Marketing Authorizations ensures that all medicinal products are assessed by a competent authority to ensure compliance with contemporary requirements of safety, quality, and efficacy. A system of manufacturing authorizations ensures that all products authorized on the European market are manufactured only by authorized manufacturers, whose activities are regularly inspected by the competent authorities. Manufacturing authorizations are required by all pharmaceutical manufacturers in the European Community whether the products are sold within or outside the Community.

Two directives laying down principles and guidelines of good manufacturing practice (GMP) for medicinal products were adopted by the Commission. Directive 2003/94/EC applies to medicinal products for human use and Directive 91/412/EEC for veterinary use. Detailed guidelines in accordance with those principles are published in the *Guide to Good Manufacturing Practice,* which will be used in assessing applications for manufacturing authorizations and as a basis for inspection of manufacturers of medicinal products.

The principles of GMP and the detailed guidelines are applicable to all operations which require the authorization referred to in Article 40 of Directive 2001/83/EC and in Article 44 of Directive 2001/82/EC, as amended by Directives 2004/27/EC and 2004/28/EC, respectively. They are also relevant for all other large-scale pharmaceutical manufacturing processes, such as that undertaken in hospitals, and for the preparation of products for use in clinical trials.

All member states and the industry agreed that the GMP requirements applicable to the manufacture of veterinary medicinal products are the same as those applicable to the manufacture of medicinal products for human use. Certain detailed adjustments to the GMP guidelines are set out in two annexes specific to veterinary medicinal products and to immunological veterinary medicinal products.

The guide is presented in two parts of basic requirements and specific annexes. Part I covers GMP principles for the manufacture of medicinal products. Part II covers GMP for active substances used as starting materials.

Chapters of Part I on "basic requirements" are headed by principles as defined in Directives 2003/94/EC and 91/412/EEC. Chapter 1 on Quality Management outlines the fundamental concept of quality assurance as applied to the manufacture of medicinal products. Thereafter, each chapter has a principle outlining the quality assurance objectives of that chapter and a text which provides sufficient detail for manufacturers to be made aware of the essential matters to be considered when implementing the principle.

Part II was established newly on the basis of a guideline developed on the level of ICH and published as ICH Q7a on "active pharmaceutical ingredients," which was implemented as GMP Annex 18 for voluntary application in 2001. According to the revised Article 47 and Article 51, respectively, of the Directive 2001/83/EC and Directive 2001/82/EC, as amended, detailed guidelines on the principles of GMP for active substances used as starting materials shall be adopted and published by the Commission. The former Annex 18 has been replaced by the new Part II of the GMP guide, which has an extended application both for the human and the veterinary sector.

In addition to the general matters of good manufacturing practice outlined in Part I and II, a series of annexes providing detail about specific areas of activity is included. For some manufacturing processes, different annexes will apply simultaneously (e.g., annex on sterile preparations and on radiopharmaceuticals and/or on biological medicinal products).

GMP Part I, Chapter 1 on Quality Management, has been revised to include aspects of quality risk management within the quality system framework. In future revisions of the guide, the opportunity will be taken to introduce quality risk management elements when appropriate.

The new GMP Annex 20, which corresponds to the ICH Q9 guideline, provides guidance on a systematic approach to quality risk management leading to compliance with GMP and other quality requirements. It includes principles to be used and options for processes, methods, and tools, which may be used when applying a formal quality risk management approach. While the GMP guide is primarily addressed to manufacturers, the ICH Q9 guideline has relevance for other quality guidelines and includes specific sections for regulatory agencies. However, for reasons of coherence and completeness the ICH Q9 guideline has been transferred completely into GMP Annex 20.

A glossary of some terms used in the guide has been incorporated after the annexes.

The guide is not intended to cover security aspects for the personnel engaged in manufacture. This may be particularly important in the manufacture of certain medicinal products such as highly active, biological and radioactive medicinal products. However, those aspects are governed by other provisions of Community or national law.

Throughout the guide it is assumed that the requirements of the Marketing Authorization relating to the safety, quality, and efficacy of the products are systematically incorporated into all the manufacturing, control, and release for sale arrangements of the holder of the manufacturing authorization.

The manufacture of medicinal products has for many years taken place in accordance with guidelines for Good Manufacturing Practice and the manufacture of medicinal products is not governed by CEN/ISO standards. Harmonized standards as adopted by the European standardization organizations CEN/ISO may be used at industry's discretion as a tool for implementing a quality system in the pharmaceutical sector. The CEN/ISO standards have been considered but the terminology of these standards has not been implemented in this edition. It is recognized that there are acceptable methods, other than those described in the guide, which are capable of achieving the principles of quality assurance. The guide is not intended to place any restraint upon the development of any new concepts or new technologies which have been validated and which provide a level of quality assurance at least equivalent to those set out in this guide. With its principles, methods, and tools, Annex 20 provides a systematic approach, which may be used to demonstrate such equivalence.

The GMP guide will be regularly revised. Revisions will be made publicly available on the Web site of the European Commission (http://ec.europa.eu/enterprise/pharmaceuticals/eudralex/homev4.htm).

Part I: Chapter 1: Quality Management

Principle

The holder of a manufacturing authorization must manufacture medicinal products so as to ensure that they are fit for their intended use, comply with the requirements of the Marketing Authorization, and do not place patients at risk due to inadequate safety, quality, or efficacy. The attainment of this quality objective is the responsibility of senior management and requires the participation and commitment by staff in many different departments and at all levels within the company, by the company's suppliers, and by the distributors. To achieve the quality objective reliably there must be a comprehensively designed and correctly implemented system of Quality Assurance incorporating Good Manufacturing Practice, Quality Control, and Quality Risk Management. It should be fully documented and its effectiveness monitored. All parts of the Quality Assurance system should be adequately resourced with competent personnel, and suitable and sufficient premises, equipment, and facilities. There are additional legal responsibilities for the holder of the manufacturing authorization and for the Qualified Person(s).

The basic concepts of Quality Assurance, Good Manufacturing Practice, Quality Control, and Quality Risk Management are interrelated. They are described here in order to emphasize their relationships and their fundamental importance to the production and control of medicinal products.

Quality Assurance

1.1 Quality Assurance is a wide-ranging concept, which covers all matters, which individually or collectively influence the quality of a product. It is the sum total of the organized arrangements made with the objective of ensuring that medicinal products are of the quality required for their intended use. Quality Assurance therefore incorporates Good Manufacturing Practice plus other factors outside the scope of this guide.

The system of Quality Assurance appropriate for the manufacture of medicinal products should ensure that

(i) medicinal products are designed and developed in a way that takes account of the requirements of GMP;
(ii) production and control operations are clearly specified and GMP adopted;
(iii) managerial responsibilities are clearly specified;
(iv) arrangements are made for the manufacture, supply, and use of the correct starting and packaging materials;
(v) all necessary controls on intermediate products, and any other in-process controls and validations are carried out;
(vi) the finished product is correctly processed and checked, according to the defined procedures;
(vii) medicinal products are not sold or supplied before a Qualified Person has certified that each production batch has been produced and controlled in accordance with the requirements of the Marketing Authorization and any other regulations relevant to the production, control, and release of medicinal products;
(viii) satisfactory arrangements exist to ensure, as far as possible, that the medicinal products are stored, distributed, and subsequently, handled so that quality is maintained throughout their shelf life; and
(ix) there is a procedure for Self-Inspection and/or quality audit, which regularly appraises the effectiveness and applicability of the Quality Assurance system.

Good Manufacturing Practice for Medicinal Products (GMP)

1.2 Good Manufacturing Practice is that part of Quality Assurance which ensures that products are consistently produced and controlled to the quality standards appropriate to their intended use and as required by the Marketing Authorization or product specification.

Good Manufacturing Practice is concerned with both production and Quality Control. The basic requirements of GMP are as follows:

(i) All manufacturing processes are clearly defined, systematically reviewed in the light of experience, and shown to be capable of consistently manufacturing medicinal products of the required quality and complying with their specifications.
(ii) Critical steps of manufacturing processes and significant changes to the process are validated.
(iii) All necessary facilities for GMP are provided including
    appropriately qualified and trained personnel;
    adequate premises and space;
    suitable equipment and services;
    correct materials, containers, and labels;
    approved procedures and instructions; and
    suitable storage and transport.
(iv) Instructions and procedures are written in an instructional form in clear and unambiguous language, specifically applicable to the facilities provided.
(v) Operators are trained to carry out procedures correctly.
(vi) Records are made, manually and/or by recording instruments, during manufacture which demonstrate that all the steps required by the defined procedures and instructions were in fact taken and that the quantity and quality of the product was as expected. Any significant deviations are fully recorded and investigated.
(vii) Records of manufacture including distribution, which enable the complete history of a batch to be traced, are retained in a comprehensible and accessible form.
(viii) The distribution (wholesaling) of the products minimizes any risk to their quality.
(ix) A system is available to recall any batch of product, from sale or supply.
(x) Complaints about marketed products are examined, the causes of quality defects investigated, and appropriate measures taken in respect of the defective products and to prevent reoccurrence.

Quality Control

1.3 Quality Control is that part of Good Manufacturing Practice which is concerned with sampling, specifications, and testing, and with the organization, documentation, and release procedures which ensure that the necessary and relevant tests are actually carried out and that materials are not released for use, nor products released for sale or supply, until their quality has been judged to be satisfactory.

The basic requirements of Quality Control are as follows:

(i) Adequate facilities, trained personnel, and approved procedures are available for sampling, inspecting, and testing starting materials, packaging materials, intermediate, bulk, and finished products, and where appropriate for monitoring environmental conditions for GMP purposes.
(ii) Samples of starting materials, packaging materials, intermediate products, bulk products, and finished products are taken by personnel and by methods approved by Quality Control.
(iii) Test methods are validated.
(iv) Records are made, manually and/or by recording instruments, which demonstrate that all the required sampling, inspecting, and testing procedures were actually carried out. Any deviations are fully recorded and investigated.
(v) The finished products contain active ingredients complying with the qualitative and quantitative composition of the Marketing Authorization, are of the purity required, and are enclosed within their proper containers and correctly labeled.
(vi) Records are made of the results of inspection and that testing of materials, intermediate, bulk, and finished products is formally assessed against specification. Product assessment includes a review and evaluation of relevant production documentation and an assessment of deviations from specified procedures.
(vii) No batch of product is released for sale or supply prior to certification by a Qualified Person that it is in accordance with the requirements of the relevant authorizations.
(viii) Sufficient reference samples of starting materials and products are retained to permit future examination of the product if necessary and that the product is retained in its final pack unless exceptionally large packs are produced.

Product Quality Review

1.4 Regular periodic or rolling quality reviews of all licensed medicinal products, including export only products, should be conducted with the objective of verifying the consistency of the existing process, the appropriateness of current specifications for both starting materials and finished product to highlight any trends, and to identify product and process improvements. Such reviews should normally be conducted and documented annually, taking into account previous reviews, and should include at least

(i) a review of starting materials including packaging materials used in the product, especially those from new sources;
(ii) a review of critical in-process controls and finished product results;
(iii) a review of all batches that failed to meet established specification(s) and their investigation;
(iv) a review of all significant deviations or nonconformances, their related investigations, and the effectiveness of resultant corrective and preventative actions taken;
(v) a review of all changes carried out to the processes or analytical methods;
(vi) a review of Marketing Authorization variations submitted/granted/refused, including those for third country (export only) dossiers;
(vii) a review of the results of the stability monitoring program and any adverse trends;
(viii) a review of all quality-related returns, complaints, and recalls and the investigations performed at the time;
(ix) a review of adequacy of any other previous product process or equipment corrective actions;
(x) for new Marketing Authorizations and variations to Marketing Authorizations, a review of postmarketing commitments;
(xi) the qualification status of relevant equipment and utilities, for example, HVAC, water, compressed gases; and
(xii) a review of any contractual arrangements as defined in Chapter 7 to ensure that they are up-to-date.

The manufacturer and Marketing Authorization holder should evaluate the results of this review, where different, and an assessment made of whether corrective and preventative action or any revalidation should be undertaken. Reasons for such corrective actions should be documented. Agreed corrective and preventative actions should be completed in a timely and effective manner. There should be management procedures for the ongoing management and review of these actions and the effectiveness of these procedures verified during self-inspection. Quality reviews may be grouped by product type, for example, solid dosage forms, liquid dosage forms, sterile products, where scientifically justified.

Where the Marketing Authorization holder is not the manufacturer, there should be a technical agreement in place between the various parties that defines their respective responsibilities in producing the quality review. The Qualified Person responsible for final batch certification together with the Marketing Authorization holder should ensure that the quality review is performed in a timely manner and is accurate.

Quality Risk Management

1.5 Quality Risk Management is a systematic process for the assessment, control, communication, and review of risks to the quality of the medicinal product. It can be applied both proactively and retrospectively.

1.6 The Quality Risk Management system should ensure that

- the evaluation of the risk to quality is based on scientific knowledge, experience with the process, and ultimately links to the protection of the patient and
- the level of effort, formality, and documentation of the Quality Risk Management process is commensurate with the level of risk.

Chapter 2: Personnel

Principle

The establishment and maintenance of a satisfactory system of Quality Assurance and the correct manufacture of medicinal products relies upon people. For this reason, there must be sufficient qualified personnel to carry out all the tasks which are the responsibility of the manufacturer. Individual responsibilities should be clearly understood by the individuals and recorded. All personnel should be aware of the principles of Good Manufacturing Practice that affect them and receive initial and continuing training, including hygiene instructions, relevant to their needs.

General

2.1 The manufacturer should have an adequate number of personnel with the necessary qualifications and practical experience. The responsibilities placed on any one individual should not be so extensive as to present any risk to quality.

2.2 The manufacturer must have an organization chart. People in responsible positions should have specific duties recorded in written job descriptions and adequate authority to carry out their responsibilities. Their duties may be delegated to designated deputies of a satisfactory qualification level. There should be no gaps or unexplained overlaps in the responsibilities of those personnel concerned with the application of Good Manufacturing Practice.

Key Personnel

2.3 Key Personnel include the head of Production, the head of Quality Control, and if at least one of these persons is not responsible for the duties described in Article 51 of Directive 2001/83/EC1, the Qualified Person(s) designated for the purpose. Normally, key posts should be occupied by full-time personnel. The heads of Production and Quality Control must be independent from each other. In large organizations, it may be necessary to delegate some of the functions listed in 2.5, 2.6, and 2.7.

2.4 The duties of the Qualified Person(s) are fully described in Article 51 of Directive 2001/83/EC, and can be summarized as follows:

(a) For medicinal products manufactured within the European Community, a Qualified Person must ensure that each batch has been produced and tested/checked in accordance with the directives and the Marketing Authorization (2).
(b) For medicinal products manufactured outside the European Community, a Qualified Person must ensure that each imported batch has undergone, in the importing country, the testing specified in paragraph 1 (b) of Article 51; Article 55 of Directive 2001/82/EC (2) According to Directive 75/319/EEC (now codified Directive 2001/83/EC) and the Ruling (Case 247/81) of the Court of Justice of the European Communities, medicinal products which have been properly controlled in the EU by a Qualified Person do not have to be recontrolled or rechecked in any other member state of the Community.
(c) A Qualified Person must certify in a register or equivalent document, as operations are carried out and before any release, that each production batch satisfies the provisions of Article 51. The persons responsible for these duties must meet the qualification requirements laid down in Article 493 of the same Directive, they shall be permanently and continuously at the disposal of the holder of the manufacturing authorization to carry out their responsibilities. Their responsibilities may be delegated, but only to other Qualified Person(s).

2.5 The head of the Production Department generally has the following responsibilities:

(i) to ensure that products are produced and stored according to the appropriate documentation in order to obtain the required quality;
(ii) to approve the instructions relating to production operations and to ensure their strict implementation;
(iii) to ensure that the production records are evaluated and signed by an authorized person before they are sent to the Quality Control Department;
(iv) to check the maintenance of his department, premises, and equipment;
(v) to ensure that the appropriate validations are done; and
(vi) to ensure that the required initial and continuing training of his department personnel is carried out and adapted according to need.

2.6 The head of the Quality Control Department generally has the following responsibilities:

(i) to approve or reject, as he sees fit, starting materials, packaging materials, and intermediate, bulk and finished products;
(ii) to evaluate batch records;
(iii) to ensure that all necessary testing is carried out;
(iv) to approve specifications, sampling instructions, test methods, and other Quality Control procedures;
(v) to approve and monitor any contract analysts;
(vi) to check the maintenance of his department, premises, and equipment;
(vii) to ensure that the appropriate validations are done; and
(viii) to ensure that the required initial and continuing training of his department personnel is carried out and adapted according to need.

Other duties of the Quality Control Department are summarized in Chapter 6.

2.7 The heads of Production and Quality Control generally have some shared, or jointly exercised, responsibilities relating to quality. These may include, subject to any national regulations,

the authorization of written procedures and other documents, including amendments;
the monitoring and control of the manufacturing environment;
plant hygiene;
process validation;
training;
the approval and monitoring of suppliers of materials;
the approval and monitoring of contract manufacturers;
the designation and monitoring of storage conditions for materials and products;
the retention of records;
the monitoring of compliance with the requirements of Good Manufacturing Practice; and
the inspection, investigation, and taking of samples, in order to monitor factors which may affect product quality.

Training

2.8 The manufacturer should provide training for all the personnel whose duties take them into production areas or into control laboratories (including the technical, maintenance, and cleaning personnel), and for other personnel whose activities could affect the quality of the product.

2.9 Besides the basic training on the theory and practice of Good Manufacturing Practice, newly recruited personnel should receive training appropriate to the duties assigned to them. Continuing training should also be given, and its practical effectiveness should be periodically assessed. Training programs should be available, approved by either the head of Production or the head of Quality Control, as appropriate. Training records should be kept.

2.10 Personnel working in areas where contamination is a hazard, for example, clean areas or areas where highly active, toxic, infectious, or sensitizing materials are handled, should be given specific training.

2.11 Visitors or untrained personnel should, preferably, not be taken into the production and Quality Control areas. If this is unavoidable, they should be given information in advance, particularly about personal hygiene and the prescribed protective clothing. They should be closely supervised.

2.12 The concept of Quality Assurance and all the measures capable of improving its understanding and implementation should be fully discussed during the training sessions.

Personnel Hygiene

2.13 Detailed hygiene programs should be established and adapted to the different needs within the factory. They should include procedures relating to the health, hygiene practices, and clothing of personnel. These procedures should be understood and followed in a very strict way by every person whose duties take him into the production and control areas. Hygiene programs should be promoted by management and widely discussed during training sessions.

2.14 All personnel should receive medical examination upon recruitment. It must be the manufacturer's responsibility that there are instructions ensuring that health conditions that can be of relevance to the quality of products come to the manufacturer's knowledge. After the first medical examination, examinations should be carried out when necessary for the work and personal health.

2.15 Steps should be taken to ensure as far as is practicable that no person affected by an infectious disease or having open lesions on the exposed surface of the body is engaged in the manufacture of medicinal products.

2.16 Every person entering the manufacturing areas should wear protective garments appropriate to the operations to be carried out.

2.17 Eating, drinking, chewing, or smoking, or the storage of food, drink, smoking materials, or personal medication in the production and storage areas should be prohibited. In general, any unhygienic practice within the manufacturing areas or in any other area where the product might be adversely affected should be forbidden.

2.18 Direct contact should be avoided between the operator's hands and the exposed product as well as with any part of the equipment that comes into contact with the products.

2.19 Personnel should be instructed to use the hand-washing facilities.

2.20 Any specific requirements for the manufacture of special groups of products, for example, sterile preparations, are covered in the annexes.

Chapter 3: Premises and Equipment

Principle

Premises and equipment must be located, designed, constructed, adapted, and maintained to suit the operations to be carried out. Their layout and design must aim to minimize the risk of errors and permit effective cleaning and maintenance in order to avoid cross-contamination, build up of dust or dirt, and in general, any adverse effect on the quality of products.

Premises

General

3.1 Premises should be situated in an environment which, when considered together with measures to protect the manufacture, presents minimal risk of causing contamination of materials or products.

3.2 Premises should be carefully maintained, ensuring that repair and maintenance operations do not present any hazard to the quality of products. They should be cleaned and, where applicable, disinfected according to detailed written procedures.

3.3 Lighting, temperature, humidity, and ventilation should be appropriate and such that they do not adversely affect, directly or indirectly, either the medicinal products during their manufacture and storage or the accurate functioning of equipment.

3.4 Premises should be designed and equipped so as to afford maximum protection against the entry of insects or other animals.

3.5 Steps should be taken in order to prevent the entry of unauthorized people. Production, storage, and Quality Control areas should not be used as a right of way by personnel who do not work in them.

Production Area

3.6 In order to minimize the risk of a serious medical hazard due to cross-contamination, dedicated and self-contained facilities must be available for the production of particular medicinal products, such as highly sensitizing materials (e.g., penicillins) or biological preparations (e.g., from live microorganisms). The production of certain additional products, such as certain antibiotics, certain hormones, certain cytotoxics, certain highly active drugs and nonmedicinal products, should not be conducted in the same facilities. For those products, in exceptional cases, the principle of campaign working in the same facilities can be accepted provided that specific precautions are taken and the necessary validations are made. The manufacture of technical poisons, such as pesticides and herbicides, should not be allowed in premises used for the manufacture of medicinal products.

3.7 Premises should preferably be laid out in such a way as to allow the production to take place in areas connected in a logical order corresponding to the sequence of the operations and to the requisite cleanliness levels.

3.8 The adequacy of the working and in-process storage space should permit the orderly and logical positioning of equipment and materials so as to minimize the risk of confusion between different medicinal products or their components, to avoid cross-contamination and to minimize the risk of omission or wrong application of any of the manufacturing or control steps.

3.9 Where starting and primary packaging materials and intermediate or bulk products are exposed to the environment, interior surfaces (walls, floors, and ceilings) should be smooth, free from cracks and open joints, and should not shed particulate matter and should permit easy and effective cleaning and, if necessary, disinfection.

3.10 Pipework, light fittings, ventilation points, and other services should be designed and sited to avoid the creation of recesses which are difficult to clean. As far as possible, for maintenance purposes, they should be accessible from outside the manufacturing areas.

3.11 Drains should be of adequate size and have trapped gullies. Open channels should be avoided where possible, but if necessary, they should be shallow to facilitate cleaning and disinfection.

3.12 Production areas should be effectively ventilated, with air-control facilities (including temperature and, where necessary, humidity and filtration) appropriate both to the products handled, to the operations undertaken within them, and to the external environment.

3.13 Weighing of starting materials usually should be carried out in a separate weighing room designed for that use.

3.14 In cases where dust is generated (e.g., during sampling, weighing, mixing and processing operations, packaging of dry products), specific provisions should be taken to avoid cross-contamination and facilitate cleaning.

3.15 Premises for the packaging of medicinal products should be specifically designed and laid out so as to avoid mix-ups or cross-contamination.

3.16 Production areas should be well lit, particularly where visual controls are carried out.

3.17 In-process controls may be carried out within the production area provided they do not carry any risk for the production.

Storage Areas

3.18 Storage areas should be of sufficient capacity to allow orderly storage of the various categories of materials and products: starting and packaging materials, intermediate, bulk and finished products, and products in quarantine, released, rejected, returned, or recalled.

3.19 Storage areas should be designed or adapted to ensure good storage conditions. In particular, they should be clean and dry and maintained within acceptable temperature limits. Where special storage conditions are required (e.g., temperature, humidity), these should be provided, checked, and monitored.

3.20 Receiving and dispatch bays should protect materials and products from the weather. Reception areas should be designed and equipped to allow containers of incoming materials to be cleaned where necessary before storage.

3.21 Where quarantine status is ensured by storage in separate areas, these areas must be clearly marked and their access restricted to authorized personnel. Any system replacing the physical quarantine should give equivalent security.

3.22 There should normally be a separate sampling area for starting materials. If sampling is performed in the storage area, it should be conducted in such a way as to prevent contamination or cross-contamination.

3.23 Segregated areas should be provided for the storage of rejected, recalled, or returned materials or products.

3.24 Highly active materials or products should be stored in safe and secure areas.

3.25 Printed packaging materials are considered critical to the conformity of the medicinal product and special attention should be paid to the safe and secure storage of these materials.

Quality Control Areas

3.26 Normally, Quality Control laboratories should be separated from production areas. This is particularly important for laboratories for the control of biologicals, microbiologicals, and radioisotopes, which should also be separated from each other.

3.27 Control laboratories should be designed to suit the operations to be carried out in them. Sufficient space should be given to avoid mix-ups and cross-contamination. There should be adequate suitable storage space for samples and records.

3.28 Separate rooms may be necessary to protect sensitive instruments from vibration, electrical interference, humidity, and so forth.

3.29 Special requirements are needed in laboratories handling particular substances, such as biological or radioactive samples.

Ancillary Areas

3.30 Rest and refreshment rooms should be separate from other areas.

3.31 Facilities for changing clothes, washing, and toilet purposes should be easily accessible and appropriate for the number of users. Toilets should not directly communicate with production or storage areas.

3.32 Maintenance workshops should as far as possible be separated from production areas. Whenever parts and tools are stored in the production area, they should be kept in rooms or lockers reserved for that use.

3.33 Animal houses should be well isolated from other areas, with separate entrance (animal access) and air-handling facilities.

Equipment

3.34 Manufacturing equipment should be designed, located, and maintained to suit its intended purpose.

3.35 Repair and maintenance operations should not present any hazard to the quality of the products.

3.36 Manufacturing equipment should be designed so that it can be easily and thoroughly cleaned. It should be cleaned according to detailed and written procedures and stored only in a clean and dry condition.

3.37 Washing and cleaning equipment should be chosen and used in order not to be a source of contamination.

3.38 Equipment should be installed in such a way as to prevent any risk of error or of contamination.

3.39 Production equipment should not present any hazard to the products. The parts of the production equipment that come into contact with the product must not be reactive, additive or absorptive to such an extent that it will affect the quality of the product and thus present any hazard.

3.40 Balances and measuring equipment of an appropriate range and precision should be available for production and control operations.

3.41 Measuring, weighing, recording, and control equipment should be calibrated and checked at defined intervals by appropriate methods. Adequate records of such tests should be maintained.

3.42 Fixed pipework should be clearly labeled to indicate the contents and, where applicable, the direction of flow.

3.43 Distilled, deionized, and, where appropriate, other water pipes should be sanitized according to written procedures that detail the action limits for microbiological contamination and the measures to be taken.

3.44 Defective equipment should, if possible, be removed from production and Quality Control areas, or at least be clearly labeled as defective.

Chapter 4: Documentation

Principle

Good documentation constitutes an essential part of the Quality Assurance system. Clearly written documentation prevents errors from spoken communication and permits tracing of batch history. Specifications, Manufacturing Formulae and instructions, procedures, and records must be free from errors and available in writing. The legibility of documents is of paramount importance.

General

4.1 *Specifications* describe in detail the requirements with which the products or materials used or obtained during manufacture have to conform. They serve as a basis for quality evaluation.

Manufacturing Formulae, Processing, and Packaging Instructions state all the starting materials used and lay down all processing and packaging operations.

Procedures give directions for performing certain operations, for example, cleaning, clothing, environmental control, sampling, testing, equipment operation.

Records provide a history of each batch of product, including its distribution, and also of all other relevant circumstances pertinent to the quality of the final product.

4.2 Documents should be designed, prepared, reviewed, and distributed with care. They should comply with the relevant parts of the manufacturing and Marketing Authorization dossiers.

4.3 Documents should be approved, signed, and dated by appropriate and authorized persons.

4.4 Documents should have unambiguous contents; title, nature, and purpose should be clearly stated. They should be laid out in an orderly fashion and be easy to check. Reproduced documents should be clear and legible. The reproduction of working documents from master documents must not allow any error to be introduced through the reproduction process.

4.5 Documents should be regularly reviewed and kept up-to-date. When a document has been revised, systems should be operated to prevent inadvertent use of superseded documents.

4.6 Documents should not be handwritten, although, where documents require the entry of data, these entries may be made in clear, legible, and indelible handwriting. Sufficient space should be provided for such entries.

4.7 Any alteration made to the entry on a document should be signed and dated; the alteration should permit the reading of the original information. Where appropriate, the reason for the alteration should be recorded.

4.8 The records should be made or completed at the time each action is taken and in such a way that all significant activities concerning the manufacture of medicinal products are traceable. They should be retained for at least one year after the expiry date of the finished product.

4.9 Data may be recorded by electronic data processing systems or photographic or other reliable means, but detailed procedures relating to the system in use should be available and the accuracy of the records should be checked. If documentation is handled by electronic data processing methods, only authorized persons should be able to enter or modify data in the computer and there should be a record of changes and deletions; access should be restricted by passwords or other means and the result of entry of critical data should be independently checked. Batch records electronically stored should be protected by backup transfer on magnetic tape, microfilm, paper, or other means. It is particularly important that the data are readily available throughout the period of retention.

4.10 There should be appropriately authorized and dated specifications for starting and packaging materials, and finished products; where appropriate, they should be also available for intermediate or bulk products.

Specifications for Starting and Packaging Materials

4.11 Specifications for starting and primary or printed packaging materials should include, if applicable,

- a description of the materials, including
- the designated name and the internal code reference;
- the reference, if any, to a pharmacopoeia monograph;
- the approved suppliers and, if possible, the original producer of the products;
- (a) specimen of printed materials, (b) directions for sampling and testing or reference to procedures, (c) qualitative and quantitative requirements with acceptance limits, and (d) storage conditions and precautions; and
- the maximum period of storage before reexamination.

Specifications for Intermediate and Bulk Products

4.12 Specifications for intermediate and bulk products should be available if these are purchased or dispatched, or if data obtained from intermediate products are used for the evaluation of the finished product. The specifications should be similar to specifications for starting materials or for finished products, as appropriate.

Specifications for Finished Products

4.13 Specifications for finished products should include (a) the designated name of the product and the code reference where applicable; (b) the formula or a reference to; (c) a description of the pharmaceutical form and package details; (d) directions for sampling and testing or a reference to procedures; e) the qualitative and quantitative requirements, with the acceptance limits; (f) the storage conditions and any special handling precautions, where applicable; and (g) the shelf-life.

Manufacturing Formula and Processing Instructions

Formally authorized Manufacturing Formula and Processing Instructions should exist for each product and batch size to be manufactured. They are often combined in one document.

4.14 The Manufacturing Formula should include (a) the name of the product, with a product reference code relating to its specification; (b) a description of the pharmaceutical form, strength of the product, and batch size; (c) a list of all starting materials to be used, with the amount of each, described using the designated name and a reference which is unique to that material; mention should be made of any substance that may disappear in the course of processing; and (d) a statement of the expected final yield with the acceptable limits, and of relevant intermediate yields, where applicable.

4.15 The Processing Instructions should include (a) a statement of the processing location and the principal equipment to be used; (b) the methods, or reference to the methods, to be used for preparing the critical equipment (e.g., cleaning, assembling, calibrating, sterilizing); (c) detailed stepwise processing instructions (e.g., checks on materials, pretreatments, sequence for adding materials, mixing times, temperatures); (d) the instructions for any in-process controls with their limits; (e) where necessary, the requirements for bulk storage of the products; including the container, labeling, and special storage conditions where applicable; and (f) any special precautions to be observed.

Packaging Instructions

4.16 There should be formally authorized Packaging Instructions for each product, pack size, and type. These should normally include, or have a reference to, the following:

(a) name of the product;
(b) description of its pharmaceutical form, and strength where applicable;

(c) the pack size expressed in terms of the number, weight, or volume of the product in the final container;
(d) a complete list of all the packaging materials required for a standard batch size, including quantities, sizes, and types, with the code or reference number relating to the specifications of each packaging material;
(e) where appropriate, an example or reproduction of the relevant printed packaging materials, and specimens indicating where to apply batch number references, and shelf life of the product;
(f) special precautions to be observed, including a careful examination of the area and equipment in order to ascertain the line clearance before operations begin;
(g) a description of the packaging operation, including any significant subsidiary operations, and equipment to be used; and
(h) details of in-process controls with instructions for sampling and acceptance limits.

Batch Processing Records

4.17 A Batch Processing Record should be kept for each batch processed. It should be based on the relevant parts of the currently approved Manufacturing Formula and Processing Instructions. The method of preparation of such records should be designed to avoid transcription errors. The record should carry the number of the batch being manufactured.

Before any processing begins, there should be recorded checks that the equipment and work station are clear of previous products, documents, or materials not required for the planned process, and that equipment is clean and suitable for use.

During processing, the following information should be recorded at the time each action is taken and, after completion, the record should be dated and signed in agreement by the person responsible for the processing operations:

(a) the name of the product;
(b) dates and times of commencement, of significant intermediate stages and of completion of production;
(c) name of the person responsible for each stage of production;
(d) initials of the operator of different significant steps of production and, where appropriate, of the person who checked each of these operations (e.g., weighing);
(e) the batch number and/or analytical control number as well as the quantities of each starting material actually weighed (including the batch number and amount of any recovered or reprocessed material added);
(f) any relevant processing operation or event and major equipment used;
(g) a record of the in-process controls and the initials of the person(s) carrying them out, and the results obtained;
(h) the product yield obtained at different and pertinent stages of manufacture; and
(i) notes on special problems including details, with signed authorization for any deviation from the Manufacturing Formula and Processing Instructions.

Batch Packaging Records

4.18 A Batch Packaging Record should be kept for each batch or part batch processed. It should be based on the relevant parts of the Packaging Instructions and the method of preparation of such records should be designed to avoid transcription errors. The record should carry the batch number and the quantity of bulk product to be packed, as well as the batch number and the planned quantity of finished product that will be obtained.

Before any packaging operation begins, there should be recorded checks that the equipment and work station are clear of previous products, documents, or materials not required for the planned packaging operations, and that equipment is clean and suitable for use.

The following information should be entered at the time each action is taken and, after completion, the record should be dated and signed in agreement by the person(s) responsible for the packaging operations:

(a) the name of the product;
(b) the date(s) and times of the packaging operations;
(c) the name of the responsible person carrying out the packaging operation;
(d) the initials of the operators of the different significant steps;
(e) records of checks for identity and conformity with the packaging instructions including the results of in-process controls;
(f) details of the packaging operations carried out, including references to equipment and the packaging lines used;
(g) whenever possible, samples of printed packaging materials used, including specimens of the batch coding, expiry dating, and any additional overprinting;
(h) notes on any special problems or unusual events including details, with signed authorization for any deviation from the Manufacturing Formula and Processing Instructions; and
(i) the quantities and reference number or identification of all printed packaging materials and bulk product issued, used, destroyed, or returned to stock and the quantities of obtained product, in order to provide for an adequate reconciliation.

Procedures and Records

Receipt

4.19 There should be written procedures and records for the receipt of each delivery of each starting and primary and printed packaging material.

4.20 The records of the receipts should include (a) the name of the material on the delivery note and the containers; (b) the "in-house" name and/or code of material (if different from a); (c) date of receipt; (d) supplier's name and, if possible, manufacturer's name; (e) manufacturer's batch or reference number; (f) total quantity, and number of containers received; (g) the batch number assigned after receipt; and (h) any relevant comment (e.g., state of the containers).

4.21 There should be written procedures for the internal labeling, quarantine and storage of starting materials, packaging materials, and other materials, as appropriate.

Sampling

4.22 There should be written procedures for sampling, which include the person(s) authorized to take samples, the methods and equipment to be used, the amounts to be taken, and any precautions to be observed to avoid contamination of the material or any deterioration in its quality (see Chapter 6, item 13).

Testing

4.23 There should be written procedures for testing materials and products at different stages of manufacture, describing the methods and equipment to be used. The tests performed should be recorded (see Chapter 6, item 17).

Other

4.24 Written release and rejection procedures should be available for materials and products, and in particular for the release for sale of the finished product by the Qualified Person(s) in accordance with the requirements of Article 51 of Directive 2001/83/EC[1].

4.25 Records should be maintained of the distribution of each batch of a product in order to facilitate the recall of the batch if necessary.

4.26 There should be written procedures and the associated records of actions taken or conclusions reached, where appropriate, for

- validation;
- equipment assembly and calibration;
- maintenance, cleaning, and sanitation;
- personnel matters including training, clothing, and hygiene;
- environmental monitoring;
- pest control;
- complaints;
- recalls; and
- returns.

4.27 Clear operating procedures should be available for major items of manufacturing and test equipment.

4.28 Logbooks should be kept for major or critical equipment recording, as appropriate, any validations, calibrations, maintenance, cleaning or repair operations, including the dates and identity of people who carried these operations out.

4.29 Logbooks should also record in chronological order the use of major or critical equipment and the areas where the products have been processed.

Chapter 5: Production

Principle

Production operations must follow clearly defined procedures; they must comply with the principles of Good Manufacturing Practice in order to obtain products of the requisite quality and be in accordance with the relevant manufacturing and Marketing Authorizations.

General

5.1 Production should be performed and supervised by competent people.

5.2 All handling of materials and products, such as receipt and quarantine, sampling, storage, labeling, dispensing, processing, packaging, and distribution should be done in accordance with written procedures or instructions and, where necessary, recorded.

5.3 All incoming materials should be checked to ensure that the consignment corresponds to the order. Containers should be cleaned where necessary and labeled with the prescribed data.

5.4 Damage to containers and any other problem which might adversely affect the quality of a material should be investigated, recorded, and reported to the Quality Control Department.

5.5 Incoming materials and finished products should be physically or administratively quarantined immediately after receipt or processing, until they have been released for use or distribution.

5.6 Intermediate and bulk products purchased as such should be handled on receipt as though they were starting materials.

5.7 All materials and products should be stored under the appropriate conditions established by the manufacturer and in an orderly fashion to permit batch segregation and stock rotation.

5.8 Checks on yields, and reconciliation of quantities, should be carried out as necessary to ensure that there are no discrepancies outside acceptable limits.

5.9 Operations on different products should not be carried out simultaneously or consecutively in the same room unless there is no risk of mix-up or cross-contamination.

5.10 At every stage of processing, products and materials should be protected from microbial and other contamination.

5.11 When working with dry materials and products, special precautions should be taken to prevent the generation and dissemination of dust. This applies particularly to the handling of highly active or sensitizing materials.

5.12 At all times during processing, all materials, bulk containers, major items of equipment, and, where appropriate, rooms used should be labeled or otherwise identified with an indication of the product or material being processed, its strength (where applicable), and batch number. Where applicable, this indication should also mention the stage of production and batch number.

5.13 Labels applied to containers, equipment, or premises should be clear, unambiguous, and in the company's agreed format. It is often helpful in addition to the wording on the labels to use colors to indicate status (e.g., quarantined, accepted, rejected, clean, under processing, etc.).

5.14 Checks should be carried out to ensure that pipelines and other pieces of equipment used for the transportation of products from one area to another are connected in a correct manner.

5.15 Any deviation from instructions or procedures should be avoided as far as possible. If a deviation occurs, it should be approved in writing by a competent person, with the involvement of the Quality Control Department when appropriate.

5.16 Access to production premises should be restricted to authorized personnel.

5.17 Normally, the production of nonmedicinal products should be avoided in areas and with the equipment destined for the production of medicinal products.

Prevention of Cross-Contamination in Production

5.18 Contamination of a starting material or of a product by another material or product must be avoided. This risk of accidental cross-contamination arises from the uncontrolled release of dust, gases, vapors, sprays, or organisms from materials and products in process, from residues on equipment, and from "operators" clothing. The significance of this risk varies with the type of contaminant and of product being contaminated. Among the most hazardous contaminants are highly sensitizing materials, biological preparations containing living organisms, certain hormones, cytotoxics, and other highly active materials. Products in which contamination is likely to be most significant are those administered by injection, those given in large doses, and/or over a long time.

5.19 Cross-contamination should be avoided by appropriate technical or organizational measures, for example, (a) production in segregated areas (required for products such as penicillins, live vaccines, live bacterial preparations, and some other biologicals), or by campaign (separation in time) followed by appropriate cleaning; (b) providing appropriate air locks and air extraction; (c) minimizing the risk of contamination caused by recirculation or reentry of untreated or insufficiently treated air; (d) keeping protective clothing inside areas where products with special risk of cross-contamination are processed; (e) using cleaning and decontamination procedures of known effectiveness, as ineffective cleaning of equipment is a common source of cross-contamination; (f) using "closed systems" of production; and (g) testing for residues and use of cleaning status labels on equipment.

5.20 Measures to prevent cross-contamination and their effectiveness should be checked periodically according to set procedures.

Validation

5.21 Validation studies should reinforce Good Manufacturing Practice and be conducted in accordance with defined procedures. Results and conclusions should be recorded.

5.22 When any new manufacturing formula or method of preparation is adopted, steps should be taken to demonstrate its suitability for routine processing. The defined process, using the materials and equipment specified, should be shown to yield a product consistently of the required quality.

5.23 Significant amendments to the manufacturing process, including any change in equipment or materials, which may affect product quality and/or the reproducibility of the process should be validated.

5.24 Processes and procedures should undergo periodic critical revalidation to ensure that they remain capable of achieving the intended results.

Starting Materials

5.25 The purchase of starting materials is an important operation which should involve staff who have a particular and thorough knowledge of the suppliers.

5.26 Starting materials should only be purchased from approved suppliers named in the relevant specification and, where possible, directly from the producer. It is recommended that the specifications established by the manufacturer for the starting materials be discussed with the suppliers. It is of benefit that all aspects of the production and control of the starting material in question, including handling, labeling, and packaging requirements, as well as complaints and rejection procedures are discussed with the manufacturer and the supplier.

5.27 For each delivery, the containers should be checked for integrity of package and seal and for correspondence between the delivery note and the supplier's labels.

5.28 If one material delivery is made up of different batches, each batch must be considered as separate for sampling, testing, and release.

5.29 Starting materials in the storage area should be appropriately labeled (see Chapter 5, item 13). Labels should bear at least the following information:

- the designated name of the product and the internal code reference where applicable;
- a batch number given at receipt;
- where appropriate, the status of the contents (e.g., in quarantine, on test, released, rejected); and
- where appropriate, an expiry date or a date beyond which retesting is necessary.

When fully computerized storage systems are used, all the above information need not necessarily be in a legible form on the label.

5.30 There should be appropriate procedures or measures to assure the identity of the contents of each container of starting material. Bulk containers from which samples have been drawn should be identified (see Chapter 6, item 13).

5.31 Only starting materials which have been released by the Quality Control Department and which are within their shelf life should be used.

5.32 Starting materials should only be dispensed by designated persons, following a written procedure, to ensure that the correct materials are accurately weighed or measured into clean and properly labeled containers.

5.33 Each dispensed material and its weight or volume should be independently checked and the check recorded.

5.34 Materials dispensed for each batch should be kept together and conspicuously labeled as such. Processing operations: intermediate and bulk products.

5.35 Before any processing operation is started, steps should be taken to ensure that the work area and equipment are clean and free from any starting materials, products, product residues, or documents not required for the current operation.

5.36 Intermediate and bulk products should be kept under appropriate conditions.

5.37 Critical processes should be validated (see "VALIDATION" in this Chapter).

5.38 Any necessary in-process controls and environmental controls should be carried out and recorded.

5.39 Any significant deviation from the expected yield should be recorded and investigated.

Packaging Materials

5.40 The purchase, handling, and control of primary and printed packaging materials shall be accorded attention similar to that given to starting materials.

5.41 Particular attention should be paid to printed materials. They should be stored in adequately secure conditions such as to exclude unauthorized access. Cut labels and other loose printed materials should be stored and transported in separate closed containers so as to avoid mix-ups. Packaging materials should be issued for use only by authorized personnel following an approved and documented procedure.

5.42 Each delivery or batch of printed or primary packaging material should be given a specific reference number or identification mark.

5.43 Outdated or obsolete primary packaging material or printed packaging material should be destroyed and this disposal recorded.

Packaging Operations

5.44 When setting up a program for the packaging operations, particular attention should be given to minimizing the risk of cross-contamination, mix-ups, or substitutions. Different products should not be packaged in close proximity unless there is physical segregation.

5.45 Before packaging operations are begun, steps should be taken to ensure that the work area, packaging lines, printing machines, and other equipment are clean and free from any products, materials, or documents previously used, if these are not required for the current operation. The line clearance should be performed according to an appropriate checklist.

5.46 The name and batch number of the product being handled should be displayed at each packaging station or line.

5.47 All products and packaging materials to be used should be checked on delivery to the packaging department for quantity, identity, and conformity with the Packaging Instructions.

5.48 Containers for filling should be clean before filling. Attention should be given to avoiding and removing any contaminants such as glass fragments and metal particles.

5.49 Normally, filling and sealing should be followed as quickly as possible by labeling. If it is not the case, appropriate procedures should be applied to ensure that no mix-ups or mislabeling can occur.

5.50 The correct performance of any printing operation (e.g., code numbers, expiry dates) to be done separately or in the course of the packaging should be checked and recorded. Attention should be paid to printing by hand which should be rechecked at regular intervals.

5.51 Special care should be taken when using cut labels and when overprinting is carried out off-line. Rollfeed labels are normally preferable to cut labels, in helping to avoid mix-ups.

5.52 Checks should be made to ensure that any electronic code readers, label counters, or similar devices are operating correctly.

5.53 Printed and embossed information on packaging materials should be distinct and resistant to fading or erasing.

5.54 Online control of the product during packaging should include at least checking the following:

(a) general appearance of the packages;
(b) whether the packages are complete;
(c) whether the correct products and packaging materials are used;
(d) whether any overprinting is correct; and
(e) correct functioning of line monitors.

Samples taken away from the packaging line should not be returned.

5.55 Products which have been involved in an unusual event should only be reintroduced into the process after special inspection, investigation, and approval by authorized personnel. Detailed record should be kept of this operation.

5.56 Any significant or unusual discrepancy observed during reconciliation of the amount of bulk product and printed packaging materials and the number of units produced should be investigated and satisfactorily accounted for before release.

5.57 Upon completion of a packaging operation, any unused batch-coded packaging materials should be destroyed and the destruction recorded. A documented procedure should be followed if uncoded printed materials are returned to stock.

Finished Products

5.58 Finished products should be held in quarantine until their final release under conditions established by the manufacturer.

5.59 The evaluation of finished products and documentation which is necessary before release of product for sale are described in Chapter 6 (Quality Control).

5.60 After release, finished products should be stored as usable stock under conditions established by the manufacturer.

Rejected, Recovered, and Returned Materials

5.61 Rejected materials and products should be clearly marked as such and stored separately in restricted areas. They should either be returned to the suppliers or, where appropriate, reprocessed or destroyed. Whatever action is taken should be approved and recorded by authorized personnel.

5.62 The reprocessing of rejected products should be exceptional. It is only permitted if the quality of the final product is not affected, if the specifications are met and if it is done in accordance with a defined and authorized procedure after evaluation of the risks involved. Record should be kept of the reprocessing.

5.63 The recovery of all or part of earlier batches which conform to the required quality by incorporation into a batch of the same product at a defined stage of manufacture should be authorized beforehand. This recovery should be carried out in accordance with a defined procedure after evaluation of the risks involved, including any possible effect on shelf life. The recovery should be recorded.

5.64 The need for additional testing of any finished product which has been reprocessed, or into which a recovered product has been incorporated, should be considered by the Quality Control Department.

5.65 Products returned from the market and which have left the control of the manufacturer should be destroyed unless without doubt their quality is satisfactory; they may be considered for resale, relabeling, or recovery in a subsequent batch only after they have been critically assessed by the Quality Control Department in accordance with a written procedure. The nature of the product, any special storage conditions it requires, its condition and history, and the time elapsed since it was issued should all be taken into account in this assessment. Where any doubt arises over the quality of the product, it should not be considered suitable for reissue or reuse, although basic chemical reprocessing to recover active ingredient may be possible. Any action taken should be appropriately recorded.

Chapter 6: Quality Control

Principle

Quality Control is concerned with sampling, specifications, and testing as well as the organization, documentation, and release procedures which ensure that the necessary and relevant tests are carried out, and that materials are not released for use, nor products released for sale or supply, until their quality has been judged satisfactory. Quality Control is not confined to laboratory operations, but must be involved in all decisions which may concern the quality of the product. The independence of Quality Control from Production is considered fundamental to the satisfactory operation of Quality Control (see also Chapter 1).

General

6.1 Each holder of a manufacturing authorization should have a Quality Control Department. This department should be independent from other departments, and under the authority of a person with appropriate qualifications and experience, who has one or several control laboratories at his disposal. Adequate resources must be available to ensure that all the Quality Control arrangements are effectively and reliably carried out.

6.2 The principal duties of the head of Quality Control are summarized in Chapter 2. The Quality Control Department as a whole will also have other duties, such as to establish, validate, and implement all Quality Control procedures, keep the reference samples of materials and products, ensure the correct labeling of containers of materials and products, ensure the monitoring of the stability of the products, participate in the investigation of complaints related to the quality of the product, and so forth. All these operations should be carried out in accordance with written procedures and, where necessary, recorded.

6.3 Finished product assessment should embrace all relevant factors, including production conditions, results of in-process testing, a review of manufacturing (including packaging) documentation, compliance with Finished Product Specification, and examination of the final finished pack.

6.4 Quality Control personnel should have access to production areas for sampling and investigation as appropriate.

Good Quality Control Laboratory Practice

6.5 Control laboratory premises and equipment should meet the general and specific requirements for Quality Control areas given in Chapter 3.

6.6 The personnel, premises, and equipment in the laboratories should be appropriate to the tasks imposed by the nature and the scale of the manufacturing operations. The use of outside laboratories, in conformity with the principles detailed in Chapter 7, Contract Analysis, can be accepted for particular reasons, but this should be stated in the Quality Control records.

Documentation

6.7 Laboratory documentation should follow the principles given in Chapter 4. An important part of this documentation deals with Quality Control and the following details should be readily available to the Quality Control Department:

- specifications;
- sampling procedures;
- testing procedures and records (including analytical worksheets and/or laboratory notebooks);
- analytical reports and/or certificates;
- data from environmental monitoring, where required;
- validation records of test methods, where applicable; and
- procedures for and records of the calibration of instruments and maintenance of equipment.

6.8 Any Quality Control documentation relating to a batch record should be retained for one year after the expiry date of the batch and at least 5 years after the certification referred to in Article 51(3) of Directive 2001/83/EC.

6.9 For some kinds of data (e.g., analytical tests results, yields, environmental controls), it is recommended that records are kept in a manner permitting trend evaluation.

6.10 In addition to the information which is part of the batch record, other original data such as laboratory notebooks and/or records should be retained and readily available.

Sampling

6.11 The sample taking should be done in accordance with approved written procedures that describe

- the method of sampling;
- the equipment to be used;
- the amount of the sample to be taken;
- instructions for any required subdivision of the sample;
- the type and condition of the sample container to be used;
- the identification of containers sampled;
- any special precautions to be observed, especially with regard to the sampling of sterile or noxious materials;
- the storage conditions; and
- instructions for the cleaning and storage of sampling equipment.

6.12 Reference samples should be representative of the batch of materials or products from which they are taken. Other samples may also be taken to monitor the most stressed part of a process (e.g., beginning or end of a process).

6.13 Sample containers should bear a label indicating the contents, with the batch number, the date of sampling, and the containers from which samples have been drawn.

6.14 Further guidance on reference and retention samples is given in Annex 19.

Testing

6.15 Analytical methods should be validated. All testing operations described in the Marketing Authorization should be carried out according to the approved methods.

6.16 The results obtained should be recorded and checked to make sure that they are consistent with each other. Any calculations should be critically examined.

6.17 The tests performed should be recorded and the records should include at least the following data: (a) name of the material or product and, where applicable, dosage form; (b) batch number and, where appropriate, the manufacturer and/or supplier; (c) references to the relevant specifications and testing procedures; (d) test results, including observations and calculations, and reference to any certificates of analysis; (e) dates of testing; (f) initials of the persons who performed the testing; (g) initials of the persons who verified the testing and the calculations, where appropriate; and (h) a clear statement of release or rejection (or other status decision) and the dated signature of the designated responsible person.

6.18 All the in-process controls, including those made in the production area by production personnel, should be performed according to methods approved by Quality Control and the results recorded.

6.19 Special attention should be given to the quality of laboratory reagents, volumetric glassware and solutions, reference standards, and culture media. They should be prepared in accordance with written procedures.

6.20 Laboratory reagents intended for prolonged use should be marked with the preparation date and the signature of the person who prepared them. The expiry date of unstable reagents and culture media should be indicated on the label, together with specific storage conditions. In addition, for volumetric solutions, the last date of standardization and the last current factor should be indicated.

6.21 Where necessary, the date of receipt of any substance used for testing operations (e.g., reagents and reference standards) should be indicated on the container. Instructions for use and storage should be followed. In certain cases it may be necessary to carry out an identification test and/or other testing of reagent materials upon receipt or before use.

6.22 Animals used for testing components, materials or products, should, where appropriate, be quarantined before use. They should be maintained and controlled in a manner that assures their suitability for the intended use. They should be identified, and adequate records should be maintained, showing the history of their use.

Ongoing Stability Program

6.23 After marketing, the stability of the medicinal product should be monitored according to a continuous appropriate program that will permit the detection of any stability issue (e.g., changes in levels of impurities or dissolution profile) associated with the formulation in the marketed package.

6.24 The purpose of the ongoing stability program is to monitor the product over its shelf life and to determine that the product remains, and can be expected to remain, within specifications under the labeled storage conditions.

6.25 This mainly applies to the medicinal product in the package in which it is sold, but consideration should also be given to the inclusion in the program of bulk product. For example, when the bulk product is stored for a long period before being packaged and/or shipped from a manufacturing site to a packaging site, the impact on the stability of the packaged product should be evaluated and studied under ambient conditions. In addition, consideration should be given to intermediates that are stored and used over prolonged periods. Stability studies on reconstituted product are performed during product development and need not be monitored on an ongoing basis. However, when relevant, the stability of reconstituted product can also be monitored.

6.26 The ongoing stability program should be described in a written protocol following the general rules of Chapter 4 and results formalized as a report. The equipment used for the ongoing stability program (stability chambers among others) should be qualified and maintained following the general rules of Chapter 3 and Annex 15.

6.27 The protocol for an ongoing stability program should extend to the end of the shelf life period and should include, but not be limited to, the following parameters:

- number of batch(es) per strength and different batch sizes, if applicable;
- relevant physical, chemical, microbiological and biological test methods;
- acceptance criteria;
- reference to test methods;
- description of the container closure system(s);
- testing intervals (time points);
- description of the conditions of storage (standardized ICH conditions for long-term testing, consistent with the product labeling, should be used); and
- other applicable parameters specific to the medicinal product.

6.28 The protocol for the ongoing stability program can be different from that of the initial long-term stability study as submitted in the Marketing Authorization dossier provided that this is justified and documented in the protocol (e.g., the frequency of testing, or when updating to ICH recommendations).

6.29 The number of batches and frequency of testing should provide a sufficient amount of data to allow for trend analysis. Unless otherwise justified, at least one batch per year of product manufactured in every strength and every primary packaging type, if relevant, should be included in the stability program (unless none are produced during that year). For products where ongoing stability monitoring would normally require testing using animals and no appropriate alternative, validated techniques are available, the frequency of testing may take account of a risk-benefit approach. The principle of bracketing and matrixing designs may be applied if scientifically justified in the protocol.

6.30 In certain situations, additional batches should be included in the ongoing stability program. For example, an ongoing stability study should be conducted after any significant change or significant deviation to the process or package. Any reworking, reprocessing, or recovery operation should also be considered for inclusion.

6.31 Results of ongoing stability studies should be made available to key personnel and, in particular, to the Qualified Person(s). Where on-going stability studies are carried out at a site other than the site of manufacture of the bulk or finished product, there should be a written agreement between the parties concerned. Results of ongoing stability studies should be available at the site of manufacture for review by the competent authority.

6.32 Out of specification or significant atypical trends should be investigated. Any confirmed out of specification result, or significant negative trend, should be reported to the relevant competent authorities. The possible impact on batches on the market should be considered in accordance with Chapter 8 of the GMP guide and in consultation with the relevant competent authorities.

6.33. A summary of all the data generated, including any interim conclusions on the program, should be written and maintained. This summary should be subjected to periodic review.

Chapter 7: Contract Manufacture and Analysis

Principle

Contract manufacture and analysis must be correctly defined, agreed, and controlled in order to avoid misunderstandings, which could result in a product or work of unsatisfactory quality. There must be a written contract between the Contract Giver and the Contract Acceptor, which clearly establishes the duties of each party. The contract must clearly state the way in which the Qualified Person releasing each batch of product for sale exercises his full responsibility.

Note: This Chapter deals with the responsibilities of manufacturers toward the competent authorities of the member states with respect to the granting of marketing and manufacturing authorizations. It is not intended in any way to affect the respective liability of contract acceptors and contract givers to consumers; this is governed by other provisions of Community and national law.

General

7.1 There should be a written contract covering the manufacture and/or analysis arranged under contract and any technical arrangements made in connection with it.

7.2 All arrangements for contract manufacture and analysis including any proposed changes in technical or other arrangements should be in accordance with the Marketing Authorization for the product concerned.

The Contract Giver

7.3 The Contract Giver is responsible for assessing the competence of the Contract Acceptor to carry out successfully the work required and for ensuring by means of the contract that the principles and guidelines of GMP as interpreted in this guide are followed.

7.4 The Contract Giver should provide the Contract Acceptor with all the information necessary to carry out the contracted operations correctly in accordance with the Marketing Authorization and any other legal requirements. The Contract Giver should ensure that the Contract Acceptor is fully aware of any problems associated with the product or the work which might pose a hazard to his premises, equipment, personnel, other materials, or other products.

7.5 The Contract Giver should ensure that all processed products and materials delivered to him by the Contract Acceptor comply with their specifications or that the products have been released by a Qualified Person.

The Contract Acceptor

7.6 The Contract Acceptor must have adequate premises and equipment, knowledge and experience, and competent personnel to carry out satisfactorily the work ordered by the Contract Giver. Contract manufacture may be undertaken only by a manufacturer who is the holder of a manufacturing authorization.

7.7 The Contract Acceptor should ensure that all products or materials delivered to him are suitable for their intended purpose.

7.8 The Contract Acceptor should not pass to a third party any of the work entrusted to him under the contract without the Contract Giver's prior evaluation and approval of the arrangements. Arrangements made between the Contract Acceptor and any third party should ensure that the manufacturing and analytical information is made available in the same way as between the original Contract Giver and Contract Acceptor.

7.9 The Contract Acceptor should refrain from any activity which may adversely affect the quality of the product manufactured and/or analyzed for the Contract Giver.

The Contract

7.10 A contract should be drawn up between the Contract Giver and the Contract Acceptor which specifies their respective responsibilities relating to the manufacture and control of the product. Technical aspects of the contract should be drawn up by competent persons suitably knowledgeable in pharmaceutical technology, analysis, and Good Manufacturing Practice. All arrangements for manufacture and analysis must be in accordance with the Marketing Authorization and agreed by both parties.

7.11 The contract should specify the way in which the Qualified Person releasing the batch for sale ensures that each batch has been manufactured and checked for compliance with the requirements of Marketing Authorization.

7.12 The contract should describe clearly who is responsible for purchasing materials, testing and releasing materials, undertaking production and Quality Controls, including in-process controls, and who has responsibility for sampling and analysis. In the case of contract analysis, the contract should state whether or not the Contract Acceptor should take samples at the premises of the manufacturer.

7.13 Manufacturing, analytical and distribution records, and reference samples should be kept by, or be available to, the Contract Giver. Any records relevant to assessing the quality of a product in the event of complaints or a suspected defect must be accessible and specified in the defect/recall procedures of the Contract Giver.

7.14 The contract should permit the Contract Giver to visit the facilities of the Contract Acceptor.

7.15 In the case of contract analysis, the Contract Acceptor should understand that he is subject to Inspection by the competent Authorities.

Chapter 8: Complaints and Product Recall

Principle

All complaints and other information concerning potentially defective products must be reviewed carefully according to written procedures. In order to provide for all contingencies, and in accordance with Article 117 of Directive 2001/83/EC and Article 84 of Directive 2001/82/EC, a system should be designed to recall, if necessary, promptly and effectively products known or suspected to be defective from the market.

Complaints

8.1 A person should be designated responsible for handling the complaints and deciding the measures to be taken together with sufficient supporting staff to assist him. If this person is not the Qualified Person, the latter should be made aware of any complaint, investigation, or recall.

8.2 There should be written procedures describing the action to be taken, including the need to consider a recall, in the case of a complaint concerning a possible product defect.

8.3 Any complaint concerning a product defect should be recorded with all the original details and thoroughly investigated. The person responsible for Quality Control should normally be involved in the study of such problems.

8.4 If a product defect is discovered or suspected in a batch, consideration should be given to checking other batches in order to determine whether they are also affected. In particular, other batches which may contain reworks of the defective batch should be investigated.

8.5 All the decisions and measures taken as a result of a complaint should be recorded and referenced to the corresponding batch records.

8.6 Complaints records should be reviewed regularly for any indication of specific or recurring problems requiring attention and possibly the recall of marketed products.

8.7 Special attention should be given to establishing whether a complaint was caused because of counterfeiting.

8.8 The competent authorities should be informed if a manufacturer is considering action following possibly faulty manufacture, product deterioration, detection of counterfeiting, or any other serious quality problems with a product

Recalls

8.9 A person should be designated as responsible for execution and coordination of recalls and should be supported by sufficient staff to handle all the aspects of the recalls with the appropriate degree of urgency. This responsible person should normally be independent of the sales and marketing organization. If this person is not the Qualified Person, the latter should be made aware of any recall operation.

8.10 There should be established written procedures, regularly checked and updated when necessary, in order to organize any recall activity.

8.11 Recall operations should be capable of being initiated promptly and at any time.

8.12 All Competent Authorities of all countries to which products may have been distributed should be informed promptly if products are intended to be recalled because they are, or are suspected of being defective.

8.13 The distribution records should be readily available to the person(s) responsible for recalls, and should contain sufficient information on wholesalers and directly supplied customers (with addresses, phone and/or fax numbers inside and outside working hours, batches, and amounts delivered), including those for exported products and medical samples.

8.14 Recalled products should be identified and stored separately in a secure area while awaiting a decision on their fate.

8.15 The progress of the recall process should be recorded and a final report issued, including a reconciliation between the delivered and recovered quantities of the products.

8.16 The effectiveness of the arrangements for recalls should be evaluated regularly.

15

EDQM Certification

The European legislation does not require mandatory routine GMP inspections for active substance manufacturers. Responsibility for using only active substances that have been manufactured in accordance with good manufacturing practice is placed on the holders of a manufacturing authorization. Art. 111 Directive 2001/83/EC (Art. 80 Directive 2001/82/EC for veterinary medicinal products), however makes provision for GMP inspections of active substance manufacturing sites to be carried out at the request of the manufacturer itself. The request for the inspection should be made to the EEA competent authority where the site is located or, in case of sites located in third countries, to a competent authority where the active substance is used as a starting material in the manufacture of medicinal products. If this is not the case, any EEA authority can be approached. There is no guarantee that such a request will be fulfilled, as the competent authorities need to balance such requests with other priorities. It should also be borne in mind that an inspection does not replace the responsibility of the manufacturing authorization holder using the active substance in question as a starting material and will not be accepted alone as adequate assurance that the manufacturing authorization holder has fulfilled its responsibilities.

Manufacturing authorization holders sometimes confuse the role of inspectorates with their own obligations but nevertheless, when inspection reports or GMP certificates issued by EEA, MRA partners, or other recognized authorities are available; these can provide useful information to manufacturing authorization holders. However, these alone cannot fulfill the statutory obligations of the manufacturing authorization holder or the requirements of section 5.25 of the GMP Guide, but the results of inspections, may be used together with other supporting information in a risk-based approach by the manufacturer in establishing priorities for its own audit program of active substance suppliers.

A GMP certificate is a certificate issued, following a GMP inspection, by the competent authority responsible for carrying out the inspection, to confirm the GMP compliance status of the inspected site. GMP certificates are site specific, but can be restricted to particular activities depending on the scope of the inspection (e.g., manufacturing activities related to a specific product). Directives 2001/82/EC and 2001/83/EC, as amended state that after every GMP inspection, and within 90 days of the inspection, a GMP certificate shall be issued to a manufacturer, if the outcome of the inspection shows that the manufacturer complies with GMP.

CMPs are product specific certificates, issued by the competent authority that granted the marketing authorization (EMEA issues CMPs on behalf of the European Commission for centrally authorized products), in the context of the WHO certification scheme on the quality of pharmaceutical products moving in international commerce, to confirm the marketing authorization status of the products. These certificates also confirm the GMP compliance status of the manufacturing site(s). CMPs are mainly used by companies to support applications to export their pharmaceutical products to countries with less developed regulatory systems.

CEPs are certificates issued by the European Directorate for the Quality of Medicines (EDQM) to confirm that a certain active substance is produced according to the requirements of the relevant monograph of the European Pharmacopoeia or of the monograph on TSE. CEPs can be used by companies when submitting an application for marketing authorization, and replaces much of the documentation required for the active substance in the marketing authorization dossier. GMP inspections of active substance manufacturers can be requested by EDQM in the context of the CEP certification scheme.

EMEA does not perform inspections; they are carried out on its behalf by the national competent authorities of the member states of the EEA, in connection with products under the centralized marketing authorization procedure. The competent authority responsible for carrying out the inspection issues the GMP certificate, or makes an entry of noncompliance into the EudraGMP Database.

The EDQM allows raw material manufacturers to submit and secure approval for their active pharmaceutical ingredients besides the approval of the finished products; such approvals are not available in the jurisdictions of the FDA. Given below is submission requirement that can be used by the manufacturers to audit for the quality of the API in those instances where such certificates and/or DMF are not available.

I. 2.3.S DRUG SUBSTANCE

A. 2.3.S.1 General Information

Use of the substance: *Route(s) of administration, maximum daily dose.*

Commercialization history: *Summarize the history based on the table in application form.*

Declarations: Summarize the declarations appended to the application form:

- *Manufacture of the substance in accordance with ICH Q7A GMP rules*
- *Commitment by the manufacturer to keep the proposed holder informed of any changes to the documentation*
- *If applicable: manufacturer's authorization for X to act as representative*
- *Willingness to be inspected (holder, manufacturers)*
- *Nonuse/use of materials of human or animal origin in the process*

1. 2.3.S.1.1 Nomenclature

(a) *Recommended International Nonproprietary name (INN)*
(b) *Chemical name(s)*
(c) *Company or laboratory code*
(d) *Other nonproprietary name(s) (e.g., national name, USAN, BAN)*
(e) *CAS No.: Molecular Formula MW*

2.3.S.1.2 General Properties

Give summarized data on

(a) *Physical description (e.g., appearance, color, physical state. . .)*
(b) *Physical form (e.g., polymorphic form, solvate, hydrate): to be commented especially if requested as grade*
(c) *Solubility and other properties as necessary*
(d) *Particle size: for example, nonmicronized, micronized, or any grade claimed as subtitle*

2.3.S.2 Manufacture

2.3.S.2.1 Manufacturer(s) (Name, Manufacturer) and Sites Involved in the Entire Process

Give the name, address, and responsibility of each manufacturer, including contractors and manufacturer and each proposed production site or facility involved in manufacture.

2.3.S.2.2 Description of Manufacturing Process and Process Controls

(a) *Give a brief narrative step-by-step description of the manufacturing process(es) and provide reference to detailed description in the documentation. Confirm the maximum batch size*
(b) *If applicable, summarize alternate processes and give a short explanation of their use*
(c) *Comment shortly on recovery of materials (solvents, reagents, and mother liquor) together with reprocessing steps and give a brief justification*

2.3.S.2.3 Control of Materials

(I) Starting material(s)
  (a) *Give summarized specifications (including impurities profile) including their justification based on studies of carry-over.*
  NB: If starting material is obtained by fermentation or is from herbal origin, summarize the information related to the nature of this material.

(II) Reagents and solvents
  Summarize the quality and controls of the materials (e.g., raw materials, solvents pure, and/or recovered, reagents, catalysts) used in the manufacture of the drug substance.

2.3.S.2.4 Controls of Critical Steps and Intermediates

Summary of the controls performed at critical steps of the manufacturing process and on intermediates, compare analytical procedures used for intermediates and final substance.

2.3.S.2.5 Process Validation and/or Evaluation

For aseptic processing and sterilization, only give the summary of process validation and/or evaluation studies.

2.3.S.3 Characterization

2.3.S.3.1 Impurities

(I) Related substances
  (a) *Fill in the following table identifying related substances, their origin, and distinguishing between potential and actual impurities and comparing with impurity section of the monograph*
  (b) Justify these specifications based on *data observed for impurities in relevant batches*
  (c) *Discuss briefly about the* suitability of the mono-graph *to control the potential impurities present in the substance (residual starting materials, reactants, and reagents etc.)*
  (d) Specific discussion on possible genotoxic impurities: *Give a brief discussion on impurities with potential genotoxicity based on the requirements of the guideline*

(II) Residual solvent(s)/reagent(s)/catalyst(s)
  (a) *Fill in the following table*
  (b) Discuss briefly the basis for setting the specification

2.3.S.4 Control of the Drug Substance

2.3.S.4.1 Specification

Give a table summarizing the proposed specifications.

2.3.S.4.2 Analytical Procedures

(a) *Summarize of the analytical procedures*

2.3.S.4.3 Validation of Analytical Procedures

Give the summary of the validation information for any in-house tests and compare shortly with the method(s) described in the monograph (cross-validation).

2.3.S.4.4 Batch Analyses

(a) *Give a short description of the batches: batch number, batch size date, and site of production*
(b) *Summarize the results for relevant batches (according to specifications and showing equivalence of any alternative supplier, process etc.)*

2.3.S.4.5 Justification of Specification

Justify the drug substance specification

2.3.S.5 Reference Standards or Materials

(a) *Give the source of primary reference standards or reference materials (e.g., Ph.Eur.) for final substance and its impurities where relevant*
(b) *Summarize characterization and evaluation of in-house standards*

Chemical Name	Ph.Eur. Impurity	Applicant's Specifications	Ph.Eur. Specifications	Origin	Levels Found	LOD of the Method	LOQ of the Method

Solvent/Reagent/Catalyst	Used in Step X/Y	Applicant's Limit	ICH Class/Limit	Levels (PPM)	LOD of the Method	LOQ of the Method

2.3.S.6 Container Closure System

(a) *Describe shortly the container closure system(s) for the storage and shipment of the drug substance, as it has to be mentioned on the CEP in case a retest period is requested (i.e.. in a clear and understandable manner)*
(b) *Summarize the specifications (description + identification)*

2.3.S.7 Stability

State retest period claimed for the substance and storage recommendations, if any.

2.3.S.7.1 Stability Summary and Conclusions

(a) *Summarize accelerated* and *long-term testing (e.g., studies conducted, protocols used, results obtained)*
(b) *Justify of the retest period claimed based on data available*

2.3.S.7.2 Postapproval Stability Protocol and Stability Commitment

Give the stability protocol for commitment batches.

16

Impurities: Guideline for Residual Solvents

I. INTRODUCTION

The objective of this guideline is to recommend acceptable amounts for residual solvents in pharmaceuticals for the safety of the patient. The guideline recommends use of less toxic solvents and describes levels considered to be toxicologically acceptable for some residual solvents.

Residual solvents in pharmaceuticals are defined here as organic volatile chemicals that are used or produced in the manufacture of drug substances or excipients, or in the preparation of drug products. The solvents are not completely removed by practical manufacturing techniques. Appropriate selection of the solvent for the synthesis of drug substance may enhance the yield, or determine characteristics such as crystal form, purity, and solubility. Therefore, the solvent may sometimes be a critical parameter in the synthetic process. This guideline does not address solvents deliberately used as excipients nor does it address solvates. However, the content of solvents in such products should be evaluated and justified.

Since there is no therapeutic benefit from residual solvents, all residual solvents should be removed to the extent possible to meet product specifications, good manufacturing practices, or other quality-based requirements. Drug products should contain no higher levels of residual solvents than can be supported by safety data. Some solvents that are known to cause unacceptable toxicities (Class 1, Table 16.1) should be avoided in the production of drug substances, excipients, or drug products unless their use can be strongly justified in a risk-benefit assessment. Some solvents associated with less severe toxicity (Class 2, Table 16.2) should be limited in order to protect patients from potential adverse effects. Ideally, less toxic solvents (Class 3, Table 16.3) should be used where practical. The complete list of solvents included in this guideline is given in Appendix 1.

The lists are not exhaustive and other solvents can be used and later added to the lists. Recommended limits of Class 1 and 2 solvents or classification of solvents may change as new safety data becomes available. Supporting safety data in a marketing application for a new drug product containing a new solvent may be based on concepts in this guideline or the concept of qualification of impurities as expressed in the guideline for drug substance (Q3A, *Impurities in New Drug Substances*) or drug product (Q3B, *Impurities in New Drug Products*), or all three guidelines.

II. SCOPE OF THE GUIDELINE

Residual solvents in drug substances, excipients, and in drug products are within the scope of this guideline. Therefore, testing should be performed for residual solvents when production or purification processes are known to result in the presence of such solvents. It is only necessary to test for solvents that are used or produced in the manufacture or purification of drug substances, excipients, or drug product. Although manufacturers may choose to test the drug product, a cumulative method may be used to calculate the residual solvent levels in the drug product from the levels in the ingredients used to produce the drug product. If the calculation results in a level equal to or below that recommended in this guideline, no testing of the drug product for residual solvents need be considered. If, however, the calculated level is above the recommended level, the drug product should be tested to ascertain whether the formulation process has reduced the relevant solvent level to within the acceptable amount. Drug product should also be tested if a solvent is used during its manufacture.

This guideline does not apply to potential new drug substances, excipients, or drug products used during the clinical research stages of development, nor does it apply to existing marketed drug products.

The guideline applies to all dosage forms and routes of administration. Higher levels of residual solvents may be acceptable in certain cases such as short term (30 days or less) or topical application. Justification for these levels should be made on a case-by-case basis.

See Appendix 2 for additional background information related to residual solvents.

III. GENERAL PRINCIPLES

A. Classification of Residual Solvents by Risk Assessment

The term "tolerable daily intake" (TDI) is used by the International Programme on Chemical Safety (IPCS) to describe exposure limits of toxic chemicals and "acceptable daily intake" (ADI) is used by the World Health Organization (WHO) and other national and international health authorities and institutes. The new term "permitted daily exposure" (PDE) is defined in the present guideline as a pharmaceutically acceptable intake of residual solvents to avoid confusion of differing values for ADIs of the same substance.

Residual solvents assessed in this guideline are listed in Appendix 1 by common names and structures. They were evaluated for their possible risk to human health and placed into one of three classes as follows:

Class 1 solvents: solvents to be avoided: Known human carcinogens, strongly suspected human carcinogens, and environmental hazards.

Class 2 solvents: solvents to be limited: Nongenotoxic animal carcinogens or possible causative agents of other irreversible toxicity such as neurotoxicity or teratogenicity. Solvents suspected of other significant but reversible toxicities.

Class 3 solvents: solvents with low toxic potential: Solvents with low toxic potential to man; no health-based exposure limit is needed. Class 3 solvents have PDEs of 50 mg or more per day.

Table 16.1 Class 1 Solvents in Pharmaceutical Products (Solvents That Should Be Avoided)

Solvent	Concentration limit (ppm)	Concern
Benzene	2	Carcinogen
Carbon tetrachloride	4	Toxic and environmental hazard
1,2-Dichloroethane	5	Toxic
1,1-Dichloroethene	8	Toxic
1,1,1-Trichloroethane	1500	Environmental hazard

Table 16.2 Class 2 Solvents in Pharmaceutical Products

Solvent	PDE (mg/day)	Concentration limit (ppm)
Acetonitrile	4.1	410
Chlorobenzene	3.6	360
Chloroform	0.6	60
Cyclohexane	38.8	3880
1,2-Dichloroethene	18.7	1870
Dichloromethane	6.0	600
1,2-Dimethoxyethane	1.0	100
N,N-Dimethylacetamide	10.9	1090
N,N-Dimethylformamide	8.8	880
1,4-Dioxane	3.8	380
2-Ethoxyethanol	1.6	160
Ethyleneglycol	6.2	620
Formamide	2.2	220
Hexane	2.9	290
Methanol	30.0	3000
2-Methoxyethanol	0.5	50
Methylbutyl ketone	0.5	50
Methylcyclohexane	11.8	1180
N-Methylpyrrolidone	48.4	4840
Nitromethane	0.5	50
Pyridine	2.0	200
Sulfolane	1.6	160
Tetralin	1.0	100
Toluene	8.9	890
1,1,2-Trichloroethene	0.8	80
Xylene[a]	21.7	2170

[a]Usually 60% *m*-xylene, 14% *p*-xylene, 9% *o*-xylene with 17% ethyl benzene.

Table 16.3 Class 3 Solvents Which Should Be Limited by GMP or Other Quality-Based Requirements

Acetic acid	Heptane
Acetone	Isobutyl acetate
Anisole	Isopropyl acetate
1-Butanol	Methyl acetate
2-Butanol	3-Methyl-1-butanol
Butyl acetate	Methylethyl ketone
tert-Butylmethyl ether	Methylisobutyl ketone
Cumene	2-Methyl-1-propanol
Dimethyl sulfoxide	Pentane
Ethanol	1-Pentanol
Ethyl acetate	1-Propanol
Ethyl ether	2-Propanol
Ethyl formate	Propyl acetate
Formic acid	Tetrahydrofuran

B. Methods for Establishing Exposure Limits

The method used to establish permitted daily exposures for residual solvents is presented in Appendix 3. Summaries of the toxicity data that were used to establish limits are published in *Pharmeuropa*, Vol. 9, No. 1, Supplement, April 1997.

C. Options for Describing Limits of Class 2 Solvents

Two options are available when setting limits for Class 2 solvents.

Option 1: The concentration limits in ppm stated in Table 16.2 can be used. They were calculated using equation (1) below by assuming a product mass of 10 g administered daily.

$$\text{Concentration (ppm)} = \frac{1000 \times \text{PDE}}{\text{dose}} \qquad (1)$$

Here, PDE is given in terms of mg/day and dose is given in g/day.

These limits are considered acceptable for all substances, excipients, or products. Therefore this option may be applied if the daily dose is not known or fixed. If all excipients and drug substances in a formulation meet the limits given in Option 1, then these components may be used in any proportion. No further calculation is necessary provided the daily dose does not exceed 10 g. Products that are administered in doses greater than 10 g/day should be considered under Option 2.

Option 2: It is not considered necessary for each component of the drug product to comply with the limits given in Option 1. The PDE in terms of mg/day as stated in Table 16.2 can be used with the known maximum daily dose and equation (1) above to determine the concentration of residual solvent allowed in drug product. Such limits are considered acceptable provided that it has been demonstrated that the residual solvent has been reduced to the practical minimum. The limits should be realistic in relation to analytical precision, manufacturing capability, reasonable variation in the manufacturing process, and the limits should reflect contemporary manufacturing standards.

Option 2 may be applied by adding the amounts of a residual solvent present in each of the components of the drug product. The sum of the amounts of solvent per day should be less than that given by the PDE.

Consider an example of the use of Option 1 and Option 2 applied to acetonitrile in a drug product. The permitted daily exposure to acetonitrile is 4.1 mg/day; thus, the Option 1 limit is 410 ppm. The maximum administered daily mass of a drug product is 5.0 g, and the drug product contains two excipients. The composition of the drug product and the calculated maximum content of residual acetonitrile are given in the following table.

Component	Amount in formulation	Acetonitrile content	Daily exposure
Drug substance	0.3 g	800 ppm	0.24 mg
Excipient 1	0.9 g	400 ppm	0.36 mg
Excipient 2	3.8 g	800 ppm	3.04 mg
Drug product	5.0 g	728 ppm	3.64 mg

Excipient 1 meets the Option 1 limit, but the drug substance, excipient 2, and drug product do not meet the Option 1 limit. Nevertheless, the product meets the Option 2 limit of 4.1 mg/day and thus conforms to the recommendations in this guideline.

Consider another example using acetonitrile as residual solvent. The maximum administered daily mass of a drug product is 5.0 g, and the drug product contains two excipients. The composition of the drug product and the calculated maximum content of residual acetonitrile is given in the following table.

Component	Amount in formulation	Acetonitrile content	Daily exposure
Drug substance	0.3 g	800 ppm	0.24 mg
Excipient 1	0.9 g	2000 ppm	1.80 mg
Excipient 2	3.8 g	800 ppm	3.04 mg
Drug Product	5.0 g	1016 ppm	5.08 mg

In this example, the product meets neither the Option 1 nor the Option 2 limit according to this summation. The manufacturer could test the drug product to determine if the formulation process reduced the level of acetonitrile. If the level of acetonitrile was not reduced during formulation to the allowed limit, then the manufacturer of the drug product should take other steps to reduce the amount of acetonitrile in the drug product. If all of these steps fail to reduce the level of residual solvent, in exceptional cases the manufacturer could provide a summary of efforts made to reduce the solvent level to meet the guideline value, and provide a risk-benefit analysis to support allowing the product to be used with residual solvent at a higher level.

D. Analytical Procedures

Residual solvents are typically determined using chromatographic techniques such as gas chromatography. Any harmonized procedures for determining levels of residual solvents as described in the pharmacopoeias should be used, if feasible. Otherwise, manufacturers would be free to select the most appropriate validated analytical procedure for a particular application. If only Class 3 solvents are present, a nonspecific method such as loss on drying may be used.

Validation of methods for residual solvents should conform to ICH guidelines Text on Validation of Analytical Procedures and Extension of the ICH Text on Validation of Analytical Procedures.

E. Reporting Levels of Residual Solvents

Manufacturers of pharmaceutical products need certain information about the content of residual solvents in excipients or drug substances in order to meet the criteria of this guideline. The following statements are given as acceptable examples of the information that could be provided from a supplier of excipients or drug substances to a pharmaceutical manufacturer. The supplier might choose one of the following as appropriate:

- Only Class 3 solvents are likely to be present. Loss on drying is less than 0.5%.
- Only Class 2 solvents X, Y,... are likely to be present. All are below the Option 1 limit. (Here the supplier would name the Class 2 solvents represented by X, Y,...).
- Only Class 2 solvents X, Y,... and Class 3 solvents are likely to be present. Residual Class 2 solvents are below the Option 1 limit and residual Class 3 solvents are below 0.5%.

If Class 1 solvents are likely to be present, they should be identified and quantified.

"Likely to be present" refers to the solvent used in the final manufacturing step and to solvents that are used in earlier manufacturing steps and not removed consistently by a validated process.

If solvents of Class 2 or Class 3 are present at greater than their Option 1 limits or 0.5%, respectively, they should be identified and quantified.

Table 16.4 Solvents for Which No Adequate Toxicological Data Was Found

1,1-Diethoxypropane	Methylisopropyl ketone
1,1-Dimethoxymethane	Methyltetrahydrofuran
2,2-Dimethoxypropane	Petroleum ether
Isooctane	Trichloroacetic acid
Isopropyl ether	Trifluoroacetic acid

IV. LIMITS OF RESIDUAL SOLVENTS

A. Solvents to Be Avoided

Solvents in Class 1 should not be employed in the manufacture of drug substances, excipients, and drug products because of their unacceptable toxicity or their deleterious environmental effect. However, if their use is unavoidable in order to produce a drug product with a significant therapeutic advance, then their levels should be restricted as shown in Table 16.1, unless otherwise justified. 1,1,1-Trichloroethane is included in Table 16.1 because it is an environmental hazard. The stated limit of 1500 ppm is based on a review of the safety data.

B. Solvents to Be Limited

Solvents in Table 16.2 should be limited in pharmaceutical products because of their inherent toxicity. PDEs are given to the nearest 0.1 mg/day, and concentrations are given to the nearest 10 ppm. The stated values do not reflect the necessary analytical precision of determination. Precision should be determined as part of the validation of the method.

C. Solvents with Low Toxic Potential

Solvents in Class 3 (shown in Table 16.3) may be regarded as less toxic and of lower risk to human health. Class 3 includes no solvent known as a human health hazard at levels normally accepted in pharmaceuticals. However, there are no long-term toxicity or carcinogenicity studies for many of the solvents in Class 3. Available data indicate that they are less toxic in acute or short-term studies and negative in genotoxicity studies. It is considered that amounts of these residual solvents of 50 mg/day or less (corresponding to 5000 ppm or 0.5% under Option 1) would be acceptable without justification. Higher amounts may also be acceptable provided they are realistic in relation to manufacturing capability and good manufacturing practice.

D. Solvents for Which No Adequate Toxicological Data Was Found

The following solvents (Table 16.4) may also be of interest to manufacturers of excipients, drug substances, or drug products. However, no adequate toxicological data on which to base a PDE was found. Manufacturers should supply justification for residual levels of these solvents in pharmaceutical products.

GLOSSARY

Genotoxic Carcinogens—Carcinogens which produce cancer by affecting genes or chromosomes.

LOEL—Abbreviation for lowest-observed effect level.

Lowest-Observed Effect Level—The lowest dose of substance in a study or group of studies that produces biologically significant increases in frequency or severity of any effects in the exposed humans or animals.

Modifying Factor—A factor determined by professional judgment of a toxicologist and applied to bioassay data to relate that data safely to humans.

Neurotoxicity—The ability of a substance to cause adverse effects on the nervous system.

NOEL—Abbreviation for no-observed-effect level.

No-Observed-Effect Level—The highest dose of substance at which there are no biologically significant increases in frequency or severity of any effects in the exposed humans or animals.

PDE—Abbreviation for permitted daily exposure.

Permitted Daily Exposure—The maximum acceptable intake per day of residual solvent in pharmaceutical products.

Reversible Toxicity—The occurrence of harmful effects that are caused by a substance and which disappear after exposure to the substance ends.

Strongly Suspected Human Carcinogen—A substance for which there is no epidemiological evidence of carcinogenesis but there are positive genotoxicity data and clear evidence of carcinogenesis in rodents.

Teratogenicity—The occurrence of structural malformations in a developing fetus when a substance is administered during pregnancy.

Appendix 1. List of Solvents Included in the Guideline

Solvent	Other names	Structure	Class
Acetic acid	Ethanoic acid	CH_3COOH	Class 3
Acetone	2-Propanone Propan-2-one	CH_3COCH_3	Class 3
Acetonitrile		CH_3CN	Class 2
Anisole	Methoxybenzene	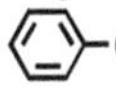 $-OCH_3$	Class 3
Benzene	Benzol		Class 1
1-Butanol	*n*-Butyl alcohol Butan-1-ol	$CH_3(CH_2)_3OH$	Class 3
2-Butanol	*sec*-Butyl alcohol Butan-2-ol	$CH_3CH_2CH(OH)CH_3$	Class 3
Butyl acetate	Acetic acid butyl ester	$CH_3COO(CH_2)_3CH_3$	Class 3
tert-Butylmethyl ether	2-Methoxy-2-methyl- propane	$(CH_3)_3COCH_3$	Class 3
Carbon tetrachloride	Tetrachloromethane	CCl_4	Class 1
Chlorobenzene		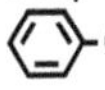 $-Cl$	Class 2
Chloroform	Trichloromethane	$CHCl_3$	Class 2
Cumene	Isopropylbenzene (1-Methyl) ethylbenzene	$-CH(CH_3)_2$	Class 3
Cyclohexane	Hexamethylene	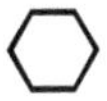	Class 2
1,2-Dichloroethane	*sym*-Dichloroethane Ethylene dichloride Ethylene chloride	CH_2ClCH_2Cl	Class 1
1,1-Dichloroethene	1,1-Dichloroethylene Vinylidene chloride	$H_2C = CCl_2$	Class 1
1,2-Dichloroethene	1,2-Dichloroethylene Acetylene dichloride	$ClHC = CHCl$	Class 2
Dichloromethane	Methylene chloride	CH_2Cl_2	Class 2
1,2-Dimethoxyethane	Ethyleneglycol dimethyl ether Monoglyme Dimethyl Cellosolve	$H_3COCH_2CH_2OCH_3$	Class 2
N,N-Dimethylacetamide	DMA	$CH_3CON(CH_3)_2$	Class 2
N,N-Dimethylformamide	DMF	$HCON(CH_3)_2$	Class 2
Dimethyl sulfoxide	Methylsulfinylmethane Methyl sulfoxide DMSO	$(CH_3)_2SO$	Class 3
1,4-Dioxane	*p*-Dioxane [1,4]Dioxane	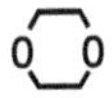 O O	Class 2
Ethanol	Ethyl alcohol	CH_3CH_2OH	Class 3
2-Ethoxyethanol	Cellosolve	$CH_3CH_2OCH_2CH_2OH$	Class 2
Ethyl acetate	Acetic acid ethyl ester	$CH_3COOCH_2CH_3$	Class 3
Ethyleneglycol	1,2-Dihydroxyethane 1,2-Ethanediol	$HOCH_2CH_2OH$	Class 2

(*continued*)

Appendix 1. List of Solvents Included in the Guideline *(Continued)*

Solvent	Other names	Structure	Class
Ethyl ether	Diethyl ether Ethoxyethane 1,1′-Oxybisethane	$CH_3CH_2OCH_2CH_3$	Class 3
Ethyl formate	Formic acid ethyl ester	$HCOOCH_2CH_3$	Class 3
Formamide	Methanamide	$HCONH_2$	Class 2
Formic acid		$HCOOH$	Class 3
Heptane	*n*-Heptane	$CH_3(CH_2)_5CH_3$	Class 3
Hexane	*n*-Hexane	$CH_3(CH_2)_4CH_3$	Class 2
Isobutyl acetate	Acetic acid isobutyl ester	$CH_3COOCH_2CH(CH_3)_2$	Class 3
Isopropyl acetate	Acetic acid isopropyl ester	$CH_3COOCH(CH_3)_2$	Class 3
Methanol	Methyl alcohol	CH_3OH	Class 2
2-Methoxyethanol	Methyl Cellosolve	$CH_3OCH_2CH_2OH$	Class 2
Methyl acetate	Acetic acid methyl ester	CH_3COOCH_3	Class 3
3-Methyl-1-butanol	Isoamyl alcohol Isopentyl alcohol 3-Methylbutan-1-ol	$(CH_3)_2CHCH_2CH_2OH$	Class 3
Methylbutyl ketone	2-Hexanone Hexan-2-one	$CH_3(CH_2)_3COCH_3$	Class 2
Methylcyclohexane	Cyclohexylmethane	CH_3	Class 2
Methylethyl ketone	2-Butanone MEK Butan-2-one	$CH_3CH_2COCH_3$	Class 3
Methylisobutyl ketone	4-Methylpentan-2-one 4-Methyl-2-pentanone MIBK	$CH_3COCH_2CH(CH_3)_2$	Class 3
2-Methyl-1-propanol	Isobutyl alcohol 2-Methylpropan-1-ol	$(CH_3)_2CHCH_2OH$	Class 3
N-Methylpyrrolidone	1-Methylpyrrolidin-2-one 1-Methyl-2-pyrrolidinone	N, O, CH_3	Class 2
Nitromethane		CH_3NO_2	Class 2
Pentane	*n*-Pentane	$CH_3(CH_2)_3CH_3$	Class 3
1-Pentanol	Amyl alcohol Pentan-1-ol Pentyl alcohol	$CH_3(CH_2)_3CH_2OH$	Class 3
1-Propanol	Propan-1-ol Propyl alcohol	$CH_3CH_2CH_2OH$	Class 3
2-Propanol	Propan-2-ol Isopropyl alcohol	$(CH_3)_2CHOH$	Class 3
Propyl acetate	Acetic acid propyl ester	$CH_3COOCH_2CH_2CH_3$	Class 3
Pyridine		N	Class 2
Sulfolane	Tetrahydrothiophene 1,1-dioxide	O, S, O	Class 2
Tetrahydrofuran	Tetramethylene oxide Oxacyclopentane	O	Class 3
Tetralin	1,2,3,4-Tetrahydro-naphthalene		Class 2
Toluene	Methylbenzene	CH_3	Class 2
1,1,1-Trichloroethane	Methylchloroform	CH_3CCl_3	Class 1
1,1,2-Trichloroethene	Trichloroethene	$HClC = CCl_2$	Class 2
Xylene[a]	Dimethybenzene Xylol	CH_3, CH_3	Class 2

[a]Usually 60% *m*-xylene, 14% *p*-xylene, 9% *o*-xylene with 17% ethyl benzene.

Appendix 2. Additional Background

A2.1 Environmental Regulation of Organic Volatile Solvents

Several of the residual solvents frequently used in the production of pharmaceuticals are listed as toxic chemicals in Environmental Health Criteria (EHC) monographs and the Integrated Risk Information System (IRIS). The objectives of such groups as the International Programme on Chemical Safety (IPCS), the United States Environmental Protection Agency (USEPA), and the United States Food and Drug Administration (USFDA) include the determination of acceptable exposure levels. The goal is the protection of human health and maintenance of environmental integrity against the possible deleterious effects of chemicals resulting from long-term environmental exposure. The methods involved in the estimation of maximum safe exposure limits are usually based on long-term studies. When long-term study data are unavailable, shorter-term study data can be used with modification of the approach such as use of larger safety factors. The approach described therein relates primarily to long-term or *lifetime exposure of the general population* in the ambient environment, that is, ambient air, food, drinking water, and other media.

A2.2 Residual Solvents in Pharmaceuticals

Exposure limits in this guideline are established by referring to methodologies and toxicity data described in EHC and IRIS monographs. However, some specific assumptions about residual solvents to be used in the synthesis and formulation of pharmaceutical products should be taken into account in establishing exposure limits. They are as follows:

(1) Patients (not the general population) use pharmaceuticals to treat their diseases or for prophylaxis to prevent infection or disease.
(2) The assumption of lifetime patient exposure is not necessary for most pharmaceutical products but may be appropriate as a working hypothesis to reduce risk to human health.
(3) Residual solvents are unavoidable components in pharmaceutical production and will often be a part of drug products.
(4) Residual solvents should not exceed recommended levels except in exceptional circumstances.
(5) Data from toxicological studies that are used to determine acceptable levels for residual solvents should have been generated using appropriate protocols such as those described, for example, by OECD, EPA, and the FDA *Red Book*.

Appendix 3. Methods for Establishing Exposure Limits

The Gaylor–Kodell method of risk assessment (Gaylor DW, Kodell RL (1980). Linear interpolation algorithm for low dose assessment of toxic substance. J Environ Pathol 4:305.) is appropriate for Class 1 carcinogenic solvents. Only in cases where reliable carcinogenicity data are available should extrapolation by the use of mathematical models be applied to setting exposure limits. Exposure limits for Class 1 solvents could be determined with the use of a large safety factor (i.e., 10,000 to 100,000) with respect to the no-observed-effect level (NOEL). Detection and quantitation of these solvents should be by state-of-the-art analytical techniques.

Acceptable exposure levels in this guideline for Class 2 solvents were established by calculation of PDE values according to the procedures for setting exposure limits in pharmaceuticals (*Pharmacopeial Forum*, Nov–Dec 1989), and the method adopted by IPCS for Assessing Human Health Risk of Chemicals (Environmental Health Criteria 170, WHO, 1994). These methods are similar to those used by the USEPA (IRIS) and the USFDA (*Red Book*) and others. The method is outlined here to give a better understanding of the origin of the PDE values. It is not necessary to perform these calculations in order to use the PDE values tabulated in section IV of this document.

PDE is derived from the no-observed-effect level (NOEL) or the lowest-observed-effect level (LOEL) in the most relevant animal study as follows:

$$\text{PDE} = \frac{\text{NOEL} \times \text{Weight Adjustment}}{\text{F1} \times \text{F2} \times \text{F3} \times \text{F4} \times \text{F5}} \quad (1)$$

The PDE is derived preferably from a NOEL. If no NOEL is obtained, the LOEL may be used. Modifying factors proposed here, for relating the data to humans, are the same kind of "uncertainty factors" used in EHC (Environmental Health Criteria 170, World Health Organization, Geneva, 1994), and "modifying factors" or "safety factors" in *Pharmacopeial Forum*. The assumption of 100% systemic exposure is used in all calculations regardless of route of administration.

The modifying factors are as follows:

F1 = A factor to account for extrapolation between species
F1 = 5 for extrapolation from rats to humans
F1 = 12 for extrapolation from mice to humans
F1 = 2 for extrapolation from dogs to humans
F1 = 2.5 for extrapolation from rabbits to humans
F1 = 3 for extrapolation from monkeys to humans
F1 = 10 for extrapolation from other animals to humans

F1 takes into account the comparative surface area:body weight ratios for the species concerned and for man. Surface area (S) is calculated as:

$$S = kM\,0.67 \quad (2)$$

in which M = body mass, and the constant k has been taken to be 10. The body weights used in the equation are those shown below in Table A3.1.

F2 = A factor of 10 to account for variability between individuals

A factor of 10 is generally given for all organic solvents, and 10 is used consistently in this guideline.

F3 = A variable factor to account for toxicity studies of short-term exposure
F3 = 1 for studies that last at least one half lifetime (1 year for rodents or rabbits; 7 years for cats, dogs, and monkeys)
F3 = 1 for reproductive studies in which the whole period of organogenesis is covered
F3 = 2 for a 6-month study in rodents or a 3.5-year study in nonrodents
F3 = 5 for a 3-month study in rodents or a 2-year study in nonrodents
F3 = 10 for studies of a shorter duration

In all cases, the higher factor has been used for study durations between the time points, for example, a factor of 2 for a 9-month rodent study.

Table A3.1 Values Used in the Calculations in This Document

Rat body weight	425 g	Mouse respiratory volume	43 L/day
Pregnant rat body weight	330 g	Rabbit respiratory volume	1440 L/day
Mouse body weight	28 g	Guinea pig respiratory volume	430 L/day
Pregnant mouse body weight	30 g	Human respiratory volume	28,800 L/day
Guinea pig body weight	500 g	Dog respiratory volume	9000 L/day
Rhesus monkey body weight	2.5 kg	Monkey respiratory volume	1150 L/day
Rabbit body weight (pregnant or not)	4 kg	Mouse water consumption	5 mL/day
Beagle dog body weight	11.5 kg	Rat water consumption	30 mL/day
Rat respiratory volume	290 L/day	Rat food consumption	30 g/day

F4 = A factor that may be applied in cases of severe toxicity, for example, nongenotoxic carcinogenicity, neurotoxicity, or teratogenicity. In studies of reproductive toxicity, the following factors are used:
F4 = 1 for fetal toxicity associated with maternal toxicity
F4 = 5 for fetal toxicity without maternal toxicity
F4 = 5 for a teratogenic effect with maternal toxicity
F4 = 10 for a teratogenic effect without maternal toxicity
F5 = A variable factor that may be applied if the no-effect level was not established

When only an LOEL is available, a factor of up to 10 could be used depending on the severity of the toxicity.

The weight adjustment assumes an arbitrary adult human body weight for either sex of 50 kg. This relatively low weight provides an additional safety factor against the standard weights of 60 kg or 70 kg that are often used in this type of calculation. It is recognized that some adult patients weigh less than 50 kg; these patients are considered to be accommodated by the built-in safety factors used to determine a PDE. If the solvent was present in a formulation specifically intended for pediatric use, an adjustment for a lower body weight would be appropriate.

As an example of the application of this equation, consider a toxicity study of acetonitrile in mice that is summarized in *Pharmeuropa*, Vol. 9, No. 1, Supplement, April 1997, page S24. The NOEL is calculated to be 50.7 mg/kg/day. The PDE for acetonitrile in this study is calculated as follows:

$$\text{PDE} = \frac{50.7\ \text{mg kg}^{-1}\ \text{day}^{-1} \times 50\ \text{kg}}{12 \times 10 \times 5 \times 1 \times 1} = 4.22\ \text{mg day}^{-1}$$

In this example,

F1 = 12 to account for the extrapolation from mice to humans
F2 = 10 to account for differences between individual humans
F3 = 5 because the duration of the study was only 13 weeks
F4 = 1 because no severe toxicity was encountered
F5 = 1 because the no-effect level was determined

The equation for an ideal gas, $PV = nRT$, is used to convert concentrations of gases used in inhalation studies from units of ppm to units of mg/L or mg/m^3. Consider as an example the rat reproductive toxicity study by inhalation of carbon tetrachloride (molecular weight 153.84) that is summarized in *Pharmeuropa*, Vol. 9, No. 1, Supplement, April 1997, page S9.

$$\frac{n}{V} = \frac{P}{RT} = \frac{300 \times 10^{-6}\ \text{atm} \times 153840\ \text{mg mol}^{-1}}{0.082\ \text{L atm K}^{-1}\ \text{mol}^{-1} \times 298\ \text{K}}$$
$$= \frac{46.15\ \text{mg}}{24.45\ \text{L}} = 1.89\ \text{mg/L}$$

The relationship 1000 L = 1 m^3 is used to convert to mg/m3.

17

Electronic Records and Signatures (CFR 21 Part 11 Compliance)

The regulations in 21 CFR part 11 set forth the criteria under which the agency (FDA) considers electronic records, electronic signatures, and handwritten signatures executed to electronic records to be trustworthy, reliable, and generally equivalent to paper records and handwritten signatures executed on paper. This chapter discusses the current revisions as of April 2008 on these compliance issues.

This part applies to records in electronic form that are created, modified, maintained, archived, retrieved, or transmitted, under any records requirements set forth in agency regulations. This part also applies to electronic records submitted to the agency under requirements of the Federal Food, Drug, and Cosmetic Act and the Public Health Service Act, even if such records are not specifically identified in agency regulations. However, this part does not apply to paper records that are, or have been, transmitted by electronic means.

Where electronic signatures and their associated electronic records meet the requirements of this part, the agency will consider the electronic signatures to be equivalent to full handwritten signatures, initials, and other general signings as required by agency regulations, unless specifically excepted by regulation(s) effective on or after August 20, 1997.

Electronic records that meet the requirements of this part may be used in lieu of paper records, in accordance with 11.2, unless paper records are specifically required.

Computer systems (including hardware and software), controls, and attendant documentation maintained under this part shall be readily available for, and subject to, FDA inspection.

This part does not apply to records required to be established or maintained by 1.326 through 1.368 of this chapter. Records that satisfy the requirements of part 1, subpart J of this chapter, but that also are required under other applicable statutory provisions or regulations, remain subject to this part.

For records required to be maintained but not submitted to the agency, persons may use electronic records in lieu of paper records or electronic signatures in lieu of traditional signatures, in whole or in part, provided that the requirements of this part are met.

For records submitted to the agency, persons may use electronic records in lieu of paper records or electronic signatures in lieu of traditional signatures, in whole or in part, provided that the requirements of this part are met and the document or parts of a document to be submitted have been identified in public docket No. 92S-0251 as being the type of submission the agency accepts in electronic form. This docket will identify specifically what types of documents or parts of documents are acceptable for submission in electronic form without paper records and the agency receiving unit(s) (e.g., specific center, office, division, branch) to which such submissions may be made. Documents to agency receiving unit(s) not specified in the public docket will not be considered as official if they are submitted in electronic form; paper forms of such documents will be considered as official and must accompany any electronic records. Persons are expected to consult with the intended agency receiving unit for details on how (e.g., method of transmission, media, file formats, and technical protocols) and whether to proceed with the electronic submission.

I. DEFINITIONS

The following definitions of terms also apply to this part:

- Act means the Federal Food, Drug, and Cosmetic Act [secs. 201–903 (21 USC 321–393)].
- Agency means the Food and Drug Administration.
- Biometrics means a method of verifying an individual's identity based on measurement of the individual's physical feature(s) or repeatable action(s) where those features and/or actions are both unique to that individual and measurable.
- Closed system means an environment in which system access is controlled by persons who are responsible for the content of electronic records that are on the system.
- Digital signature means an electronic signature based upon cryptographic methods of originator authentication, computed by using a set of rules and a set of parameters such that the identity of the signer and the integrity of the data can be verified.
- Electronic record means any combination of text, graphics, data, audio, pictorial, or other information representation in digital form that is created, modified, maintained, archived, retrieved, or distributed by a computer system.
- Electronic signature means a computer data compilation of any symbol or series of symbols executed, adopted, or authorized by an individual to be the legally binding equivalent of the individual's handwritten signature.
- Handwritten signature means the scripted name or legal mark of an individual handwritten by that individual and executed or adopted with the present intention to authenticate a writing in a permanent form. The act of signing with a writing or marking instrument such as a pen or stylus is preserved. The scripted name or legal mark, while conventionally applied to paper, may also be applied to other devices that capture the name or mark.
- Open system means an environment in which system access is not controlled by persons who are responsible for the content of electronic records that are on the system.

II. ELECTRONIC RECORDS—CONTROLS FOR CLOSED SYSTEMS

Persons who use closed systems to create, modify, maintain, or transmit electronic records shall employ procedures and controls designed to ensure the authenticity, integrity, and, when appropriate, the confidentiality of electronic records, and to ensure that the signer cannot readily repudiate the signed record as not genuine. Such procedures and controls shall include the following:

- Validation of systems to ensure accuracy, reliability, consistent intended performance, and the ability to discern invalid or altered records.
- The ability to generate accurate and complete copies of records in both human readable and electronic form suitable for inspection, review, and copying by the agency. Persons should contact the agency if there are any questions regarding the ability of the agency to perform such review and copying of the electronic records.
- Protection of records to enable their accurate and ready retrieval throughout the records retention period.
- Limiting system access to authorized individuals.
- Use of secure, computer-generated, time-stamped audit trails to independently record the date and time of operator entries and actions that create, modify, or delete electronic records. Record changes shall not obscure previously recorded information. Such audit trail documentation shall be retained for a period at least as long as that required for the subject electronic records and shall be available for agency review and copying.
- Use of operational system checks to enforce permitted sequencing of steps and events, as appropriate.
- Use of authority checks to ensure that only authorized individuals can use the system, electronically sign a record, access the operation or computer system input or output device, alter a record, or perform the operation at hand.
- Use of device (e.g., terminal) checks to determine, as appropriate, the validity of the source of data input or operational instruction.
- Determination that persons who develop, maintain, or use electronic record/electronic signature systems have the education, training, and experience to perform their assigned tasks.
- The establishment of, and adherence to, written policies that hold individuals accountable and responsible for actions initiated under their electronic signatures, in order to deter record and signature falsification.
- Use of appropriate controls over systems documentation including
  - adequate controls over the distribution of, access to, and use of documentation for system operation and maintenance and
  - revision and change control procedures to maintain an audit trail that documents time-sequenced development and modification of systems documentation.

III. CONTROLS FOR OPEN SYSTEMS

Persons who use open systems to create, modify, maintain, or transmit electronic records shall employ procedures and controls designed to ensure the authenticity, integrity, and, as appropriate, the confidentiality of electronic records from the point of their creation to the point of their receipt. Such procedures and controls shall include those identified above, as appropriate, and additional measures such as document encryption and use of appropriate digital signature standards to ensure, as necessary under the circumstances, record authenticity, integrity, and confidentiality.

A. Signature Manifestations

- Signed electronic records shall contain information associated with the signing that clearly indicates all of the following:
  - The printed name of the signer;
  - The date and time when the signature was executed; and
  - The meaning (such as review, approval, responsibility, or authorship) associated with the signature.
- The items identified in paragraphs above this section shall be subject to the same controls as for electronic records and shall be included as part of any human readable form of the electronic record (such as electronic display or printout).

B. Signature/Record Linking

Electronic signatures and handwritten signatures executed to electronic records shall be linked to their respective electronic records to ensure that the signatures cannot be excised, copied, or otherwise transferred to falsify an electronic record by ordinary means.

C. Electronic Signatures

- Each electronic signature shall be unique to one individual and shall not be reused by, or reassigned to, anyone else.
- Before an organization establishes, assigns, certifies, or otherwise sanctions an individual's electronic signature, or any element of such electronic signature, the organization shall verify the identity of the individual.
- Persons using electronic signatures shall, prior to or at the time of such use, certify to the agency that the electronic signatures in their system, used on or after August 20, 1997, are intended to be the legally binding equivalent of traditional handwritten signatures.
  - The certification shall be submitted in paper form and signed with a traditional handwritten signature, to the Office of Regional Operations (HFC-100), 5600 Fishers Lane, Rockville, MD 20857.
  - Persons using electronic signatures shall, upon agency request, provide additional certification or testimony that a specific electronic signature is the legally binding equivalent of the signer's handwritten signature.

IV. ELECTRONIC SIGNATURE COMPONENTS AND CONTROLS

- Electronic signatures that are not based upon biometrics shall:
  - employ at least two distinct identification components such as an identification code and password.
- When an individual executes a series of signings during a single, continuous period of controlled system access, the first signing shall be executed using all electronic signature components; subsequent signings shall be executed using at least one electronic signature component that is only executable by, and designed to be used only by, the individual.
- When an individual executes one or more signings not performed during a single, continuous period of controlled system access, each signing shall be executed using all of the electronic signature components.
  - Be used only by their genuine owners; and
  - Be administered and executed to ensure that attempted use of an individual's electronic signature by anyone

other than its genuine owner requires collaboration of two or more individuals.

- Electronic signatures based upon biometrics shall be designed to ensure that they cannot be used by anyone other than their genuine owners.

V. CONTROLS FOR IDENTIFICATION CODES/PASSWORDS

Persons who use electronic signatures based upon use of identification codes in combination with passwords shall employ controls to ensure their security and integrity. Such controls shall include:

- Maintaining the uniqueness of each combined identification code and password, such that no two individuals have the same combination of identification code and password.
- Ensuring that identification code and password issuances are periodically checked, recalled, or revised (e.g., to cover such events as password aging).
- Following loss management procedures to electronically deauthorize lost, stolen, missing, or otherwise potentially compromised tokens, cards, and other devices that bear or generate identification code or password information, and to issue temporary or permanent replacements using suitable, rigorous controls.
- Use of transaction safeguards to prevent unauthorized use of passwords and/or identification codes, and to detect and report in an immediate and urgent manner any attempts at their unauthorized use to the system security unit, and, as appropriate, to organizational management.
- Initial and periodic testing of devices, such as tokens or cards, that bear or generate identification code or password information to ensure that they function properly and have not been altered in an unauthorized manner.

VI. EXPLICATORY NOTES ABOUT 21 CFR PART 11 COMPLIANCE

The guidance described above is intended to describe the Food and Drug Administration's (FDA's) current thinking (as of April 2008) regarding the scope and application of part 11 of Title 21 of the Code of Federal Regulations; Electronic Records; Electronic Signatures (21 CFR part 11).

Given below is a discussion on how to implement systems that would fulfill the requirements in the above guidance. This pertains mostly to persons who maintain records or submit information to FDA and have chosen to maintain the records or submit designated information electronically and, as a result, have become subject to part 11. Part 11 applies to records in electronic form that are created, modified, maintained, archived, retrieved, or transmitted under any records requirements set forth in Agency regulations. Part 11 also applies to electronic records submitted to the Agency under the Federal Food, Drug, and Cosmetic Act (the Act) and the Public Health Service Act (the PHS Act), even if such records are not specifically identified in Agency regulations (§ 11.1). The underlying requirements set forth in the Act, PHS Act, and FDA regulations (other than part 11) are referred to in this guidance document as predicate rules.

As an outgrowth of its current good manufacturing practice (CGMP) initiative for human and animal drugs and biologics, FDA continuously reexamines how part 11 applies to all FDA regulated products. In making rules based on the guidance, FDA interprets the scope of part 11 rather narrowly. The FDA does not currently exercise enforcement discretion with respect to certain part 11 requirements to enforce compliance with the validation, audit trail, record retention, and record copying requirements of part 11. However, records must still be maintained or submitted in accordance with the underlying predicate rules, and the Agency can take regulatory action for noncompliance with such predicate rules.

The FDA does not intend to take (or recommend) action to enforce any part 11 requirements with regard to systems that were operational before August 20, 1997, the effective date of part 11 (commonly known as legacy systems).

A. Overall Approach to Part 11 Requirements

As described in more detail below, the approach outlined in this guidance is based on three main elements:

- Part 11 will be interpreted narrowly and FDA offers clarification on which record are considered subject to part 11.
- For those records that remain subject to part 11, FDA exercises enforcement discretion with regard to part 11 requirements for validation, audit trails, record retention, and record copying in the manner described in this guidance and with regard to all part 11 requirements for systems that were operational before the effective date of part 11 (also known as legacy systems).
- FDA will enforce all predicate rule requirements, including predicate rule record and record-keeping requirements.

It is important to note that FDA's exercise of enforcement discretion as described in this guidance is limited to specified part 11 requirements (setting aside legacy systems, as to which the extent of enforcement discretion, under certain circumstances, will be more broad). FDA enforces all other provisions of part 11 including, but not limited to, certain controls for closed systems in § 11.10. For example, we intend to enforce provisions related to the following controls and requirements:

- limiting system access to authorized individuals
- use of operational system checks
- use of authority checks
- use of device checks
- determination that persons who develop, maintain, or use electronic systems have the education, training, and experience to perform their assigned tasks
- establishment of and adherence to written policies that hold individuals accountable for actions initiated under their electronic signatures
- appropriate controls over systems documentation
- controls for open systems corresponding to controls for closed systems bulleted above (§ 11.30)
- requirements related to electronic signatures (e.g., §§ 11.50, 11.70, 11.100, 11.200, and 11.300)

The FDA expects compliance with these provisions, and enforces them. Furthermore, persons must comply with applicable predicate rules, and records that are required to be maintained or submitted must remain secure and reliable in accordance with the predicate rules.

B. Details of Approach—Scope of Part 11

The FDA interprets part 11 rather narrowly since broad interpretations could lead to unnecessary controls and costs and could discourage innovation and technological advances without providing added benefit to the public health. Under the narrow interpretation of the scope of part 11, with respect to records required to be maintained under predicate rules or submitted to FDA, when persons choose to use records in electronic format in place of paper format, part 11 would apply. On the other hand, when persons use computers to generate paper printouts of electronic records, and those paper records meet all the requirements of the applicable predicate rules and persons rely on the paper records to perform their regulated activities, FDA would generally not consider persons to be "using electronic records in lieu of paper records" under §§ 11.2(a) and 11.2(b). In these instances, the use of computer systems in the generation of paper records would not trigger part 11.

C. Definition of Part 11 Records

Under this narrow interpretation, FDA considers part 11 to be applicable to the following records or signatures in electronic format (part 11 records or signatures):

- Records that are required to be maintained under predicate rule requirements and that are maintained in electronic format in place of paper format. On the other hand, records (and any associated signatures) that are not required to be retained under predicate rules, but that are nonetheless maintained in electronic format, are not part 11 records. It is recommended that firms determine, based on the predicate rules, whether specific records are part 11 records and document such decisions.
- Records that are required to be maintained under predicate rules, that are maintained in electronic format in addition to paper format, and that are relied on to perform regulated activities. In some cases, actual business practices may dictate whether firms are using electronic records instead of paper records under § 11.2(a). For example, if a record is required to be maintained under a predicate rule and you use a computer to generate a paper printout of the electronic records, but the firm nonetheless relies on the electronic record to perform regulated activities, the Agency may consider you to be using the electronic record instead of the paper record. That is, the Agency may take your business practices into account in determining whether part 11 applies. Accordingly, FDA recommends that for each record required to be maintained under predicate rules, you determine in advance whether you plan to rely on the electronic record or paper record to perform regulated activities. We recommend that you document this decision [e.g., in a standard operating procedure (SOP), or specification document].
- Records submitted to FDA, under predicate rules (even if such records are not specifically identified in Agency regulations) in electronic format (assuming the records have been identified in docket number 92S-0251 as the types of submissions the Agency accepts in electronic format). However, a record that is not itself submitted, but is used in generating a submission, is not a part 11 record unless it is otherwise required to be maintained under a predicate rule and it is maintained in electronic format.
- Electronic signatures that are intended to be the equivalent of handwritten signatures, initials, and other general signings required by predicate rules. Part 11 signatures include electronic signatures that are used, for example, to document the fact that certain events or actions occurred in accordance with the predicate rule (e.g., approved, reviewed, and verified).

D. Approach to Specific Part 11 Requirements

1. Validation: The Agency exercises enforcement discretion regarding specific part 11 requirements for validation of computerized systems [§ 11.10(a) and corresponding requirements in § 11.30]. Although persons must still comply with all applicable predicate rule requirements for validation [e.g., 21 CFR 820.70(i)], this guidance should not be read to impose any additional requirements for validation. It is suggested that a firm's decision to validate computerized systems, and the extent of the validation, take into account the impact the systems have on its ability to meet predicate rule requirements. Firms should also consider the impact those systems might have on the accuracy, reliability, integrity, availability, and authenticity of required records and signatures. Even if there is no predicate rule requirement to validate a system, in some instances it may still be important to validate the system. It is also recommended that firms base their approach on a justified and documented risk assessment and a determination of the potential of the system to affect product quality and safety, and record integrity. For instance, validation would not be important for a word processor used only to generate SOPs.
2. Audit Trail: The Agency exercises enforcement discretion regarding specific part 11 requirements related to computer-generated, time-stamped audit trails [§ 11.10 (e), (k)(2) and any corresponding requirement in § 11.30]. Persons must still comply with all applicable predicate rule requirements related to documentation of, for example, date [e.g., § 58.130(e)], time, or sequencing of events, as well as any requirements for ensuring that changes to records do not obscure previous entries. Even if there are no predicate rule requirements to document, for example, date, time, or sequence of events in a particular instance, it may nonetheless be important to have audit trails or other physical, logical, or procedural security measures in place to ensure the trustworthiness and reliability of the records. It is recommended that firms base their decision on whether to apply audit trails, or other appropriate measures, on the need to comply with predicate rule requirements, a justified and documented risk assessment, and a determination of the potential effect on product quality and safety and record integrity. It is also recommended that firms apply appropriate controls based on such an assessment. Audit trails can be particularly appropriate when users are expected to create, modify, or delete regulated records during normal operation.
3. Legacy Systems: The Agency exercises enforcement discretion with respect to all part 11 requirements for systems that otherwise were operational prior to August 20, 1997, the effective date of part 11, under the circumstances specified below. This means that the Agency does not intend to take enforcement action to enforce compliance with any part 11 requirements if all the following criteria are met for a specific system:
   a. The system was operational before the effective date.
   b. The system met all applicable predicate rule requirements before the effective date.
   c. The system currently meets all applicable predicate rule requirements.
   d. Firm has documented evidence and justification that the system is fit for its intended use (including having an acceptable level of record security and integrity, if applicable).
   e. If a system has been changed since August 20, 1997, and if the changes would prevent the system from meeting predicate rule requirements, part 11 controls should be applied to part 11 records and signatures pursuant to the enforcement policy expressed in this guidance.

E. Copies of Records

The Agency exercises enforcement discretion with regard to specific part 11 requirements for generating copies of records [§ 11.10 (b) and any corresponding requirement in § 11.30]. Firms should provide an investigator with reasonable and useful access to records during an inspection. All records held by firms are subject to inspection in accordance with predicate rules [e.g., §§ 211.180(c), (d), and 108.35(c)(3)(ii)].

It is recommend that firms supply copies of electronic records by

- producing copies of records held in common portable formats when records are maintained in these formats;
- Using established automated conversion or export methods, where available, to make copies in a more common format (examples of such formats include, but are not limited to, PDF, XML, or SGML).

In each case, it is recommended that the copying process used produces copies that preserve the content and meaning of the record. If you have the ability to search, sort, or trend part 11 records, copies given to the Agency should provide the same capability if it is reasonable and technically feasible. You should allow inspection, review, and copying of records in a human readable form at your site using your hardware and following your established procedures and techniques for accessing records.

F. Record Retention

The Agency exercises enforcement discretion with regard to the part 11 requirements for the protection of records to enable their accurate and ready retrieval throughout the records retention period [§ 11.10 (c) and any corresponding requirement in § 11.30]. Persons must still comply with all applicable predicate rule requirements for record retention and availability [e.g., §§ 211.180(c),(d), 108.25(g), and 108.35(h)]. It is suggested that firm's decision on how to maintain records be based on predicate rule requirements and that the firm bases its decision on a justified and documented risk assessment and a determination of the value of the records over time.

FDA does not object if firms decide to archive required records in electronic format to nonelectronic media such as microfilm, microfiche, and paper, or to a standard electronic file format (examples of such formats include, but are not limited to, PDF, XML, or SGML). Persons must still comply with all predicate rule requirements, and the records themselves and any copies of the required records should preserve their content and meaning. As long as predicate rule requirements are fully satisfied and the content and meaning of the records are preserved and archived, you can delete the electronic version of the records. In addition, paper and electronic record and signature components can coexist (i.e., a hybrid situation) as long as predicate rule requirements are met and the content and meaning of those records are preserved.

VII. ESTABLISHING A COMPLIANCE PLAN

A large number of vendors are available to assist companies in identifying the level of compliance, building software control systems and auditing facilities to assure continued compliance. However, it is not possible for any vendor to offer a "turnkey" solution since compliance requires both procedural controls (i.e., notification, training, SOPs, administration) and administrative controls to be put in place by the user in addition to the technical controls that the vendor can offer. Vendors should be relied only for supply of application containing the required technical requirements of a compliant system.

In keeping records, question often arises on the type of media used to store data, particularly the type that is alterable such as flash memory or memory buffer. Generally, this is not the main concern how the data are stored, the important thing for the FDA to consider is whether the operator can manipulate the data before they are printed. The real problem is that most of this equipment does not have functions as required by part 11.

Often firms use a hybrid system who have not yet developed confidence in electronic database management. A "Hybrid System" is defined as an environment consisting of both Electronic and Paper-based Records (Frequently Characterized by Handwritten Signatures Executed on Paper). A very common example of a Hybrid System is one in which the system user generates an electronic record using a computer-based system (e-batch records, analytical instruments, etc.) and then is require to sign that record as per the Predicate Rules (GLP, GMP. GCP). However, the system does not have an electronic signature option, so the user has to print out the report and sign the paper copy. Now he has an electronic record and a paper/handwritten signature. The "system" has an electronic and a paper component, hence the term, hybrid. Since part 11 does not require that electronic records be signed using electronic signatures, e-records may be signed with handwritten signatures that are applied to electronic records or handwritten signatures that are applied to a piece of paper. If the handwritten signature is applied to a piece of paper, it must link to the electronic record. The FDA will publish guidance on how to achieve this link in the future, but for now it is suggested that firms include in the paper as much information as possible to accurately identify the unique electronic record (e.g., at least file name, size in bytes, creation date, and a hash or checksum value.) Hoverer, the master record is still the electronic record. Thus, signing a printout of an electronic record does not exempt the electronic record from part 11 compliance. There is no deadline for converting to electronic signatures. Having handwritten signatures on paper is acceptable if signature are linked to electronic records so signers cannot repudiate records.

Audio recordings of regulated patient information or experimental observations are infrequent, but sometimes acquired. Also, audio conferences discussing projects, reports, data are common in the pharma industry. If the data therein is required to be maintained by predicate rules, and the audio file is saved to durable media, part 11 would apply.

An audit trail initiation requirements differ for data versus textual materials. For data: if you are generating, retaining, importing, or exporting any electronic data, the Audit Trail begins from the instant the data hits the durable media. For textual documents: if the document is subject to approval and review, the Audit Trail begins upon approval and release of the document. The execution of a signature is also part of audit trail. When using e-mails as recorded data, then the e-mails have to be managed in a compliant way.

The restrictions regarding login are specific and enforceable. A single restricted login does not suffice as an electronic signature. The operator has to indicate intent when signing something, and he has to reenter the user ID/password (shows awareness that he is executing a signature) and give the meaning for the e-sig. To support this, part 11 § 11.50, states that signed e-records shall contain information associated with the signing that indicates the printed name of the signer, the date/time, and the meaning, and that these items shall be included in any human readable form of the record. The predicate rules mandate when a regulated document needs to be signed. It is however not necessary for a firm to certify that every associate's electronic signature is legally binding. The required one-time e-sig certification is for an organization as a whole. Its intent is to certify that a company recognizes that its e-signatures are equivalent to their handwritten signatures.

The Agency has recently reconsidered its position on local date and time stamp requirements. The draft guidance document reflects their current thinking, and supersedes the position with respect to the time zone that should be recorded. The document states, "You should implement time stamps with a clear understanding of what time zone reference you use. Systems documentation should explain time zone references as well as zone acronyms or other naming conventions."

According to the Rule, the definition of closed system is "an environment in which system access is controlled by persons who are responsible for the content of electronic records that are on the system." The agency agrees that the most important factor in classifying a system as closed or open is whether the persons responsible for the content of the electronic records control access to the system containing those records. A system is closed if persons responsible for the content of the records control access. If those persons do not control such access, then the system is open because the records may be read, modified, or compromised by others to the possible detriment of the persons responsible for record content. Hence, those responsible for the records would need to take appropriate additional measures in an open system to protect those records from being read, modified, destroyed, or otherwise compromised by unauthorized and potentially unknown parties.

Part 11 sec. 11.70 states that electronic signatures and handwritten signatures executed to electronic records must be linked (i.e., verifiably bound) to their respective records to ensure that signatures could not be excised, copied, or otherwise transferred to falsify another electronic record. The agency does not, however, intend to mandate use of any particular "linking" technology. FDA recognizes that, because it is relatively easy to copy an electronic signature to another electronic record and thus compromise or falsify that record, a technology-based link is necessary. The agency does not believe that procedural or administrative controls alone are sufficient to ensure that objective because such controls could be more easily circumvented than a straightforward technology-based approach.

A predicate rule is any requirements set forth in the Act (Federal Food, Drug and Cosmetic Act), the PHS Act (Public Health Service Act), or any FDA regulation (GxP: GLP, GMP, GCP, etc.). The predicate rules mandate what records must be maintained; the content of records; whether signatures are required; how long records must be maintained, etc. If there is no FDA requirement that a particular record be created or retained, then 21 CFR part 11 most likely does not apply to the record.

To make sure that e-records are still readable throughout the retention period (with focus on the formats), there are several possible solutions being considered include data migration, data emulation, and system "Time Capsules". As of today, there are no set standards, or widely accepted procedures to ensure long-term data viability.

Meta data is defined as "data about data". In practical terms, the types of metadata that can be associated with an electronic record may include the following: details of the record's creation, author, creation date, ownership, searchable keywords that can be used to classify the document, details of the type of data found in the document, and the relationships between different data components. Metadata must be stored as an integral part of the electronic document it describes.

The use of Electronic Signatures implies that your system is an Electronic Record system and, therefore, must be in compliance with all provisions of 21 CFR part 11. For the exact wording for the e-sig certification, please consult the FDA website at www.fda.gov. One can also find wording for the certification in the preamble of the final Rule. The response to comment #120 is "...The final rule instructs persons to send certifications to FDA's Office of Regional Operations (HFC-100), 5600 Fishers Lane, Rockville, MD 20857. Persons outside the United States may send their certifications to the same office. The agency offers, as guidance, an example of an acceptable sec. 11.100(c) certification: Pursuant to section 11.100 of title 21 of the Code of Federal Regulations, this is to certify that (name of organization) intends that all electronic signatures executed by our employees, agents, or representatives, located anywhere in the world, are the legally binding equivalent of traditional handwritten signatures."

In an effort to remain technologically neutral, the FDA does not specify the kind of media that one must use for archiving. There are studies currently underway from independent sources that are trying to test the "lifetime" of such media as CD-ROM, although there is no set standard lifetime for such media. Some companies are doing their own tests on media lifetime.

Whether part 11 applies to instruments that are not connected to computers but that have microprocessors within depends whether such a system generates electronic records according to the definition of e-records in part 11 (data starting its life written to durable media), and/or these e-records are not subject to the GxP regulations, then part 11 does not apply.

The "Predicate Rules" (GxP) regulations determine what records must be signed, not part 11. Not all e-records need to be signed. Check your predicate rules for what records must be signed, when and by whom.

In order for a system to comply with part 11, both the hardware and the software should be under controlled access. This is necessary to monitor who is signing the documents.

Although it is not specified in part 11, most software programs that execute e-sigs and that have notification capabilities report attempts via an e-mail notice to a database administrator for any forgery attempts.

The audit trail for Excel should capture changes to both the data and to formulas. Things like formatting changes (alignment/font) to cells do not have to be audit trailed.

Hashing can be used for accessing data or for data security. A hash is a number generated from a string of text. The hash is substantially smaller than the text itself and is generated by a formula in such a way that it is unlikely that some other text will produce the same hash value. Hashes play a role in security systems where they are used to ensure that transmitted messages have not been tampered with. The sender generates a hash of the message, encrypts it, and sends it with the message itself. The recipient then decrypts both the message and the hash, produces another hash from the received message, and compares the two hashes. If they are the same, there is a very high probability that the message was transmitted intact.

In part 11.300, controls for identification codes/passwords usage is listed under.

The controls for password/user ID usage apply across the board for ERES systems. They apply to the proper management of electronic records in addition to executing compliant electronic signatures.

For part 11, data integrity is related to the trustworthiness of the electronic records generated/managed by critical systems. The FDA is most concerned about systems that are involved with drug distribution, drug approval, manufacturing, and quality assurance because these systems pose the most risk in terms of product quality and/or public safety.

What type of "reporting" capability on audit trail data should be supported?

According to part 11 § 11.10 (e) audit trails must be secure, computer-generated and time-stamped to independently record the date and time of operator entries and actions that create, modify, or delete electronic records. Such audit trail documentation shall be retained for a period at least as long as that required for the subject electronic records and shall be available for agency review and copying. Audit trails should say "who did what to your records and when (why for GLP)". Part 11 does not specify the format for audit trials. This should be discussed in a forthcoming FDA guidance document for part 11 audit trails.

A digital signature is computed using a set of rules and a mathematical algorithm such that the identity of the signatory and integrity of the data can be verified. Signature generation makes use of a private key to generate a digital signature. Signature verification makes use of a public key that corresponds to, but is not the same as, the private key. Each user possesses a private and public key pair. Public keys are obviously known to the public, while private keys are never shared. Anyone can verify the signature of a user by employing that user's public key. Only the possessor of the user's private key can perform signature generation. A hash function is used in the signature generation process to obtain a condensed version of data, called a message digest. The message digest is then incorporated into the mathematical algorithm to generate the digital signature. The digital signature is sent to the intended verifier along with the signed message. The verifier of the message and signature verifies the signature by using the sender's public key. The same hash function must also be used in the verification process. The hash function is specified in a separate standard.

For an analytical instrument, any information that is captured by a computerized workstation is considered either data or metadata. (Metadata is described as data-about-data. It is what puts the real data into logical context.) The second that any information hits the "durable media" it then becomes an electronic record. Parameters that are typically captured by an HPLC system (i.e., flow rate, sample lot #, etc.) are considered metadata. This information should be saved and protected as part of the official electronic record.

VIII. SOFTWARE AND SYSTEMS SUPPORT

The Food and Drug Administration (FDA) in the United States designed part 11 of title 21 of the Code of Federal Regulations (21 CFR part 11) to help ensure that life sciences companies can use electronic records and signatures that are equivalent to those based on paper and ink. However, initiating and maintaining part 11 compliance can be complex and costly. Many excellent fully validated software systems are available for all levels of investment. Most notably, SAP and Oracle systems now provide full integration of all recommendations made in part 11. On the other end of the cost of deployment, the 2007 Microsoft Office system simplifies compliance with support for the complete document lifecycle. In fact, much of the functionality necessary for part 11 compliance is built into the Office system, including workflow, audit trails, digital signatures, and full versioning support.

The life sciences industry is challenged with increasingly stringent regulations, requiring enormous volumes of documentation. Electronic document management has helped to streamline these documentation processes. However, in the life sciences industry, the way in which this documentation is managed comes with its own specific regulations, known as 21 CFR part 11.

These FDA regulations establish criteria under which electronic records and signatures can be considered equivalent to paper-based records and handwritten signatures. Without a part 11-compliant document management environment, life sciences companies that fail to meet compliance regulations are subject to substantial fines or the shutdown of operations. Technology requirements pertaining to part 11 compliance include the following:

- Security controls to prevent unauthorized access to documents
- Time and date-stamped audit trails recording changes to records
- Electronic signatures on documents with name, date, and purpose of signature
- Policies that hold users accountable for documents

Although many systems exist that claim to be part 11-compliant, they are often too complex to be effective. Common complaints include the following:

- The inability to collaborate efficiently on documentation while maintaining competitive speed-to-market
- Difficulty locating files across multiple databases and applications
- Lack of understanding and use of compliant enterprise content management systems
- Bottlenecks resulting from having only one "expert" appointed to post documents into a repository

The 2007 Microsoft Office system provides easy-to-use document management tools that can help life science companies of all sizes achieve part 11 compliance quickly and cost-effectively. Following are the key features that address specific part 11 requirements:

- Document security. Apply restrictions to individual documents and across entire libraries in order to more easily control who can open, copy, print, or forward information. A records vault prevents direct tampering of documents and helps ensure the protection of original versions. Portal access is password-protected, and access to specific content can be restricted based on role.
- Detailed auditing. Powerful document tracking functionality provides a detailed, time-stamped audit trail of document management activity.
- Digital signatures. The applications of the 2007 Microsoft Office system automatically assess the authenticity of digital signatures and signed documents and alert the administrator if there are any discrepancies.
- Automated workflow and policies. Managers can easily configure templates so that all the elements required for compliance (such as specific content fields, digital signature fields, and policy requirements) can be built directly

into a Microsoft Office Word 2007 or Microsoft Office Excel 2007 file. This helps support compliant practices and helps ensure that documents are automatically assigned to the right people for review and approval.

By adopting a 21 CFR part 11 solution based on the 2007 Microsoft Office system, life sciences companies can

- dramatically simplify the document management processes required for compliance;
- reduce errors by using predefined templates;
- encourage compliant document management practices through familiar, easy-to-use Microsoft technologies;
- minimize compliance-related headcount;
- reduce compliance and infrastructure costs by leveraging investments in Microsoft products; and
- implement a solution quickly without disrupting the organization.

To rapidly address 21 CFR part 11 challenges, the 2007 Microsoft Office system is the ideal choice. New technologies built into the 2007 Microsoft Office system can help in the following ways:

- Simplify the management of complex compliance process
- Users can easily initiate a wide range of automated workflows directly from Microsoft Office Word 2007 or Microsoft Office Excel 2007, including reviews, approvals, edits, requests for digital signatures, and feedback
- Administrators can track each workflow and monitor how it performs overall, as well as drill down into specific instances of a workflow
- Content types allow administrators and compliance managers to predefine templates so that all new documents of a given type are automatically assigned the appropriate policies, such as workflow, resulting actions, and expiration
- Perform detailed audit analysis
- Microsoft Office SharePoint Server 2007 allows administrators to audit key events within document libraries and monitor global events on a site (such as search, user changes, and changes in content types and columns), which creates evidence of who accessed which resources at what time
- A central administration site makes it easy to configure various settings for auditing, such as selecting specific events to audit
- Auditing functionality can be extended using a Web service or by using the audit log service object model, so other applications can provide a full audit when their files are stored on a SharePoint site
- Protect data with more powerful security features
- Users of the portal are authenticated automatically based on their role and user information from Active Directory
- Information Rights Management (IRM) policies can be applied to both individual documents and entire libraries, making it easier to get consistent use of IRM across a set of documents without creating extra work for individual users
- The applications of the 2007 Microsoft Office system automatically assess the authenticity of digital signatures and signed documents, and alert the administrator if there are any discrepancies
- A records repository facilitates security-enhanced document management processes, including content collection, consistent policy enforcement, item retention and holds in response to external events, and content expiration
- Reduce administrative costs with new tools and formats
- New, XML-based file formats for Microsoft Office Word 2007, Microsoft Office Excel 2007, and Microsoft Office PowerPoint 2007 can allow these documents to easily integrate with existing and future line-of-business systems
- Office Open XML Formats use ZIP compression technology, so documents take up far less space than the previous formats, which means shorter transmission times and a smaller impact on storage
- The Office Customization Tool simplifies customization simple and efficient by replacing the many wizards that were necessary in previous releases of the Microsoft Office
- Leverage deployed Microsoft technologies
- Roll out a 21 CFR part 11 solution quickly, with minimal training, leveraging the familiar Microsoft products you have already installed
- Maintain a low total cost of ownership by extending investments in Microsoft products
- Take advantage of a rich network of technology partners who are well-versed in Microsoft Office technologies and 21 CFR part 11 implementations

The 2007 Microsoft Office system is an integrated set of products, technologies, and services that enable customers to increase their organizational, team, and personal productivity. A 21 CFR part 11-compliant solution often uses these products and technologies:

Microsoft Office SharePoint Server 2007
Microsoft Office Word 2007
Microsoft Office Excel 2007
Microsoft Office InfoPath 2007

In addition to Microsoft products, many companies have partnered with Microsoft to offer very affordable solutions to part 11 compliance. Some of these include the following:

- NextDocs Corporation: NextDocs Document Management. NextDocs DM is an enterprise document and records management solution.
- QualityDocs is end-to-end quality management system that enables management of quality documents and processes.
- EmployeeDocs is a robust tracking and employee record management system.
- ProjectDocs provides turnkey project level document management.
- ThoughtBridge, LLC: Engineering Change Orders (ECOs). ThoughtBridge has created an automated, systematic approach to driving the ECO process—and customized it for the life sciences industry using the 2007 Microsoft Office System. ECOs help companies monitor and track activities associated with any changes to its products.
- Zorch Software: Zorch DM/Zorch Submission Manager. Zorch Software provides comprehensive Microsoft-based document management and submission management solutions.
- Clusterseven Ltd: Enterprise Spreadsheet Management Software is a complete solution to support the use of Excel spreadsheets as operational applications in business-critical processes. It delivers auditability, regulatory compliance (e.g., SOX), reduced risk, change management and transparency of data and activity. It does all this without reducing the flexibility and familiarity that makes Excel so powerful at delivering fast, competitive and cost-effective solutions to changing business needs.
- Perficient: Collaborative Document Generation and Workflow. The Collaborative Document Generation and

Workflow solution is a comprehensive Document Creation application that automatically generates word documents for very complex documents with a high degree of business rules and processing.

- Newtech Global Solutions LLC: NGS's SPLGen. A quality process that lighten the need for companies to undertake significant internal review prior to submission in preparing and validating the SPL XML data. The ability to keep labeling documents within Microsoft Share Point Electronic Document Management System, so it meets document compliance and record management requirements. SPLGen has an option to import SPL compliant XML data files from other systems like DailyMed.
- Strategic Thought Group PLC: Active Risk Manager. Providing compliance, project, operational and corporate risk, control, opportunity, and issue management. Fully integrated to the MS Project Server family of products and MS SharePoint. Delivers value streams for projects, assets, processes, organization, key performance indicators and financial accounts.
- Workshare USA: Workshare Professional. Workshare Professional is an Outbound Content Security and Document Integrity solution that eliminates the risk of content leaks and inaccuracies, enabling the safe, compliant and high speed information exchange needed in today's competitive business environment.
- Workshare, an information security company, delivers Secure Content Compliance solutions ensuring safe information exchange without business disruption. SourceCode – K2.net Workflow: K2.net BlackPearl (K2.net 2007).

BIBLIOGRAPHY

Glossary of Computerized System and Software Development Terminology (Division of Field Investigations, Office of Regional Operations, Office of Regulatory Affairs, FDA 1995) (http://www.fda.gov/ora/inspect_ref/igs/gloss.html)

General Principles of Software Validation; Final Guidance for Industry and FDA Staff (FDA, Center for Devices and Radiological Health, Center for Biologics Evaluation and Research, 2002) (http://www.fda.gov/cdrh/comp/guidance/938.html)

Guidance for Industry, FDA Reviewers, and Compliance on Off-The-Shelf Software Use in Medical Devices (FDA, Center for Devices and Radiological Health, 1999) (http://www.fda.gov/cdrh/ode/guidance/585.html)

Pharmaceutical CGMPs for the 21st Century: A Risk-Based Approach; A Science and Risk-Based Approach to Product Quality Regulation Incorporating an Integrated Quality Systems Approach (FDA 2002) (http://www.fda.gov/oc/guidance/gmp.html)

The Good Automated Manufacturing Practice (GAMP) Guide for Validation of Automated Systems, GAMP 4 (ISPE/GAMP Forum, 2001) (http://www.ispe.org/gamp/).

ISO/IEC 17799:2000 (BS 7799:2000) Information technology – Code of practice for information security management (ISO/IEC, 2000).

ISO 14971:2002 Medical Devices – Application of risk management to medical devices (ISO, 2001)

18

GMP Audit Template, EU Guidelines (http://ec.europa.eu/enterprise/pharmaceuticals/eudralex/vol4_en.htm)

		Compliance 1 2 3[a]	Remarks	EU Guide
1	**PERSONNEL**			
1.1	Qualified personnel available?	☐ ☐ ☐		2.1
1.2	Organization charts available?	☐ ☐ ☐		2.2
1.3	Job descriptions available?	☐ ☐ ☐		2.2
1.4	Responsibilities clearly defined?	☐ ☐ ☐		2.2
	Key personnel			
	Responsible persons designated for			
1.5	• production?	☐ ☐ ☐		2.5
1.6	• quality control?	☐ ☐ ☐		2.6
1.7	Are they independent from each other?	☐ ☐ ☐		2.3
1.8	Are joint functions clearly defined?	☐ ☐ ☐		2.7
1.9	Are the responsible persons working full time?	☐ ☐ ☐		2.3
1.10	Do the responsible persons have the appropriate formation, knowledge, and experience?	☐ ☐ ☐		2.1/2.2
1.11	Do the relevant departments have enough personnel?	☐ ☐ ☐		2.1
	Training			
1.12	Continuous training programs for the production and QC staff?	☐ ☐ ☐		2.8
1.13	Initial job training for all employees?	☐ ☐ ☐		2.9
1.14	Teaching aids (videos, slides, and brochures) available?	☐ ☐ ☐		2.9
1.15	External training courses for the staff?	☐ ☐ ☐		2.9
1.16	Training records?	☐ ☐ ☐		2.9
1.17	Special training in sensitive areas? (sterile prod. and toxic subs.)	☐ ☐ ☐		2.10
1.18	Information for visitors to the manufacturing area?	☐ ☐ ☐		2.11
2	**HYGIENE**			
	Personnel hygiene			
	Detailed written hygiene programs for			
2.1	• clothing?	☐ ☐ ☐		2.13
2.2	• use of washrooms?	☐ ☐ ☐		2.13
2.3	• behavior in production areas?	☐ ☐ ☐		2.13
2.4	Precautions against sick or personnel with open wounds in production?	☐ ☐ ☐		2.14
	Medical examination:			
2.5	• on recruitment?	☐ ☐ ☐		2.15
2.6	• regular reexaminations?	☐ ☐ ☐		2.15

		Compliance 1 2 3[a]	Remarks	EU Guide
	Duty of notification after:			
2.7	• trips to tropical countries?	☐ ☐ ☐		2.15
2.8	• cases of contagious illness in the family?	☐ ☐ ☐		2.15
2.9	Instructions for appropriate working clothes?	☐ ☐ ☐		2.16
2.10	Absence of food and drinks (chewing gum!) in the working area?	☐ ☐ ☐		2.17
2.11	Measures against contact with open product (gloves etc.)?	☐ ☐ ☐		2.18
2.12	Instructions for hand washing in production?	☐ ☐ ☐		2.19
2.13	Change of clothes when entering and leaving the production area?	☐ ☐ ☐		5.19
2.14	Change rooms and toilets easily within reach?	☐ ☐ ☐		3.31
2.15	Toilets and restrooms sufficiently separated from production areas?	☐ ☐ ☐		3.30/3.31
2.16	Workshops separate from production areas?	☐ ☐ ☐		3.32
2.17	Laboratory animal rooms totally segregated from production rooms?	☐ ☐ ☐		3.33
3	**WAREHOUSE**			
	Rooms, general			
3.1	Suitable for the intended use?	☐ ☐ ☐		3
3.2	• adequate size?	☐ ☐ ☐		3
3.3	• clean?	☐ ☐ ☐		3
3.4	Located and designed to exclude external contamination?	☐ ☐ ☐		3.1
3.5	Appropriate level of maintenance?	☐ ☐ ☐		3.2
3.6	Maintenance works possible without contamination risk?	☐ ☐ ☐		3.2
3.7	Appropriate lighting and air-conditioning?	☐ ☐ ☐		3.3
3.8	Recording of temperature and humidity?	☐ ☐ ☐		
3.9	Protection against the entry of insects or other animals?	☐ ☐ ☐		3.4
3.10	Controlled access for authorized personnel only?	☐ ☐ ☐		3.5
	Rooms, special requirements			
	Type of warehousing:			
3.11	Separation of goods sufficient?	☐ ☐ ☐		3.18
3.12	Provision for different storage temperatures?	☐ ☐ ☐		3.19
3.13	Goods receiving zone weather protected?	☐ ☐ ☐		3.20
3.14	Cleaning zone for incoming goods?	☐ ☐ ☐		3.20
3.15	Separate quarantine area with controlled access?	☐ ☐ ☐		3.21
3.16	Separate, protected sampling area?	☐ ☐ ☐		3.22
	Separate and safe storage of			
3.17	• returned goods?	☐ ☐ ☐		3.23
3.18	• rejected goods?	☐ ☐ ☐		3.23
3.19	Separate and safe storage of highly active, toxic, or dangerous substances?	☐ ☐ ☐		3.24
3.20	Safe storage of narcotics?	☐ ☐ ☐		3.24
3.21	Safe storage of printed packaging materials?	☐ ☐ ☐		3.25
3.22	Security measurements against theft?	☐ ☐ ☐		3.25
3.23	Smoke detectors?	☐ ☐ ☐		3.25
3.24	Fire extinguishing system?	☐ ☐ ☐		3.25

		Compliance 1 2 3[a]	Remarks	EU Guide
	Operations			
3.25	Reception, sampling, and labeling according to written procedures?	☐ ☐ ☐		5.2
3.26	Is a sampling plan available?	☐ ☐ ☐		Suppl. 4
3.27	Cleaning of incoming containers?	☐ ☐ ☐		5.3
3.28	Investigation and recording of damaged deliveries?	☐ ☐ ☐		5.4
3.29	FIFO principle?	☐ ☐ ☐		5.7
3.30	Inventory system?	☐ ☐ ☐		5.8
3.31	The location of materials can be detected at all times?	☐ ☐ ☐		
3.32	Incoming goods: containers and seals intact?	☐ ☐ ☐		5.27
3.33	Incoming goods: conformity with bill of delivery?	☐ ☐ ☐		5.27
	Labeling of incoming containers with			
3.34	• internal name and code?	☐ ☐ ☐		5.29
3.35	• allocated batch number?	☐ ☐ ☐		5.29
3.36	• quarantine status?	☐ ☐ ☐		5.29
3.37	• expiry date or reanalysis date?	☐ ☐ ☐		5.29
3.38	Identity test for each incoming container?	☐ ☐ ☐		5.29
3.39	Are the sampled containers marked?	☐ ☐ ☐		5.30
3.40	Are reference samples taken?	☐ ☐ ☐		5.30
3.41	Safe storage of printed packaging materials?	☐ ☐ ☐		5.41
3.42	Lot tracing of all packaging materials possible?	☐ ☐ ☐		5.42
3.43	Are excessive packaging materials destroyed?	☐ ☐ ☐		5.43
	Release of starting materials by			
	Physical/inventory checks on raw materials, packaging materials, and finished goods:			

	Item:	Stocks: Physical:	Stocks: Inventory:	Storage conditions:	

4	**DISPENSING/ASSEMBLING**			
	Rooms, general			
4.1	Suitable for the intended use?	☐ ☐ ☐		3
4.2	• adequate size?	☐ ☐ ☐		3
4.3	• clean?	☐ ☐ ☐		3
4.4	Located and designed to exclude external contamination?	☐ ☐ ☐		3.1
4.5	Appropriate level of maintenance?	☐ ☐ ☐		3.2
4.6	Maintenance works possible without contamination risk?	☐ ☐ ☐		3.2

		Compliance 1 2 3[a]	Remarks	EU Guide
4.7	Appropriate lighting and air-conditioning?	☐ ☐ ☐		3.3
4.8	Recording of temperature and humidity?	☐ ☐ ☐		
4.9	Protection against the entry of insects or other animals?	☐ ☐ ☐		3.4
4.10	Controlled access for authorized personnel only?	☐ ☐ ☐		3.5
	Rooms, special requirements			
4.11	Segregated from production and warehouse?	☐ ☐ ☐		3.13
4.12	Separate weighing cabins?	☐ ☐ ☐		3.13
4.13	Separate AHU for each cabin?	☐ ☐ ☐		3.12
	Air pressure gradient from weighing cabin → corridor:			3.3
4.14	Dust extraction systems available?	☐ ☐ ☐		5.11
	Operations			
4.15	Balances regularly calibrated?	☐ ☐ ☐		3.41
4.16	Only pharmaceutical raw materials in this area?	☐ ☐ ☐		5.17
4.17	Check on remains from previous materials before entering of new materials into a weighing cabin?	☐ ☐ ☐		5.9/5.35
4.18	Only one material in one cabin?	☐ ☐ ☐		5.9
4.19	Are dispensed materials correct labeled?	☐ ☐ ☐		5.29
4.20	Only released products in the dispensing?	☐ ☐ ☐		5.31
4.21	Cleaning SOP's for the dispensing?	☐ ☐ ☐		4.28
4.22	Previously dispensed material recorded on weighing protocol?	☐ ☐ ☐		4.8
4.23	Safety measures against mix-ups during assembling (e.g., cage pallets)?	☐ ☐ ☐		5.32/5.34
5	**SOLIDS MANUFACTURING**			
	Field of activity:			
	• granulation	☐		
	• compression	☐		
	• encapsulation	☐		
	• film and sugar coating	☐		
	• visual inspection (capsules, tablets, etc.)	☐		
	• premix (human)	☐		
	Rooms, general			
5.1	Suitable for the intended use?	☐ ☐ ☐		3
5.2	• adequate size?	☐ ☐ ☐		3
5.3	• clean?	☐ ☐ ☐		3
5.4	Located and designed to exclude external contamination?	☐ ☐ ☐		3.1
5.5	Appropriate level of maintenance?	☐ ☐ ☐		3.2
5.6	Maintenance works possible without contamination risk?	☐ ☐ ☐		3.2
5.7	Appropriate lighting and air-conditioning?	☐ ☐ ☐		3.3
5.8	Recording of temperature and humidity?	☐ ☐ ☐		
5.9	Protection against the entry of insects or other animals?	☐ ☐ ☐		3.4
5.10	Controlled access for authorized personnel only?	☐ ☐ ☐		3.5
	Rooms, special requirements			
5.11	Separate manufacturing area for penicillins/cephalosporins or highly sensitizing substances?	☐ ☐ ☐		3.6

		Compliance 1 2 3[a]	Remarks	EU Guide
5.12	Only for processing of pharmaceuticals?	☐ ☐ ☐		3.6
5.13	Logical flow of materials?	☐ ☐ ☐		3.7
5.14	Walls, floors, and ceilings: smooth surface and free of cracks?	☐ ☐ ☐		3.8
5.15	Easy cleaning possible?	☐ ☐ ☐		3.10
5.16	Adequate drains with traps and grilles?	☐ ☐ ☐		3.11
5.17	Appropriate air-handling system?	☐ ☐ ☐		3.12
	Air pressure gradient from working bay → corridor:			
	Classification according to EC guide?			
5.18	Appropriate dust extraction system?	☐ ☐ ☐		3.14
5.19	Appropriate lighting?	☐ ☐ ☐		3.16
5.20	Separate rest rooms?	☐ ☐ ☐		3.30
5.21	Changing rooms designed to avoid contamination?	☐ ☐ ☐		3.31
5.22	Toilets segregated from manufacturing areas?	☐ ☐ ☐		3.31
	Equipment			
5.23	Suitable for the intended use?	☐ ☐ ☐		3.34
5.24	Well maintained?	☐ ☐ ☐		3.34
5.25	Written & validated cleaning procedures?	☐ ☐ ☐		3.36
5.26	Maintenance without contamination risk (sep. area)?	☐ ☐ ☐		3.35
5.27	Equipment in contact with product: suitable materials quality?	☐ ☐ ☐		3.39
5.28	Machinery equipped with measuring and control devices?	☐ ☐ ☐		3.40
5.29	Calibration in fixed intervals acc. to written procedures?	☐ ☐ ☐		3.41
5.30	Calibration records available?	☐ ☐ ☐		3.41
5.31	Contents and flow direction marked on pipes?	☐ ☐ ☐		3.42
5.32	Pipes for distilled and demineralized water regularly monitored and sanitized?	☐ ☐ ☐		3.43
5.33	Not functioning equipment in the production area (if yes: clearly marked)?	Y N ☐ ☐ ☐		3.44
5.34	Status of cleanliness indicated?	☐ ☐ ☐		5.13
5.35	Previous product indicated?	☐ ☐ ☐		5.13
	Operations			
5.36	Are written and validated procedures for all manufacturing steps available?	☐ ☐ ☐		5.2
5.37	Are all manufacturing steps recorded with actual parameters?	☐ ☐ ☐		5.2
5.38	Check of each single container of the starting materials (contents, weight, and identity)?	☐ ☐ ☐		5.3
5.39	Limits for yields?	☐ ☐ ☐		5.8
5.40	Only one batch of one product processed?	☐ ☐ ☐		5.9
5.41	Protection against microbial contamination?	☐ ☐ ☐		5.10
5.42	Appropriate measures against generation of dust (e.g. closed systems)?	☐ ☐ ☐		5.11
	Correct labeling of containers, materials, equipment, and rooms with			5.12

		Compliance 1 2 3[a]	Remarks		EU Guide
5.43	• product name and batch no.	☐ ☐ ☐			5.12
5.44	• quarantine status?	☐ ☐ ☐			5.12
5.45	Deviations from standard procedures recorded and signed by the supervisor?	☐ ☐ ☐			5.14
5.46	Special procedures for the production of antibiotics, hormones, etc.?	☐ ☐ ☐			5.19
5.47	• Campaign production?	☐ ☐ ☐			5.19
5.48	• Special monitoring?	☐ ☐ ☐			5.19
5.49	• Validated decontamination procedure?	☐ ☐ ☐			5.19
5.50	Double check on weight?	☐ ☐ ☐			5.34
5.51	Line clearance before start of production?	☐ ☐ ☐			5.35
5.52	Investigation of deviations in yields?	☐ ☐ ☐			5.39
5.53	Validated procedures for reworking of rejected batches?	☐ ☐ ☐			5.62
5.54	Detailed procedures for the addition of previous batches?	☐ ☐ ☐			5.63
5.55	Special release procedure (QA) for those batches?	☐ ☐ ☐			5.64
5.56	Use of protective clothing (hair cover, shoes, masks, and gloves)?	☐ ☐ ☐			2.16
5.57	Clothing regulation for visitors?	☐ ☐ ☐			2.11
	IPC				5.38
	Who performs IPC?				
5.58	Are IPC methods approved by QC?	☐ ☐ ☐			6.18
	Performance of IPCs:	During Start-up? **Yes No**	Frequency	Automatic data recording? **Yes No**	
	Tablets/kernels				
5.59	Individual weights	☐ ☐		☐ ☐	
5.60	Disintegration	☐ ☐		☐ ☐	
5.61	Thickness	☐ ☐		☐ ☐	
5.62	Hardness	☐ ☐		☐ ☐	
5.63	Friability/Abrasion	☐ ☐		☐ ☐	
	Sugar-/film-coated tablets				
5.64	Weights	☐ ☐		☐ ☐	
5.65	Disintegration	☐ ☐		☐ ☐	
5.66	Residual absolute humidity (IR or)	☐ ☐		☐ ☐	
	Capsules				
5.67	Individual weights	☐ ☐		☐ ☐	
5.68	Disintegration	☐ ☐		☐ ☐	
	Validation				
5.69	Validation according to fixed procedures?	☐ ☐ ☐			5.21
5.70	New procedures released only after validation?	☐ ☐ ☐			5.22
	Validation of changes of				
5.71	• processes?	☐ ☐ ☐			5.23
5.72	• starting materials?	☐ ☐ ☐			5.23
5.73	• equipment?	☐ ☐ ☐			5.23

		Compliance 1 2 3[a]	Remarks	EU Guide
5.74	Revalidation in fixed intervals?	☐ ☐ ☐		5.24
5.75	Procedures for the retrospective validation of old procedures?	☐ ☐ ☐		
6	**LIQUIDS MANUFACTURING**			
	Operations carried out:			
	• Dispensing (if different from solid)	☐ ☐ ☐		
	• Syrups and suspensions	☐ ☐ ☐		
	• Drops	☐ ☐ ☐		
	• Ointment manufacture	☐ ☐ ☐		
	• Ointment filling	☐ ☐ ☐		
	• Ampoule solution manufacture	☐ ☐ ☐		
	• Sterile or aseptic ampoule filling	☐ ☐ ☐		
	• Sterile freeze drying	☐ ☐ ☐		
	• Sterile powder filling	☐ ☐ ☐		
	Rooms, general			
6.1	Suitable for the intended use?	☐ ☐ ☐		3
6.2	• adequate size?	☐ ☐ ☐		3
6.3	• clean?	☐ ☐ ☐		3
6.4	Located and designed to exclude external contamination?	☐ ☐ ☐		3.1
6.5	Appropriate level of maintenance?	☐ ☐ ☐		3.2
6.6	Maintenance works possible without contamination risk?	☐ ☐ ☐		3.2
6.7	Appropriate lighting and air-conditioning?	☐ ☐ ☐		3.3
6.8	Recording of temperature and humidity?	☐ ☐ ☐		
6.9	Protection against the entry of insects or other animals?	☐ ☐ ☐		3.4
6.10	Controlled access for authorized personnel only?	☐ ☐ ☐		3.5
	Rooms, special requirements			
6.11	Separate manufacturing area for penicillins/cephalosporins or highly sensitizing substances?	☐ ☐ ☐		3.6
6.12	Only for processing of pharmaceuticals?	☐ ☐ ☐		3.6
6.13	Logical flow of materials?	☐ ☐ ☐		3.7
6.14	Walls, floors, and ceilings: smooth surface and free of cracks?	☐ ☐ ☐		3.8
6.15	Easy cleaning possible?	☐ ☐ ☐		3.10
6.16	Adequate drains with traps and grilles?	☐ ☐ ☐		3.11
6.17	Appropriate air-handling system with filtered air where open products are exposed to the environment?	☐ ☐ ☐		3.12
	Air pressure gradient from working bay → corridor:			
	Classification according to EC guide?			
6.18	Appropriate lighting?	☐ ☐ ☐		3.16
6.19	Separate rest rooms?	☐ ☐ ☐		3.30
6.20	Changing rooms designed to avoid contamination?	☐ ☐ ☐		3.31
6.21	Toilets segregated from manufacturing areas?	☐ ☐ ☐		3.31
	Equipment			
6.22	Suitable for the intended use?	☐ ☐ ☐		3.34
6.23	Well maintained?	☐ ☐ ☐		3.34
6.24	Tanks, containers, pipework, and pumps designed for easy cleaning and sanitation (dead legs!)?	☐ ☐ ☐		Suppl. 2

		Compliance 1 2 3[a]	Remarks	EU Guide
6.25	Written & validated cleaning procedures?	☐ ☐ ☐		3.36
6.26	Maintenance without contamination risk (sep. area)?	☐ ☐ ☐		3.35
6.27	Equipment in contact with product: suitable materials quality?	☐ ☐ ☐		3.39
6.28	Machinery equipped with measuring and control devices?	☐ ☐ ☐		3.40
6.29	Calibration in fixed intervals acc. to written procedures?	☐ ☐ ☐		3.41
6.30	Calibration records available?	☐ ☐ ☐		3.41
6.31	Contents and flow direction marked on pipes?	☐ ☐ ☐		3.42
6.32	Pipes for distilled and demineralized water regularly monitored and sanitized?	☐ ☐ ☐		3.43
6.33	Not functioning equipment in the production area (if yes: clearly marked)?	Y N ☐ ☐ ☐		3.44
6.34	Status of cleanliness indicated?	☐ ☐ ☐		5.13
6.35	Previous product indicated?	☐ ☐ ☐		5.13
	Operations			
6.36	Are written and validated procedures for all manufacturing steps available?	☐ ☐ ☐		5.2
6.37	Are all manufacturing steps recorded with actual parameters?	☐ ☐ ☐		5.2
6.38	Check of each single container of the starting materials (contents, weight, and identity)?	☐ ☐ ☐		5.3
6.39	Limits for yields?	☐ ☐ ☐		5.8
6.40	Only one batch of one product processed?	☐ ☐ ☐		5.9
6.41	Protection against microbial contamination?	☐ ☐ ☐		5.10
	Correct labeling of containers, materials, equipment, and rooms with			5.12
6.42	• product name and batch no.	☐ ☐ ☐		5.12
6.43	• quarantine status?	☐ ☐ ☐		5.12
6.44	Deviations from standard procedures recorded and signed by the supervisor?	☐ ☐ ☐		5.14
6.45	Special procedures for the production of antibiotics, hormones, etc.?	☐ ☐ ☐		5.19
6.46	• Campaign production?	☐ ☐ ☐		5.19
6.47	• Special monitoring?	☐ ☐ ☐		5.19
6.48	• Validated decontamination procedure?	☐ ☐ ☐		5.19
6.49	Double check on weight?	☐ ☐ ☐		5.34
6.50	Line clearance before start of production?	☐ ☐ ☐		5.35
6.51	Investigation of deviations in yields?	☐ ☐ ☐		5.39
6.52	Specification of max. storage time and storage conditions if products are not immediately filled or packaged?	☐ ☐ ☐		Suppl. 9
6.53	Validated procedures for reworking of rejected batches?	☐ ☐ ☐		5.62
6.54	Detailed procedures for the addition of previous batches?	☐ ☐ ☐		5.63
6.55	Special release procedure (QA) for those batches?	☐ ☐ ☐		5.64
6.56	Use of protective clothing (hair cover, shoes, masks, and gloves)?	☐ ☐ ☐		2.16
6.57	Clothing regulation for visitors?	☐ ☐ ☐		2.11

		Compliance 1 2 3[a]	Remarks	EU Guide
	Water			
6.58	Loop system for purified water?	☐ ☐ ☐		Suppl. 4
6.59	Antimicrobial treatment of purified water?	☐ ☐ ☐		Suppl. 4
6.60	Loop system for water for injection?	☐ ☐ ☐		Suppl. 4
	Storage temperature of water for injection:			Suppl. 4
6.61	Loop system constructed to avoid deadlegs?	☐ ☐ ☐		Suppl. 4
6.62	Regular microbiological monitoring?	☐ ☐ ☐		Suppl. 4
6.63	Regular endotoxin control?	☐ ☐ ☐		Suppl. 4
	Special requirements for sterile and aseptic products			**Suppl.**
	Rooms and equipment			
6.64	Access of staff and materials to clean areas *only* through air locks?	☐ ☐ ☐		1
6.66	Rooms classified according EC guide?	☐ ☐ ☐		3
	Classification for products to be sterilized:			
6.67	• Solution preparation (EC: class C, with special precautions class D):	Class:		5
6.68	• Filling (EC: under LF in class C):	Class:		5
	Classification for aseptic products:			
6.69	• Handling of starting materials that can be sterile filtered (EC: class C):	Class:		6
6.70	• Handling of starting materials that cannot be sterile filtered (EC: class A in class B):	Class:		6
6.71	• Handling and filling of bulk (EC: class A in Class B):	Class:		6
6.72	All rooms easy to clean disinfect?	☐ ☐ ☐		17
6.73	Doors, windows, frames, lighting, etc. without edges?	☐ ☐ ☐		18
6.74	Suspended ceilings (if yes: sealed?)?	☐ ☐ ☐		19
6.75	Traps constructed to avoid microb. contamination?	☐ ☐ ☐		21
6.76	Appropriate constructed changing rooms?	☐ ☐ ☐		22
6.77	Measures against opening of both doors of air locks?	☐ ☐ ☐		23
6.78	Overpressure gradient from cleanest areas to others?	☐ ☐ ☐		24
6.79	AHU validated and regularly revalidated?	☐ ☐ ☐		25
6.80	Control instruments for pressure gradient?	☐ ☐ ☐		26
6.81	Warning system for errors in air supply?	☐ ☐ ☐		26
6.82	Recording of pressure gradients?	☐ ☐ ☐		26
6.83	Do conveyor belts leave sterile areas?	☐ ☐ ☐		28
6.84	Maintenance works outside from clean areas possible?	☐ ☐ ☐		28
6.85	Cleaning and disinfection procedure after maintenance works?	☐ ☐ ☐		29
6.86	Regular revalidation of all equipment and systems?	☐ ☐ ☐		30
6.87	Water prepared, circulated, and stored to exclude microb. contamination?	☐ ☐ ☐		31
6.88	Cleaning and disinfection of rooms according to validated SOPs rooms?	☐ ☐ ☐		32
	• Disinfection methods?			
6.89	Microb. monitoring of cleaning and disinfection agents?	☐ ☐ ☐		33

		Compliance 1 2 3[a]	Remarks	EU Guide
6.90	Microb. monitoring program of production areas?	☐ ☐ ☐		35
6.91	Results recorded and considered for the release?	☐ ☐ ☐		35
	Personnel and hygiene			
6.92	Minimal no. of personnel in clean areas?	☐ ☐ ☐		7
6.93	Special and regular training?	☐ ☐ ☐		8
6.94	Regular medical examinations?	☐ ☐ ☐		10
6.95	Appropriate clean room clothes (material, design)?	☐ ☐ ☐		12
6.96	Protective clothes worn correctly?	☐ ☐ ☐		12
6.97	Prohibition of cosmetics, jewellery, and watches?	☐ ☐ ☐		13
6.98	New clean room clothes for each working cycle?	☐ ☐ ☐		15
6.99	Appropriate washing and sterilization of clothes?	☐ ☐ ☐		16
	Operations			
6.100	Validation (media filling) in regular intervals?	☐ ☐ ☐		38
	Monitoring of water preparation system, frequency:			
6.101	• microbiological:			40
6.102	• chemical:			40
6.103	• particles:			40
6.104	• endotoxins:			40
6.105	Microbiological monitoring of starting materials?	☐ ☐ ☐		42
6.106	Max. storage times defined for sterilized equipment?	☐ ☐ ☐		45
6.107	Max. storage time defined between solution preparation and filtration?	☐ ☐ ☐		46
6.108	Material transfer to clean areas through double door autoclaves?	☐ ☐ ☐		48
	Sterilization processes			
6.109	All processes validated?	☐ ☐ ☐		50
6.110	Sterilized and nonsterilized materials clearly separated?	☐ ☐ ☐		54
	Trays and boxes clearly labeled with			
6.111	• product name and code	☐ ☐ ☐		54
6.112	• batch no.	☐ ☐ ☐		54
6.113	• status: sterilized or not sterilized	☐ ☐ ☐		54
	Sterilizers:			
6.114	• Recording of temp., pressure, and time?	☐ ☐ ☐		55
6.115	• Coldest point determined?	☐ ☐ ☐		55
6.116	• Independent counter check probe?	☐ ☐ ☐		55
6.117	• Heat-up time for each product determined?	☐ ☐ ☐		56
6.118	• Sterile cooling media?	☐ ☐ ☐		57
6.119	• Tightness tests for vacuum autoclaves?	☐ ☐ ☐		58
6.120	• Clean steam for steam autoclaves?	☐ ☐ ☐		58
6.121	• Circulated air with overpressure?	☐ ☐ ☐		61
6.122	• Recirculated air: sterile filtered?	☐ ☐ ☐		61
6.123	• Ethylene oxide autoclaves: humidity, temp., and time recorded?	☐ ☐ ☐		69
6.124	• Ethylene oxide autoclaves: use of bioindicators?	☐ ☐ ☐		70

		Compliance 1 2 3[a]	Remarks	EU Guide
	Filtration			
6.125	Double filtration?	☐ ☐ ☐		75
6.126	Integrity testing of filters immediately after use?	☐ ☐ ☐		77
6.127	Are results part of the batch protocol?	☐ ☐ ☐		77
6.128	Optical control of each single container of ampoules, vials, and infusions?	☐ ☐ ☐		82
	IPC			
6.129	Written IPC procedures and SOPs?	☐ ☐ ☐		
	Particle testing of			
6.130	• rooms	☐ ☐ ☐		
6.131	• primary packaging materials	☐ ☐ ☐		
6.132	• system of warning and action limits?	☐ ☐ ☐		
	Microbiological monitoring of:			
6.133	• rooms			
6.134	• personnel			
6.135	• equipment			
6.136	Residual O_2 of ampoules, infusions, and syrups?	☐ ☐ ☐		
6.137	Endotoxin testing of water and packaging materials?	☐ ☐ ☐		
6.138	Calibration of equipment?	☐ ☐ ☐		
6.139	Regular revalidation of equipment?	☐ ☐ ☐		
7	**PACKAGING**			
	Operations carried out: • Blistering • Foil-packaging • Filling into tablet glasses • Effervescent packaging • Powder filling • Syrup/drops filling • Ointment filling	 ☐ ☐ ☐ ☐ ☐ ☐ ☐		
	Rooms			
7.1	Suitable for the intended use?	☐ ☐ ☐		3
7.2	• adequate size?	☐ ☐ ☐		3
7.3	• clean?	☐ ☐ ☐		3
7.4	Located and designed to exclude external contamination?	☐ ☐ ☐		3.1
7.5	Appropriate level of maintenance?	☐ ☐ ☐		3.2
7.6	Maintenance works possible without contamination risk?	☐ ☐ ☐		3.2
7.7	Appropriate lighting and air-conditioning?	☐ ☐ ☐		3.3
7.8	Recording of temperature and humidity?	☐ ☐ ☐		
7.9	Protection against the entry of insects or other animals?	☐ ☐ ☐		3.4
7.10	Controlled access for authorized personnel only?	☐ ☐ ☐		3.5
7.11	Adequate separation of the packaging lines?	☐ ☐ ☐		3.15
	Operations			
7.12	Only *one* product per line?	☐ ☐ ☐		5.44

		Compliance 1 2 3[a]	Remarks	EU Guide
7.13	Check list for clearance before processing a new product/new batch?	☐ ☐ ☐		5.45
7.14	Adequate labeling of the lines (product name and code)?	☐ ☐ ☐		5.46
7.15	Check of all materials delivered to the line (quantity, identity, and conformity with order)?	☐ ☐ ☐		5.47
7.16	Cleaning of primary packaging materials?	☐ ☐ ☐		5.48
7.17	Immediate labeling after filling?	☐ ☐ ☐		5.49
7.18	Careful check of all printing processes (code and expiry date)?	☐ ☐ ☐		5.50
7.19	Special safety measures for off-line printing?	☐ ☐ ☐		5.51
7.20	Regular checks of all control devices (code reader, counter, etc.)?	☐ ☐ ☐		5.52
7.21	Printings clear and durable?	☐ ☐ ☐		5.53
7.22	Balancing of printed packaging materials and bulk?	☐ ☐ ☐		5.56
7.23	Destruction of excessive coded packaging material after completion of an order?	☐ ☐ ☐		5.57
7.24	Are the finished products kept in quarantine until final release?	☐ ☐ ☐		5.58
7.25	Appropriate storage after release?	☐ ☐ ☐		5.60
	IPC			
7.26	Checks on identity of bulk and packaging materials?	☐ ☐ ☐		5.47
	Regular line checks on:			
7.27	• aspect of the packages	☐ ☐ ☐		5.54a
7.28	• completeness	☐ ☐ ☐		5.54b
7.29	• conformity of quantity and quality of materials with packaging order	☐ ☐ ☐		5.54c
7.30	• correct imprint	☐ ☐ ☐		5.54d
7.31	• correct function of control devices	☐ ☐ ☐		5.54d
	Are the following IPC checks performed?			
7.32	• Leaking	☐ ☐ ☐		
7.33	• Release torque of screw caps	☐ ☐ ☐		
7.34	• pH, density, drop weight, viscosity, and sedimentation	☐ ☐ ☐		
8	**DOCUMENTATION**			
	Specifications			
8.1	Specifications for raw/packaging materials available?	☐ ☐ ☐		4.10
	Do they include			
8.2	• internal name and code	☐ ☐ ☐		4.11
8.3	• name of supplier and/or manufacturer?	☐ ☐ ☐		4.11
8.4	• reference sample (printed pack.mat.)?	☐ ☐ ☐		4.11
8.5	• sampling procedure?	☐ ☐ ☐		4.11
8.6	• qualitative/quantitative specifications with limits?	☐ ☐ ☐		4.11
8.7	• storage conditions?	☐ ☐ ☐		4.11
8.8	• maximum storage period?	☐ ☐ ☐		4.11
	Goods receiving?			
8.9	Written procedures for the reception of deliveries?	☐ ☐ ☐		4.19

		Compliance 1 2 3[a]	Remarks	EU Guide
	Do records receipt include			
8.10	• product name on labels and delivery note?	☐ ☐ ☐		4.20
8.11	• internal name and code?	☐ ☐ ☐		4.20
8.12	• receiving date?	☐ ☐ ☐		4.20
8.13	• name of supplier and/or manufacturer?	☐ ☐ ☐		4.20
8.14	• batch number of supplier?	☐ ☐ ☐		4.20
8.15	• total quantity and number of containers?	☐ ☐ ☐		4.20
8.16	• allocated internal batch number?	☐ ☐ ☐		4.20
8.17	SOPs for labeling, quarantine, and storage conditions of all incoming goods available?	☐ ☐ ☐		4.21
	Sampling procedures (SOPs) include:			
8.18	• authorized sampling personnel?	☐ ☐ ☐		4.22
8.19	• methods, equipment, and quantities?	☐ ☐ ☐		4.22
8.20	• safety measures?	☐ ☐ ☐		4.22
	Master formulae			
8.21	Are master formulae for each product and batch size available?	☐ ☐ ☐		4.3
8.22	Is the master formula approved and signed by the authorized persons?	☐ ☐ ☐		4.3
	The master formula includes			
8.23	• product name and code?	☐ ☐ ☐		4.14a
8.24	• description of galenical form, dosage, and batch size?	☐ ☐ ☐		4.14b
8.25	• all active ingredients with name, code, and weight?	☐ ☐ ☐		4.14c
8.26	• all excipients used during manufacture with name, code, and weight?	☐ ☐ ☐		4.14c
8.27	• yields with limits?	☐ ☐ ☐		4.14d
	Does the working procedure include			
8.28	• the production line?	☐ ☐ ☐		4.15a
8.29	• equipment to be used?	☐ ☐ ☐		4.15a
8.30	• reference to methods for cleaning, assembling, and calibration of machines?	☐ ☐ ☐		4.15b
8.31	• detailed stepwise manufacturing prescription?	☐ ☐ ☐		4.15c
8.32	• IPCs to be performed with limits?	☐ ☐ ☐		4.15d
8.33	• precautions to be followed?	☐ ☐ ☐		4.15e
8.34	Are batch records kept for each batch processed?	☐ ☐ ☐		4.17
	Do batch records include			
8.35	• protocol of line clearance?	☐ ☐ ☐		4.17
8.36	• name of the product and batch no.?	☐ ☐ ☐		4.17a
8.37	• date and time of start and end of production?	☐ ☐ ☐		4.17b
8.38	• name and initials of responsible workers for each step?	☐ ☐ ☐		4.17c, d
8.39	• batch and analytical no. and actual weight of all starting materials?	☐ ☐ ☐		4.17e
8.40	• equipment used?	☐ ☐ ☐		4.17f
8.41	• results of IPCs with initials of person who carries them out?	☐ ☐ ☐		4.17g
8.42	• yields of the relevant manufacturing steps?	☐ ☐ ☐		4.17h
8.43	• detailed notes on problems and process deviations?	☐ ☐ ☐		4.17i

		Compliance 1 2 3[a]	Remarks	EU Guide
8.44	Records on reprocessing of batches?	☐ ☐ ☐		
	Packaging instructions			
8.45	Packaging instructions for each product, package size, and presentation?	☐ ☐ ☐		4.16
	Do they include			
8.46	• product name?	☐ ☐ ☐		4.16a
8.47	• description of galenical form and strength?	☐ ☐ ☐		4.16b
8.48	• package size?	☐ ☐ ☐		4.17c
8.49	• list of all packaging materials with code for a standard batch size?	☐ ☐ ☐		4.17d
8.50	• samples of printed packaging materials?	☐ ☐ ☐		4.17e
8.51	• special precautions?	☐ ☐ ☐		4.17f
8.52	• description of the process and equipment?	☐ ☐ ☐		4.17g
8.53	• IPCs to be performed with sampling instruction?	☐ ☐ ☐		4.17h
8.54	Are packaging batch records kept for each batch or part batch?	☐ ☐ ☐		4.18
	Do the packaging batch records include			
8.55	• protocol of line clearance?	☐ ☐ ☐		4.18
8.56	• name of the product?	☐ ☐ ☐		4.18a
8.57	• date and time when operations have been performed?	☐ ☐ ☐		4.18b
8.58	• name of the responsible person?	☐ ☐ ☐		4.18c
8.59	• initials of workers carrying out operations?	☐ ☐ ☐		4.18d
8.60	• notes on identity checks and conformity with packaging instructions?	☐ ☐ ☐		4.18e
8.61	• results of IPCs	☐ ☐ ☐		4.18e
8.62	• details of operations and equipment used?	☐ ☐ ☐		4.18f
8.63	• samples of printed packaging materials with codes (MFD, EXP, Batch no., etc.)?	☐ ☐ ☐		4.18g
8.64	• record of problems and process deviations?	☐ ☐ ☐		4.18h
8.65	• quantities of packaging materials delivered, used, destroyed, or returned?	☐ ☐ ☐		4.18i
8.66	• no. of packs consumed?	☐ ☐ ☐		4.18j
	Testing			
	Do the written testing procedures include			
8.67	• test methods?	☐ ☐ ☐		4.23
8.68	• equipment for testing?	☐ ☐ ☐		4.23
8.69	Tests documented?	☐ ☐ ☐		4.23
	Others			
8.70	Procedures for release and rejection of materials and finished products?	☐ ☐ ☐		4.24
8.71	Final release by authorized person?	☐ ☐ ☐		4.24
8.72	Records about distribution of each batch?	☐ ☐ ☐		4.25
	Procedures and protocols about			
8.73	• validation?	☐ ☐ ☐		4.26

		Compliance 1 2 3[a]	Remarks	EU Guide
8.74	• set up and calibration of equipment?	☐ ☐ ☐		4.26
8.75	• maintenance, cleaning, and disinfection?	☐ ☐ ☐		4.26
8.76	• training records?	☐ ☐ ☐		4.26
8.77	• environmental monitoring of production areas?	☐ ☐ ☐		4.26
8.78	• pest control?	☐ ☐ ☐		4.26
8.79	• complaints?	☐ ☐ ☐		4.26
8.80	• recalls?	☐ ☐ ☐		4.26
8.81	• returned goods?	☐ ☐ ☐		4.26
8.82	Instructions for use of manufacturing and testing equipment?	☐ ☐ ☐		4.27
	Logbooks for major equipment incl. date and name of persons who performed			
8.83	• validation?	☐ ☐ ☐		4.28
8.84	• calibration?	☐ ☐ ☐		4.28
8.85	• maintenance, cleaning, and repair works?	☐ ☐ ☐		4.28
8.86	Chronological records of use of major equipment and manufacturing areas?	☐ ☐ ☐		4.29
9	**QUALITY CONTROL**			6
	General requirements			
9.1	Independent QC department available?	☐ ☐ ☐		6.1
9.2	Head of QC well qualified and sufficiently experienced?	☐ ☐ ☐		6.1
9.3	Qualified personnel available?	☐ ☐ ☐		2.1
9.4	Organization charts available?	☐ ☐ ☐		2.2
9.5	Job descriptions available?	☐ ☐ ☐		2.2
9.6	Responsibilities clearly defined?	☐ ☐ ☐		2.2
9.7	Continuous training programs for QC staff?	☐ ☐ ☐		2.2
9.8	Initial job training for all employees?	☐ ☐ ☐		2.9
9.9	Training records?	☐ ☐ ☐		
9.10	QC personnel admitted to the production rooms for sampling etc.?	☐ ☐ ☐		
	QC Laboratories			
9.11	Suitable for the intended use?	☐ ☐ ☐		3.26
9.12	Laboratories of adequate size?	☐ ☐ ☐		3.26
9.13	Appropriate level of maintenance?	☐ ☐ ☐		3.1
9.14	Adequate separation from the production area?	☐ ☐ ☐		3.26
9.15	Controlled access of authorized personnel only?	☐ ☐ ☐		3.5
9.16	Special laboratory to handle biological samples available?	☐ ☐ ☐		3.29
9.17	Special laboratory to handle radioactive material available?	☐ ☐ ☐		3.29
9.18	Separate recreation rooms for the personnel available?	☐ ☐ ☐		3.30
9.19	Animal laboratories present?	☐ ☐ ☐		3.33
9.20	Animal laboratories separated from other areas?	☐ ☐ ☐		3.33
9.21	Animal laboratories equipped with a separate air-handling system?	☐ ☐ ☐		3.33

		Compliance 1 2 3[a]	Remarks	EU Guide
	QC Documentation			
9.22	Do procedures exist for			
	self inspection?	☐ ☐ ☐		
	release or rejection of products or raw material?	☐ ☐ ☐		
	product complaints?	☐ ☐ ☐		
	product recalls?	☐ ☐ ☐		
	local stability testing?	☐ ☐ ☐		
	storage of reference samples?	☐ ☐ ☐		
	validation of analytical procedures?	☐ ☐ ☐		
9.23	Specifications available for	☐ ☐ ☐		6.7
	raw materials?	☐ ☐ ☐		
	bulk products?	☐ ☐ ☐		
	packaging materials?	☐ ☐ ☐		
9.24	Analytical procedures for every product?	☐ ☐ ☐		
9.25	Are Basel methods followed?	☐ ☐ ☐		
9.26	Validation of locally developed test methods?	☐ ☐ ☐		
9.27	Sampling procedures available for			6.7
	raw materials?	☐ ☐ ☐		
	bulk products?	☐ ☐ ☐		
	packaging materials?	☐ ☐ ☐		
9.28	Suppliers certificates available?	☐ ☐ ☐		6.7
9.29	Calibration program for analytical instruments installed?	☐ ☐ ☐		6.7
9.30	Maintenance program for analytical instruments?	☐ ☐ ☐		6.7
9.31	Retention system for QC records?	☐ ☐ ☐		6.8
9.32	Batch documents stored for expiry + 1 year or 5 years (EEC 75/319, article 22) minimum?	☐ ☐ ☐		6.8
9.33	Are original data like notebooks stored in addition to the batch documents?	☐ ☐ ☐		6.10
9.34	Can the original data be traced back easily and quickly from the analytical report number or batch number?	☐ ☐ ☐		6.10
9.35	Are trend analyses being performed for			6.9
	analytical results?	☐ ☐ ☐		
	yields?	☐ ☐ ☐		
	environmental monitoring data?	☐ ☐ ☐		
	Sampling			
9.36	Written procedures for taking samples?	☐ ☐ ☐		6.11
9.37	Do procedures define			
	method of sampling?	☐ ☐ ☐		
	necessary equipment?	☐ ☐ ☐		
	quantity of the sample?	☐ ☐ ☐		
	subdivision of the sample?	☐ ☐ ☐		
	sample container?	☐ ☐ ☐		
	labeling of samples?	☐ ☐ ☐		
	storage conditions?	☐ ☐ ☐		
	cleaning and storage of sampling equipment?	☐ ☐ ☐		
	identification of containers sampled	☐ ☐ ☐		
9.38	Are samples representative for the batch they are taken from? (sampling plan)	☐ ☐ ☐		6.12
9.39	Are critical steps being surveilled and validated by additional sampling (e.g., beginning or end of a process)?	☐ ☐ ☐		6.12

		Compliance 1 2 3[a]	Remarks	EU Guide
9.40	Sample containers labeled with			6.13
	name of the content	☐ ☐ ☐		
	batch number	☐ ☐ ☐		
	date of sampling	☐ ☐ ☐		
	batch containers sampled	☐ ☐ ☐		
9.41	Are samples taken by QC/QA?	☐ ☐ ☐		
9.42	Reference samples retained for validity plus 1 year?	☐ ☐ ☐		6.14
9.43	Storage of reference samples under the recommended storage conditions?	☐ ☐ ☐		6.14
9.44	Finished products stored in the final packaging?	☐ ☐ ☐		6.14
9.45	Quantity of the reference sample makes 1 (better 2) complete reanalysis possible?	☐ ☐ ☐		6.14
9.46	Sample room secure?	☐ ☐ ☐		
9.47	Sample room neatly organized and not overcrowded?	☐ ☐ ☐		
	Testing			
9.48	Are the applied analytical methods validated?	☐ ☐ ☐		6.15
9.49	Analytical methods in compliance with the registration?	☐ ☐ ☐		6.16
9.50	Are all results recorded and checked for correctness?	☐ ☐ ☐		6.16
9.51	Are all calculations checked?	☐ ☐ ☐		6.16
9.52	Do the testing protocols contain			6.17
	name and galenical form of material?	☐ ☐ ☐		
	batch number?	☐ ☐ ☐		
	supplier if applicable?	☐ ☐ ☐		
	specification reference?	☐ ☐ ☐		
	method reference?	☐ ☐ ☐		
	analytical results?	☐ ☐ ☐		
	reference to analytical certificates?	☐ ☐ ☐		
	date of the analysis?	☐ ☐ ☐		
	name of the analyst?	☐ ☐ ☐		
	name of the person verifying the data?	☐ ☐ ☐		
	statement of release or rejection?	☐ ☐ ☐		
	date and sign of the release person?	☐ ☐ ☐		
9.53	Are all IPC methods in production approved by QC?	☐ ☐ ☐		6.18
9.54	Are written methods available for the preparation of reagents and volumetric solutions?	☐ ☐ ☐		6.19
9.55	Is a record maintained of standardization of volumetric solutions?	☐ ☐ ☐		6.2
9.56	Are reagents for prolonged use labeled with			6.20
	date of the preparation?	☐ ☐ ☐		
	sign of the preparator?	☐ ☐ ☐		
9.57	Are unstable reagents labeled with;			6.20
	expiry date?	☐ ☐ ☐		
	storage conditions?	☐ ☐ ☐		
9.58	Are volumetric solutions labeled with			6.20
	the last date of standardization?	☐ ☐ ☐		
	last current factor?	☐ ☐ ☐		
9.59	Are reference standards labeled with			6.21
	name and potency	☐ ☐ ☐		
	suppliers reference	☐ ☐ ☐		
	date of receipt	☐ ☐ ☐		
	date of expiry	☐ ☐ ☐		

		Compliance 1 2 3[a]	Remarks	EU Guide
9.60	Are reference standards stored properly and under the control of a designated person?	☐ ☐ ☐		
9.61	Are animals used for testing of components, materials, or products; quarantined before use? checked for suitability? Are records maintained showing the history of their use?	 ☐ ☐ ☐ ☐ ☐ ☐ ☐ ☐ ☐		
10	**COMPLAINTS AND PRODUCT RECALLS**			**8**
	Complaints			8.1
10.1	Does a written complaint procedure exist?	☐ ☐ ☐		8.2
10.2	Are product complaints carefully reviewed?	☐ ☐ ☐		8.1
10.3	Is a person designated to handle complaints and to decide on measures to be taken?	☐ ☐ ☐		8.1
10.4	Is each complaint concerning a product recorded with all original details?	☐ ☐ ☐		8.3
10.5	Are product complaints thoroughly investigated?	☐ ☐ ☐		8.3
10.6	Is a responsible person of QC involved in the study?	☐ ☐ ☐		8.3
10.7	Is it considered that other batches might be concerned as well?	☐ ☐ ☐		8.4
10.8	Are decisions and measures as a result recorded?	☐ ☐ ☐		8.5
10.9	Is this record added to the corresponding batch documents?	☐ ☐ ☐		8.5
10.10	Are the complaint records regularly revised with respect to specific or recurring problems?	☐ ☐ ☐		8.6
10.11	Are the authorities informed of serious quality problems with a product?	☐ ☐ ☐		8.7
	Recalls			8.8
10.12	Does a written recall procedure exist?	☐ ☐ ☐		8.9
10.13	Is a person nominated responsible for the execution and coordination of a recall?	☐ ☐ ☐		8.8
10.14	Responsible person independent of the marketing and sales organization?	☐ ☐ ☐		8.8
10.15	Are the competent authorities informed of an imminent recall?	☐ ☐ ☐		8.11
10.16	Does the person responsible for a recall have access to the distribution records?	☐ ☐ ☐		8.12
10.17	Do the distribution records contain sufficient information on customers with addresses? Phone numbers inside or outside working hours? Batches and amounts delivered? Medical samples?	☐ ☐ ☐ ☐ ☐ ☐ ☐ ☐ ☐ ☐ ☐ ☐		8.12
10.18	Are recalled products stored separately in a secure area?	☐ ☐ ☐		8.13
10.19	Is a final record made including a reconciliation between the delivered and recovered quantities?	☐ ☐ ☐		8.14
10.20	Is the effectiveness of the arrangements for recalls checked critically from time to time?	☐ ☐ ☐		8.15
11	**SELF-INSPECTION**			**9**
11.1	Does a self-inspection procedure exist which defines frequency and program?	☐ ☐ ☐		9.1
11.2	Are self-inspections carried out to check compliance with GMP rules?	☐ ☐ ☐		9.1

		Compliance 1 2 3[a]	Remarks	EU Guide
11.3	Are self-inspections conducted in an independent and detailed way? by designated competent persons from the company or external experts?	☐ ☐ ☐ ☐ ☐ ☐		9.2
11.4	Are self-inspections recorded?	☐ ☐ ☐		9.3
11.5	Do reports contain the observations made during a self-inspection? proposals for corrective measures?	☐ ☐ ☐ ☐ ☐ ☐		9.3
11.6	Are actions subsequently taken recorded?	☐ ☐ ☐		9.3
12	**CONTRACT MANUFACTURE AND ANALYSIS**			**7**
12.1	Written contract between contract giver and contract acceptor available?	☐ ☐ ☐		7.1
12.2	Are responsibilities and duties clearly defined?	☐ ☐ ☐		7
12.3	All arrangements in accordance with the marketing authorization of the product concerned?	☐ ☐ ☐		7.2
	The contract giver			
12.4	Competence of the acceptor to carry out the work successful and according to GMP assessed?	☐ ☐ ☐		7.3
12.5	Acceptor provided with all the informations necessary to carry out the contract work?	☐ ☐ ☐		7.4
12.6	Acceptor informed of safety aspects?	☐ ☐ ☐		7.4
12.7	Conformance of products supplied by the acceptor ensured?	☐ ☐ ☐		7.5
12.8	Product released by a qualified person on the acceptor's side?	☐ ☐ ☐		7.5
	The contract acceptor			
12.9	Does the acceptor have adequate premises and equipment? Knowledge and experience? Competent personnel? A manufacturing authorization?	☐ ☐ ☐ ☐ ☐ ☐ ☐ ☐ ☐ ☐ ☐ ☐		7.6
12.10	Does the acceptor ensure that all products or materials delivered to him are suitable?	☐ ☐ ☐		7.7
12.11	There must be no work passed to a third party without the permission of the giver.	☐ ☐ ☐		7.8
12.12	If a third party is involved, it must have the necessary manufacturing and analytical information.	☐ ☐ ☐		7.8
	The contract			
12.13	Does the written contract specify the responsibilities?	☐ ☐ ☐		7.10
12.14	Have technical aspects been drawn up by competent persons?	☐ ☐ ☐		7.10
12.15	Release of material and check for compliance with the marketing authorization defined?	☐ ☐ ☐		7.11
12.16	Is it defined who is responsible for purchasing of materials? IPC controls Testing and release of materials? Manufacturing and quality control? Sampling? Storage of batch documentation?	 ☐ ☐ ☐ ☐ ☐ ☐ ☐ ☐ ☐ ☐ ☐ ☐ ☐ ☐ ☐ ☐ ☐ ☐		7.12
12.17	Are manufacturing, analytical, and distribution records available to the contract giver?	☐ ☐ ☐		7.13
12.18	Contract permits the giver to visit the facilities of the acceptor?	☐ ☐ ☐		7.14

		Compliance 1 2 3[a]	Remarks	EU Guide
12.19	In the case of contract analysis: Does the contract acceptor understand that he is subject to inspection by the competent authorities?	☐ ☐ ☐		7.15
13	**AUDIT OF SUPPLIERS**			**2.7**
13.1	Supplier audits performed for excipients? Active substances? Packaging material?	☐ ☐ ☐ ☐ ☐ ☐ ☐ ☐ ☐		

[a] 1. Fulfilled or available; 2. partially fulfilled; 3. not fulfilled or not available.

GLOSSARY

Acceptance Criteria—Numerical limits, ranges, or other suitable measures for acceptance of test results.

Active Pharmaceutical Ingredient (API) (or Drug Substance)—Any substance or mixture of substances intended to be used in the manufacture of a drug (medicinal) product and that, when used in the production of a drug, becomes an active ingredient of the drug product. Such substances are intended to furnish pharmacological activity or other direct effect in the diagnosis, cure, mitigation, treatment, or prevention of disease or to affect the structure and function of the body.

Air lock—An enclosed space with two or more doors, which is interposed between two or more rooms, for example, of differing classes of cleanliness, for the purpose of controlling the airflow between those rooms when they need to be entered. An air lock is designed for use either by people or for goods and/or equipment.

API Starting Material—A raw material, intermediate, or an API that is used in the production of an API and that is incorporated as a significant structural fragment into the structure of the API. An API Starting Material can be an article of commerce, a material purchased from one or more suppliers under contract or commercial agreement, or produced in-house. API Starting Materials are normally of defined chemical properties and structure.

Authorized Person—The person recognized by the national regulatory authority as having the responsibility for ensuring that each batch of finished product has been manufactured, tested, and approved for release in compliance with the laws and regulations in force in that country.

Batch (or Lot)—A specific quantity of material produced in a process or series of processes so that it is expected to be homogeneous within specified limits. In the case of continuous production, a batch may correspond to a defined fraction of the production. The batch size can be defined either by a fixed quantity or by the amount produced in a fixed time interval. A defined quantity of starting material, packaging material, or product processed in a single process or series of processes so that it is expected to be homogeneous. It may sometimes be necessary to divide a batch into a number of sub-batches, which are later brought together to form a final homogeneous batch. In the case of terminal sterilization, the batch size is determined by the capacity of the autoclave. In continuous manufacture, the batch must correspond to a defined fraction of the production, characterized by its intended homogeneity. The batch size can be defined either as a fixed quantity or as the amount produced in a fixed time interval.

Batch Number (or Lot Number)—A unique combination of numbers, letters, and/or symbols that identifies a batch (or lot) and from which the production and distribution history can be determined. A distinctive combination of numbers and/or letters which uniquely identifies a batch on the labels, its batch records and corresponding certificates of analysis, etc.

Batch Records—All documents associated with the manufacture of a batch of bulk product or finished product. They provide a history of each batch of product and of all circumstances pertinent to the quality of the final product.

Bioburden—The level and type (e.g., objectionable or not) of microorganisms that can be present in raw materials, API starting materials, intermediates, or APIs. Bioburden should not be considered contamination unless the levels have been exceeded or defined objectionable organisms have been detected.

Bulk Product—Any product that has completed all processing stages up to, but not including, final packaging.

Calibration—The demonstration that a particular instrument or device produces results within specified limits by comparison with those produced by a reference or traceable standard over an appropriate range of measurements. The set of operations that establish, under specified conditions, the relationship between values indicated by an instrument or system for measuring (especially weighing), recording, and controlling, or the values represented by a material measure, and the corresponding known values of a reference standard. Limits for acceptance of the results of measuring should be established.

Clean Area—An area with defined environmental control of particulate and microbial contamination, constructed and used in such a way as to reduce the introduction, generation, and retention of contaminants within the area.

Computer System—A group of hardware components and associated software, designed and assembled to perform a specific function or group of functions. A process or operation integrated with a computer system.

Consignment (or delivery)—The quantity of a pharmaceutical(s), made by one manufacturer and supplied at one time in response to a particular request or order. A consignment may comprise one or more packages or containers and may include material belonging to more than one batch.

Contamination—The undesired introduction of impurities of a chemical or microbiological nature, or of foreign matter, into or on to a starting material or intermediate during production, sampling, packaging or repackaging, and storage or transport.

Contract Manufacturer—A manufacturer performing some aspect of manufacturing on behalf of the original manufacturer.

Critical—Describes a process step, process condition, test requirement, or other relevant parameter or item that must be controlled within predetermined criteria to ensure that the API meets its specification.

Critical Operation—An operation in the manufacturing process that may cause variation in the quality of the pharmaceutical product.

Cross-Contamination—Contamination of a material or product with another material or product. Contamination of a starting material, intermediate product, or finished product with another starting material or product during production.

Deviation—Departure from an approved instruction or established standard.

Drug (Medicinal) Product—The dosage form in the final immediate packaging intended for marketing. (Reference Q1A).

Drug Substance—See Active Pharmaceutical Ingredient.

Expiry Date (or Expiration Date)—The date placed on the container/labels of an API designating the time during which the API is expected to remain within established shelf-life specifications if stored under defined conditions, and after which it should not be used.

Finished Product—A finished dosage form that has undergone all stages of manufacture, including packaging in its final container and labeling.

Impurity—Any component present in the intermediate or API that is not the desired entity.

Impurity Profile—A description of the identified and unidentified impurities present in an API.

In-Process Control (or Process Control)—Checks performed during production in order to monitor and, if appropriate, to adjust the process and/or to ensure that the intermediate or API conforms to its specifications.

In-Process Control—Checks performed during production in order to monitor and, if necessary, to adjust the process to ensure that the product conforms to its specifications. The control of the environment or equipment may also be regarded as a part of in-process control.

Intermediate—A material produced during steps of the processing of an API that undergoes further molecular change or purification before it becomes an API. Intermediates may or may not be isolated. Partly processed product that must undergo further manufacturing steps before it becomes a bulk product.

Large-Volume Parenterals—Sterile solutions intended for parenteral application with a volume of 100 mL or more in one container of the finished dosage form.

Lot—See Batch

Lot Number—See Batch Number

Manufacture—All operations of receipt of materials, production, packaging, repackaging, labeling, relabeling, quality control, release, storage, and distribution of APIs and related controls.

Manufacturer—A company that carries out operations such as production, packaging, repackaging, labeling, and relabeling of pharmaceuticals.

Marketing Authorization (Product License, Registration Certificate)—A legal document issued by the competent drug regulatory authority that establishes the detailed composition and formulation of the product and the pharmacopoeial or other recognized specifications of its ingredients and of the final product itself, and includes details of packaging, labeling, and shelf life.

Master Formula—A document or set of documents specifying the starting materials with their quantities and the packaging materials, together with a description of the procedures and precautions required to produce a specified quantity of a finished product as well as the processing instructions, including the in-process controls.

Master Record—A document or set of documents that serve as a basis for the batch documentation (blank batch record).

Material—A general term used to denote raw materials (starting materials, reagents, and solvents), process aids, intermediates, APIs, and packaging and labeling materials.

Mother Liquor—The residual liquid which remains after the crystallization or isolation processes. A mother liquor may contain unreacted materials, intermediates, levels of the API, and/or impurities. It may be used for further processing.

Packaging—All operations, including filling and labeling, that a bulk product has to undergo in order to become a finished product. Filling of a sterile product under aseptic conditions or a product intended to be terminally sterilized would not normally be regarded as part of packaging.

Packaging Material—Any material intended to protect an intermediate or API during storage and transport. Any material, including printed material, employed in the packaging of a pharmaceutical, but excluding any outer packaging used for transportation or shipment. Packaging materials are referred to as primary or secondary according to whether or not they are intended to be in direct contact with the product.

Pharmaceutical Product—Any material or product intended for human or veterinary use presented in its finished dosage form or as a starting material for use in such a dosage form, that is subject to control by pharmaceutical legislation in the exporting state and/or the importing state.

Procedure—A documented description of the operations to be performed, the precautions to be taken, and measures to be applied directly or indirectly related to the manufacture of an intermediate or API.

Process Aids—Materials, excluding solvents, used as an aid in the manufacture of an intermediate or API that do not themselves participate in a chemical or biological reaction (e.g., filter aid, activated carbon).

Process Control—See In-Process Control.

Production—All operations involved in the preparation of a pharmaceutical product, from receipt of materials, through processing, packaging and repackaging, and labeling and relabeling, to completion of the finished product.

Qualification—Action of proving and documenting that equipment or ancillary systems are properly installed, work correctly, and actually lead to the expected results. Qualification is part of validation, but the individual qualification steps alone do not constitute process validation.

Quality Assurance (QA)—The sum total of the organised arrangements made with the object of ensuring that all APIs are of the quality required for their intended use and that quality systems are maintained.

Quality Control (QC)—Checking or testing that specifications are met.

Quality Unit(s)—An organizational unit independent of production, which fulfills both Quality Assurance and Quality Control responsibilities. This can be in the form of separate QA and QC units or a single individual or group, depending upon the size and structure of the organization.

Quarantine—The status of materials isolated physically or by other effective means pending a decision on their subsequent approval or rejection.

Quarantine—The status of starting or packaging materials, intermediates, or bulk or finished products isolated physically or by other effective means while a decision is awaited on their release, rejection, or reprocessing.

Raw Material—A general term used to denote starting materials, reagents, and solvents intended for use in the production of intermediates or APIs.

Reconciliation—A comparison between the theoretical quantity and the actual quantity.

Recovery—The introduction of all or part of previous batches (or of redistilled solvents and similar products) of the required quality into another batch at a defined stage of manufacture. It includes the removal of impurities from waste to obtain a pure substance or the recovery of used materials for a separate use.

Reference Standard, Primary—A substance that has been shown by an extensive set of analytical tests to be authentic material that should be of high purity.

Reference Standard, Secondary—A substance of established quality and purity, as shown by comparison to a primary reference standard, used as a reference standard for routine laboratory analysis.

Reprocessing—Subjecting all or part of a batch or lot of an in-process drug, bulk process intermediate (final biological bulk intermediate), or bulk product of a single batch/lot to a previous step in the validated manufacturing process due to failure to meet predetermined specifications. Reprocessing procedures are foreseen as occasionally necessary for biological drugs and, in such cases, are validated and preapproved as part of the marketing authorization.

Retest Date—The date when a material should be reexamined to ensure that it is still suitable for use.

Reworking—Subjecting an intermediate or API that does not conform to standards or specifications to one or more processing steps that are different from the established manufacturing process to obtain acceptable quality intermediate or API (e.g., recrystallizing with a different solvent).

Reworking—Subjecting an in-process or bulk process intermediate (final biological bulk intermediate) or final product of a single batch to an alternate manufacturing process due to a failure to meet predetermined specifications. Reworking is an unexpected occurrence and is not preapproved as part of the marketing authorization.

Self-Contained Area—Premises which provide complete and total separation of all aspects of an operation, including personnel and equipment movement, with well-established procedures, controls, and monitoring. This includes physical barriers as well as separate air-handling systems, but does not necessarily imply two distinct and separate buildings.

Signature (Signed)—See definition for signed.

Signed (Signature)—The record of the individual who performed a particular action or review. This record can be initials, full handwritten signature, personal seal, or authenticated and secure electronic signature.

Solvent—An inorganic or organic liquid used as a vehicle for the preparation of solutions or suspensions in the manufacture of an intermediate or API.

Specification—A list of tests, references to analytical procedures, and appropriate acceptance criteria that are numerical limits, ranges, or other criteria for the test described. It establishes the set of criteria to which a material should conform to be considered acceptable for its intended use. "Conformance to specification" means that the material, when tested according to the listed analytical procedures, will meet the listed acceptance criteria.

Specification—A list of detailed requirements with which the products or materials used or obtained during manufacture have to conform. They serve as a basis for quality evaluation.

Standard Operating Procedure (SOP)—An authorized written procedure giving instructions for performing operations not necessarily specific to a given product or material (e.g., equipment operation, maintenance, and cleaning; validation; cleaning of premises and environmental control; sampling and inspection). Certain SOPs may be used to supplement product-specific master and batch production documentation.

Starting Material—Any substance of a defined quality used in the production of a pharmaceutical product, but excluding packaging materials.

Validation—A documented program that provides a high degree of assurance that a specific process, method, or system will consistently produce a result meeting predetermined acceptance criteria. Action of proving, in accordance with the principles of GMP, that any procedure, process, equipment, material, activity, or system actually leads to the expected results (see also qualification).

Validation Protocol—A written plan stating how validation will be conducted and defining acceptance criteria. For example, the protocol for a manufacturing process identifies processing equipment, critical process parameters/operating ranges, product characteristics, sampling, test data to be collected, number of validation runs, and acceptable test results.

Yield, Expected—The quantity of material or the percentage of theoretical yield anticipated at any appropriate phase of production based on previous laboratory, pilot scale, or manufacturing data.

Yield, Theoretical—The quantity that would be produced at any appropriate phase of production, based upon the quantity of material to be used, in the absence of any loss or error in actual production.

19

Bioequivalence Testing Protocols

To receive approval for an ANDA, applicants generally must demonstrate, among other things, that their product has the same active ingredient, dosage form, strength, route of administration and conditions of use as the listed drug, and that the proposed drug product is BE to the reference listed drug [21 USC 355(j)(2)(A); 21 CFR 314.94(a)]. BE drug products show no significant difference in the rate and extent of absorption of the therapeutic ingredient [21 USC 355(j)(8); 21 CFR 320.1(e)]. BE studies are undertaken in support of ANDA submissions with the goal of demonstrating BE between a proposed generic drug product and its reference listed drug. The regulations governing BE are provided at 21 CFR in part 320.

The U.S. FDA has recently begun to promulgate individual bioequivalence requirements. To streamline the process for making guidance available to the public on how to design product-specific BE studies, the U.S. FDA will be issuing product-specific BE recommendations (www.fda.gov/cder/ogd/index.htm). Given below are the current recommendations for the products of relevance to this specific volume of the book:

Amoxicillin; Clavulanate Potassium Suspension/Oral. *Recommended studies*: Three studies. (1) *Type of study*: Fasting. *Design*: Single-dose, two-way crossover in vivo. *Strength*: 600 mg/EQ 42.9 mg (base)/5 mL. *Subjects*: Normal healthy males and females, general population. *Additional comments*: (2) *Type of study*: Fed. *Design*: Single-dose, two-way crossover in vivo. *Strength*: 600 mg/EQ 42.9 mg (base)/ 5 mL. *Subjects*: Normal healthy males and females, general population. *Additional comments*: (3) *Type of study*: Fasting. *Design*: Single-dose, two-way crossover in vivo. *Strength*: 400 mg/EQ 57 mg (base)/5 mL. *Subjects*: Normal healthy males and females, general population. *Additional comments*: *Analytes to measure*: Amoxicillin and clavulanate potassium in plasma. *Bioequivalence based on (90% CI)*: Amoxicillin and clavulanate potassium. *Waiver request of in vivo testing*: 200 mg/EQ 28.5 mg (base)/5 mL based on (i) acceptable bioequivalence studies on the 400 mg/EQ 57 mg (base)/5-mL strength, (ii) proportional similarity of the 200 mg/EQ 28.5 mg (base)/5 mL and 400 mg/EQ 57 mg (base)/5-mL strengths, and (iii) acceptable in vitro dissolution testing of the 200 mg/EQ 28.5 mg (base)/5 mL and 400 mg/EQ 57 mg (base)/5-mL strengths.

Carbamazepine Suspension/Oral. *Recommended studies*: Two studies. (1) *Type of study*: Fasting. *Design*: Single-dose, two-way crossover in vivo. *Strength*: 100 mg/5 mL. *Subjects*: Normal healthy males and females, general population. *Additional comments*: (2) *Type of study*: Fed. *Design*: Single-dose, two-way crossover in vivo. *Strength*: 100 mg/5 mL. *Subjects*: Normal healthy males and females, general population. *Additional comments*: *Analytes to measure (in appropriate biological fluid)*: Carbamazepine in plasma. *Bioequivalence based on (90% CI)*: Carbamazepine. *Waiver request of in vivo testing*: Not applicable.

Cefixime Suspension/Oral. *Recommended studies*: Two studies. (1) *Type of study*: Fasting. *Design*: Single-dose, two-way crossover in vivo. *Strength*: 200 mg/5 mL. *Subjects*: Normal healthy males and females, general population. *Additional comments*: Females should not be pregnant or lactating, and if applicable, should practice abstention or contraception during the study. (2) *Type of Study*: Fed. *Design*: Single-dose, two-way crossover in vivo. *Strength*: 200 mg/5 mL. *Subjects*: Normal healthy males and females, general population. *Additional comments*: Please see comment above. *Analytes to measure (in appropriate biological fluid)*: Cefixime in plasma. *Bioequivalence based on (90% CI)*: Cefixime. *Waiver request of in vivo testing*: 100 mg/5 mL based on (i) acceptable bioequivalence studies on the 200-mg strength /5-mL strength, (ii) proportional similarity of the formulations across all strengths, and (iii) acceptable in vitro dissolution testing of all strengths. A dosage unit for a suspension is the labeled strength (5 mL). A total of 12 units from 12 different bottles should be used.

Clarithromycin Granules for Suspension/Oral. *Recommended studies*: Two studies. (1) *Type of study*: Fasting. *Design*: Single-dose, two-way crossover in vivo. *Strength*: 250 mg/5 mL. *Subjects*: Normal healthy males and females, general population. *Additional comments*: (2) *Type of study*: Fed. *Design*: Single-dose, two-way crossover in vivo. *Strength*: 250 mg/5 mL. *Subjects*: Normal healthy males and females, general population. *Additional comments*: *Analytes to measure*: Clarithromycin in plasma. *Bioequivalence based on (90% CI)*: Clarithromycin. *Waiver request of in vivo testing*: 125 mg/5 mL based on (i) acceptable bioequivalence studies on the 250-mg strength/5-mL strength, (ii) proportional similarity of the formulations across all strengths, and (iii) acceptable in vitro dissolution testing of all strengths.

Deferasirox Tablets for Oral Suspension. *Recommended studies*: One study. *Type of study*: Fasting. *Design*: Single-dose, two-way crossover in vivo. *Strength*: 500 mg. *Subjects*: Normal healthy males and females, general population. *Additional comments*: The following passage is reproduced from the Dosage and Administration section of the labeling: Tablets should be completely dispersed by stirring in water, orange juice, or apple juice until a fine suspension is obtained. Doses of <1 g should be dispersed in 3.5 oz of liquid and doses of >1 g in 7.0 oz of liquid. After swallowing the suspension, any residue should be resuspended in a small volume of liquid and swallowed. Tablets should not be chewed or swallowed whole. *Analytes to measure (in appropriate biological fluid)*: Deferasirox in plasma. *Bioequivalence based on (90% CI)*: Deferasirox. *Waiver request of in vivo testing*: 250- and 125-mg tablets based on (i) acceptable bioequivalence studies on the 500-mg strength, (ii) proportionally similar across all strengths, and (iii) acceptable in vitro dissolution testing of all strengths.

Dextromethorphan Polistirex Extended-Release Oral Suspension/Oral. *Recommended studies*: Two studies. (1) *Type of study*: Fasting. *Design*: Single-dose, two-way crossover in vivo. *Strength*: 30 mg/5 mL. *Subjects*: Normal healthy males and females, general population. *Additional comments*: (2) *Type of study*: Fed. *Design*: Single-dose, two-way crossover in vivo. *Strength*: 30 mg/5 mL. *Subjects*: Normal healthy males and females, general population. *Additional comments*: *Analytes to measure (in appropriate biological fluid)*: Dextromethorphan and its metabolite. Dextrorphan in plasma. *Bioequivalence based on (90% CI)*: Dextromethorphan. Please submit the metabolite data as supportive evidence of comparable therapeutic outcome. For the metabolite, the following data should be submitted: individual and mean concentrations, individual and mean pharmacokinetic parameters, and geometric means and ratios of means for AUC and Cmax. *Waiver request of in vivo testing*: Not applicable. A dosage unit for a suspension is the labeled strength (5 mL). A total of 12 units from 12 different bottles should be used. In addition to the method above, for modified-release products, dissolution profiles on 12 dosage units each of test and reference products generated using USP apparatus I at 100 rpm and/or apparatus II at 50 rpm in at least three dissolution media (pH 1.2, 4.5, and 6.8 buffer) should be submitted in the application. Agitation speeds may have to be increased, if appropriate. It is acceptable to add a small amount of surfactant, if necessary. Please include early sampling times of 1, 2, and 4 hours and continue every 2 hours until at least 80% of the drug is released, to provide assurance against premature release of drug (dose dumping) from the formulation.

Felbamate Oral Suspension/Oral. *Recommended studies*: One study. *Type of study*: Fasting. *Design*: Multiple-dose, two-way steady-state crossover in vivo. *Strength*: 600 mg/5 mL. *Subjects*: Male and nonpregnant female epilepsy patients. *Additional comments*: Please also consider the following additional safety monitoring: (a) If any evidence of bone marrow (hematologic) depression occurs, felbamate treatment should be discontinued and a hematologist consulted to ensure appropriate medical care. (b) Additional criteria for exclusion from the study relative to baseline be practiced including (i) twofold increase in the highest, 2-day prestudy seizure frequency, (ii) single, generalized, tonic–clonic seizure if none occurred during pretreatment screening, and/or, (iii). significant prolongation of generalized, tonic–clonic seizures. *Analytes to measure*: Felbamate in plasma. (1) Measurements of felbamate are requested on at least two consecutive days immediately prior to PK-analysis, days 7 and 14 to confirm steady-state concentrations of felbamate (i.e., additional consecutive measures on days 5, 6 and 12, 13). (2) Because felbamate is rapidly absorbed and reaches a peak plasma concentration within 1 to 3 hours post consumption, please also include blood sampling at 0.25 hours after drug dosing to accurately measure the absorption/distribution phases of the felbamate PK profile. (3) Patients who receive multiples of 600 mg of felbamate per day (1200–4800 mg/day) would be eligible for the study by continuing their established maintenance dose. Because patients will be administered different dosing regimens, the dose needs to be included in the analysis of variance (ANOVA) statistical model. Dose normalization is not advised. (4) No washout period is necessary between treatment periods. (5) You are encouraged to submit protocols for the in vivo bioequivalence studies to be conducted at steady state in patients already taking the RLD at a therapeutic dose for review prior to initiating the studies. *Bioequivalence based on (90% CI)*: Felbamate. *Waiver request of in vivo testing*: Not applicable of all strengths of the test and reference products. A dosage unit for a suspension is the labeled strength (5 mL). A total of 12 units from 12 different bottles should be used.

Fosamprenavir Calcium Suspension/Oral. *Recommended studies*: Two studies. (1) *Type of study*: Fasting. *Design*: Single-dose, two-treatment, two-period crossover in vivo. *Strength*: EQ 50 mg Base/mL (Dose = 28 mL corresponding to a dose of 1400 mg). *Subjects*: Normal healthy males and females, general population. *Additional comments*: Females should not be pregnant or lactating, and if applicable, should practice abstention or contraception during the study. Bottle should be shaken well before drug administration. (2) *Type of Study*: Fed. *Design*: Single-dose, two-treatment, two-period crossover in vivo. *Strength*: EQ 50 mg Base/mL (Dose = 28 mL corresponding to a dose of 1400 mg). *Subjects*: Normal healthy males and females, general population. *Additional comments*: Please see comment above. *Analytes to measure (in appropriate biological fluid)*: Amprenavir, the active metabolite of fosamprenavir, in plasma. *Bioequivalence based on (90% CI)*: Amprenavir. *Waiver request of in vivo testing*: Not applicable.

Ibuprofen and Pseudoephedrine Hydrochloride Suspension/Oral. *Recommended studies*: Two studies. (1) *Type of study*: Fasting. *Design*: Single-dose, two-way crossover in vivo. *Strength*: 100 mg/5 mL and 15 mg/5 mL. *Subjects*: Normal healthy males and females, general population. *Additional comments*: (2) *Type of study*: Fed. *Design*: Single-dose, two-way crossover in vivo. *Strength*: 100 mg/5 mL and 15 mg/5 mL. *Subjects*: Normal healthy males and females, general population. *Additional comments*: *Analytes to measure*: Ibuprofen and pseudoephedrine in plasma. *Bioequivalence based on (90% CI)*: Ibuprofen and pseudoephedrine. *Waiver request of in vivo testing*: Not applicable of all strengths of the test and reference products. A dosage unit for a suspension is the labeled strength (5 mL). A total of 12 units from 12 different bottles should be used.

Meloxicam Suspension/Oral. *Recommended studies*: Two studies. (1) *Type of study*: Fasting. *Design*: Single-dose, two-way crossover in vivo dose and suspension. *Strength*: 5 mL of 7.5 mg/5 mL. *Subjects*: Normal healthy males and females, general population. *Additional comments*: Females should not be pregnant, and if applicable, should practice abstinence or contraception during the study. (2) *Type of study*: Fed. *Design*: Single-dose, two-way crossover in vivo dose and suspension. *Strength*: 5 mL of 7.5 mg/5 mL. *Subjects*: Normal healthy males and females, general population. *Additional comments*: Please see comment above. *Analytes to measure (in appropriate biological fluid)*: Meloxicam in plasma. *Bioequivalence based on (90% CI)*: Meloxicam. *Waiver request of in vivo testing*: Not applicable.

Nelfinavir Mesylate Suspension/Oral. *Recommended studies*: Two studies. (1) *Type of study*: Fasting. *Design*: Single-dose, two-treatment, two-period crossover in vivo. *Strength*: 50 mg/scoopful. *Subjects*: Normal healthy males and females, general population. *Additional comments*: (2) *Type of study*: Fed. *Design*: Single-dose, two-treatment, two-period crossover in vivo. *Strength*: 50 mg/scoopful. *Subjects*: Normal healthy males and females, general population. *Additional comments*: *Analytes to measure (in appropriate biological fluid)*: Nelfinavir in plasma. *Bioequivalence based on (90% CI)*: Nelfinavir. *Waiver request of in vivo testing*: Not applicable.

Nevirapine Suspension/Oral. *Recommended studies*: Two studies. (1) *Type of study*: Fasting. *Design*: Single-dose, one-period parallel in vivo. *Strength*: 50 mg/5 mL. *Subjects*:

Normal healthy males and females, general population. *Additional comments*: Because of safety concerns of sever life-threatening skin reactions and hepatotoxicity, single-dose parallel study designs in normal healthy subjects are recommended. (2) *Type of study*: Fed. *Design*: Single-dose, one-period parallel in vivo. *Strength*: 50 mg/5 mL. *Subjects*: Normal healthy males and females, general population. *Additional comments*: Please see comments above. *Analytes to measure (in appropriate biological fluid)*: Nevirapine in plasma. *Bioequivalence based on (90% CI)*: Nevirapine. *Waiver request of in vivo testing*: Not applicable.

Omeprazole Powder for Suspension/Oral. *Recommended studies*: One study. *Type of study*: Fasting. *Design*: Single-dose, two-treatment, two-period crossover in vivo. *Strength*: 40 mg/packet. *Subjects*: Normal healthy males and females, general population. *Additional comments*: *Analytes to measure*: Omeprazole in plasma. *Bioequivalence based on (90% CI)*: Omeprazole. *Waiver request of in vivo testing*: 20 mg/packet based on (i) acceptable bioequivalence study on the 40-mg strength, (ii) proportional similarity of the formulations across all strengths, and (iii) acceptable in vitro dissolution testing of all strengths. Since omperazole powder for oral suspension, 20 mg/packet and 40 mg/packet, are subject to two separate New Drug Applications, two separate Abbreviated New Drug Application must be submitted. A waiver of in vivo bioequivalence testing is available.

Oxcarbazepine Suspension/Oral. *Recommended studies*: Two studies. 1. *Type of study*: Fasting. *Design*: Single-dose, two-treatment, two-period crossover in vivo. *Strength*: 300 mg/5 mL (600-mg dose). *Subjects*: Normal healthy males and females, general population. *Additional comments*: (2) *Type of study*: Fed. *Design*: Single-dose, two-treatment, two-period crossover in vivo. *Strength*: 300 mg/5 mL (600-mg dose). *Subjects*: Normal healthy males and females, general population. *Additional comments*: *Analytes to measure (in appropriate biological fluid)*: Oxcarbazepine and its 10-hydroxy metabolite (monohydroxy derivative, MHD) in plasma using an achiral assay. *Bioequivalence based on (90% CI)*: Oxcarbazepine. Please submit the metabolite data as supportive evidence of comparable therapeutic outcome. For the metabolite, the following data should be submitted: individual and mean concentrations, individual and mean pharmacokinetic parameters, and geometric means and ratios of means for AUC and Cmax. *Waiver request of in vivo testing*: Not applicable product at this Web site. Please note that a dosage unit for a suspension is the labeled strength (5 mL). A total of 12 units from 12 different bottles should be used.

Phenytoin Suspension/Oral. *Recommended studies*: Two studies. (1) *Type of study*: Fasting. *Design*: Single-dose, two-way crossover in vivo. *Strength*: 125 mg/5 mg (dose of 300 mg). *Subjects*: Normal healthy males and females, general population. *Additional comments*: Washout period of at least 14 days. The single-dose studies for fasting and fed can be conducted as single dose, two-treatment, four periods, replicated design. The strength(s) designated in the Orange Book as the RLD should be used in the studies. (2) *Type of study*: Fed. *Design*: Single-dose, two-way crossover in vivo. *Strength*: 125 mg/5 mg (dose of 300 mg). *Subjects*: Normal healthy males and females, general population. *Additional comments*: Please see comments above. *Analytes to measure*: Phenytoin in plasma. *Bioequivalence based on (90% CI)*: Phenytoin. *Waiver request of in vivo testing*: Not applicable. Please conduct comparative dissolution testing on 12 dosage units of all strengths of the test and reference products using the USP method. A dosage unit for a suspension is the labeled strength (5 mL). A total of 12 units from 12 different bottles should be used.

Posaconazole Suspension/Oral. *Recommended studies*: Two studies. (1) *Type of study*: Fasting. *Design*: Single-dose, two-treatment, two-period crossover in vivo. *Strength*: 40 mg/mL (dose of 400 mg). *Subjects*: Normal healthy males and females, general population. *Additional comments*: Females must have a negative baseline pregnancy test within 24 hours prior to receiving the drug. Females should not be pregnant or lactating, and if applicable, should practice abstention or contraception during the study. (2) *Type of study*: Fed. *Design*: Single-dose, two-treatment, two-period crossover in vivo. *Strength*: 40 mg/mL (dose of 400 mg). *Subjects*: Normal healthy males and females, general population. *Additional comments*: Please see comment above. *Analytes to measure (in appropriate biological fluid)*: Posaconazole in plasma. *Bioequivalence based on (90% CI)*: Posaconazole. *Waiver request of in vivo testing*: Not applicable product at this Web site. Please note that a dosage unit for a suspension is the labeled strength (mL). A total of 12 units from 12 different bottles should be used. Specifications

Sulfamethoxazole; Trimethoprim Suspension/Oral. *Recommended studies*: One study. *Type of study*: Fasting. *Design*: Single-dose, two-treatment, two-period crossover in vivo. *Strength*: 200 mg/40 mg per 5 mL. *Subjects*: Normal healthy males and females, general population. *Additional comments*: *Analytes to measure (in appropriate biological fluid)*: Sulfamethoxazole and trimethoprim in plasma. *Bioequivalence based on (90% CI)*: Sulfamethoxazole and trimethoprim. *Waiver request of in vivo testing*: Not applicable.

Voriconazole Suspension/Oral. *Recommended studies*: One study. *Type of study*: Fasting. *Design*: Single-dose, two-way crossover in vivo. *Strength*: 200 mg/5 mL. *Subjects*: Normal healthy males and females, general population. Females should not be pregnant, and if applicable, should practice abstention or contraception during the study. *Additional comments*: *Analytes to measure (in appropriate biological fluid)*: Voriconazole in plasma. *Bioequivalence based on (90% CI)*: Voriconazole. *Waiver request of in vivo testing*: Not applicable.

20

Dissolution Testing of Liquid Dosage Forms

Drug Name	Dosage Form	USP Apparatus	Speed (RPMs)	Medium	Volume (mL)	Recommended Sampling Times (min)	Date Updated
Acyclovir	Suspension	II (Paddle)	50	0.1 N HCl	900	10, 20, 30, 45, and 60	02/20/2004
Amoxicillin/clavulanate potassium	Suspension	II (Paddle)	75	Water (deaerated)	900	5, 10, 15, and 30	01/14/2004
Carbamazepine	Suspension	II (Paddle)	50	Water (deaerated)	900	10, 20, 30, 45, and 60	01/20/2004
Cefadroxil	Suspension	II (Paddle)	25	Water	900	5, 10, 15, 30, and 45	07/25/2007
Cefdinir	Suspension	II (Paddle)	50	0.05 M phosphate buffer, pH 6.8	900	10, 20, 30, and 45	04/09/2007
Cefixime	Suspension	II (Paddle)	50	0.05 M phosphate buffer, pH 7.2	900	10, 20, 30, and 45	04/09/2007
Cefpodoxime proxetil	Suspension	II (Paddle)	50	0.04 M glycine buffer, pH 3.0	900	10, 20, 30, and 45	12/20/2005
Cefprozil monohydrate	Suspension	II (Paddle)	25	Water (deaerated)	900	5, 10, 15, and 30	01/21/2004
Ceftibuten dihydrate	Suspension	II (Paddle)	50	0.05 M phosphate buffer, pH 7.0	1000	10, 20, 30, and 45	01/21/2004
Cephalexin	Suspension	II (Paddle)	25	Water	900	5, 10, 20, and 30	07/25/2007
Clarithromycin	Suspension	II (Paddle)	50	0.05 M phosphate buffer, pH 6.8	900	10, 20, 30, 45, and 60	01/23/2004
Dextromethorphan polistirex	Suspension	II (Paddle)	50	0.1 N HCl	500	30, 60, 90, and 180	03/04/2006
Erythromycin ethylsuccinate	Suspension	II (Paddle)	75	Monobasic sodium phosphate, pH 6.8 buffer with 1% SLS buffer w/1% SLS	900	10, 20, 30, 45, and 60	01/27/2004
Felbamate	Suspension	II (Paddle)	50	Water (deaerated)	900	5, 10, 15, and 30	01/28/2004
Fluconazole (200 mg/5 mL)	Suspension	II (Paddle)	50	Water (deaerated)	900	10, 20, 30, and 45	01/30/2004
Fluconazole (50 mg/5 mL)	Suspension	II (Paddle)	50	Water (deaerated)	500	10, 20, 30, and 45	01/30/2004
Griseofulvin	Suspension	II (Paddle)	50	0.54% SLS	1000	10, 20, 30, and 45	04/09/2007
Ibuprofen/pseudoephedrine HCl	Suspension	II (Paddle)	50	0.05 M phosphate buffer, pH 7.2	900	5, 10, 15, and 30	02/04/2004
Linezolid	Suspension	II (Paddle)	50	0.05 M phosphate buffer, pH 6.8	900	10, 20, 30, and 45	01/14/2008
Meloxicam	Suspension	II (Paddle)	25	Phosphate buffer at pH 7.5	900	5, 10, 15, and 30	01/26/2006

Drug Name	Dosage Form	USP Apparatus	Speed (RPMs)	Medium	Volume (mL)	Recommended Sampling Times (min)	Date Updated
Mycophenolate mofetil	Suspension	II (Paddle)	40	0.1 N HCl	900	5, 10, 20, and 30	02/10/2004
Nevirapine	Suspension	II (Paddle)	25	0.1 N HCl	900	10, 20, 30, 45, and 60	02/11/2004
Oxcarbazepine	Suspension	II (Paddle)	75	1% SDS in water	900	10, 20, 30, and 45	02/12/2004
Paroxetine HCl	Suspension	II (Paddle)	100	SGF without enzyme	900	10, 20, 30, and 45	02/13/2004
Phenytoin	Suspension			Refer to USP			06/18/2007
Sucralfate	Suspension	II (Paddle)	75	0.1 N HCl/0.067 M KCl, pH 1.0	900	10, 20, 30, and 45	03/04/2006
Sulfamethoxazole/trimethoprim	Suspension	II (Paddle)	50	1 mL of 0.2 N HCl in water	900	10, 20, 30, 45, 60, and 90	02/25/2004
Voriconazole	Suspension	II (Paddle)	50	0.1 N HCl	900	10, 20, 30, and 45	01/03/2007
Azithromycin	Suspension oral	II (Paddle)	50	Phosphate buffer, pH 6.0	900	10, 20, 30, and 45	08/17/2006
Fosamprenavir calcium	Suspension oral	II (Paddle)	25	10 mM HCl	900	5, 10,15, and 20	12/03/2007
Posaconazole	Suspension oral	II (Paddle)	25	0.3% SLS	900	10, 20, 30, and 45	12/03/2007
Sulfisoxazole acetyl	Suspension oral (pediatric)	II (Paddle)	30	1% SLS in 0.1 N HCl	900	15, 30, 45, 60, and 90	08/17/2006
Ampicillin/ampicillin trihydrate	Suspension oral, powder	II (Paddle)	25	Water (deaerated)	900	5, 10, 15, 20	01/03/2007
Mesalamine enema	Suspension, enema	II (Paddle)	50	Phosphate buffer, pH 7.2	900	5, 10, 15, and 30	06/18/2007

21

Approved Excipients in Liquid Forms

Ingredient	Dosage Form	Qty	Unit
1-o-tolylbiguanide	Topical; solution	0.0125	%
Acesulfame potassium	Oral; suspension, liquid	0.15	%
Acesulfame potassium	Oral; solution	0.5	%
Acetic acid	Topical; suspension	0.04	%
Acetic acid, glacial	Oral; solution, syrup	0.1	%
Acetic acid, glacial	Oral; solution, elixir	0.1067	%
Acetone	Topical; solution	12.69	%
Acetone	Topical; shampoo	13	%
Acetylated monoglycerides	Oral; solution	24	%
Alcohol	Rectal; suspension	0.35	%
Alcohol	Oral; suspension	7.25	%
Alcohol	Topical; shampoo	10	%
Alcohol	Oral; solution, liquid, concentrate, oral	15.068	%
Alcohol	Topical; emulsion, aerosol foam	58.21	%
Alcohol	Oral; solution	66	%
Alcohol	Oral; concentrate	71.6	%
Alcohol	Oral; syrup	75	%
Alcohol	Topical; solution	91.07	%
Alcohol	Oral; solution, elixir	94.7	%
Alcohol, dehydrated	Oral; aerosol, metered	0.4716	%
Alcohol, dehydrated	Topical; swab	0.695	ML
Alcohol, dehydrated	Sublingual; spray, metered	0.95	%
Alcohol, dehydrated	Oral; suspension	1.75	%
Alcohol, dehydrated	Rectal; gel	11.224	%
Alcohol, dehydrated	Oral; solution, elixir	20	%
Alcohol, dehydrated	Topical; solution, liquid	25	%
Alcohol, dehydrated	Oral; syrup	29	%
Alcohol, dehydrated	Oral; solution	35.63	%
Alcohol, dehydrated	Topical; aerosol	60.39	%
Alcohol, dehydrated	Topical; emulsion, aerosol foam	60.43	%
Alcohol, dehydrated	Topical; solution	96.67	%
Alcohol, denatured	Oral; syrup	7	%
Alcohol, denatured	Topical; solution	60.16	%
Alcohol, denatured	Topical; aerosol	68	%
Alcohol, denatured	Topical; swab	75	ML
Alcohol, diluted	Oral; syrup	1.5	%

Ingredient	Dosage Form	Qty	Unit
Alcohol, diluted	Oral; solution, elixir	20	%
Alcohol, diluted	Topical; aerosol	68.5	%
Alkyl aryl sodium sulfonate	Topical; shampoo, suspension	2.5	%
Aluminum acetate	Topical; shampoo	0.1	%
Amerchol C	Topical; emulsion	0.1	%
Ammonia solution	Oral; suspension	0.015	%
Ammonium chloride	Oral; syrup	7	%
Ammonium glycyrrhizate	Oral; solution	0.8	%
Ammonium lauryl sulfate	Topical; emulsion	39.75	%
Ammonyx	Topical; aerosol, metered	3	%
Ammonyx	Topical; solution	3.5	%
Amphoteric-2	Topical; shampoo, suspension	5	%
Anethole	Oral; solution, elixir	0.003	%
Anethole	Oral; syrup	0.046	%
Anise	Oral; solution, elixir	0.009	%
Anise extract	Oral; solution, elixir	0.015	%
Anise oil	Oral; suspension	0.05	%
Anise oil	Oral; solution	0.14	%
Anise oil	Rectal; solution	0.14	%
Anise oil	Oral; solution, elixir	15	%
Arlacel	Topical; emulsion	5.5	%
Ascorbic acid	Topical; solution	0.044	%
Ascorbic acid	Oral; suspension	0.2	%
Ascorbic acid	Oral; concentrate	0.6	%
Ascorbic acid	Oral; syrup	1.25	%
Ascorbyl palmitate	Topical; solution	0.0044	%
Aspartame	Oral; syrup	0.0125	%
Aspartame	Oral; suspension	40.244	%
Beheneth-10	Topical; solution	1.5	%
Bentonite	Oral; suspension	1.3	%
Bentonite	Topical; shampoo, suspension	4	%
Benzaldehyde	Oral; suspension	0.06	%
Benzalkonium chloride	Topical; solution	0.005	%
Benzalkonium chloride	Topical; solution, drops	0.0075	%
Benzalkonium chloride	Topical; suspension	0.01	%
Benzalkonium chloride	Topical; shampoo	0.2	%
Benzoic acid	Oral; suspension	0.1	%
Benzoic acid	Rectal; suspension	0.1	%
Benzoic acid	Topical; solution	0.1	%
Benzoic acid	Rectal; gel	0.14	%
Benzoic acid	Oral; solution	0.5	%
Benzoic acid	Oral; solution, elixir	0.5	%
Benzoic acid	Oral; syrup	0.753	%

Ingredient	Dosage Form	Qty	Unit
Benzoic acid	Oral; concentrate	1.25	%
Benzyl alcohol	Oral; suspension	1	%
Benzyl alcohol	Topical; suspension	1	%
Benzyl alcohol	Rectal; gel	1.55	%
Benzyl alcohol	Topical; solution	2	%
Benzyl alcohol	Oral; solution	5	%
Boric acid	Topical; solution, drops	0.12	%
Boric acid	Topical; suspension	0.6	%
Boric acid	Topical; emulsion	1.3	%
Boric acid	Topical; shampoo	2	%
Butane	Sublingual; aerosol, metered	2.1998	%
Butyl alcohol	Topical; solution	0.0786	%
Butyl ester of PVM/MA copolymer	Topical; solution	30	%
Butylated hydroxyanisole	Oral; concentrate	0.0075	%
Butylated hydroxyanisole	Oral; solution	0.0189	%
Butylated hydroxyanisole	Oral; suspension	0.05	%
Butylated hydroxytoluene	Oral; solution, liquid, concentrate, oral	0.01	%
Butylated hydroxytoluene	Oral; solution	0.0189	%
Butylated hydroxytoluene	Topical; solution	0.088	%
Butylated hydroxytoluene	Topical; emulsion, aerosol foam	0.1	%
Butylated hydroxytoluene	Topical; shampoo	0.1	%
Butylparaben	Oral; syrup	0.0075	%
Butylparaben	Oral; drops	0.1	%
Butylparaben	Oral; solution	0.5	%
Butylparaben	Rectal; solution	0.5	%
Butylparaben	Oral; suspension	0.8	%
C20-40 pareth-24	Topical; solution	0.25	%
Calcium chloride	Oral; concentrate	0.008	%
Calcium chloride	Oral; suspension	0.05	%
Calcium phosphate, dibasic	Topical; shampoo	54.8	%
Calcium salicylate	Oral; solution, elixir	0.2487	%
Caprylic/capric triglyceride	Oral; solution	2.62	%
Caprylic/capric triglyceride	Topical; solution	50	%
Caprylic/capric/succinic triglyceride	Sublingual; aerosol, metered	1.0359	%
Capsicum oleoresin	Oral; syrup	0.0011	%
Captan	Topical; shampoo, suspension	1	%
Caramel	Oral; solution	0.008	%
Caramel	Oral; syrup	2.4	%
Caramel	Oral; suspension	11.112	%
Carbomer 934	Topical; solution	0.15	%
Carbomer 934	Oral; suspension	1	%
Carbomer 934	Rectal; enema	14.4	%
Carbomer 934P	Rectal; enema	0.075	%

Ingredient	Dosage Form	Qty	Unit
Carbomer 934P	Topical; solution	0.18	%
Carbomer 934P	Oral; suspension	1.4	%
Carbomer 940	Topical; emulsion	0.6	%
Carboxymethylcellulose	Oral; suspension	6.4	%
Carboxymethylcellulose sodium	Oral; suspension, drops	0.1	%
Carboxymethylcellulose sodium	Oral; drops	0.514	%
Carboxymethylcellulose sodium	Oral; syrup	2.65	%
Carboxymethylcellulose sodium	Oral; solution	3.5	%
Carboxymethylcellulose sodium	Oral; suspension	3.75	%
Cardamom	Oral; solution, elixir	0.25	%
Carmine	Oral; suspension	1.008	%
Cedar leaf oil	Topical; shampoo	30	%
Cellulose microcrystalline/carboxymethylcellulose sodium	Oral; suspension, drops	0.76	%
Cellulose microcrystalline/carboxymethylcellulose sodium	Oral; suspension	3	%
Cellulose microcrystalline/carboxymethylcellulose sodium	Oral; suspension, liquid	3	%
Cellulose, microcrystalline	Oral; suspension	1.45	%
Cellulose, microcrystalline	Oral; mucilage	63	MG
Cellulose, microcrystalline	Oral; dispersible tablet	253.2	MG
Cetearyl alcohol	Topical; suspension	2.5	%
Ceteth-20	Topical; solution	2	%
Ceteth-20	Topical; solution, liquid	2	%
Cetyl alcohol	Rectal; aerosol, metered	0.162	%
Cetyl alcohol	Topical; aerosol	1.16	%
Cetyl alcohol	Topical; suspension	2.013	%
Cetyl alcohol	Topical; emulsion, aerosol foam	3.226	%
Cetyl alcohol	Topical; aerosol, metered	10	%
Cetyl palmitate	Topical; solution	0.05	%
Chlorobutanol	Topical; solution	0.3	%
Choleth-24	Topical; emulsion	5	%
Cinnamaldehyde	Oral; suspension	0.01	%
Cinnamon	Oral; solution, elixir	1.05	%
Cinnamon oil	Oral; syrup	0.005	%
Cinnamon oil	Oral; suspension	0.0204	%
Cinnamon oil	Oral; solution, elixir	55	%
Citrate	Oral; syrup	1.2	%
Citric acid	Oral; suspension, for inhalation	0.028	%
Citric acid	Topical; aerosol	0.08	%
Citric acid	Topical; emulsion	0.11	%
Citric acid	Topical; emulsion, aerosol foam	0.11	%
Citric acid	Oral; drops	0.18	%
Citric acid	Oral; suspension, liquid	0.18	%

Ingredient	Dosage Form	Qty	Unit
Citric acid	Oral; suspension, drops	0.24	%
Citric acid	Oral; suspension, sustained action	0.5	%
Citric acid	Oral; solution, liquid	0.7	%
Citric acid	Oral; solution	0.8	%
Citric acid	Topical; shampoo, suspension	1	%
Citric acid	Oral; liquid	1.35	%
Citric acid	Oral; suspension	1.4065	%
Citric acid	Oral; concentrate	1.85	%
Citric acid	Oral; solution, elixir	2	%
Citric acid	Topical; shampoo	2.3	%
Citric acid	Topical; solution	40	%
Citric acid	Topical; swab	40	MG
Citric acid	Oral; syrup	72.2	%
Citric acid monohydrate	Topical; solution	0.188	%
Citric acid monohydrate	Topical; shampoo	0.24	%
Citric acid monohydrate	Oral; suspension	0.3	%
Citric acid monohydrate	Oral; solution	0.5	%
Citric acid monohydrate	Oral; syrup	0.96	%
Citric acid monohydrate	Oral; suspension, sustained action	14.08	%
Citric acid, hydrous	Oral; syrup	0.26	%
Citric acid, hydrous	Oral; suspension	0.75	%
Clove oil	Oral; suspension	0.01	%
Clove oil	Oral; solution, elixir	40	%
Cocamide diethanolamine	Topical; aerosol, metered	3	%
Cocamide diethanolamine	Topical; shampoo	3.5	%
Cocamide diethanolamine	Topical; solution	4	%
Cocamide diethanolamine	Topical; suspension	4	%
Cocamide ether sulfate	Topical; shampoo	5	%
Cocamine oxide	Topical; shampoo	2	%
Coco betaine	Topical; shampoo	6	%
Cocoa bean	Oral; suspension	24.666	%
Coconut oil	Topical; solution	15.5	%
Coriander oil	Oral; solution, elixir	15	%
Corn glycerides	Oral; solution	31.885	%
Corn oil	Oral; suspension	50	%
Corn syrup	Oral; solution	15	%
Corn syrup	Oral; solution, elixir	30.4	%
Corn syrup	Oral; suspension	34.2	%
Corn syrup	Oral; syrup	65.78	%
Crospovidone	Oral; suspension	0.05	%
Crospovidone	Topical; emulsion	1	%
Crospovidone	Oral; mucilage	9	MG
Crospovidone	Oral; suspension, sustained action	18.68	%

Ingredient	Dosage Form	Qty	Unit
Crospovidone	Oral; dispersible tablet	340	MG
Cyclomethicone	Topical; emulsion, aerosol foam	5.26	%
D&C Red No. 19	Topical; emulsion	0.0007	%
D&C Red No. 28	Topical; aerosol	0.0007	%
D&C Red No. 28	Oral; suspension	0.05	%
D&C Red No. 33	Oral; solution, elixir	0.0007	%
D&C Red No. 33	Oral; suspension, liquid	0.0013	%
D&C Red No. 33	Topical; shampoo	0.002	%
D&C Red No. 33	Oral; concentrate	0.0022	%
D&C Red No. 33	Oral; suspension	0.0025	%
D&C Red No. 33	Oral; solution	0.005	%
D&C Red No. 33	Oral; syrup	0.006	%
D&C Red No. 33	Oral; suspension, sustained action	0.4	%
D&C Yellow No. 10	Rectal; solution	0.0007	%
D&C Yellow No. 10	Oral; solution, liquid	0.0008	%
D&C Yellow No. 10	Oral; suspension, liquid	0.0008	%
D&C Yellow No. 10	Topical; shampoo	0.001	%
D&C Yellow No. 10	Oral; concentrate	0.0025	%
D&C Yellow No. 10	Topical; shampoo, suspension	0.005	%
D&C Yellow No. 10	Oral; solution, elixir	0.03	%
D&C Yellow No. 10	Oral; syrup	0.05	%
D&C Yellow No. 10	Oral; suspension	2	%
D&C Yellow No. 10	Oral; solution	5	%
D&C Yellow No. 6 Lake	Oral; solution	0.005	%
Denatonium benzoate	Topical; solution	0.0003	%
Dextrin	Topical; shampoo	5	%
Dextrose	Oral; syrup	27	%
Dichlorodifluoromethane	Topical; emulsion, aerosol foam	8	%
Dichlorodifluoromethane	Rectal; aerosol, metered	13.5	%
Dichlorofluoromethane	Oral; aerosol, metered	35	%
Dichlorotetrafluoroethane	Rectal; aerosol, metered	9	%
Diethyl sebacate	Topical; solution	24	%
Diisopropyl adipate	Topical; solution	17	%
Diisopropyl dimerate	Topical; solution	1	%
Dimethicone 350	Topical; solution	0.5	%
Disodium edisylate	Oral; solution	0.02	%
Disodium laureth sulfosuccinate	Topical; shampoo	15	%
Disodium lauryl sulfosuccinate	Topical; shampoo	15	%
Docosanol	Topical; solution	1.1	%
Docusate sodium	Oral; suspension, sustained action	0.077	%
Docusate sodium	Oral; suspension	0.115	%
Docusate sodium	Topical; shampoo	2	%
Dye blue 1	Oral; solution	0.0753	%

Ingredient	Dosage Form	Qty	Unit
Dye caramel 105	Oral; syrup	0.0052	%
Dye caramel acid proof 100	Oral; solution, elixir	0.005	%
Dye caramel acid proof 100	Oral; syrup	0.048	%
Dye FDC blue 10	Oral; syrup	0.0001	%
Dye wild cherry 7598	Oral; syrup	0.0035	%
Dye yellow 10	Oral; solution	0.006	%
Edamine	Oral; solution	0.37	%
Edetate calcium disodium	Oral; concentrate	0.025	%
Edetate calcium disodium	Oral; solution, elixir	0.1	%
Edetate disodium	Oral; suspension, for inhalation	0.01	%
Edetate disodium	Topical; solution	0.01	%
Edetate disodium	Topical; suspension	0.01	%
Edetate disodium	Oral; suspension, drops	0.04	%
Edetate disodium	Rectal; solution	0.04	%
Edetate disodium	Oral; liquid	0.05	%
Edetate disodium	Rectal; enema	0.1	%
Edetate disodium	Topical; emulsion	0.1107	%
Edetate disodium	Oral; suspension	0.2497	%
Edetate disodium	Oral; concentrate	0.3	%
Edetate disodium	Oral; solution	0.5	%
Edetate disodium	Oral; syrup	0.5	%
Edetic acid	Topical; suspension	0.0633	%
Edetic acid	Topical; shampoo	0.2	%
Edetic acid	Topical; solution	0.5	%
Epilactose	Oral; solution	1.3333	%
Epilactose	Rectal; solution	1.3333	%
Essence fritzbro orange	Oral; suspension	2.01	%
Essence lemon	Oral; syrup	0.25	%
Essence orange	Oral; syrup	1	%
Ethyl acetate	Topical; solution	31	%
Ethyl hexanediol	Topical; solution	0.25	%
Ethyl maltol	Oral; solution	0.05	%
Ethyl maltol	Oral; solution, elixir	0.06	%
Ethyl maltol	Oral; syrup	3.05	%
Ethyl vanillin	Oral; suspension	0.008	%
Ethylene glycol	Topical; shampoo, suspension	1	%
Eucalyptus oil	Oral; syrup	0.014	%
Fatty acid glycerides	Sublingual; spray, metered	0.096	%
Fatty acids	Topical; solution	13.58	%
FD&C Blue No. 1	Oral; solution, elixir	0.0005	%
FD&C Blue No. 1	Oral; suspension, liquid	0.0007	%
fd&c Blue No. 1	Oral; suspension	0.0015	%
fd&c Blue No. 1	Topical; shampoo	0.0036	%

Ingredient	Dosage Form	Qty	Unit
FD&C Blue No. 1	Oral; syrup	0.004	%
FD&C Blue No. 1	Oral; solution	0.0753	%
FD&C Blue No. 1	Rectal; solution	0.0753	%
FD&C Blue No. 1-Aluminum Lake	Oral; syrup	0.0013	%
FD&C Green No. 3	Oral; syrup	0.075	%
FD&C Red No. 3	Oral; solution, elixir	0.0008	%
FD&C Red No. 3	Oral; drops	0.005	%
FD&C Red No. 3	Oral; syrup	0.015	%
FD&C Red No. 3	Oral; suspension	0.02	%
FD&C Red No. 33	Oral; solution	0.0011	%
FD&C Red No. 33	Oral; syrup	0.002	%
FD&C Red No. 33	Oral; solution, elixir	2.75	%
FD&C Red No. 3-Aluminum Lake	Topical; solution	0.006	%
FD&C Red No. 4	Topical; solution	0.0005	%
FD&C Red No. 40	Oral; drops	0.001	%
FD&C Red No. 40	Oral; concentrate	0.0035	%
FD&C Red No. 40	Topical; shampoo	0.004	%
FD&C Red No. 40	Oral; suspension, liquid	0.005	%
FD&C Red No. 40	Oral; suspension, drops	0.016	%
FD&C Red No. 40	Oral; solution	0.04	%
FD&C Red No. 40	Oral; syrup	2	%
FD&C Red No. 40	Oral; suspension	10	%
FD&C Red No. 40	Oral; solution, elixir	12.5	%
FD&C Red No. 40-Aluminum Lake	Oral; solution	0.007	%
FD&C Red No. 40-Aluminum Lake	Oral; suspension	0.04	%
FD&C Yellow No. 10	Oral; suspension	0.01	%
FD&C Yellow No. 10	Oral; syrup	0.025	%
FD&C Yellow No. 5	Oral; syrup	0.0015	%
FD&C Yellow No. 5	Oral; solution, elixir	0.002	%
FD&C Yellow No. 5	Topical; solution	0.0055	%
FD&C Yellow No. 5	Oral; solution	0.1	%
FD&C Yellow No. 6	Oral; concentrate	0.003	%
FD&C Yellow No. 6	Oral; suspension, liquid	0.01	%
FD&C Yellow No. 6	Oral; suspension, sustained action	0.0115	%
FD&C Yellow No. 6	Oral; suspension	0.1	%
FD&C Yellow No. 6	Oral; syrup	0.4	%
FD&C Yellow No. 6	Oral; solution, elixir	4	%
FD&C Yellow No. 6	Oral; solution	20	%
FD&C Yellow No. 6	Rectal; solution	20	%
Ferric oxide red	Oral; suspension, sustained action	0.27	%
Flavor anise 29653	Oral; solution	0.0186	%
Flavor apple watermelon PFC 9887	Oral; syrup	0.51	%
Flavor apricot 23067	Oral; suspension	0.0963	%

Ingredient	Dosage Form	Qty	Unit
Flavor apricot 24829	Oral; solution	0.2	%
Flavor apricot peach	Oral; syrup	0.52	%
Flavor banana 74546	Oral; suspension	0.21	%
Flavor BBA-47769	Oral; drops	0.23	%
Flavor berry citrus blend 8409	Oral; concentrate	0.8	%
Flavor berry citrus blend 8409	Oral; solution	5	%
Flavor berry citrus blend 9621	Oral; solution	5.125	%
Flavor bitter mask 9885	Oral; solution	0.5	%
Flavor bitterness modifier 36734	Oral; syrup	0.1	%
Flavor bitterness modifier 367343	Oral; syrup	0.5	%
Flavor blood orange SA	Oral; syrup	0.021	%
Flavor bubble gum 15864	Oral; syrup	0.1	%
Flavor bubble gum 175303	Oral; solution	0.1234	%
Flavor bubble gum 3266P	Oral; syrup	0.05	%
Flavor bubble gum mc-4938	Oral; suspension	0.36	%
Flavor butterscotch F-1785	Oral; syrup	35	%
Flavor C&K mixed fruit A13688	Oral; solution	2.5	%
Flavor candied sugar 510155U	Oral; syrup	0.7223	%
Flavor cheri beri PCD-5580	Oral; syrup	5	%
Flavor cheri beri PFC-8580	Oral; solution	0.05	%
Flavor cheri beri PFC-8580	Oral; syrup	5	%
Flavor cherry 104613	Oral; syrup	0.0002	%
Flavor cherry 107026	Oral; syrup	0.1	%
Flavor cherry 1566	Oral; solution	0.15	%
Flavor cherry 213	Oral; syrup	0.07	%
Flavor cherry 3321	Oral; syrup	0.15	%
Flavor cherry 349	Oral; solution	1.645	%
Flavor cherry 500910U	Oral; suspension	0.04	%
Flavor cherry 57.679/A	Oral; suspension	5	%
Flavor cherry 590271A	Oral; suspension	0.0061	%
Flavor cherry 598384	Oral; syrup	0.14	%
Flavor cherry 825.476WC	Oral; solution	0.3	%
Flavor cherry 842	Oral; syrup	0.5	%
Flavor cherry 8513	Oral; syrup	0.022	%
Flavor cherry berry F-1194	Oral; suspension, liquid	0.4	%
Flavor cherry burgundy 11650	Oral; solution	0.3	%
Flavor cherry cream 14850	Oral; suspension	0.0715	%
Flavor cherry DP300684	Oral; syrup	0.35	%
Flavor cherry E.P.modified 151	Oral; concentrate	0.1	%
Flavor cherry F-232	Oral; concentrate	0.1	%
Flavor cherry F-232	Oral; suspension	0.1	%
Flavor cherry F-232	Oral; solution	1.5	%
Flavor cherry FMC 8513	Oral; solution	0.05	%

Ingredient	Dosage Form	Qty	Unit
Flavor cherry FMC 8513	Oral; syrup	0.08	%
Flavor cherry FONA 825.662	Oral; suspension, liquid	0.205	%
Flavor cherry IFF 13530912	Oral; solution, elixir	0.005	%
Flavor cherry MINT 5073A	Oral; solution	0.5	%
Flavor cherry PFC-9768	Oral; concentrate	0.7	%
Flavor cherry PFC-9768	Oral; solution	2	%
Flavor cherry PFC-9768	Oral; syrup	2	%
Flavor cherry pistachio PFC-8450	Oral; concentrate	0.9	%
FLAVOR cherry vanilla compound A77487	Oral; syrup	0.1057	%
Flavor cherry wixon 3566	Oral; syrup	1	%
Flavor cherry WL-1093	Oral; syrup	0.08	%
Flavor cherry WL-4658	Oral; solution	0.65	%
Flavor cherry anise PFC-9758	Oral; syrup	0.5313	%
Flavor coconut toasted 1323PG	Oral; solution	0.06	%
Flavor cola FMC 15740	Oral; solution, elixir	1.5	%
Flavor cotton candy 30-92-0011	Oral; solution	1.02	%
Flavor cotton candy F-9967	Oral; solution	0.7	%
Flavor cough syrup 110257	Oral; solution	0.1	%
Flavor cough syrup 134681	Oral; syrup	0.6	%
Flavor cough syrup 819	Oral; syrup	0.15	%
Flavor creamy vanilla 16345	Oral; solution	0.2	%
Flavor creme de menthe 14677	Oral; suspension	0.0003	%
Flavor creme de menthe 14677	Oral; solution	0.3	%
Flavor creme de vanilla 28156	Oral; drops	0.16	%
Flavor E-472	Oral; concentrate	0.4	%
Flavor F-5397A	Oral; concentrate	8	%
Flavor F-9843	Oral; suspension	0.05	%
Flavor felton 6-R-9	Oral; syrup	0.15	%
Flavor fritzsche 73959	Oral; syrup	0.5	%
Flavor fritzsche 78087	Oral; syrup	0.1	%
Flavor fruit 01-10428	Oral; concentrate	0.025	%
Flavor fruit punch 28140	Oral; suspension	0.75	%
Flavor fruit TAK 20008	Oral; concentrate	0.1	%
Flavor grape 501040A	Oral; solution	0.03	%
Flavor grape 6175	Oral; suspension	0.2	%
Flavor grape firmenich 587.444	Oral; suspension, liquid	0.37	%
Flavor grape firmenich 597.303/C	Oral; suspension, liquid	0.133	%
Flavor grape givaudan 433160	Oral; suspension, liquid	0.37	%
Flavor grape manheimer 522463	Oral; suspension	0.5	%
Flavor grape nector PFC-8599	Oral; syrup	0.2	%
Flavor grape PFC 8439	Oral; syrup	1.003	%
Flavor grape PFC-9711	Oral; syrup	0.0015	%
Flavor grape PFC-9924	Oral; solution	0.4	%

Ingredient	Dosage Form	Qty	Unit
Flavor guarana FMC-15417	Oral; suspension	0.756	%
Flavor lemon 812	Oral; suspension	0.176	%
Flavor lemon FMC-10471	Oral; syrup	0.5	%
Flavor lemon givaudan 74940-74	Oral; suspension, liquid	9	%
Flavor lemon mint 862.547	Oral; solution	0.12	%
Flavor lemon mint fritzsche 54369	Oral; syrup	0.1	%
Flavor magnasweet 110	Oral; solution	2.95	%
Flavor mixed fruit PFC-9970	Oral; syrup	0.235	%
Flavor orange 7679	Oral; solution	0.4	%
Flavor orange 7679	Oral; syrup	1.25	%
Flavor orange 607217	Oral; syrup	0.5	%
Flavor orange givaudan 74388-74	Oral; suspension, liquid	0.02	%
Flavor orange PFW-730016U	Oral; suspension, sustained action	1.5	%
Flavor orange pineapple FV-43	Oral; solution, elixir	0.2454	%
Flavor orange WONF 608352	Oral; solution	0.01	%
Flavor peach 10457	Oral; solution	0.06	%
Flavor peach 13503584	Oral; syrup	0.308	%
Flavor peach 302789	Oral; solution	0.12	%
Flavor peach mint fritzsche 106109	Oral; syrup	0.1	%
Flavor peach pineapple FMC 14258	Oral; solution	0.0003	%
Flavor peach pineapple FMC 14258	Oral; suspension	0.0003	%
Flavor peppermint 104	Oral; solution	0.05	%
Flavor peppermint 104	Oral; suspension	0.2	%
Flavor peppermint 894.143	Oral; solution	0.03	%
Flavor peppermint PFC 9927	Oral; solution	0.07	%
Flavor pharmasweet 10772900	Oral; syrup	0.2	%
Flavor pineapple N-2766	Oral; syrup	1	%
Flavor punch WL-7126	Oral; suspension	0.3	%
Flavor raspberry 1840	Oral; solution, elixir	0.125	%
Flavor raspberry 21028d	Oral; solution	0.044	%
Flavor raspberry 21028d	Oral; syrup	0.5	%
Flavor raspberry 28106	Oral; drops	0.5	%
Flavor raspberry 50776	Oral; syrup	0.05	%
Flavor raspberry 65934	Oral; solution	0.075	%
Flavor raspberry 8456	Oral; syrup	0.336	%
Flavor raspberry 998	Oral; solution	0.75	%
Flavor raspberry 998	Oral; syrup	1	%
Flavor raspberry A11693	Oral; syrup	0.075	%
Flavor raspberry arome PFC-9908	Oral; syrup	0.5	%
Flavor raspberry D9599	Oral; suspension	0.2	%
Flavor raspberry F-1784	Oral; solution	1	%
Flavor raspberry F-1784	Oral; syrup	7	%
Flavor raspberry F-1840	Oral; solution	0.25	%

Ingredient	Dosage Form	Qty	Unit
Flavor raspberry F-1840	Oral; syrup	0.6	%
Flavor raspberry PFC-8407	Oral; solution, elixir	0.025	%
Flavor raspberry POLAK 5000064	Oral; solution	0.0001	%
Flavor strawberry 14953	Oral; solution	0.3	%
Flavor strawberry 17C56217	Oral; solution	0.3	%
Flavor strawberry 5210(FD&D)	Oral; syrup	0.078	%
Flavor strawberry 523121a	Oral; suspension	4.2	%
Flavor strawberry 55058	Oral; concentrate	0.1	%
Flavor strawberry 55058	Oral; syrup	0.1	%
Flavor strawberry 5951	Oral; drops	0.2	%
Flavor strawberry 9843	Oral; syrup	0.1	%
Flavor strawberry FN-13819	Oral; solution	0.87	%
Flavor strawberry PFC-9626	Oral; syrup	1.5795	%
Flavor strawberry trusil windsor 2373031	Oral; suspension, sustained action	2.21	%
Flavor sweet tone 28837	Oral; solution	0.05	%
Flavor sweet-AM 918.005	Oral; solution	0.04	%
Flavor sweetness enhancer 5401b	Oral; syrup	0.3	%
Flavor tangerine fritzsche 51465	Oral; syrup	0.05	%
Flavor tetrarome	Oral; suspension	0.01	%
Flavor TM 313298	Oral; suspension	0.075	%
Flavor TPF 135	Oral; suspension	0.007	%
Flavor TPF 143	Oral; suspension	0.13	%
Flavor tropical blend FV-50	Oral; solution, elixir	0.2999	%
Flavor tropical fruit punch 1591	Oral; solution	0.8	%
Flavor tropical fruit punch N&A 50432	Oral; syrup	0.52	%
Flavor tropical fruit punch N&A 50432	Oral; solution	18.2	%
Flavor tutti frutti 0002028	Oral; suspension	0.35	%
Flavor tutti frutti 51.880/AP05.51	Oral; suspension	0.05	%
Flavor vanilla 323453	Oral; solution	0.156	%
Flavor vanilla 33869	Oral; solution	1.27	%
Flavor vanilla beck C7984	Oral; syrup	0.6	%
Flavor vanilla F-6257	Oral; solution	0.6	%
Flavor vanilla PFC-8541	Oral; concentrate	0.01	%
Flavor vanilla PFC-9772	Oral; concentrate	1	%
Flavor wild cherry 29653	Oral; solution	0.04	%
Flavor wild cherry 695047u	Oral; concentrate	1	%
Flavor wild cherry PFC-14783	Oral; suspension	0.037	%
Flavor wild cherry PFC-14783	Oral; syrup	0.4	%
Flavor wild cherry WL-1093 florasynth	Oral; syrup	0.25	%
Flavor wintergreen PFC-8421	Oral; solution	0.0001	%
Flavor yellow plum lemon 39K 020	Oral; suspension	0.05	%
Florasynth	Oral; solution	0.5	%
Formaldehyde	Topical; solution	0.2	%

Ingredient	Dosage Form	Qty	Unit
Fragrance 3949-5	Topical; shampoo, suspension	0.4	%
Fragrance 91-122	Topical; shampoo, suspension	3	%
Fragrance felton 066M	Topical; solution	0.12	%
Fragrance firmenich 47373	Topical; solution	0.1	%
Fragrance givaudan ESS 9090/1C	Topical; solution	0.101	%
Fragrance herbal 10396	Topical; shampoo	0.3	%
Fragrance P O FL-147	Topical; aerosol, metered	0.1	%
Fragrance P O FL-147	Topical; solution	0.13	%
Fragrance P O FL-147	Topical; aerosol	0.274	%
Fragrance P O FL-147	Topical; emulsion	0.274	%
Fragrance PA 52805	Topical; solution	5	%
Fragrance PA 52805	Topical; swab	50	MG
Fragrance pera derm D	Topical; solution	0.0217	%
Fragrance RBD-9819	Topical; solution	0.025	%
Fragrance RBD-9819	Topical; emulsion, aerosol foam	0.1	%
Fragrance shaw mudge U-7776	Topical; solution	0.01	%
Fragrance TF 044078	Topical; solution	0.5	%
Fragrance ungerer honeysuckle K 2771	Topical; shampoo	1	%
Fructose	Rectal; solution	0.6667	%
Fructose	Oral; suspension	2	%
Fructose	Oral; solution	35	%
Fumaric acid	Oral; syrup	0.075	%
Fumaric acid	Oral; suspension	0.5	%
Galactose	Rectal; solution	14.6667	%
Galactose	Oral; solution	14.7	%
Gelatin	Oral; solution	3.48	%
Ginger fluidextract	Oral; solution, elixir	1	%
Ginger fluidextract	Oral; syrup	1	%
Gluconolactone	Topical; aerosol, metered	0.25	%
Gluconolactone	Topical; solution	0.25	%
Glucose, liquid	Oral; solution	49.78	%
Glucose, liquid	Oral; syrup	62	%
Glycerin	Topical; emulsion, aerosol foam	2.11	%
Glycerin	Topical; suspension	5	%
Glycerin	Oral; drops	10	%
Glycerin	Oral; suspension, drops	10	%
Glycerin	Oral; suspension, liquid	10	%
Glycerin	Oral; solution, concentrate	20	%
Glycerin	Oral; solution, syrup	20	%
Glycerin	Oral; liquid	22	%
Glycerin	Topical; solution	50	%
Glycerin	Oral; solution, elixir	62.3	%
Glycerin	Oral; concentrate	75	%

Ingredient	Dosage Form	Qty	Unit
Glycerin	Oral; syrup	77	%
Glycerin	Oral; suspension	79	%
Glycerin	Oral; solution	94	%
Glyceryl caprylate	Oral; solution	34.91	%
Glyceryl palmitostearate	Oral; suspension	3	%
Glyceryl ricinoleate	Topical; shampoo, suspension	2	%
Glyceryl stearate SE	Topical; suspension	1.25	%
Glycine	Oral; suspension	2	%
Glycine	Oral; solution	5	%
Glycine	Rectal; solution	5	%
Glycol distearate	Topical; shampoo	1.25	%
Glycol stearate	Topical; shampoo, suspension	1	%
Glycol stearate	Topical; shampoo	3	%
Glycyrrhizic acid	Oral; syrup	0.125	%
Glycyrrhizin, ammoniated	Oral; syrup	0.125	%
Glycyrrhizin, ammoniated	Oral; solution	0.13	%
Guar gum	Oral; suspension	0.493	%
Hexylene glycol	Topical; solution	12	%
High fructose corn syrup	Oral; solution	16.86	%
Histidine	Oral; suspension	0.5	%
Hydrocarbon	Rectal; aerosol, metered	5.21	%
Hydrochloric acid	Oral; syrup	0.203	%
Hydrochloric acid	Topical; solution	1.24	%
Hydrochloric acid	Oral; concentrate	3.1	%
Hydrochloric acid	Topical; shampoo	4	%
Hydrochloric acid	Oral; solution	9.51	%
Hydrochloric acid	Oral; suspension	10	%
Hydrochloric acid, diluted	Topical; shampoo	2.35	%
Hydrochloric acid, diluted	Oral; solution	2.75	%
Hydrochloric acid, diluted	Topical; solution	5.55	%
Hydroxyethyl cellulose	Oral; suspension	0.1	%
Hydroxyethyl cellulose	Topical; suspension	0.686	%
Hydroxyethyl cellulose	Oral; solution	0.75	%
Hydroxyethyl cellulose	Topical; solution	0.75	%
Hydroxyethyl cellulose	Oral; syrup	10	%
Hydroxymethyl cellulose	Topical; solution	0.909	%
Hydroxypropyl cellulose	Topical; solution	0.6	%
Hydroxypropyl methylcellulose 100	Oral; syrup	0.25	%
Hydroxypropyl methylcellulose 100	Oral; suspension	5	%
Hydroxypropyl methylcellulose 2910	Oral; syrup	0.45	%
Hydroxypropyl methylcellulose 2910	Oral; suspension	0.5	%
Hydroxypropyl methylcellulose 4000	Oral; suspension	2	%
Hydroxypropyl methylcellulose 603	Oral; suspension	2.3	%

Ingredient	Dosage Form	Qty	Unit
Hydroxypropyl-*b*-cyclodextrin	Oral; solution	40	%
Imidurea	Topical; shampoo	0.4	%
Invert sugar	Oral; syrup	77	%
Isobutane	Topical; aerosol	6	%
Isoceteth-20	Topical; solution	2.3	%
Isopropyl alcohol	Topical; aerosol, metered	4	%
Isopropyl alcohol	Topical; aerosol, spray	10	%
Isopropyl alcohol	Topical; solution	51.5	%
Isopropyl myristate	Topical; emulsion, aerosol foam	7.9	%
Isostearyl alcohol	Topical; suspension	2.5	%
Kaolin	Oral; syrup	1	%
Kola nut extract	Oral; solution	2	%
Kola nut extract	Rectal; solution	2	%
Kola nut extract	Oral; concentrate	24.72	%
Lactic acid	Topical; suspension	0.7	%
Lactic acid	Topical; emulsion, aerosol foam	1.05	%
Lactic acid	Oral; concentrate	5	%
Lactic acid	Topical; solution	18.06	%
D-Tagatose	Topical; solution	7.4	%
Lactose	Rectal; solution	8	%
Lactose	Oral; solution	11.2133	%
Lactose monohydrate	Oral; dispersible tablet	543.6	MG
Laneth	Topical; solution	0.5	%
Lauramine oxide	Topical; solution	4.8	%
Laurdimonium hydrolyzed animal collagen	Topical; shampoo	1	%
Laureth-23	Topical; aerosol	0.45	%
Laureth-23	Topical; emulsion	0.45	%
Laureth-23	Topical; emulsion, aerosol foam	1.075	%
Laureth-4	Topical; solution	5.22	%
Lauric diethanolamide	Topical; suspension	0.475	%
Lauric diethanolamide	Topical; solution	1.4167	%
Lauric diethanolamide	Topical; shampoo, suspension	4	%
Lauric diethanolamide	Topical; emulsion	15	%
Lauric diethanolamide	Topical; shampoo	20	%
Lauryl sulfate	Topical; shampoo, suspension	25	%
Lecithin	Topical; solution	1.4	%
Lecithin	Oral; suspension	11	%
Lecithin, soybean	Oral; suspension	0.2	%
Levomenthol	Sublingual; aerosol, metered	0.002	%
Light mineral oil	Topical; emulsion, aerosol foam	5.26	%
Lithium hydroxide monohydrate	Oral; syrup	33.7	%
Magnasweet 110	Oral; solution	0.8	%
Magnasweet 180	Oral; solution	0.13	%

Ingredient	Dosage Form	Qty	Unit
Magnesium aluminum silicate	Oral; drops	0.166	%
Magnesium aluminum silicate	Topical; shampoo, suspension	0.85	%
Magnesium aluminum silicate	Rectal; suspension	1	%
Magnesium aluminum silicate	Oral; suspension	6.4	%
Magnesium aluminum silicate hydrate	Topical; shampoo	0.5	%
Magnesium aluminum silicate hydrate	Rectal; suspension	1	%
Magnesium aluminum silicate hydrate	Oral; syrup	10	%
Magnesium aluminum silicate hydrate	Oral; suspension	10.6	%
Magnesium aluminum silicate hydrate	Oral; concentrate	41	%
Magnesium stearate	Oral; suspension, sustained action	2.7	%
Magnesium stearate	Oral; mucilage	4.5	MG
Magnesium stearate	Oral; suspension	5.756	%
Maleic acid	Oral; syrup	0.0345	%
Malic acid	Oral; solution	0.042	%
Malic acid, DL-	Oral; solution	0.33	%
Maltitol	Oral; solution	65	%
Maltol	Oral; concentrate	0.01	%
Maltol	Oral; solution	0.01	%
Mannitol	Topical; solution, drops	1.6	%
Medical antifoam emulsion C	Oral; suspension	0.0528	%
Menthol	Oral; concentrate	0.005	%
Menthol	Oral; suspension	0.041	%
Menthol	Oral; solution, liquid, concentrate, oral	0.05	%
Menthol	Oral; solution	0.075	%
Menthol	Topical; solution	0.08	%
Menthol	Oral; syrup	0.4	%
Methyl alcohol	Oral; concentrate	4.42	%
Methyl gluceth-120 dioleate	Topical; shampoo	1.8	%
Methylcellulose	Oral; suspension	0.025	%
Methylparaben	Rectal; aerosol, metered	0.09	%
Methylparaben	Oral; solution, concentrate	0.1	%
Methylparaben	Rectal; suspension	0.1	%
Methylparaben	Topical; solution	0.1	%
Methylparaben	Topical; emulsion, aerosol foam	0.108	%
Methylparaben	Topical; shampoo, suspension	0.15	%
Methylparaben	Oral; solution, syrup	0.18	%
Methylparaben	Topical; shampoo	0.18	%
Methylparaben	Oral; concentrate	0.2	%
Methylparaben	Oral; suspension, liquid	0.2	%
Methylparaben	Topical; emulsion	0.2	%
Methylparaben	Topical; suspension	0.3	%
Methylparaben	Oral; solution, elixir	0.5	%
Methylparaben	Oral; liquid	0.5	%

Ingredient	Dosage Form	Qty	Unit
Methylparaben	Oral; suspension, sustained action	0.75	%
Methylparaben	Oral; suspension	1	%
Methylparaben	Oral; syrup	5	%
Methylparaben	Rectal; enema	10.8	%
Methylparaben	Oral; solution	13	%
Methylparaben	Rectal; solution	13	%
Methylparaben sodium	Oral; suspension	0.13	%
Mineral oil	Topical; suspension	2.013	%
Myristyl alcohol	Topical; suspension	1.05	%
N,N-dimethyl lauramine oxide	Topical; solution	3.5	%
Nipasept	Oral; syrup	0.1	%
Nonoxynol iodine	Topical; solution	15.11	%
Nonoxynol-15	Topical; solution	5.05	%
Nonoxynol-9	Topical; solution	0.01	%
Norflurane	Oral; aerosol, metered	5.4234	%
Norflurane	Oral; suspension, for inhalation	7.5	%
Nutmeg oil, expressed	Oral; solution, elixir	0.45	%
Oatmeal	Topical; shampoo	8	%
Octoxynol-9	Topical; solution	22	%
Octyldodecanol	Topical; suspension	2.013	%
Oleic acid	Topical; solution	7.4	%
Olive oil	Topical; solution	0.6	%
Olive oil	Oral; solution	42.5	%
Opadry oy-ls-58900 white	Oral; solution	0.3	%
Opadry ys-1-7003 white	Oral; mucilage	27	MG
Orange juice	Oral; solution	0.01	%
Orange oil	Oral; suspension	0.054	%
Orange oil	Oral; solution, elixir	0.12	%
Orange oil, terpeneless	Oral; syrup	0.0005	%
Orange oil, terpeneless	Oral; suspension	0.264	%
Orange peel extract	Oral; syrup	0.9	%
Orvus K liquid	Topical; aerosol	39.75	%
Palmitamine oxide	Topical; solution	3.75	%
Parabens	Topical; aerosol, metered	10	%
Peg-8 caprylic/capric glycerides	Oral; solution	6.12	%
Peglicol-5-oleate	Oral; solution	31.9	%
Peppermint oil	Oral; concentrate	0.005	%
Peppermint oil	Sublingual; aerosol, metered	0.0222	%
Peppermint oil	Sublingual; spray, metered	0.0345	%
Peppermint oil	Oral; solution	0.35	%
Peppermint oil	Oral; suspension	10	%
Peppermint oil	Oral; syrup	60	%
Perfume bouquet	Topical; shampoo	0.2	%

Ingredient	Dosage Form	Qty	Unit
Perfume W-1952-1	Topical; solution	10	%
Petrolatum	Topical; emulsion	5.3	%
Petrolatum, white	Topical; emulsion, aerosol foam	7.9	%
Phenoxyethanol	Topical; emulsion, aerosol foam	1.05	%
Phosphoric acid	Topical; solution	0.027	%
Phosphoric acid	Oral; solution	0.1282	%
Pineapple	Oral; concentrate	0.1	%
Polacrilin potassium	Oral; suspension, liquid	0.4	%
Poloxamer 124	Oral; suspension	0.009	%
Poloxamer 188	Oral; concentrate	0.025	%
Poloxamer 188	Oral; suspension	0.6	%
Poloxamer 188	Oral; solution	10	%
Poloxamer 331	Oral; suspension	1.25	%
Poloxamer 407	Oral; solution	1	%
Polyethylene glycol 1000	Oral; concentrate	10	%
Polyethylene glycol 1000	Oral; solution	20	%
Polyethylene glycol 1450	Oral; solution	20	%
Polyethylene glycol 1540	Oral; solution	3.364	%
Polyethylene glycol 1540	Topical; solution	29.7	%
Polyethylene glycol 200	Oral; solution	20	%
Polyethylene glycol 300	Topical; solution	29.7	%
Polyethylene glycol 3350	Oral; suspension	4.5	%
Polyethylene glycol 400	Oral; syrup	0.05	%
Polyethylene glycol 400	Oral; suspension	5	%
Polyethylene glycol 400	Oral; concentrate	60	%
Polyethylene glycol 400	Oral; solution	60	%
Polyethylene glycol 400	Topical; solution	69.9	%
Polyethylene glycol 600	Topical; solution	0.3	%
Polyethylene glycol 600	Oral; solution	65	%
Polyethylene glycol 900	Topical; solution	0.95	%
Polyglyceryl-10 oleate	Oral; solution	19	%
Polyglyceryl-3 oleate	Oral; solution	31	%
Polyoxyl 150 distearate	Topical; solution	1.25	%
Polyoxyl 20 cetostearyl ether	Topical; emulsion, aerosol foam	4.74	%
Polyoxyl 35 castor oil	Oral; suspension	0.04	%
Polyoxyl 35 castor oil	Oral; solution	51.5	%
Polyoxyl 40 hydrogenated castor oil	Oral; solution	45	%
Polyoxyl 40 stearate	Topical; emulsion, aerosol foam	1.075	%
Polyoxyl 6 laurate	Topical; shampoo	2	%
Polyoxyl 75 lanolin	Topical; solution	1	%
Polyoxyl 75 lanolin	Topical; aerosol	1.5	%
Polyoxyl 75 lanolin	Topical; emulsion	1.5	%
Polyoxyl 8 laurate	Topical; suspension	0.633	%

Ingredient	Dosage Form	Qty	Unit
Polyoxyl 8 stearate	Oral; suspension	0.085	%
Polyoxyl 8 stearate	Oral; concentrate	2.5	%
Polyoxyl lanolin	Topical; solution	0.94	%
Polypropylene glycol	Oral; solution	20	%
Polyquaternium-1	Topical; solution, drops	0.0005	%
Polyquaternium-10	Topical; shampoo	2	%
Polyquaternium-7	Topical; shampoo	1	%
Polysorbate 20	Oral; suspension	0.5	%
Polysorbate 20	Topical; emulsion	2	%
Polysorbate 20	Topical; solution	15	%
Polysorbate 40	Oral; solution, elixir	0.005	%
Polysorbate 40	Oral; suspension	0.5	%
Polysorbate 60	Topical; aerosol	0.42	%
Polysorbate 60	Topical; emulsion, aerosol foam	0.42	%
Polysorbate 60	Oral; suspension	0.5	%
Polysorbate 60	Topical; suspension	2.85	%
Polysorbate 60	Topical; shampoo	15	%
Polysorbate 80	Oral; solution, elixir	0.0167	%
Polysorbate 80	Oral; suspension, for inhalation	0.02	%
Polysorbate 80	Oral; concentrate	0.1	%
Polysorbate 80	Oral; suspension, liquid	0.1	%
Polysorbate 80	Oral; drops	0.2	%
Polysorbate 80	Oral; suspension, sustained action	0.25	%
Polysorbate 80	Oral; suspension, drops	0.3	%
Polysorbate 80	Rectal; enema	0.6	%
Polysorbate 80	Oral; suspension	3	%
Polysorbate 80	Rectal; solution	10	%
Polysorbate 80	Oral; solution	12.6	%
Potash	Topical; solution	15	%
Potassium acetate	Rectal; enema	0.41	%
Potassium bicarbonate	Oral; solution	2.5	%
Potassium carbonate	Oral; solution	0.62	%
Potassium citrate	Topical; emulsion, aerosol foam	0.17	%
Potassium citrate	Topical; aerosol	0.26	%
Potassium hydroxide	Topical; solution	14.02	%
Potassium metabisulfite	Rectal; enema	0.468	%
Potassium phosphate, dibasic	Oral; solution	1.2	%
Potassium phosphate, dibasic	Oral; syrup	2.2	%
Potassium phosphate, monobasic	Oral; syrup	0.2732	%
Potassium phosphate, monobasic	Oral; solution	0.4	%
Potassium phosphate, monobasic	Oral; suspension	1	%
Potassium soap	Topical; solution	32.8	%
Potassium sorbate	Oral; concentrate	0.01	%

Ingredient	Dosage Form	Qty	Unit
Potassium sorbate	Rectal; solution	0.1067	%
Potassium sorbate	Oral; solution	0.15	%
Potassium sorbate	Topical; solution	0.47	%
Potassium sorbate	Oral; suspension	0.65	%
Potassium sorbate	Oral; syrup	0.65	%
Povidone acrylate copolymer	Topical; solution, liquid	6	%
Povidone K25	Oral; solution	50	%
Povidone K29-32	Oral; solution	3.05	%
Povidone K30	Oral; liquid	5	%
Povidone K30	Oral; dispersible tablet	51.2	MG
Povidone K90	Topical; solution	0.25	%
Primary taste modifier 29275	Oral; syrup	0.2	%
Product wat	Topical; aerosol	10.78	%
Promulgen G	Topical; shampoo	4	%
Propyl gallate	Oral; concentrate	0.02	%
Propylene glycol	Oral; drops	0.1252	%
Propylene glycol	Topical; shampoo, suspension	2	%
Propylene glycol	Topical; aerosol	2.11	%
Propylene glycol	Topical; shampoo	3.5	%
Propylene glycol	Oral; suspension, liquid	5	%
Propylene glycol	Rectal; suspension	5	%
Propylene glycol	Topical; solution, liquid	5	%
Propylene glycol	Topical; suspension	5.275	%
Propylene glycol	Topical; emulsion	8	%
Propylene glycol	Oral; solution, syrup	10	%
Propylene glycol	Oral; suspension, sustained action	15	%
Propylene glycol	Rectal; aerosol, metered	18	%
Propylene glycol	Topical; emulsion, aerosol foam	21.05	%
Propylene glycol	Topical; swab	25	ML
Propylene glycol	Rectal; gel	41.44	%
Propylene glycol	Oral; solution, elixir	45	%
Propylene glycol	Oral; solution	55	%
Propylene glycol	Oral; liquid	61	%
Propylene glycol	Topical; solution	61.5	%
Propylene glycol	Oral; concentrate	70	%
Propylene glycol	Oral; suspension	89.02	%
Propylene glycol	Oral; syrup	92	%
Propylene glycol—lecithin	Oral; solution	99.32	%
Propylene glycol ricinoleate	Topical; shampoo, suspension	2	%
Propylene glycol/diazolidinyl urea/methylparaben/propylparben	Topical; aerosol, metered	12.5	%
Propylparaben	Rectal; aerosol, metered	0.009	%
Propylparaben	Topical; emulsion, aerosol foam	0.011	%
Propylparaben	Oral; solution, concentrate	0.02	%

Ingredient	Dosage Form	Qty	Unit
Propylparaben	Oral; solution, syrup	0.02	%
Propylparaben	Oral; liquid	0.02	%
Propylparaben	Topical; shampoo	0.03	%
Propylparaben	Topical; solution	0.033	%
Propylparaben	Rectal; suspension	0.05	%
Propylparaben	Oral; suspension, liquid	0.06	%
Propylparaben	Topical; emulsion	0.06	%
Propylparaben	Oral; suspension, sustained action	0.15	%
Propylparaben	Oral; concentrate	0.25	%
Propylparaben	Oral; solution, elixir	0.3	%
Propylparaben	Rectal; solution	1.5	%
Propylparaben	Oral; solution	10	%
Propylparaben	Oral; suspension	20	%
Propylparaben	Oral; syrup	36	%
Propylparaben sodium	Oral; suspension	0.02	%
Propylparaben sodium	Oral; solution	0.0225	%
Prosweet	Oral; suspension	1	%
Prosweet	Oral; solution	5.275	%
Prosweet 604	Oral; syrup	0.5	%
Prosweet K	Oral; syrup	0.4	%
Rhodigel-23	Oral; suspension	0.0008	%
Rhodigel-23	Oral; suspension, drops	0.16	%
Saccharin	Oral; syrup	0.1	%
Saccharin	Oral; solution	1	%
Saccharin	Oral; suspension	1	%
Saccharin calcium	Oral; syrup	0.05	%
Saccharin calcium	Oral; solution	1.75	%
Saccharin sodium	Rectal; suspension	0.02	%
Saccharin sodium	Oral; suspension, liquid	0.05	%
Saccharin sodium	Oral; liquid	0.06	%
Saccharin sodium	Rectal; solution	0.085	%
Saccharin sodium	Oral; concentrate	0.15	%
Saccharin sodium	Oral; suspension	1.4	%
Saccharin sodium	Oral; solution, elixir	3	%
Saccharin sodium	Oral; solution	5	%
Saccharin sodium	Oral; syrup	5	%
Saccharin sodium, anhydrous	Oral; syrup	0.0793	%
Saccharin sodium, anhydrous	Oral; suspension	0.333	%
Saccharin sodium, anhydrous	Oral; solution	66.7	%
Saccharin sodium, anhydrous	Rectal; solution	66.7	%
SD alcohol 3A	Topical; solution, liquid	1.2	%
SD alcohol 40	Topical; emulsion, aerosol foam	46	%
SD alcohol 40-2	Topical; aerosol	57.65	%

Ingredient	Dosage Form	Qty	Unit
SD alcohol 40B	Topical; solution	26.14	%
SD alcohol 40B	Topical; emulsion, aerosol foam	56.09	%
Silicon dioxide, colloidal	Oral; suspension	1.113	%
Silicon dioxide, colloidal	Oral; suspension, sustained action	2.16	%
Silicon dioxide, colloidal	Oral; dispersible tablet	3.6	MG
Silicone emulsion	Oral; suspension	0.1	%
Simethicone	Topical; suspension	0.1055	%
Simethicone	Oral; suspension	0.2	%
Simethicone	Oral; suspension, liquid	0.2	%
Simethicone emulsion	Oral; suspension, liquid	0.01	%
Simethicone emulsion	Oral; suspension	0.5	%
Sipon I-20	Topical; emulsion	38	%
Sodium acetate	Topical; suspension	0.03	%
Sodium acetate	Oral; solution, syrup	0.11	%
Sodium acetate, anhydrous	Oral; solution	17.7	%
Sodium alginate	Oral; suspension	0.123	%
Sodium alginate	Oral; syrup	0.3	%
Sodium benzoate	Oral; solution, liquid	0.1	%
Sodium benzoate	Rectal; enema	0.1	%
Sodium benzoate	Oral; concentrate	0.2	%
Sodium benzoate	Oral; suspension, liquid	0.2	%
Sodium benzoate	Oral; suspension, drops	0.24	%
Sodium benzoate	Oral; drops	0.3	%
Sodium benzoate	Oral; solution, elixir	0.5	%
Sodium benzoate	Oral; liquid	0.5	%
Sodium benzoate	Oral; solution	1.08	%
Sodium benzoate	Oral; suspension	3.788	%
Sodium benzoate	Oral; syrup	5	%
Sodium bisulfate	Oral; concentrate	0.095	%
Sodium bisulfite	Oral; suspension	0.04	%
Sodium bisulfite	Oral; concentrate	0.0499	%
Sodium bisulfite	Topical; solution	0.055	%
Sodium bisulfite	Oral; solution	0.1	%
Sodium chloride	Oral; solution, elixir	0.1	%
Sodium chloride	Oral; syrup	0.3	%
Sodium chloride	Topical; suspension	0.53	%
Sodium chloride	Topical; solution	0.6	%
Sodium chloride	Oral; suspension, for inhalation	0.85	%
Sodium chloride	Oral; solution	1.9	%
Sodium chloride	Topical; shampoo	2.25	%
Sodium chloride	Oral; suspension	4.112	%
Sodium citrate	Oral; solution, concentrate	0.05	%
Sodium citrate	Oral; suspension, for inhalation	0.05	%

Ingredient	Dosage Form	Qty	Unit
Sodium citrate	Oral; suspension, liquid	0.1	%
Sodium citrate	Topical; solution	0.1	%
Sodium citrate	Topical; solution, drops	0.294	%
Sodium citrate	Oral; solution, elixir	0.45	%
Sodium citrate	Oral; concentrate	0.507	%
Sodium citrate	Oral; solution, liquid	0.7087	%
Sodium citrate	Oral; solution	1.1	%
Sodium citrate	Oral; drops	2	%
Sodium citrate	Oral; suspension, sustained action	2.35	%
Sodium citrate	Topical; shampoo	2.6	%
Sodium citrate	Oral; suspension	8	%
Sodium citrate	Oral; syrup	32.5	%
Sodium citrate hydrous	Oral; solution, elixir	0.03	%
Sodium citrate hydrous	Oral; suspension	0.3176	%
Sodium citrate hydrous	Oral; syrup	1.1048	%
Sodium citrate, anhydrous	Oral; suspension	0.15	%
Sodium citrate, anhydrous	Oral; syrup	0.159	%
Sodium cyclamate	Oral; suspension	0.5	%
Sodium hydroxide	Topical; solution	0.021	%
Sodium hydroxide	Topical; emulsion	0.2	%
Sodium hydroxide	Rectal; enema	0.44	%
Sodium hydroxide	Rectal; solution	0.629	%
Sodium hydroxide	Oral; concentrate	1	%
Sodium hydroxide	Oral; syrup	1.42	%
Sodium hydroxide	Oral; solution	8	%
Sodium hydroxide	Oral; suspension	40	%
Sodium hypochlorite	Oral; suspension	0.3	%
Sodium iodide	Topical; solution, liquid	0.74	%
Sodium lactate	Topical; solution	1.62	%
Sodium lactate	Oral; suspension	2	%
Sodium laureth sulfate	Topical; shampoo	27	%
Sodium laureth-2 sulfate	Topical; shampoo	36	%
Sodium laureth-5 sulfate	Topical; shampoo	38	%
Sodium lauroyl sarcosinate	Topical; suspension	0.75	%
Sodium lauryl sulfate	Oral; suspension	0.15	%
Sodium lauryl sulfate	Oral; dispersible tablet	8.4	MG
Sodium lauryl sulfate	Topical; shampoo, suspension	40	%
Sodium lauryl sulfoacetate	Topical; shampoo	3	%
Sodium metabisulfite	Oral; suspension	0.1	%
Sodium metabisulfite	Oral; syrup	0.1	%
Sodium metabisulfite	Oral; liquid	0.1	%
Sodium metabisulfite	Oral; concentrate	0.2	%
Sodium metabisulfite	Topical; suspension	0.3165	%

Ingredient	Dosage Form	Qty	Unit
Sodium phosphate	Topical; shampoo	0.667	%
Sodium phosphate	Oral; solution	1.25	%
Sodium phosphate, dibasic	Oral; syrup	1.37	%
Sodium phosphate, dibasic	Oral; concentrate	1.7	%
Sodium phosphate, dibasic	Oral; solution	2.06	%
Sodium phosphate, dibasic, anhydrous	Oral; suspension	0.1371	%
Sodium phosphate, dibasic, anhydrous	Oral; syrup	0.35	%
Sodium phosphate, dibasic, anhydrous	Oral; solution	3.82	%
Sodium phosphate, dibasic, heptahydrate	Oral; syrup	0.02	%
Sodium phosphate, dibasic, heptahydrate	Topical; solution	0.035	%
Sodium phosphate, dibasic, heptahydrate	Oral; suspension	0.45	%
Sodium phosphate, dibasic, heptahydrate	Oral; solution	2	%
Sodium phosphate, monobasic	Topical; shampoo, suspension	1	%
Sodium phosphate, monobasic	Oral; solution	1.37	%
Sodium phosphate, monobasic, anhydrous	Oral; syrup	0.07	%
Sodium phosphate, monobasic, anhydrous	Topical; solution	0.17	%
Sodium phosphate, monobasic, anhydrous	Topical; shampoo, suspension	1	%
Sodium phosphate, monobasic, anhydrous	Oral; solution	4	%
Sodium phosphate, monobasic, dihydrate	Oral; suspension	2	%
Sodium phosphate, monobasic, monohydrate	Oral; suspension	0.05	%
Sodium phosphate, monobasic, monohydrate	Topical; solution	0.09	%
Sodium phosphate, monobasic, monohydrate	Oral; solution	0.8	%
Sodium phosphate, monobasic, monohydrate	Oral; syrup	2.06	%
Sodium propionate	Oral; syrup	0.8	%
Sodium sulfite	Oral; concentrate	0.03	%
Sodium thiosulfate	Oral; solution	0.0093	%
Sodium thiosulfate, anhydrous	Oral; solution	0.2	%
Sodium xylenesulfonate	Topical; solution	4.6	%
Solulan	Topical; aerosol, metered	1.5	%
Solulan	Topical; solution	1.5	%
Somay 44	Topical; solution	0.1	%
Sorbic acid	Oral; concentrate	0.01	%
Sorbic acid	Oral; suspension	0.01	%
Sorbic acid	Oral; solution	0.1	%
Sorbic acid	Oral; syrup	0.5	%
Sorbitan monolaurate	Oral; suspension	0.25	%
Sorbitan monolaurate	Topical; emulsion, aerosol foam	4.74	%
Sorbitan monooleate	Oral; solution	15	%
Sorbitan monostearate	Oral; suspension	1.25	%
Sorbitan monostearate	Topical; suspension	2.15	%
Sorbitol	Oral; drops	3	%
Sorbitol	Topical; emulsion	7	%
Sorbitol	Oral; solution, elixir	20	%

Ingredient	Dosage Form	Qty	Unit
Sorbitol	Oral; solution	30	%
Sorbitol	Rectal; suspension	33.3333	%
Sorbitol	Oral; concentrate	40	%
Sorbitol	Oral; syrup	75	%
Sorbitol	Oral; suspension	91.283	%
Sorbitol anhydride	Oral; solution, elixir	60	%
Sorbitol solution	Oral; drops	5	%
Sorbitol solution	Oral; suspension, drops	10	%
Sorbitol solution	Oral; solution, concentrate	30	%
Sorbitol solution	Rectal; suspension	46.1817	%
Sorbitol solution	Oral; concentrate	60	%
Sorbitol solution	Oral; suspension	71.4	%
Sorbitol solution	Oral; syrup	75	%
Sorbitol solution	Oral; solution, elixir	83.33	%
Sorbitol solution	Oral; solution	90	%
Soybean flour	Topical; emulsion	3	%
Soybean oil	Topical; solution	5.82	%
Spearmint extract	Oral; solution	3.5	%
Spearmint oil	Oral; suspension	0.0029	%
Spearmint oil	Oral; solution	0.05	%
Spearmint oil	Oral; syrup	2	%
Squalane	Topical; solution	1	%
Starch	Oral; suspension	0.4	%
Starch, corn	Oral; suspension	7.25	%
Starch, pregelatinized	Oral; drops	1.2	%
Starch, pregelatinized	Oral; suspension, liquid	1.5	%
Starch, pregelatinized	Oral; suspension, sustained action	12.5	%
Steareth-10	Rectal; aerosol, metered	0.225	%
Steareth-10	Topical; aerosol, metered	6.25	%
Stearic acid	Topical; suspension	1.75	%
Stearic acid	Oral; suspension	86.184	%
Stearyl alcohol	Topical; aerosol	0.53	%
Stearyl alcohol	Topical; emulsion, aerosol foam	0.53	%
Stearyl alcohol	Topical; suspension	2.013	%
Strawberry	Oral; syrup	0.05	%
Succinic acid	Oral; concentrate	0.6	%
Sucralose	Oral; solution	0.8	%
Sucralose	Oral; suspension	1.1	%
Sucrose	Oral; drops	30.22	%
Sucrose	Oral; suspension, drops	50	%
Sucrose	Oral; suspension	55.5	%
Sucrose	Oral; solution	60	%
Sucrose	Oral; suspension, sustained action	60	%

Ingredient	Dosage Form	Qty	Unit
Sucrose	Oral; solution, elixir	61.3	%
Sucrose	Oral; concentrate	67	%
Sucrose	Oral; liquid	72	%
Sucrose	Oral; syrup	82.105	%
Sucrose syrup	Oral; suspension	33.4	%
Sucrose syrup	Oral; syrup	85.46	%
Sugar liquid type 0	Oral; syrup	0.375	%
Sugar/starch insert granules	Oral; suspension	45.048	%
Sulfacetamide sodium	Topical; emulsion, aerosol foam	3.013	%
Surfactol QS	Topical; solution	2	%
Tagatose, D-	Oral; solution	1.3333	%
Tagatose, D-	Rectal; solution	1.3333	%
Talc	Oral; solution, elixir	0.09	%
Talc	Oral; mucilage	1.53	MG
Talc	Topical; shampoo	24	%
Tallow glycerides	Topical; aerosol	2.55	%
Tallow glycerides	Topical; emulsion	2.55	%
Tartaric acid	Oral; solution	0.75	%
Tartaric acid, DL-	Oral; syrup	0.2	%
T-butyl hydroperoxide	Topical; solution	0.2	%
Titanium dioxide	Oral; suspension	2.215	%
Titanium dioxide	Topical; shampoo, suspension	3	%
Tocophersolan	Topical; solution, drops	0.5	%
Tocophersolan	Oral; solution	12	%
Tragacanth	Oral; suspension	1.33	%
Tragacanth	Oral; suspension, sustained action	2.25	%
Trichloromonofluoromethane	Oral; aerosol, metered	65	%
Trideceth-10	Topical; aerosol, metered	4	%
Trideceth-10	Topical; solution	4	%
Triglycerides, medium chain	Sublingual; spray, metered	3.6695	%
Triglycerides, medium chain	Oral; solution	94.46	%
Trisodium citrate dihydrate	Oral; suspension	0.1	%
Trisodium citrate dihydrate	Oral; solution	0.15	%
Trisodium hedta	Topical; solution	0.4	%
Triton X-200 sodium salt of alkylauryl polyether sulfonate	Topical; emulsion	40.3	%
Triton X-200 sodium salt of alkylauryl polyether sulfonate	Topical; shampoo	54	%
Trolamine	Topical; aerosol, metered	1	%
Trolamine lauryl sulfate	Topical; emulsion	10.78	%
Trolamine lauryl sulfate	Topical; shampoo	77.8	%
Tromethamine	Topical; solution	8.4	%
Tyloxapol	Topical; suspension	0.05	%
Vanillin	Oral; solution, elixir	0.0003	%

Ingredient	Dosage Form	Qty	Unit
Vanillin	Oral; solution	0.05	%
Vanillin	Oral; suspension	0.1	%
Vitamin E	Oral; solution	0.105	%
Wax, emulsifying	Rectal; aerosol, metered	1.5	%
Wax, emulsifying	Topical; aerosol, metered	20	%
Xanthan gum	Topical; suspension	0.1055	%
Xanthan gum	Oral; suspension, liquid	0.23	%
Xanthan gum	Rectal; enema	0.25	%
Xanthan gum	Oral; drops	0.29	%
Xanthan gum	Oral; suspension	1.2	%
Xanthan gum	Oral; suspension, sustained action	18.68	%
Xylitol	Oral; solution	30	%
Xylitol	Oral; suspension	67.09	%
Zarzarol	Oral; suspension	24.48	%
Zarzarol	Oral; solution	67.4	%
Zinc acetate	Topical; solution	0.0012	%
Zinc acetate	Topical; swab	12000	mg

Part II

Manufacturing Formulations

Manufacturing Formulations

Abacavir Sulfate Oral Solution

Ziagen oral solution is for oral administration. One milliliter of Ziagen oral solution contains abacavir sulfate equivalent to 20 mg of abacavir (20 mg/mL) in an aqueous solution and the inactive ingredients artificial strawberry and banana flavors, citric acid (anhydrous), methyl paraben and propyl paraben (added as preservatives), propylene glycol, saccharin sodium, sodium citrate (dihydrate), and sorbitol solution.

Abacavir Sulfate Oral Solution

Bill of Materials			
Scale (mg/mL)	Item	Material Name	Qty/L (g)
20.00	1	Abacavir, use abacavir hemisulfate	23.40
344.40	2	Sorbitol 70%	344.40
0.30	3	Sodium saccharin	0.30
2.00	4	Strawberry flavor	2.00
2.00	5	Banana flavor	2.00
QS	6	Sodium citrate dihydrate for pH adjustment	10.00
QS	7	Citric acid anhydrous for pH adjustment	7.00
1.50	8	Methyl paraben	1.50
0.18	9	Propyl paraben	0.18
50.00	10	Propylene glycol	50.00
QS	11	Hydrochloric acid dilute for pH adjustment to 4.0	QS
QS	12	Sodium hydroxide for pH adjustment	QS

Manufacturing Directions

1. The pH range for this solution is from 3.8 to 4.5.
2. Charge 40% of the propylene glycol to an appropriately sized stainless steel and add methyl paraben and propyl paraben with mixing and mix until dissolved.
3. Charge purified water into a stainless steel manufacturing tank equipped with a suitable mixer to approximately 40% of final batch volume.
4. Add sorbitol solution to the manufacturing tank.
5. While mixing, add item 1 and mix until dissolved.
6. While continuing to mix the solution, the paraben/glycol solution, the remaining propylene glycol, artificial strawberry flavor, artificial banana flavor, saccharin sodium, citric acid anhydrous, and sodium citrate dihydrate are added and mixed until dissolved.
7. Turn off the mixer and bring the solution to a volume of 500 L and mix until a homogeneous solution is achieved.
8. Measure and adjust pH to 3.8 to 4.5 with sodium hydroxide or hydrochloric acid.
9. Filter the solution through a clarifying filter into an appropriately sized receiving vessel.

Acetaminophen, Chlorpheniramine, and Pseudoephedrine Syrup

Bill of Materials			
Scale (mg/mL)	Item	Material Name	Qty/L (g)
24.00	1	Acetaminophen (fine powder)	24.00
3.00	2	Pseudoephedrine HCl	3.00
0.44	3	Chlorpheniramine maleate (10% excess)	0.44
14.00	4	Ascorbic acid	14.00
2.40	5	Sodium hydroxide	2.40
1.00	6	Edetate disodium (sodium EDTA)	1.00
0.50	7	Saccharin sodium	0.50
2.00	8	Sodium metabisulfite (sodium disulfite)	2.00
80.00	9	Alcohol (ethanol, 95%)	80.00
100.00	10	Propylene glycol	100.00
100.00	11	Sorbitol (70% solution)	100.00
250.00	12	Glycerin (glycerol)	250.00
300.00	13	Sucrose	300.00
0.04	14	Quinoline yellow	0.04
0.25	15	Pineapple flavor	0.25
QS	16	Purified water	QS to 1 L

Manufacturing Directions

1. Add 200 g of item 16 to the manufacturing vessel and heat to 90°C to 95°C.
2. Add item 13 while mixing at slow speed at a temperature of 90°C to 95°C.
3. Mix for 1 hour at high speed.
4. Add items 10, 11, and 12 to the manufacturing vessel while mixing at high speed. Mix for 10 minutes.
5. Cool the temperature to 50°C while mixing at slow speed.
6. Add 70 g of item 9 to the syrup solution while mixing at slow speed.
7. Load item 1 into the manufacturing vessel while mixing at high speed.
8. Mix for 30 minutes to obtain a clear solution. Check the clarity of the solution.
9. Flush the solution with nitrogen gas for 5 minutes at 1 bar.
10. Add items 2, 4, 6, and 8 to the manufacturing vessel while mixing at slow speed.
11. Dissolve item 3 in 2 g of item 16 (25°C) and check that the solution is complete.
12. Add the solution to the manufacturing vessel while mixing at slow speed.
13. Dissolve item 15 in 10 g of item 9 in a stainless steel container and add to the manufacturing vessel while mixing at slow speed.
14. Dissolve items 5 and 7 in 20 g of item 16 (25°C) and add to the manufacturing vessel while mixing at slow speed.
15. Dissolve item 14 in 2 g of item 16 (25°C).
16. Transfer the color solution to the manufacturing vessel while mixing at slow speed.
17. Rinse the container of color solution with 2 g of item 16 (25°C), then transfer the rinsing to the manufacturing vessel and mix for 5 minutes at high speed.
18. Bring the volume up to 1 L with item 16 and finally mix for 15 to 20 minutes at high speed.
19. Check and record the pH (limit: 5.1–5.2). If required, adjust pH with 10% citric acid or 10% sodium citrate solution.
20. Assemble the filter press with 13.1 T-1000 12 sheets (K 800 14 sheets). Use changeover plate. Wash the filters using purified water (25°C) by passing through filters at 0.2 bar; discard the washings. Filter the syrup at 1.5 bar. Recirculate about 20 to 30 mL syrup.
21. Connect the hose to the manufacturing vessel and transfer the filtered syrup to the storage vessel.

Acetaminophen Drops

Bill of Materials			
Scale (mg/mL)	Item	Material Name	Qty/L (g)
739.00	1	Propylene glycol	739.00
90.00	2	Acetaminophen	90.00
17.50	3	Saccharin sodium	17.50
8.75	4	Sodium chloride	8.75
0.05	5	FD&C red dye No. 40[a]	0.05
2.50	6	Purified water, USP	2.50
2.00	7	Wild cherry artificial flavor	2.00
65.00	8	Alcohol (ethanol; 190 proof; Nonbeverage), USP	65.00
QS	9	Deionized purified water, USP	QS to 1 L

[a]Check for local regulatory allowance to use red dyes.

Manufacturing Directions

Caution: Ensure that the solution in the tank never exceeds 65°C.

1. Add 739 g of propylene glycol to jacketed mixing tank and start heating with slow mixing.
2. Dissolve dye in 2.5 mL of purified water and add to tank while mixing.
3. Rinse container with small amount of purified water and add to tank.
4. While mixing, add acetaminophen, saccharin sodium, and sodium chloride.
5. Hold at 60°C to 65°C with continued moderate mixing until all are in solution.
6. Force cool to less than 30°C with slow mixing.
7. Blend flavor with alcohol and add to tank with slow mixing.
8. Add purified water with mixing QS to make 1 L.
9. Mix well with moderate agitation until uniform.
10. Filter through an 8-μm millipore membrane (or equivalent).

Acetaminophen Oral Suspension

Bill of Materials			
Scale (mg/5 mL)	Item	Material Name	Qty/L (g)
250.00	1	Acetaminophen (micronized) (2.0% excess)	51.00
2500.00	2	Sucrose	500.00
5.00	3	Methyl paraben	1.00
1.50	4	Propyl paraben	0.30
0.30	5	Sodium citrate	0.06
35.00	6	Glycerin (glycerol)	7.00
400.00	7	Glycerin (glycerol)	80.00
2000.00	8	Sorbitol (70%)	400.00
10.00	9	Xanthan gum (Keltrol® F)	2.00
0.50	10	Dye	0.10
22.50	11	Flavor	4.50
3.50	12	Strawberry flavor	0.70
–	13	Purified water	QS to 1 L

Manufacturing Directions

Note: Acetaminophen dispersion should be uniformly mixed. If acetaminophen dispersion is either added to hot syrup base or homogenized for a long time, flocculation may appear. While handling the syrup or mucilage or drug dispersion, the handling loss should not be more than 1%. If it exceeds 1%, a poor suspension may result.

1. Add 180 g of purified water to the mixer and heat to 90°C.
2. Dissolve items 3 and 4 while mixing.
3. Add and dissolve item 2 while mixing.
4. Cool down to approximately 50°C to 55°C.
5. Add and dissolve item 5 while mixing.
6. Filter the syrup through T-1500 filters washed with purified water.
7. Collect the syrup in a clean stainless steel tank.
8. Disperse item 9 in item 6 in a separate stainless steel container.
9. Add 40 g of hot purified water (90°C) at once while mixing.
10. Mix for 20 minutes to make a homogeneous smooth mucilage.
11. Mix item 7 in 10 g of purified water (25°C) in a separate stainless steel container.
12. Add item 1 while mixing with stirrer.
13. Mix for 25 minutes to make uniform suspension.
14. Add sugar syrup and mucilage to the mixer.
15. Rinse the container of mucilage with 15 g of purified water and add the rinsings to the mixer.
16. Cool to 25°C while mixing.
17. Add item 1 dispersion to the mixer.
18. Rinse the container of dispersion with 15 g of purified water and add rinsings to the mixer.
19. Check the suspension for uniformity of dispersion.
20. Mix for additional 5 minutes at 18 rpm and a vacuum of 0.5 bar, if required.
21. Add item 8 to the mixer and mix for 10 minutes.
22. Dissolve item 10 in 7 g of purified water and add to the mixer.
23. Disperse item 11 in 7 g of purified water and add to the mixer.
24. Add item 12 to the mixer.
25. Add cold purified water (25°C) to bring the volume up to 1 L.
26. Homogenize for 5 minutes at low speed under a vacuum of 0.5 bar, 18 rpm, and temperature of 25°C.
27. Check the dispersion for uniformity.
28. Check the pH (limit: 5.7 ± 0.5 at 25°C). If required, adjust the pH with a 20% solution of citric acid or sodium citrate.
29. Transfer the suspension through a 630-μm sieve to the stainless steel storage tank, after mixing for 5 minutes at 18 to 20 rpm at room temperature.

Acetaminophen Rectal Solution

Bill of Materials			
Scale (mg/mL)	Item	Material Name	Qty/L (g)
QS	1	Vehicle (pluronic P105 44.21%, propylene glycol 52.635, water 3.16%)	QS to 1 L
50.00	2	Acetaminophen micronized	50.00

Manufacturing Directions

1. Mill and screen the acetaminophen to further reduce the particle size.
2. Add the acetaminophen into a clean vessel.
3. Add propylene glycol to the vessel.
4. Subsequently add the poloxamer and water to the vessel. Mix until uniform.

Acetaminophen Suspension

Bill of Materials			
Scale (mg/10 mL)	Item	Material Name	Qty/L (g)
500.00	1	Acetaminophen (powder)	50.00
50.00	2	Citric acid (powder)	5.00
50.00	3	Sodium citrate	5.00
500.00	4	Kollidon® CL-M	50.00
10.00	5	Orange flavor	1.00
3000.00	6	Dextrose	300.00
QS	7	Water	589.00

Manufacturing Directions

1. Prepare the solution of dextrose in water and add the other solid ingredients with stirring in the following sequence: citric acid, sodium citrate, orange flavor, Kollidon CL-M, and acetaminophen.
2. A white homogeneous suspension is obtained that is a practically tasteless, stable suspension showing almost no sedimentation over 24 hours and good redispersibility (easily homogenized by shaking 2–3 times).

Acetaminophen Syrup

Bill of Materials			
Scale (mg/mL)	Item	Material Name	Qty/L (g)
569.00	1	Sucrose (granulated sugar), NF	560.000
2.00	2	Sodium citrate (dihydrate powder), USP	2.000
1.00	3	Citric acid (anhydrous powder), USP	1.000
1.00	4	Saccharin sodium (powder), USP	1.000
1.00	5	Sodium chloride (powder), USP	1.000
204.00	6	Propylene glycol, USP	204.000
35.00	7	Acetaminophen, USP	35.000
77.11	8	Alcohol (ethanol; 190 proof), USP	77.112
0.12	9	Cherry flavor (artificial), N59456/A	0.120
0.12	10	FD&C red dye No. 40	0.100
QS	11	Deionized purified water, USP	400.000
–	12	HyFlo filter aid	QS

Manufacturing Directions

1. Add 300 mL of purified water to a jacketed stainless steel mixing tank. Start heating.
2. Add sugar with mixing.
3. Heat to 60°C to 65°C and hold. Mix for complete solution.
4. Add, while mixing, sodium citrate, citric acid, saccharine sodium, and sodium chloride. Mix for complete solution.
5. Add propylene glycol with mixing.
6. Add acetaminophen powder with moderate mixing.
7. Continue mixing at 60°C to 65°C for complete solution.
8. Force cool to 25°C to 30°C with slow mixing.
9. Blend cherry flavor with approximately twice its volume of alcohol and add with mixing.
10. Rinse the container with several portions of alcohol and add. Mix until uniform.
11. Dissolve red dye in approximately 4 g of slightly warmed (50–60°C) purified water and add with mixing.
12. Rinse the container twice with approximately 1.5 g purified water and add. Mix until uniform.
13. Adjust volume to 1 L with purified water. Mix well.
14. Add a small amount of HyFlo filter aid to the mixing tank and continue to mix slowly while filtering.
15. Filter through press until sparkling clear.
16. Use clarifying pad backed by lint-free filter paper.

Acetaminophen Syrup

Bill of Materials			
Scale (mg/mL)	Item	Material Name	Qty/L (g)
50.00	1	Acetaminophen (Merck)	50.00
50.00	2	Sorbitol (crystalline)	50.00
40.00	3	Cyclamate sodium	40.00
1.00	4	Strawberry flavor	1.00
200.00	5	Kollidon® 25	200.00
150.00	6	Glycerol	150.00
200.00	7	1,2-Propylene glycol	200.00
310.00	8	Water	310.00

Manufacturing Directions

1. First dissolve Kollidon 25 and then the other solid components in the solvent mixture of glycerol, propylene glycol, and water.
2. The clear solution has a slightly bitter taste.
3. The solution remains clear for more than 1 week at 6°C and for more than 3 months at 25°C and 40°C.
4. The color of the solution changes only a little during 3 months at 25°C and 40°C.
5. To prevent discoloration during storage, 0.2% to 0.5% of cysteine could be added as antioxidant.

Acetaminophen Syrup for Children

Bill of Materials			
Scale (mg/mL)	Item	Material Name	Qty/L (g)
25.00	1	Acetaminophen (crystalline)	25.00
300.00	2	Kollidon® 25 or Kollidon® 30	300.00
60.00	3	Glycerol	600.00
40.00	4	Sodium cyclamate	40.00
QS	5	Orange flavor	<01.0
QS	6	Raspberry flavor	2.00
QS	7	Water	575.00

Manufacturing Directions

1. Dissolve Kollidon in water, add acetaminophen and cyclamate, heat to 50°C, and stir to obtain a clear solution.
2. Dissolve the flavors and mix with glycerol.
3. The obtained syrup is a viscous, clear, sweet, and only slightly bitter liquid.

Acetaminophen Syrup

Bill of Materials			
Scale (mg/mL)	Item	Material Name	Qty/L (g)
50.0	1	Acetaminophen (Merck)	50.0
50.0	2	Sorbitol, crystalline	50.0
40.0	3	Cyclamate sodium	40.0
1.0	4	Strawberry flavor	1.0
200.0	5	Kollidon 25	200.0
150.0	6	Glycerol	150.0
200.0	7	1,2-Propylene glycol	200.0
310.0	8	Water	310.0

Manufacturing Directions

1. Dissolve first Kollidon 25 and then the other solid components in the solvent mixture of glycerol, propylene glycol, and water.
2. The result is a clear solution of certain viscosity having only a slightly bitter taste. To prevent discoloration during storage, 0.2% to 0.5% cysteine could be added as an antioxidant.

Acetaminophen Syrup

Bill of Materials			
Scale (mg/mL)	Item	Material Name	Qty/L (g)
569.00	1	Sucrose (sugar granulated)	560.000
2.00	2	Sodium citrate dihydrate powder	2.000
1.00	3	Acid citric anhydrous powder	1.000
1.00	4	Saccharin sodium powder	1.000
1.00	5	Sodium chloride powder	1.000
204.00	6	Propylene glycol	204.000
35.00	7	Acetaminophen	35.000
77.11	8	Alcohol (ethanol) 190 proof	77.112
0.12	9	Flavor cherry artifical N59456/A	0.1200
0.12	10	Dye red FD&C N40	0.1000
QS	11	Water purified	400.000
QS	12	Filter aid HyFlo	QS

Manufacturing Directions

1. Add 300 mL purified water to a jacketed stainless steel mixing tank. Start heating.
2. Add sugar with mixing.
3. Heat to 60°C to 65°C and hold. Mix for complete solution.
4. Add, while mixing, sodium citrate, citric acid, sodium saccharine, and sodium chloride. Mix for complete solution. Add propylene glycol by mixing.
5. Add acetaminophen powder with moderate mixing. Continue mixing at 60°C to 65°C for complete solution. Force cool to 25°C to 30°C with slow mixing.
6. Blend cherry flavor with approximately twice its volume of alcohol and add with mixing. Rinse the container with several portions of alcohol and add. Mix until uniform.
7. Dissolve red dye in approximately 4 g of slightly warmed (50–60°C) purified water and add by mixing. Rinse the container twice with approximately 1.5 g purified water and add to step 6.
8. Mix until uniform. Adjust volume to 1 L with purified water. Mix well.
9. Add a small amount of HyFlo filter aid to the mixing tank and continue to mix slowly while filtering.
10. Filter through press until sparkling clear. Use clarifying pad backed by lint-free filter paper.

Acne Scrub

Bill of Materials			
Scale (mg/g)	Item	Material Name	Qty/kg (g)
20.00	1	Magnesium aluminum silicate magnabrite HV	20.00
582.00	2	Water	582.00
100.00	3	Propylene glycol	100.00
150.00	4	Mineral oil and acetylated lanolin alcohol	150.00
30.00	5	Glyceryl stearate and PEG-100 stearate	30.00
14.00	6	Myristyl propionate	14.00
100.00	7	PEG-600	100.00
4.00	8	Eucalyptus oil	4.00
QS	9	Preservatives	QS

Manufacturing Directions

1. Slowly sift item 1 into water, mixing until smooth.
2. Heat to 75°C.
3. Heat items 3 to 6 separately; mix and heat to 70°C.
4. Add this portion to item 1 dispersion and mix well until smooth.
5. Add item 7 to mixture and mix.
6. Finally, add items 8 and 9 and mix until cool.
7. If using parabens, prepare a solution in a portion of water and add before adding item 8 and after allowing parabens to cool to 50°C.

Acyclovir Oral Suspension (2% = 200 mg/10 mL)

Formulation

Acyclovir, 2 g; Kollidon CL-M [1], 6 g; Kollidon 30 [1], 3 g; sorbitol [10], 28 g; citric acid, 0.5 g; preservative, QS; water, 60.5 g.

Manufacturing Directions

Suspend acyclovir and Kollidon CL-M in the solution of the other components under vigorous stirring.

Acyclovir Oral Suspension

Scale (mg/5 mL)	Item	Material Name	Qty/L (g)
215.00	1	Acyclovir	43.00
5.00	2	Methyl paraben	1.00
1.00	3	Propyl paraben	0.20
75.00	4	Microcrystalline cellulose (Avicel RC-591)	15.00
750.00	5	Glycerin (glycerol)	150.00
2250.00	6	Sorbitol (70% solution)	450.00
20.00	7	Orange, banana dry flavor	4.00
–	8	Water purified	QS to 1 L

Manufacturing Directions

1. Disperse item 1 in item 6. Keep stirring for 1 hour.
2. Heat 333.33 g of item 8 in mixer to 90°C to 95°C. Dissolve items 2 and 3 while mixing. Cool to 30°C.
3. Disperse items 4 and 5 in a stainless steel container and keep stirring for 1 hour.
4. Add step 3 into step 2 at 30°C. Mix and homogenize for 5 minutes at high speed under vacuum 0.5 bar.
5. Add step 1 in to step 2 and mix for 5 minutes.
6. Disperse item 7 in 13.33 g of item 8. Add into step 2.
7. Make up the volume with item 8. Finally homogenize for 5 minutes at high speed under vacuum 0.5 bar.

Acyclovir Oral Suspension

Bill of Materials			
Scale (mg/mL)	Item	Material Name	Qty/L (g)
20.00	1	Acyclovir	20.00
60.00	2	Kollidon CL-M	60.00
30.00	3	Kollidon 30	30.00
28.00	4	Sorbitol	28.00
0.50	5	Citric acid	0.50
QS	6	Preservative	QS
QS	7	Water purified	QS to 1 L

Manufacturing Directions

1. Suspend item 1 and item 2 in the solution of items 3 through 7.
2. Mix vigorously to suspend.
3. Fill.

Adapalene Solution

Differin® solution, containing adapalene, is used for the topical treatment of acne vulgaris. Each milliliter of Differin solution contains adapalene 0.1% (1 mg) in a vehicle consisting of polyethylene glycol 400 and SD alcohol 40-B, 30% (w/v).

Bill of Materials			
Scale (mg/mL)	Item	Material Name	Qty/L (g)
1.00	1	Adapalene	1.00
700.00	2	Polyethylene glycol 400	700.00
QS	3	Alcohol	QS to 1 L

Manufacturing Directions

1. Add and dissolve item 1 and mix.
2. Charge items 1 and 2 in a suitable mixing vessel. Stir.

Albendazole Oral Suspension

Bill of Materials			
Scale (mg/5 mL)	Item	Material Name	Qty/L (g)
100.000	1	Albendazole	20.00
7.500	2	Saccharin sodium	1.50
7.500	3	Potassium sorbate	1.50
550.000	4	Propylene glycol	110.00
15.000	5	Xanthan gum	3.00
2.500	6	Passion fruit flavor 502010A	0.50
7.500	7	Polysorbate 80 (Tween 80)	1.50
2.000	8	Citric acid	0.40
2.500	9	Vanilla dry flavor	0.50
2.500	10	Blood orange dry flavor	0.50
QS to 5 mL	11	Water purified	QS to 1 L

Manufacturing Directions

This product dispersion should be uniformly mixed and levigated. Xanthan gum dispersion should be uniform and smooth.

1. Disperse items 1 and 6 in 100 g of item 4 in a stainless steel container, using stirrer.
2. Dissolve item 7 in 100 g of item 11 (50–60°C) in a stainless steel container while stirring with the stirrer. Cool to 25°C to 30°C. Add in to step 1 while mixing.
3. Levigate to make smooth slurry and keep aside for 2 hours.
4. Make slurry of item 5 in 10 g of item 4 in a stainless steel container while stirring with the stirrer. Add 200 g of item 11 (25–30°C) while stirring and continue stirring for 30 minutes.
5. Dissolve item 8 in 10 g of item 11 (25–30°C) in a stainless steel container using a spatula.
6. Add 500 g of item 11 (25–30°C) into mixer. Dissolve items 2 and 3 while mixing.
7. Add the content from steps 1, 2, and 3 into step 4. Mix and homogenize at 25°C to 30°C, mixer speed 18 rpm, homogenizer high speed, and vacuum 0.4 to 0.6 bar for 10 minutes.
8. Add items 9 and 10 in step 4.
9. Mix and homogenize at 25°C to 30°C, mixer speed 18 rpm, homogenizer at high speed, and vacuum 0.4 to 0.6 bar for 15 minutes.
10. Make up the volume with item 11. Mix for 20 minutes.
11. Check the suspension for homogeneity. Transfer the suspension through a 630-micron sieve to stainless steel storage tank. It is important that you do not store the bulk suspension more than 48 hours in the storage tank without stirring. Before sending for filling in packaging, stir no fewer than 30 minutes for uniform dispersion to avoid the problem of content uniformity.

Albendazole Suspension

Bill of Materials			
Scale (mg/5 mL)	Item	Material Name	Qty/L (g)
200.00	1	Albendazole	40.00
1.25	2	Simethicone	0.24
5.00	3	Tween 80	1.00
15.00	4	Xanthan gum	3.00
1950.00	5	Sucrose	390.00
650.00	6	Sorbitol	130.00
20.00	7	Sodium benzoate	4.00
20.00	8	Potassium sorbate	4.00
3.00	9	Citric acid	0.60
QS	10	Flavor	QS
QS	11	Water purified	QS to 1 L

Manufacturing Directions

1. Charge in a tank 20% of item 11 and heat to 90°C.
2. Add and dissolve item 7; reduce temperature to 40°C and add item 3.
3. In a separate vessel, add and dissolve item 9 in a portion of item 11.
4. Add step 3 to step 2.
5. In a separate vessel, disperse item 4 in 40% of item 11 at 65°C and allow to hydrate to make it into a paste. Cool to room temperature.
6. Add to step 3 through a stainless steel filter.
7. In a separate vessel, add and make a paste of items 1 (passed through No. 100 mesh), 3, and 6. Add to step above.
8. Add item 2. Stir well.
9. Add flavor and item 11 to make up the volume.

Albuterol Inhalation Solution

Each milliliter of Proventil inhalation solution 0.083% contains 0.83 mg albuterol (as 1 mg albuterol sulfate) in an isotonic aqueous solution containing sodium chloride and benzalkonium chloride; sulfuric acid is used to adjust the pH between 3 and 5. The 0.083% solution requires no dilution before administration by nebulization. Proventil inhalation solution 0.083% contains no sulfiting agents. It is supplied in 3-mL high-density polyethylene (HDPE) bottles for unit-dose dispensing. AccuNeb (albuterol sulfate) inhalation solution is supplied in two strengths in unit-dose vials. Each unit-dose vial contains either 0.75 mg of albuterol sulfate (equivalent to 0.63 mg of albuterol) or 1.50 mg of albuterol sulfate (equivalent to 1.25 mg of albuterol) with sodium chloride and sulfuric acid in a 3-mL isotonic, sterile aqueous solution. Sodium chloride is added to adjust isotonicity of the solution and sulfuric acid is added to adjust the pH of the solution to 3.5.

Albuterol Inhalation Solution

Bill of Materials			
Scale (mg/mL)	Item	Material Name	Qty/L (g)
1.25	1	(R)-Albuterol, use albuterol sulfate	1.50
27.00	2	Sodium chloride	27.00
QS	3	Sulfuric acid	QS
QS	4	Water purified	QS to 1 L

Manufacturing Directions

1. Charge all items in a suitable stainless steel vessel and mix. Keep nitrogen flushing throughout and also into item 4 before adding other ingredients.
2. Check and adjust pH, using sulfuric acid, to 3.5.
3. Fill.

Alginic Acid + Aluminium Hydroxide + Magnesium Silicate Tablets (500 mg + 100 mg + 25 mg)

Bill of Materials			
Scale (mg/tablet)	Item	Material Name	Qty/1000 Tablets (g)
500.00	1	Alginic acid	500.00
100.00	2	Aluminum hydroxide dried gel (Giulini)	100.00
25.00	3	Magnesium trisilicate	25.00
170.00	4	Sodium bicarbonate	170.00
160.00	5	Sorbitol crystalline	160.00
627.00	6	Sucrose crystalline	627.00
900.00	7	Ludipress	900.00
70.00	8	Kollidon VA 64	70.00
50.00	9	Magnesium stearate	50.00
5.00	10	Vanillin	5.00

1. Manufacturing Directions

Pass all components through a 0.8-mm sieve. Mix and press with high compression force.

Alpha-Bisabolol Aqueous Mouthwash Solution

Bill of Materials			
Scale (mg/g)	Item	Material Name	Qty/kg (g)
2.00.00	1	Alpha-bisabolol, natural (BASF)	2.00
QS	2	Flavor	QS
25.00	3	Cremophor RH 40	25.00
50.00	4	Glycerol	50.00
1.00	5	Saccharin sodium	1.00
QS	6	Preservative	QS
922.00	7	Water	922.00

2. Manufacturing Directions

1. Heat mixture of items 1 to 3 to approximately 60°C and slowly add the warm solution of items 4 to 7 (60°C).
2. The clear, colorless liquid has a low viscosity.

Alpha-Bisabolol Buccal or Topical Solution

Bill of Materials			
Scale (mg/mL)	Item	Material Name	Qty/L (g)
1.20	1	Alpha-bisabolol (racemic) (BASF)	1.20
10.00	2	Cremophor RH 40	10.00
0.10	3	Butylhydroxytoluene (BHT)	0.10
QS	4	Preservative	QS
990.00	5	Water	990.00

3. Manufacturing Directions

Heat mixture of items 1 to 3 to approximately 60°C, stir well, and slowly add the warm solution of items 4 in 5 to obtain a clear solution.

Alpha-Bisabolol Ethanolic Mouthwash Solution

Bill of Materials			
Scale (mg/mL)	Item	Material Name	Qty/L (g)
10.00	1	Alpha-bisabolol, racemic (BASF)	10.00
100.00	2	Flavor	100.00
60.00	3	Cremophor RH 40	60.00
10.00	4	Glycerol	10.00
2.00	5	Saccharin sodium	2.00
818.00	6	Ethanol, 96%	818.00

4. Manufacturing Directions

1. Heat mixture of items 1 to 3 to approximately 60°C and slowly add the warm solution of items 4 to 6.
2. The clear, colorless liquid can be diluted with water.

Alpha-Bisabolol Mouthwash Solution

Bill of Materials			
Scale (mg/mL)	Item	Material Name	Qty/L (g)
5.00	1	(-)Alpha-Bisabolol, natural (BASF)	5.00
50.00	2	Lutrol F 127 [1]	50.00
QS	3	Flavor	QS
100.00	4	Propylene glycol (pharma)	100.00
300.00	5	Ethanol 96%	300.00
545.00	6	Water	545.00

5. Manufacturing Directions

1. Prepare solution of items 1 through 5 and slowly add the water.
2. The clear, colorless solution should have a pH of 8. Do not adjust.

Aluminium Hydroxide + Magnesium Silicate Chewable Tablets (120 mg + 250 mg)

Bill of Materials			
Scale (mg/tablet)	Item	Material Name	Qty/1000 Tablets (g)
120.00	1	Aluminum hydroxide dried gel (Giulini)	120.00
250.00	2	Magnesium trisilicate	250.00
232.00	3	Ludipress	232.00
6.00	4	Aerosil 200	6.00
6.00	5	Magnesium stearate	6.00
12.00	6	Cyclamate sodium	12.00
1.50	7	Menthol	1.50

6. Manufacturing Directions

Mix all components, pass through a 0.8-mm sieve, and press with a compression force of 20 kN at 640 mg.

Aluminum Chloride Solution

Aluminum chloride (hexahydrate) 6.25% (w/v) in anhydrous ethyl alcohol (SD alcohol 40) 96% (v/v).

Bill of Materials			
Scale (mg/mL)	Item	Material Name	Qty/L (g)
62.50	1	Aluminum chloride hexahydrate	62.50
QS	2	Alcohol anhydrous	QS to 1 L

Manufacturing Directions

1. Charge items 1 and 2 in a suitable stainless steel container and mix.
2. Fill.

Aluminum Hydroxide and Magnesium Carbonate Dry Syrup

Bill of Materials			
Scale (mg/g)	Item	Material Name	Qty/kg (g)
200.00	1	Aluminum hydroxide dry gel (Giulini)	200.00
200.00	2	Basic magnesium carbonate	200.00
240.00	3	Kollidon® CL-M	240.00
211.50	4	Sorbitol (crystalline)	211.50
41.30	5	Orange flavor	41.30
82.60	6	Kollidon® 30	82.60
3.30	7	Coconut flavor	3.30
4.13	8	Banana flavor	4.13
4.13	9	Saccharin sodium	4.13
8.26	10	Water	8.26

Manufacturing Directions

1. Granulate mixture of items 1 to 5 with solution of items 6 to 10, pass through a sieve, and dry.
2. Shake 58 g of the granules with 100 mL of water.
3. Product remains homogeneous and without sedimentation for more than 24 hours.

Aluminum Hydroxide and Magnesium Carbonate Dry Syrup

Bill of Materials			
Scale (mg/g)	Item	Material Name	Qty/kg (g)
200.00	1	Aluminum hydroxide dry gel (Giulini)	200.00
200.00	2	Basic magnesium carbonate	200.00
240.00	3	Kollidon CL-M	240.00
211.50	4	Sorbitol, crystalline	211.50
41.30	5	Orange flavor	41.3
82.60	6	Kollidon 30	82.6
3.30	7	Coconut flavor	3.30
4.13	8	Banana flavor	4.13
4.13	9	Saccharin sodium	4.13
8.26	10	Water	8.26

Manufacturing Directions

1. Granulate mixture of items 1 to 5 with solution of items 6 to 10.
2. Pass through a sieve and dry.
3. Shake 58 g of the granules with 100 mL of water. Homogenize.

Aluminum Hydroxide and Magnesium Hydroxide Antacid Suspension

Bill of Materials			
Scale (mg/mL)	Item	Material Name	Qty/L (g)
5.00	1	Purified bentonite (Veegum® HS)	5.00
2.00	2	Xanthan gum (Rhodigel)	2.00
401.00	3	Water	401.00
200.00	4	Sorbitol (70%)	200.00
360.00	5	Aluminum hydroxide gel	360.00
320.00	6	Magnesium hydroxide, USP	320.00
QS	7	Preservative, flavor	QS

Manufacturing Directions

1. Slowly add a dry blend of item 1 and 2 to item 3, agitating with maximum available shear until a smooth and uniform mix is obtained.
2. Mix items 4 to 6 together in another vessel until uniform and then add to previous mix.
3. Agitate until uniform.
4. Add item 7 and mix until uniform.

Aluminum Hydroxide and Magnesium Hydroxide Antacid Suspension

Bill of Materials			
Scale (mg/mL)	Item	Material Name	Qty/L (g)
200.00	1	Magnesium aluminum silicate (Magnabrite S) (5% suspension)	200.00
2.00	2	Methyl paraben	2.00
1.00	3	Propyl paraben	1.00
0.50	4	Saccharin sodium	0.50
500.00	5	Aluminum hydroxide/Magnesium hydroxide fluid gel	500.00
3.00	6	Polysorbate 80	3.00
2.00	7	Flavor	2.00
291.50	8	Deionized water	291.50

Manufacturing Directions

1. Add the parabens and saccharin to item 1 with stirring until dissolved (may heat to 80°C to dissolve).
2. Add item 5 with mixing.
3. Finally, add item 6 and 7. Mix well.

Aluminum Hydroxide and Magnesium Hydroxide Suspension

Bill of Materials			
Scale (mg/5 mL)	Item	Material Name	Qty/L (g)
405.000	1	Aluminum hydroxide gel	290.0000
100.000	2	Magnesium hydroxide paste 30%	67.0000
0.210	3	Ammonia solution 25%	0.0420
0.053	4	Ammonia solution 25%	0.0106
10.000	5	Methyl paraben	2.0000
0.250	6	Menthol	0.0500
3.000	7	Propyl paraben	0.6000
1.000	8	Peppermint oil	0.2000
50.000	9	Propylene glycol	10.0000
1.250	10	Saccharin sodium	0.2500
150.00	11	Sorbitol (70% solution)	30.0000
4.500	12	Sodium hypochlorite 5%	0.9000
1.250	13	Sodium hypochlorite 5%	0.2500
15.000	14	Magnesium aluminum silicate (Veegum HV)	3.0000
–	15	Water purified	QS to 1 L

Note. Quantity of the sodium hypochlorite solution to be adjusted according to the assay.

Manufacturing Directions

1. Disperse item 14 in 60 g of hot item 15 (70–80°C) in stainless steel vessel, using stirrer.
2. Continue stirring for 30 minutes.
3. Transfer the dispersion into mixer (e.g., Krieger) vessel by vacuum and mix for 30 minutes at mixer speed 16/32.
4. Cool down to 30°C. Add 200 g of hot item 15 (70–80°C) into the mixer.
5. Mix and homogenize at rpm 1420 mixer speed 16/32, vacuum 0.5 bar for 30 minutes.
6. Cool down to 30°C.
7. Add 1 kg of item 15 (70°C) to a suitable vessel and heat to 85°C to 90°C for 1 hour.
8. Cool to 20°C to 25°C.
9. Mix items 4 and 13 and immediately add to item 15 (20–25°C) in the storage vessel.
10. Mix for 2 minutes. Store in a previously cleaned storage vessel.
11. Load item 2 and 100 g of item 15 (25–30°C) in a stainless steel mixing vessel with lid and stirrer.
12. Mix for 5 minutes at medium speed.
13. Transfer by vacuum into mixer. Load 80 g of item 1 and 80 g of item 15 (25–30°C) from step above in a stainless steel mixing vessel with lid and stirrer.
14. Mix for 5 minutes at medium speed. Transfer by vacuum into mixer.
15. Load 80 g of item 1 and 80 g of item 15 (25–30°C) from step above in a stainless steel mixing vessel with lid and stirrer. Mix for 5 minutes at medium speed. Transfer by vacuum into mixer.
16. Load 80 g of item 1 and 80 g of item 15 (25–30°C) from step above in a stainless steel mixing vessel with lid and stirrer.
17. Mix for 5 minutes at medium speed. Transfer by vacuum into mixer. Load 50 g of item 1 and 50 g of item 15 (25–30°C) from step above in a stainless steel mixing vessel with lid and stirrer.
18. Mix for 5 minutes at medium speed. Transfer by vacuum into mixer. Transfer item 11 into mixer by vacuum.
19. Dissolve item 10 in 2 g of item 15 (25–30°C) and transfer into mixer. Mix and homogenize for 30 minutes at 1420 rpm under vacuum 0.5 bar.
20. Dissolve items 5 and 7 in item 9 (50–60°C) by stirring in stainless steel container in a water bath.
21. Dissolve items 8 and 6 and add it to parabens–glycol solution.
22. Mix well; add to mixer. Mix and homogenize for 10 minutes under vacuum 0.5 bars.
23. Mix items 3, 12, and 2 g of item 15 and immediately add to the mixer. Mix for 10 minutes without vacuum.
24. Add cold item 15 to make up the volume up to 1 L. Mix for 15 minutes.
25. Transfer the suspension through 630-micron sieve to the stainless steel storage tank. Final pH 7.5 to 8.0, density 1.04 to 1.06.

Aluminum Hydroxide and Magnesium Hydroxide Suspension

Bill of Materials			
Scale (mg/5 mL)	Item	Material Name	Qty/L (g)
200.00	1	Aluminum hydroxide gel	214.00
80.00	2	Magnesium hydroxide paste 30%	54.20
150.00	3	Sorbitol (70% solution)	30.00
10.00	4	Methyl paraben	2.00
1.00	5	Propyl paraben	0.20
2.00	6	Saccharin sodium	0.40
15.00	7	Magnesium aluminum silicate (Veegum HV)	3.00
0.20	8	Ammonia solution 25%	0.04
4.50	9	Sodium hypochlorite 5%	0.90
100.00	10	Propylene glycol	20.00
0.75	11	Lemon-mint flavor	0.15
–	12	Water purified	QS to 1 L

Manufacturing Directions

See previous entry for manufacturing directions for Aluminum Hydroxide and Magnesium Hydroxide Suspension.

Aluminum Hydroxide and Magnesium Hydroxide Suspension

Bill of Materials			
Scale (mg/mL)	Item	Material Name	Qty/L (g)
5.00	1	Purified bentonite (Veegum HS)	5.00
2.00	2	Xanthan gum (Rhodigel)	2.00
401.00	3	Water	401.00
200.00	4	Sorbitol 70%	200.00
360.00	5	Aluminum hydroxide gel	360.00
320.00	6	Magnesium hydroxide	320.00
QS	7	Preservative, flavor	QS

Manufacturing Directions

1. Add a dry blend of items 1 and 2 to item 3 slowly, agitating with maximum available shear until a smooth and uniform mix is obtained.
2. Mix together items 4 to 6 in another vessel until uniform and then add to the above mix and agitate until uniform.
3. Add item 7 and mix until uniform.

Aluminum Hydroxide and Magnesium Hydroxide Suspension

Bill of Materials			
Scale (mg/mL)	Item	Material Name	Qty/L (g)
40.0	1	Aluminum hydroxide	40.0
40.0	2	Magnesium hydroxide	40.0
50.0 g	3	Cremophor RH 40	50.0
1.0	4	Silicon oil DC 200 (Serva)	1.0
100.0	5	Kollidon CL-M	100.0
QS	6	Water	76.9

Manufacturing Directions

1. Mix Cremophor RH 40 well with the silicon oil.
2. Add the water and suspend the solid substances.

Aluminum Hydroxide and Magnesium Hydroxide Suspension

Bill of Materials			
Scale (mg/mL)	Item	Material Name	Qty/L (g)
200.0	1	Magnesium aluminum silicate (Magnabrite S) 5% suspension	200.0
2.0	2	Methyl paraben	2.0
1.0	3	Propyl paraben	1.0
0.5	4	Saccharin sodium	0.5
500.0	5	Aluminum hydroxide-magnesium hydroxide fluid gel	500.0
3.0	6	Polysorbate 80	3.0
2.0	7	Flavor	2.0
291.5	8	Water purified	291.5

Manufacturing Directions

1. Add the parabens and saccharin to item 1 with stirring until dissolved (may heat to 80°C to dissolve).
2. Add item 5 with mixing. Finally, add items 6 and 7.
3. Mix well.

Aluminum Hydroxide and Magnesium Hydroxide Suspension

Bill of Materials			
Scale (mg/mL)	Item	Material Name	Qty/L (g)
405.00	1	Aluminum hydroxide gel	290.00
100.00	2	Magnesium hydroxide paste (30%)	67.00
0.21	3	Ammonia solution (25%)	0.04
0.05	4	Ammonia solution (25%)	0.01
10.00	5	Methyl paraben	2.00
0.25	6	Menthol	0.05
3.00	7	Propyl paraben	0.60
1.00	8	Peppermint oil	0.20
50.00	9	Propylene glycol	10.00
1.25	10	Saccharin sodium	0.25
150.00	11	Sorbitol (70% solution)	30.00
4.50	12	Sodium hypochlorite (5%)	0.90
1.25	13	Sodium hypochlorite (5%)	0.25
15.00	14	Magnesium aluminum silicate (Veegum® HV)	3.00
QS	15	Purified water	QS to 1 L

Note: The quantity of the sodium hypochlorite solution should be adjusted according to the assay.

Manufacturing Directions

1. Disperse item 14 in 60 g of hot purified water (70–80°C) in stainless steel vessel using a stirrer. Continue stirring for 30 minutes.
2. Transfer the dispersion into mixer (e.g., Krieger) vessel by vacuum and mix for 30 minutes at 16/32 mixer speed.
3. Cool down to 30°C.
4. Add 200 g of hot purified water (70–80°C) to the mixer.
5. Mix and homogenize at 1420 rpm, mixer speed of 16/32, and vacuum of 0.5 bar for 30 minutes.
6. Cool down to 30°C.
7. Add 1 kg of purified water (70°C) to a suitable vessel and heat to 85°C to 90°C for 1 hour.
8. Cool to 20°C to 25°C.
9. Mix items 13 and 4 and immediately add to purified water (20–25°C) in the storage vessel.
10. Mix for 2 minutes. Store in a previously cleaned storage vessel.
11. Load item 2 and 100 g of purified water (25–30°C) in a stainless steel mixing vessel with lid and stirrer.
12. Mix for 5 minutes at medium speed.
13. Transfer by vacuum into mixer.
14. Load 80 g of item 1 and 80 g of purified water (25–30°C) from step above in a stainless steel mixing vessel with lid and stirrer. Mix for 5 minutes at medium speed. Transfer by vacuum into mixer.
15. Load 50 g of item 1 and 50 g of purified water (25–30°C) from step above in a stainless steel mixing vessel with lid and stirrer.
16. Mix for 5 minutes at medium speed. Transfer by vacuum into mixer.
17. Transfer item 11 into mixer by vacuum.
18. Dissolve item 10 in 2 g of purified water (25–30°C) and transfer to mixer.
19. Mix and homogenize for 30 minutes at 1420 rpm under vacuum of 0.5 bar.
20. Dissolve items 5 and 7 in item 9 (50–60°C) by stirring in stainless steel container in a water bath.
21. Dissolve items 8 and 6 and add to parabens/glycol solution. Mix well and add to mixer.
22. Mix and homogenize for 10 minutes under vacuum of 0.5 bars.
23. Mix items 12 and 3 and 2 g of purified water and immediately add to the mixer.
24. Mix for 10 minutes without vacuum.
25. Add cold purified water to bring the volume up to 1 L. Mix for 15 minutes.
26. Transfer the suspension through 630-μm sieve to the stainless steel storage tank. Final pH is 7.5 to 8.0 and density is 1.04 to 1.06.

Aluminum Hydroxide and Magnesium Hydroxide Suspension

Bill of Materials			
Scale (mg/5mL)	Item	Material Name	Qty/L (g)
200.00	1	Aluminum hydroxide gel	214.00
80.00	2	Magnesium hydroxide paste (30%)	54.20
150.00	3	Sorbitol (70% solution)	30.00
10.00	4	Methyl paraben	2.00
1.00	5	Propyl paraben	0.20
2.00	6	Saccharin sodium	0.40
15.00	7	Magnesium aluminum silicate (Veegum® HV)	3.00
0.20	8	Ammonia solution (25%)	0.04
4.50	9	Sodium hypochlorite (5%)	0.90
100.00	10	Propylene glycol	20.00
0.75	11	Lemon-mint flavor	0.15
QS	12	Purified water	QS to 1 L

Manufacturing Directions

See previous entry for manufacturing directions for Aluminum Hydroxide and Magnesium Hydroxide Suspension.

Aluminum Hydroxide and Magnesium Hydroxide Suspension

Bill of Materials			
Scale (mg/mL)	Item	Material Name	Qty/L (g)
40.00	1	Aluminum hydroxide	40.00
40.00	2	Magnesium hydroxide	40.00
50.00 g	3	Cremophor RH 40	50.00
1.00	4	Silicon oil DC 200 (Serva)	1.00
100.00	5	Kollidon® CL-M	100.00
QS	6	Water	76.90

Manufacturing Directions

Mix Cremophor RH 40 well with the silicon oil, add the water, and suspend the solid substances.

Aluminum Hydroxide, Magnesium Hydroxide, and Simethicone Suspension

Bill of Materials			
Scale (g/5 mL)	Item	Material Name	Qty/L (g)
215.00	1	Aluminum hydroxide gel	217.00
80.00	2	Magnesium hydroxide paste (30%)	56.00
25.00	3	Simethicone emulsion (simethicone antifoam M30)	18.50
150.00	4	Sorbitol (70% solution)	30.00
0.20	5	Ammonia solution 25%	0.04
10.00	6	Methyl paraben	2.00
1.00	7	Propyl paraben	0.20
28.00	8	Methylcellulose 4000 (Methocel A4M)	5.60
2.00	9	Saccharin sodium	0.40
4.50	10	Sodium hypochlorite (5%)	0.90
1.00	11	Lemon-mint flavor	0.20
QS	12	Purified water	QS to 1 L

Manufacturing Directions

See manufacturing directions for Aluminum Hydroxide and Magnesium Hydroxide Suspension.

Aluminum Hydroxide, Magnesium Hydroxide, and Simethicone Suspension

Bill of Materials			
Scale (mg/mL)	Item	Material Name	Qty/L (g)
27.00	1	Simethicone 30%	27.00
30.00	2	Cremophor RH 40	30.00
70.00	3	Water	70.00
80.00	4	Aluminum hydroxide dry gel (Giulini)	80.00
80.00	5	Magnesium hydroxide	80.00
90.00	6	Kollidon® CL-M	90.00
100.00	7	Sorbitol (crystalline)	100.00
4.00	8	Banana flavor	4.00
5.00	9	Coconut flavor	5.00
1.00	10	Saccharin sodium	1.00
QS	11	Water	QS to 1 L
QS	12	Citric acid (to adjust pH)	QS

Manufacturing Directions

1. Mix Cremophor RH 40 with simethicone and heat to about 50°C, stirring well.
2. Add warm water.
3. Dissolve the flavors and saccharin in water and suspend aluminum hydroxide, magnesium hydroxide, and Kollidon CL-M.
4. Add emulsion of items 1 to 3 to the stirred suspension of items 4 to 11 and adjust the pH to about 9 with item 12, if needed.

Aluminum Hydroxide, Magnesium Hydroxide, and Simethicone Suspension

Bill of Materials			
Scale (mg/5 mL)	Item	Material Name	Qty/L (g)
215.00	1	Aluminum hydroxide gel	217.00
80.00	2	Magnesium hydroxide paste 30%	56.00
25.00	3	Simethicone emulsion (simethicone antifoam M30)	18.50
150.00	4	Sorbitol (70% solution)	30.00
0.20	5	Ammonia solution 25%	0.04
10.00	6	Methyl paraben	2.00
1.00	7	Propyl paraben	0.20
28.00	8	Methylcellulose 4000 (Methocel A4M)	5.60
2.00	9	Saccharin sodium	0.40
4.50	10	Sodium hypochlorite 5%	0.90
1.00	11	Lemon-mint flavor	0.20
–	12	Water purified	QS to 1 L

Manufacturing Directions

See previous entry for manufacturing directions for Aluminum Hydroxide, Magnesium Hydroxide, and Simethicone Suspension.

Aluminum Hydroxide, Magnesium Hydroxide, and Simethicone Suspension

Bill of Materials			
Scale (mg/mL)	Item	Material Name	Qty/L (g)
27.00	1	Simethicone 30%	27.00
30.00	2	Cremophor RH 40	30.00
70.00	3	Water	70.00
80.00	4	Aluminum hydroxide dry gel (Giulini)	80.00
80.00	5	Magnesium hydroxide	80.00
90.00	6	Kollidon CL-M	90.00
100.00	7	Sorbitol, crystalline	100.00
4.00	8	Banana flavor	4.00
5.00	9	Coconut flavor	5.00
1.00	10	Saccharin sodium	1.00
QS	11	Water	QS to 1 L
QS	12	Citric acid to adjust pH to 9	QS

Manufacturing Directions

1. Mix Cremophor RH 40 with simethicone, heat to about 50°C, stirring well.
2. Add the warm water.
3. Dissolve the flavors and saccharin in water and suspend aluminum hydroxide, magnesium hydroxide and Kollidon CL-M.
4. Add emulsion of items 1 to 3 to the stirred suspension of items 4 to 11 and adjust pH to about 9 with item 12 if needed.

Aluminum Hydroxide, Magnesium Hydroxide, and Simethicone Tablets

Bill of Materials			
Scale (mg/tablet)	Item	Material Name	Qty/1000 Tablets (g)
200.00	1	Aluminum hydroxide gel (dried)	260.00
200.00	2	Magnesium hydroxide powder	200.00
200.00	3	Mannitol	200.00
45.00	4	Sorbitol powder	45.00
65.00	5	Dextrose (glucose) monohydrate	65.00
16.50	6	Povidone (PVP K-30)	16.50
2.50	7	Saccharin sodium	2.50
1.00	8	FD&C yellow dye No.10 lake	1.00
2.50	9	Mint flavor (dry)	2.50
1.50	10	Lemon flavor (dry)	1.50
25.00	11	Simethicone GS granules	84.00
315.00	12	Dextrates (Emdex®)	315.00
1.00	13	Colloidal silicon dioxide (Aerosil® 200)	1.00
6.00	14	Magnesium stearate	6.00
–	15	Purified water	160.00

Manufacturing Directions

1. Processing should be done at relative humidity of 50% ± 5% and temperature of 26°C ± 1°C.
2. Dissolve items 4, 5, and 7 in cold purified water (25–30°C) by using stirrer, then add item 6 while mixing.
3. Add item 8 and disperse the color completely.
4. Check final weight; if required, adjust with purified water.
5. Load items 1, 2, and 3 into mixer and mix for 5 minutes using mixer and chopper at high speed.
6. Add binding solution at a rate of 16 to 20 g/min to the dry powders in mixer while mixing at low speed. Mix for 2 to 3 minutes. Scrape the sides, blade, and lid of the mixer.
7. Mix and chop at low speed for an additional 2 to 3 minutes or until the granules stop flying around the chopper. Add extra purified water if required and continue mixing until a satisfactory mass is obtained. Record extra quantity of purified water added.
8. Unload the wet mass into clean Aeromatic bowl for drying.
9. Avoid big lump formation as this leads to nonuniform drying.
10. Dry the wet mass in an Aeromatic fluid bed dryer at 60°C for 90 minutes.
11. After 30 minutes of drying, scrape the semidried granules to break up the lumps to promote uniform drying.
12. Pass the dried granules through a 1.5-mm sieve using a granulator at medium speed. Collect in stainless steel drums.
13. Load the granules into blender.
14. Add items 11 and 12 to stainless steel drum and mix for 2 minutes using drum mixer, then load into the blender and mix along with the granules for 2 minutes.
15. Pass items 9, 10, 13, and 14 through sifter using 250-μm sieve.
16. Load the sieved material into blender and mix for 2 minutes. Unload into stainless steel drums.
17. Check temperature and humidity of the room before beginning compression.
18. Compress 1.2 g per tablet using 15.8-mm flat punch at relative humidity of 50% ± 5% at a temperature of 26°C ± 1°C.

Aminacrine Hydrochloride Topical Solution

Bill of Materials			
Scale (mg/mL)	Item	Material Name	Qty/L (g)
1.00	1	Aminacrine hydrochloride	1.00
60.00	2	Thymol	60.00
100.00	3	Glyceryl monostearate	100.00
30.00	4	Cetostearyl alcohol	30.00
20.00	5	Polyoxyl 40 stearate	20.00
100.00	6	Liquid paraffin	100.00
5.00	7	Cetrimide	5.00
1.50	8	Isopropyl alcohol	1.50
QS	9	Water purified	QS to 1 L

Manufacturing Directions

1. Charge item 6 in a suitable stainless steel vessel and add and dissolve item 1 by heating to 65°C.
2. Charge items 3 to 5, 7, and 9 in a separate vessel and mix.
3. Add above items to step 1.
4. On cooling, add items 8 and 2 and mix.
5. Fill.

Aminolevulinic Acid HCl for Topical Solution (20%)

Aminolevulinic acid HCl for topical solution, 20%, contains the hydrochloride salt of aminolevulinic acid, an endogenous 5-carbon aminoketone. The stick for topical application is a two-component system consisting of a plastic tube containing two sealed glass ampules and an applicator tip. One ampule contains 1.5 mL of solution vehicle comprising alcohol (ethanol content = 48% v/v), water, laureth-4, isopropyl alcohol, and polyethylene glycol. The other ampule contains 354 mg of aminolevulinic acid hydrochloride as a dry solid. The applicator tube is enclosed in a protective cardboard sleeve and cap. The 20% topical solution is prepared just before the time of use by breaking the ampules and mixing the contents by shaking the stick applicator.

Amoxicillin Powder for Suspension

Bill of Materials			
Scale (mg/5 mL)[a]	Item	Material Name	Qty/5 L (g)
125.00	1	Amoxicillin, USE amoxicillin trihydrate, 8% excess	143.50
1.04	2	Simethicone A	1.04
111.11	3	Castor sugar	111.11
444.44	4	Castor sugar	444.44
2479.86	5	Castor sugar	2479.86
23.33	6	Sodium citrate	23.33
1.67	7	Xanthan gum	1.67
13.33	8	Blood orange dry flavor	13.33
0.74	9	Vanilla dry flavor	0.74
4.44	10	Orange, banana dry flavor	4.44
14.44	11	Aerosil 200	14.44

[a] After reconstitution

Manufacturing Directions

1. Charge items 3 and 2 in a mixer and mix for 2 minutes.
2. Add item 4 and items 6 to 11 and mix for 5 minutes.
3. Pass through Fitz mill, impact forward at high speed using sieve 24228.
4. In a separate mixer, charge items 5 and 1 and mix well, passing through a sifter.
5. Add to step 3 and mix for 20 minutes.
6. Fill 65 g for 100 mL and 39 g for 60-mL pack size.

Amoxicillin–Clavulanate Syrup

Bill of Materials			
Scale (g/60 mL volume)	Item	Material Name	Qty/kg (g)
1.500	1	Amoxicillin (1.25 g/60 mL),[a] USE amoxicillin trihydrate	215.67
0.393	2	Potassium clavulanate (equivalent to clavulanic acid 0.312 g)	56.59
0.150	3	Xanthan gum	21.56
1.800	4	Hydroxy propyl methyl cellulose	258.80
0.150	5	Saccharin sodium	21.56
0.300	6	Colloidal silica	43.13
0.010	7	Succinic acid	1.44
1.500	8	Silica gel	215.67
0.180	9	Peach dry flavor	26.39
0.230	10	Strawberry dry flavor	33.99
0.730	11	Lemon dry flavor	105.16

[a]6.955 g/60 mL: 156 mg/5 mL syrup 60 mL (125 mg amoxicillin and 31.25 mg clavulanic acid).

Manufacturing Directions

Throughout the process of manufacturing and filling, maintain relative humidity of NMT 40%.

1. Mill 50% of amoxicillin trihydrate, saccharin sodium (dried to NMT 2% moisture by Karl Fischer method), and succinic acid through a No. 100 mesh sieve using Fitz mill or equivalent with blades forward.
2. Transfer to a blending mixer and mix for 15 minutes.
3. Mill remaining amoxicillin trihydrate through a No. 100 mesh using Fitz mill or equivalent and mix with above screened powders; mix for 15 minutes.
4. Mill xanthan gum, hydroxypropylmethylcellulose (dried to NMT 2% moisture dried at 105°C for 2 hours), colloidal silica, and silica gel through a No. 100 screen using Fitz mill or equivalent with knives forward. Add to above mixture in step 2 and mix for 15 minutes at medium speed.
5. Screen all dry flavors through a No. 100 mesh screen and add to above mixture.
6. Fill dry powder approximately 7 g in dry 60-mL glass bottles at a fill weight based on the assay of the active constituent.

Amoxicillin–Clavulanate Syrup

Bill of Materials			
Scale (mg/5 mL)	Item	Material Name	
400.00	1	Amoxicillin as trihydrate	
57.00	2	Clavulanic acid as potassium salt	
2.69	3	Citric acid	
8.33	4	Sodium citrate	
28.10	5	Microcrystalline cellulose and sodium carboxymethylcellulose	
10.00	6	Xanthan gum	
16.67	7	Colloidal silicon dioxide	
216.60	8	Silicon dioxide	
13.30	9	Strawberry flavor	
15.00	10	Caramel flavor	
6.70	11	Saccharin sodium	
QS	12	Cellulose microcrystalline[a]	

[a]Total amount filled per bottle to deliver 12 doses is 15 g for 400 and 600 mg label of amoxicillin; For 200- and 300-mg amoxicillin label, the total fill weight is 12 g; adjust using item 12. Use method above to manufacture the final product.

Ampicillin Powder for Suspension

Bill of Materials			
Scale (mg/5 mL)	Item	Material Name	Qty/5 L (g)
125.00	1	Ampicillin, USE ampicillin trihydrate, 8% excess	144.25
1.00	2	Simethicone A	1.00
138.90	3	Castor sugar	138.90
27.44	4	Sodium citrate	27.44
7.00	5	Xanthan gum	7.00
15.00	6	Blood orange dry flavor	15.00
0.78	7	Vanilla dry flavor	0.78
7.55	8	Strawberry dry flavor	7.55
10.00	9	Aerosil 200	10.00
138.90	10	Castor sugar	138.90
2747.90	11	Castor sugar	2747.90

Manufacturing Directions

1. All operations to be completed in relative humidity 45% to 55% and temperature 23°C to 25°C.
2. Charge items 2 and 3 in a suitable blender and mix for 5 minutes.
3. Charge in a separate mixer items 1, 4 to 10 and mix for 5 minutes.
4. Add step 2 into step 3 and mix for 10 minutes.
5. Add item 11 and mix for 10 minutes.
6. Fill 65 g for 100-mL pack and 39 g for 60-mL pack. For 250-mg strength, adjust active ingredient and adjust with item 11.

Ampicillin Powder for Suspension

Bill of Materials			
Scale (mg/g)	Item	Material Name	Qty/kg (g)
50.00	1	Ampicillin trihydrate	50.00
50.00	2	Sodium citrate	50.00
21.00	3	Citric acid crystalline	21.00
50.00	4	Sodium gluconate	50.00
400.00	5	Sorbitol crystalline	400.00
60.00	6	Kollidon CL-M	60.00
15.00	7	Orange flavor	15.00
5.00	8	Lemon flavor	5.00
4.00	9	Saccharin sodium	4.00

Manufacturing Directions

Mix all components and fill appropriate amount.

Ampicillin and Cloxacillin Oily Suspension

Bill of Materials			
Scale (mg/mL)	Item	Material Name	Qty/L (g)
15.00	1	Ampicillin sodium	15.00
40.00	2	Cloxacillin sodium	40.00
30.00	3	Lutrol F 68	30.00
QS	4	Antioxidant	QS
915.00	5	Castor oil	915.00

Manufacturing Directions

1. Charge items 4 and 5 in a suitable stainless steel jacketed vessel; heat to 50°C. Do not overheat as castor oil may decompose.
2. Add and dissolve item 3.
3. Add and dissolve items 1 and 2.
4. Homogenize and fill.

Amprenavir Capsules

Bill of Materials			
Scale (mg/mL)	Item	Material Name	Qty/L (g)
150.00	1	Amprenavir	150.00
400.00	2	D-alpha-tocopheryl polyethylene glycol 1000 succinate (TPGS)	400.00
200.50	3	Polyethylene glycol 400	200.50
39.40	4	Polyethylene glycol 400	39.50

Manufacturing Directions

1. Charge item 2 in a suitable stainless steel-jacketed vessel and heat to 50°C until liquefied.
2. Add item 3 (90%) at 50°C and mix until homogenous solution obtained.
3. Increase temperature to 65°C, add item 1, and stir to dissolve.
4. Add item 4 and balance of item 2, cool to room temperature, apply vacuum to remove air entrapped.
5. Fill in size 12 oblong, white opaque soft gelatin capsules using a capsule-filling machine.
6. Dry the capsule shells to moisture of 3% to 6% water and a shell hardness of 7 to 10 N and pack in a suitable container.

Amprenavir Capsules

The capsules are available for oral administration in strengths of 50 and 150 mg. Each 50-mg capsule contains the inactive ingredients: D-alpha-tocopheryl polyethylene glycol 1000 succinate (TPGS), polyethylene glycol 400 (PEG 400) 246.7 mg, and propylene glycol 19 mg. Each 150-mg capsule contains the inactive ingredients: TPGS, PEG 400 740 mg, and propylene glycol 57 mg. The capsule shell contains the inactive ingredients: D-sorbitol and sorbitans solution, gelatin, glycerin, and titanium dioxide. The soft gelatin capsules are printed with edible red ink. Each 150-mg capsule contains 109 U vitamin E in the form of TPGS. The total amount of vitamin E in the recommended daily adult dose is 1744 U.

Amprenavir Oral Solution

One milliliter of Agenerase oral solution contains 15 mg of amprenavir in solution and the inactive ingredients acesulfame potassium, artificial grape bubble-gum flavor, citric acid (anhydrous), D-alpha-tocopheryl polyethylene glycol 1000 succinate (TPGS), menthol, natural peppermint flavor, polyethylene glycol 400 (PEG 400) (170 mg), propylene glycol (550 mg), saccharin sodium, sodium chloride, and sodium citrate (dihydrate). Solutions of sodium hydroxide and/or diluted hydrochloric acid may have been added to adjust pH. Each milliliter of Agenerase oral solution contains 46 U vitamin E in the form of TPGS. Propylene glycol is in the formulation to achieve adequate solubility of amprenavir.

Anise Oil Solution

Bill of Materials			
Scale (mg/mL)	Item	Material Name	Qty/L (g)
10.00	1	Anise oil	10.00
17.00	2	Cremophor RH 40	17.00
340.00	3	Ethanol	340.00
QS	4	Preservatives	QS
633.00	5	Water	633.00

Manufacturing Directions

1. Mix the anise oil with Cremophor RH 40, heat to approximately 65°C.
2. Stir vigorously and slowly add the hot solution of items 3 to 5 to produce a clear or slightly opalescent, colorless liquid.

Antipyrine and Benzocaine Elixir

Each milliliter contains antipyrine 54 mg, benzocaine 14 mg, and glycerin anhydrous QS to volume (also contains oxyquinoline sulfate).

Antiseptic Wet Wipes

Bill of Materials			
Scale (mg/mL)	Item	Material Name	Qty/L (g)
3.75	1	Cetrimonium bromide	3.75
0.15	2	Chlorhexidine gluconate	0.15
10.0–20.0	3	Polysorbate 20	10.0–20.0
10.0–20.0	4	Glycerin	10.0–20.0
QS	5	Deionized water	QS to 1 L

Manufacturing Directions

1. Preblend Polysorbate 20 and perfume.
2. Combine remaining components with stirring, add perfume/Polysorbate 20, blend.
3. Stir until clear.
4. Package in wipes.

Apraclonidine Hydrochloride Ophthalmic Solution

Each milliliter of Iopidine® 0.5% ophthalmic solution contains apraclonidine hydrochloride 5.75 mg equivalent to apraclonidine base 5 mg, benzalkonium chloride 0.01%, sodium chloride, sodium acetate, sodium hydroxide or hydrochloric acid (pH 4.4–7.8), and purified water.

Ascorbic Acid Solution

Bill of Materials			
Scale (mg/mL)	Item	Material Name	Qty/L (g)
100.00	1	Ascorbic acid	100.00
QS	2	Propylene glycol	QS to 1 L

Manufacturing Directions

Keep under CO_2 protection at all times. Avoid contact with iron. Use stainless steel or glass-lined equipment only. Propylene glycol must be water white.

1. Load 86.8 g propylene glycol into a glass-lined or suitable stainless steel-jacketed tank. While mixing, heat to 70°C to 80°C. Bubble CO_2 gas into the propylene glycol from the bottom of the tank.
2. Add and dissolve the ascorbic acid into the propylene glycol with a minimum of stirring under CO_2 protection.
3. When the ascorbic acid is in solution, immediately cool to approximately 25°C while continuing to mix. Also, while cooling, change CO_2 addition from tank bottom to tank top.
4. QS to 1 L using propylene glycol and mix for at least 10 minutes.
5. Use a prefilter pad and a lint-free filter paper, E&D No. 950 or its equivalent; alternatively, a Sparkler filter (or equivalent) may be used.
6. Recirculate the product through the filter press until sparkling clear.
7. Flush a suitable storage tank with CO_2 gas and continue CO_2 gas protection while product is being collected.
8. Filter the product into the storage tank and hold under CO_2 protection.
9. Flush headspace of storage tank with CO_2 gas protection.

Atovaquone Suspension

Mepron suspension is a formulation of microfine particles of atovaquone. The atovaquone particles, reduced in size to facilitate absorption, are significantly smaller than those in the previously marketed tablet formulation. Mepron suspension is for oral administration and is bright yellow with a citrus flavor. Each teaspoonful (5 mL) contains 750 mg of atovaquone and the inactive ingredients benzyl alcohol, flavor, poloxamer 188, purified water, saccharin sodium, and xanthan gum.

Atovaquone Suspension

Bill of Materials			
Scale (mg/mL)	Item	Material Name	Qty/L (g)
150.00	1	Atovaquone microflulidized[a]	150.00
5.00	2	Poloxamer 188	5.00
10.00	3	Benzyl alcohol	10.00
QS	4	Water purified	QS to 1 L

[a]Preparation of microfluidized particles of atovaquone: 600 mL of a mixture consisting of 2.5% w/v atovaquone in 0.25% w/v aqueous Celacol M2500 and passed through fluidizer such as model 120B Microfluidizer connected to a 90-psi pneumatic supply and adjusted to produce a fluid pressure of 15000 psi. Recirculate continuously through the interaction chamber for at least 45 minutes (65–77 passes) to achieve particle size less than 3 microns.

Manufacturing Directions

1. Charge items 4 and 3 in a suitable stainless steel vessel and mix well.
2. Add and mix item 2 with gentle mixing.
3. Add gradually item 1 and mix; pass through homogenizer.

Azelastine Hydrochloride Nasal Spray

Astelin nasal spray contains 0.1% azelastine hydrochloride in an aqueous solution at pH 6.8 ± 0.3. It also contains benzalkonium chloride (125 µg/mL), edetate disodium (EDTA), hydroxypropylmethylcellulose, citric acid, dibasic sodium phosphate, sodium chloride, and purified water.

Azelastine Hydrochloride Nasal Spray

Bill of Materials			
Scale (mg/mL)	Item	Material Name	Qty/L (g)
1.00	1	Azelastine hydrochloride	1.00
0.50	2	Edetic acid disodium dehydrate	0.50
6.80	3	Sodium chloride	6.80
0.125	4	Benzalkonium chloride	0.125
0.44	5	Citric acid	0.44
6.48	6	Sodium monohydrogen phosphase 12 H_2O	6.48
1.00	7	Hydroxypropyl methyl cellulose-Methocel E4M	1.00
QS	8	Water purified	QS to 1 L

Manufacturing Directions

1. Charge 90% of item 8 in a suitable stainless steel vessel.
2. Dissolve in the following order: azelastine hydrochloride, edetic acid, sodium chloride, benzalkonium chloride, citric acid, and sodium monohydrogenphosphate, and mix well.
3. Bring to volume with item 8.
4. Pass the solution through a membrane filter of pore size 0.22 microns.
5. The filtrate has a pH value of 6.8 ± 0.3.
6. Fill in plastic bottles that are closed with a conventional spray insert or into plastic or glass bottles that are closed with a conventional pump sprayer. In the latter case, pumps with nasal spray inserts are, for example, used that spray approximately 0.14 mL of solution per actuation. In this manner, 0.14 mg of azelastine hydrochloride is sprayed into the nose per actuation in the form of the solution.

Azithromycin Suspension

Bill of Materials			
Scale (mg/5 mL)	Item	Material Name	Qty/L (g)
200.0000	1	Azithromycin, USE azithromycin dehydrate	69.30
4.4100	2	Sucrose	883.00
0.0650	3	Sodium phosphate 12 hydrate	13.00
0.0075	4	Xanthan gum	1.50
0.0200	5	Sodium cyclamate	4.00
0.0200	6	Sodium saccharin	2.00
0.0250	7	Glycamil	5.00
0.5000	8	Starch pregelatinized	100.00
0.0200	9	Flavor	4.00
0.0550	10	Flavor	11.00
0.0400	11	Flavor	8.00
0.7500	12	Sorbitol 70%	150.00
0.7500	13	Propylene glycol	140.00
0.0075	14	Methyl paraben	1.50
0.0015	15	Propyl paraben	0.30
QS	16	Water purified	QS to 1 L

Manufacturing Directions

1. Charge in a suitable stainless steel double-cone blender sucrose, sodium phosphate, xanthan gum, sodium cyclamate, sodium saccharin, glycamil, and starch pregelatinized.
2. Mix for 15 minutes.
3. Mill the mixture in step 2 using a hammer mill (hammer forward) equipped with a 2-mm screen at high speed.
4. Charge into a double-cone mixer the mixture from step 3 and add azithromycin and flavors.
5. Mix for 15 minutes.
6. Fill 11.01 g per bottle. The bottle must be reconstituted with 10 mL of the diluent (see step below) to obtain 16.5 mL of suspension with concentration of 200 mg/5 mL.
7. Prepare the diluent by first dissolving items 14 and 15 in item 13 at 69°C to 70°C, then mix with items 12 and 16.

Azithromycin Suspension

Bill of Materials			
Scale (mg/mL)	Item	Material Name	Qty/L (g)
50.00	1	Azithromycin dihydrate	50.00
50.00	2	Sodium citrate	50.00
20.00	3	Citric acid	20.00
600.00	4	Sucrose	600.00
90.00	5	Kollidon CL-M	90.00
5.00	6	Cremophor RH 40	5.00
2.00	7	Chocolate flavor	2.00
100.00	8	Water purified	100.00
QS	9	Water purified	QS to 1 L

Manufacturing Directions

1. Charge items 1 to 5 in a suitable mixing vessel and mix.
2. In a separate vessel, add and mix items 6 to 8 and add to step 1. Mix.
3. Bring to volume. Homogenize and fill.

Azulene Solution

Bill of Materials			
Scale (mg/mL)	Item	Material Name	Qty/L (g)
10.00	1	Azulene	10.00
30.00	2	Cremophor RF 40	30.00
QS	3	Water purified	QS to 1 L

Manufacturing Directions

1. Charge items 1 and 2 in a suitable mixing vessel and heat to 60°C.
2. In a separate vessel, heat item 3 to 60°C and then add to step 1. Mix well for a clear solution.

Azulene Solution (1%)

Manufacturing Directions

1. Mix 1 g azulene, 3 g Cremophor RH 40, and heat to approximately 60°C.
2. Add slowly the water (60°C) to 100 mL and cool to room temperature.

Barium Sulfate Oral Suspension

Bill of Materials			
Scale (mg/mL)	Item	Material Name	Qty/L (g)
230.00	1	Barium sulfate	230.00
11.50	2	Kollidon 90F	11.50
0.92	3	Carboxymethylcellulose sodium	0.92
0.70	4	Sodium bisulfite	0.70
QS	5	Preservatives	QS
QS	6	Water purified	QS to 1 L

Manufacturing Directions

1. Charge 90% of item 6 in a suitable jacketed vessel.
2. Add and mix preservatives and item 3. Mix well. Allow to hydrate.
3. Add item 2 and mix well until clear solution is obtained.
4. Add item 1 and mix to a smooth suspension. Homogenize if necessary.

Beclomethasone Dipropionate Inhalation Aerosol

It is a pressurized, metered-dose aerosol intended for oral inhalation only. Each unit contains a solution of beclomethasone dipropionate in propellant HFA-134a (1,1,1,2 tetrafluoroethane) and ethanol. The 40-μg strength delivers 40 μg of beclomethasone dipropionate from the actuator and 50 μg from the valve. The 80-μg strength delivers 80 μg of beclomethasone dipropionate from the actuator and 100 μg from the valve. It is a metered-dose manual-pump spray unit containing a suspension of beclomethasone dipropionate, monohydrate equivalent to 0.084% w/w, beclomethasone dipropionate in an aqueous medium containing microcrystalline cellulose, carboxymethylcellulose sodium, dextrose, benzalkonium chloride, polysorbate 80, and phenylethyl alcohol. The suspension is formulated at a target pH of 6.4 with a range of 5.5 to 6.8 over its shelf life.

Beclomethasone Dipropionate Inhalation Aerosol

Bill of Materials			
Scale (μg/mg)	Item	Material Name	Qty/kg (g)
1.60	1	Beclomethasone dipropionate	1.60
35.20	2	Ethanol	35.20
0.16	3	Oleic acid	0.16
960.00	4	HFA 227	960.00

Manufacturing Directions

1. Charge beclomethasone dipropionate into a pressure addition vessel and dissolve with stirring in ethanol in which oleic acid has been previously dissolved.
2. After sealing and evacuation of step 1, add item 4, which has previously been aerated with carbon dioxide and adjusted to a pressure of 6.5 bar (20°C), in another pressure vessel with stirring. The solution obtained is dispensed into aluminum containers sealed with metered valves by means of the pressure-filling technique (e.g., units from Pamasol W. Maeder, Pfaffikon, Switzerland).

Beclomethasone Dipropionate and Salbutamol Sulfate Nasal Spray

Dissolve 15.6 g of beclomethasone dipropionate in 811 g of ethanol, which contains 3 g of oleic acid. The clear solution is mixed with 7.3 kg of HFA 227. The mixture obtained is added to 9.4 g of initially introduced salbutamol sulfate and adequately homogenized. After conclusion of the homogenization, the mixture is diluted with 2 kg of HFA 227 that has been aerated with carbon dioxide and adjusted to a pressure of 5 bar (20°C), diluted, and finally homogenized. The finished preparation is dispensed into aluminum containers sealed with metering valves by means of the pressure-filling technique.

Benzethonium Chloride Solution

Benzethonium chloride 1%, water, amphoteric 2, aloe vera gel, DMDM hydantoin, citric acid.

Benzethonium Chloride and Benzocaine Topical Anesthetic

Benzethonium chloride 0.2%, benzocaine 20%; inactive ingredients: acetulan, aloe vera oil, menthol, methyl paraben, *N*-butane/P152a (65:35), PEG 400, monolaurate, polysorbate 85.

Benzocaine and Tetracaine Topical Solution

Bill of Materials			
Scale (g/100 mL)	Item	Material Name	Qty/L (g)
14.00	1	Benzocaine	140.00
2.00	2	Butyl aminobenzoate	20.00
2.00	3	Tetracaine hydrochloride	20.00
0.50	4	Benzalkonium chloride	5.00
0.005	5	Cetyl dimethyl ethyl ammonium bromide	0.05
QS	6	Water purified	QS to 1 L

Benzyl Benzoate Solution

Bill of Materials			
Scale (mg/mL)	Item	Material Name	Qty/L (g)
100.00	1	Benzyl benzoate	100.00
220.00	2	Cremophor RH 40	220.00
410.00	3	Ethanol (96%)	410.00
270.00	4	Water	270.00

Manufacturing Directions

1. Heat the mixture of benzyl benzoate and Cremophor RH 40 to approximately 60°C.
2. Stir strongly and slowly add the water.
3. Finally, add the ethanol to produce a clear, colorless liquid.

Beta-Estradiol Vaginal Solution

Bill of Materials			
Scale (mg/mL)	Item	Material Name	Qty/L (g)
QS	1	Vehicle (pluronic P105 45%, propylene glycol 48%, water 7%)	QS to 1 L
0.10	2	Beta-estradiol	0.10
QS	3	Perfumes	QS

Manufacturing Directions

1. Add the beta-estradiol and propylene glycol into a clean vessel.
2. Subsequently add the poloxamer and water to the vessel.
3. Mix until uniform.

Betamethasone Syrup

Celestone syrup contains 0.6 mg betamethasone in each 5 mL. The inactive ingredients for celestone syrup include alcohol; cellulose, powdered; citric acid, anhydrous; FD&C red No. 40; FD&C yellow No. 6; flavor cherry artificial 13506457 IFF; flavor orange natural terpeneless 73502530 IFF; propylene glycol; sodium benzoate; sodium chloride; sorbitol solution; sugar, granulated; and water, purified.

Bismuth Carbonate Suspension

Bill of Materials			
Scale (mg/mL)	Item	Material Name	Qty/L (g)
266.66 mg	1	Light kaolin	266.66
8.30 mg	2	Pectin	8.30
6.70 mg	3	Bismuth carbonate	6.70
9.40 mg	4	Cellulose (microcrystalline; Avicel™ RC-591)	9.40
1.40 mg	5	Methyl paraben	1.40
0.20 mg	6	Saccharin sodium	0.20
0.40 mg	7	Aspartame	0.40
40.00 mL	8	Sorbitol	40.00 mL
5.00 mL	9	Ethanol	5.00 mL
QS	10	Deionized water	QS to 1 L

Manufacturing Directions

1. Dissolve item 2 in hot water.
2. Disperse item 1 in 75 mL of item 10 at room temperature.
3. With constant agitation, add item 3 and continue stirring.
4. Mix and cool to room temperature.
5. Disperse item 4 in item 10 and add it to the batch.
6. Dissolve item 2 in item 1 dispersion and add to the batch.
7. Dissolve items 6 and 7 in water and add to the batch.
8. Add flavor, color, and water to volume.
9. Pass through homogenizer or colloid mill if necessary.

Bismuth Subsalicylate Suspension

Bill of Materials			
Scale (mg/mL)	Item	Material Name	Qty/L (g)
15.00	1	Magnesium aluminum silicate (Magnabrite K)	15.00
1.50	2	Methylcellulose	1.50
910.00	3	Deionized water	910.00
0.50	4	Saccharin sodium	0.50
30.00	5	Bismuth subsalicylate	30.00
4.00	6	Salicylic acid	4.00
10.00	7	Sodium salicylate	10.00
29.00	8	Ethanol	29.00
QS	9	Preservatives	QS
QS	10	Colorings	QS

Manufacturing Directions

1. Dry blend items 1 and 2 and slowly add them to item 3, agitating until smooth.
2. Add items 4 to 7 to this dispersion, gradually mixing well each time.
3. Finally, add items 8 to 10 to smooth mix.

Bromazepam Drops

Bill of Materials			
Scale (mg/mL)	Item	Material Name	Qty/L (g)
2.50	1	Bromazepam	2.50
5.00	2	Saccharin sodium	5.00
0.10	3	Sequestrene disodium	0.10
5.00	4	Flavor	5.00
25.00	5	Flavor	25.00
QS	6	Sodium hydroxide for pH adjustment	QS
50.00	7	Water purified	50.00
QS	8	Propylene glycol	QS to 1 L

Manufacturing Directions

1. Charge item 8 in a suitable stainless steel mixing vessel and, while stirring, add item 3 and dissolve.
2. Add item 7 and stir continuously. Add item 2 and then item 1 and stir to dissolve.
3. Add flavors and mix.
4. Check and adjust pH to 5, if necessary, using item 5.
5. Make up volume with item 8.

Bromhexine Hydrochloride Syrup

Bill of Materials			
Scale (mg/5 mL)	Item	Material Name	Qty/L (g)
4.00	1	Bromhexine HCl	0.80
1000.00	2	Glycerin (glycerol)	200.00
10.00	3	Benzoic acid	2.00
1.70	4	All fruits flavor	0.34
5.00	5	Tartaric acid	1.00
151.58	6	Alcohol (ethanol, 95%)	30.31
2857.00	7	Sorbitol (70% solution)	571.40
10.00	8	Sodium carboxymethyl cellulose (sodium CMC)	2.00
0.72	9	Sodium hydroxide pellets	0.14
QS	10	Purified water	QS to 1 L

Manufacturing Directions

1. Add 250 g of item 10 to the manufacturing vessel and heat to 65°C to 70°C.
2. Add 20 g of item 2 in a separate stainless steel container and mix item 8 using an Ekato stirrer, carefully avoiding lump formation.
3. Transfer the slurry to the manufacturing vessel and continue mixing to make a clear mucilage. Avoid air entrapment.
4. Cool to 30°C while mixing at slow speed. Transfer the mucilage to container.
5. Load 100 g of item 2 to the manufacturing vessel.
6. Add item 6 in a separate stainless steel container and dissolve item 3 using stirrer.
7. Add 60 g of item 2 to the container while mixing at slow speed.
8. Add and dissolve item 1 to the container while mixing at slow speed. Avoid splashing of the solution. Ensure bromhexine is dissolved completely.
9. Add item 4 to the container and mix well.
10. Transfer the solution to the manufacturing vessel while mixing at high speed.
11. Rinse the container with 20 g of item 2 and transfer the rinsing to the manufacturing vessel while mixing.
12. Rinse the container with 20 g of item 10 and transfer the rinsing to the manufacturing vessel while mixing.
13. Add 15 g of item 10 in a separate stainless steel container.
14. Dissolve item 5 using a stirrer and transfer it to the manufacturing vessel while mixing. Check for clarity of the solution in the manufacturing vessel. The solution must be clear without any undissolved particles of the drug.
15. Add item 7 to the manufacturing vessel while mixing at high speed.
16. Transfer the cooled mucilage of item 8 to the manufacturing vessel used above while mixing at slow speed.
17. Check and record the pH of the solution (limit: 3.3–3.6).
18. Dissolve item 9 in 5 g of cooled item 10 (30°C) in a separate stainless steel container.
19. Adjust the pH of the syrup in the manufacturing vessel using the sodium hydroxide solution.
20. Add sodium hydroxide solution, small portions at a time. Mix well and check the pH after every addition. Adjust the pH to 3.5 (limit: 3.3–3.6).
21. Bring the volume up to 1 L with item 10 and finally mix for 15 to 20 minutes at high speed.
22. Check and record the pH (limit: 3.3–3.6).
23. Filter the syrup at 1.5 bar.
24. Recirculate.

Bromhexine Hydrochloride Syrup—Alcohol Free

Bill of Materials			
Scale (mg/5 mL)	Item	Material Name	Qty/L (g)
4.00	1	Bromhexine HCl	0.80
1000.00	2	Glycerin (glycerol)	200.00
12.00	3	Sodium benzoate	2.40
1.70	4	All fruit flavor	0.34
17.00	5	Tartaric acid	3.40
2250.00	6	Sorbitol (70% solution)	450.00
10.00	7	Sodium carboxymethyl cellulose (sodium CMC)	2.00
QS	8	Purified water	QS to 1 L

Manufacturing Directions

1. Add 240 g of item 8 (25°C) to the manufacturing vessel.
2. Add item 5 and mix for 20 minutes at high speed.
3. Load 180 g of item 2 into the manufacturing vessel and mix for 3 minutes.
4. Add item 1 to the manufacturing vessel and mix for 30 minutes at high speed.
5. Add 20 g of item 2 in a suitable vessel and levigate item 7 using stirrer, carefully avoiding lump formation.
6. Add 40 g of item 8 (70°C) to the stainless steel container while mixing to make a clear mucilage; mix for 15 minutes. Avoid air entrapment.
7. Cool down to 25°C to 30°C while mixing at slow speed.
8. Transfer the mucilage to the manufacturing vessel.
9. Rinse the vessel with 10 g of item 8 and transfer to the manufacturing vessel.
10. Mix at slow speed for 20 minutes.
11. Transfer item 6 to the manufacturing vessel while mixing. Mix at low speed for 5 minutes.
12. Add 20 g of item 8 (25°C) in a separate stainless steel container and dissolve item 3 using an Ekato stirrer until a clear solution is obtained.
13. Transfer this solution to the manufacturing vessel and mix at low speed for 3 minutes.
14. Add item 4 to the manufacturing vessel and mix at low speed for 3 minutes.
15. Record the pH of the solution (limit: 3.3–3.7). Adjust the pH of the solution with 10% solution of sodium hydroxide, if required.
16. Make the volume up to 1 L with item 8 (25°C) and finally mix for 15 to 20 minutes at high speed.
17. Filter the syrup at 1.5 bar.
18. Recirculate.

Bromhexine Hydrochloride Syrup

Bill of Materials			
Scale (mg/5 mL)	Item	Material Name	Qty/L (g)
4.00	1	Bromhexine HCl	0.80
1000000	2	Glycerin (glycerol)	200.00
10.00	3	Benzoic acid	2.00
1.00	4	All fruits flavor	0.34
5000	5	Tartaric acid	1.00
151.50	6	Alcohol (ethanol 95%)	30.31
2857000	7	Sorbitol (70% solution)	571.40
10.00	8	Carboxymethylcellulose sodium (sodium CMC)	2.00
0.70	9	Sodium hydroxide pellets	0.14
QS	10	Water purified	QS to 1 L

Manufacturing Directions

1. Add 250 g of item 10 to a suitable stainless steel manufacturing vessel and heat to 65°C to 70°C.
2. Add 20 g of item 2 in a separate stainless steel container and mix item 8 using Ekato stirrer, carefully avoiding lump formation.
3. Transfer the slurry to the manufacturing vessel while continuing to mix to make a clear mucilage. Avoid air entrapment.
4. Cool down to 30°C while mixing at slow speed.
5. Transfer the mucilage to container. Load 100 g of item 2 to the manufacturing vessel.
6. Add item 6 in a separate stainless steel container and dissolve item 3 using stirrer.
7. Add 60 g of item 2 to the container while mixing at slow speed.
8. Add and dissolve item 1 to the container while mixing at slow speed. Avoid splashing of the solution. Check that bromhexine is dissolved completely.
9. Add item 4 to the container and mix well. Transfer the solution to the manufacturing vessel while mixing at high speed.
10. Rinse the container with 20 g of item 2 and transfer the rinsing to the manufacturing vessel while mixing.
11. Rinse the container with 20 g of item 10 and transfer the rinsing to the manufacturing vessel while mixing. Add 15 g of item 10 in a separate stainless steel container and dissolve item 5 using stirrer and transfer to the manufacturing vessel while mixing.
12. Check clarity of the solution in manufacturing vessel. The solution must be clear without any undissolved particles of the drug.
13. Add item 7 to the manufacturing vessel while mixing at high speed.
14. Transfer the cooled mucilage of item 8 to the manufacturing vessel used above while mixing at slow speed.
15. Check and record the pH of the solution (limit: 3.3–3.6).
16. Dissolve item 9 in 5 g of cooled item 10 (30°C) in a separate stainless steel container.
17. Adjust the pH of the syrup in manufacturing vessel using the sodium hydroxide solution. Add sodium hydroxide solution in small portions at a time. Mix well and check the pH after every addition. Adjust the pH to 3.5 (limit: 3.3–3.6).
18. Make up the volume up to 1 L with item 10 and, finally, mix for 15 to 20 minutes at high speed. Check and record the pH (limit: 3.3–3.6). Filter the syrup at 1.5 bar. Recirculate.

Budesonide Inhaler

Bill of Materials			
Scale (mg/g)	Item	Material Name	Qty/kg (g)
20.00	1	Budesonide	20.00
1190.00	2	Oleic acid	1190.00
1372.00	3	Trichloromonofluoromethane (propellant 11)	1372.00
2745.00	4	Dichlorodifluoremethane (propellant 12)	2745.00
1373.00	5	Dichlorotetrafluoroethane (propellant 114)	1373.00

Manufacturing Directions

1. Mix oleic acid in trichloromonofluoromethane in a suitable mixer.
2. Suspend budesonide in step 1 while mixing. Homogenize for 10 minutes.
3. On quality control release, fill the suspension 2.582 g in aluminum containers.
4. Crimp the valve and pressurize with the mixture of dichlorodifluoromethane and dichlorotetrafluoromethane, 4.118 g per container.

Butamirate Citrate Syrup

Bill of Materials			
Scale (mg/5 mL)	Item	Material Name	Qty/5 L (g)
4.00	1	Butamirate citrate	4.00
12.50	2	Citric acid monohydrate	12.50
1750.00	3	Sorbitol	1750.00
1250.00	4	Glycerin	1250.00
6.25	5	Saccharin sodium	6.25
5.00	6	Sodium benzoate	5.00
10.00	7	Lemon flavor	10.00
QS	8	Sodium hydroxide	2.50
QS	9	Water purified	QS to 5 L

Manufacturing Directions

1. Dissolve items 2 to 4 in item 9 (90%).
2. Add and dissolve item 1.
3. Add items 5 to 7.
4. Add item 8.
5. Bring to volume.

Caffeine Citrate Oral Solution

Bill of Materials			
Scale (mg/mL)	Item	Material Name	Qty/L (g)
10.00	1	Caffeine, USE caffeine citrate	20.00
5.00	2	Citric acid monohydrate	5.00
8.30	3	Sodium citrate monohydrate	8.30
QS	4	Water purified	QS to 1 L

Manufacturing Directions

1. Dissolve item 1 in a solution of items 2 and 3 in item 4.
2. Adjust pH to 4.7

Calcipotriene Solution

Dovonex® (calcipotriene solution) scalp solution 0.005% is a colorless topical solution containing 0.005% calcipotriene in a vehicle of isopropanol (51% v/v) propylene glycol, hydroxypropyl cellulose, sodium citrate menthol, and water.

Calcitonin Nasal Spray

Calcitonin-salmon, 2200 U/mL (corresponding to 200 U/0.09 mL actuation), sodium chloride, benzalkonium chloride, nitrogen, hydrochloric acid (added as necessary to adjust pH), and purified water.

Calcitonin Nasal Spray

Bill of Materials			
Scale (mg/mL)	Item	Material Name	Qty/L (g)
0.1375	1	Salmon calcitonin, 10% excess	0.152
7.500	2	Sodium chloride	7.500
0.100	3	Benzalkonium chloride	0.100
QS	4	Hydrochloric acid (1 N) to adjust pH	QS
QS	5	Water purified	QS to 1 L

Manufacturing Directions

1. Charge items 1 (90%), 2, and 3 in a suitable stainless steel mixing vessel under protection of nitrogen gas and mix well.
2. Measure and adjust pH to 3.7 using item 4.
3. Filter through 0.20-micron filter.
4. Add balance of item 1 in item 5 to step 3. Mix.
5. Fill into a spray nasal dispenser with a solution volume of 2 mL. The composition comprises approximately 550 MRC units active ingredient per milliliter and the applicator delivers a quantity comprising 55 units per actuation.

Calcium Carbonate and Guar Gum Suspension

Bill of Materials			
Scale (mg/5 mL)	Item	Material Name	Qty/L (g)
400.000	1	Calcium carbonate	80.000
3935.000	2	Water purified	787.000
1000.000	3	Sorbitol solution (70%)	200.000
13.000	4	Xanthan gum	2.600
5.000	5	Hydroxyethyl cellulose	1.000
120.000	6	Magnesium hydroxide	24.000
25.000	7	Flavor strawberry[a]	5.000
1.425	8	Saccharin sodium	0.285
100.000	9	Guar gum	20.000

[a]Powder flavor is used; can change according to requirement.

Manufacturing Directions

This is a preservative-free formula; shelf life stability is achieved by maintaining pH of the suspension above 9 through the addition of magnesium hydroxide. Absence of preservatives makes it a more palatable formula but requires extra care in the manufacturing process. Rigidly control the microbial specification of all ingredients. Thoroughly clean all equipment and rinse with 1% sodium hypochlorite solution before use. Finally, rinse with purified water.

1. In a clean vessel, heat item 2°C to 90°C and maintain for 20 minutes. Cool to room temperature.
2. In approximately 90% of the quantity of item 2, add item 3 to step 1 and mix well. Set aside the balance of quantity of item 2 for bringing to volume the suspension in the step 8.
3. Add by sprinkling items 3, 4, and 9, gradually mixing aggressively to ensure fine dispersion; the powders may be passed through an appropriate sieve to break any lumps.
4. Mix for 30 minutes.
5. Add and mix item 1 for 15 minutes after passing through a fine mesh to break any lumps.
6. Add item 6 after passing through 100-mesh screen and mix for 15 minutes.
7. Add flavor and sweetener and stir for another 15 minutes. Bring to volume (if necessary) and mix for 10 minutes.
8. Check the pH of suspension to 9 and above. Add small quantity of magnesium hydroxide if needed to bring pH to above 9.
9. Heat the suspension in a covered container for 30 minutes at 68°C (maintain 68°C for 30 minutes); this is a pasteurizing step to reduce microbial load.
10. Fill in clean bottles tested for microbial contamination.

Calcium Iodide and Ascorbic Acid Syrup

Bill of Materials			
Scale (mg/mL)	Item	Material Name	Qty/L (g)
311.60	1	Glucose liquid (corn syrup)	311.60
53.90	2	Glycerin (96%)	53.90
30.00	3	Anhydrous calcium iodide; use calcium iodide solution 27% w/w	111.11
1.00	4	Ascorbic acid (white powder)	1.00
485.30	5	Sucrose (granulated sugar)	485.30
0.80	6	Saccharin sodium (powder)[a]	0.80
8.00	7	Sodium cyclamate (XIII powder)	8.00
1.31	8	Honey artificial flavor, AU-73	1.31
0.33	9	Floral mint artificial flavor	0.33
51.53	10	Alcohol (ethanol; 190 proof)	51.53
0.60	11	Isoproterenol sulfate (powder)	0.60
0.05	12	FD&C yellow dye No. 5	
0.25	13	Caramel (acid proof)	0.25
QS	14	Water purified	~344.0 mL

[a]Use 1.2 g of saccahrin to replace cyclamate; adjust balance with sucrose.

Manufacturing Directions

Isoproterenol is toxic; wear a dust mask and avoid contact. The product is sensitive to oxidation. Manufacture under N_2 protection and protect product from light and heat; all water must be boiled, cooled, and gassed with nitrogen.

1. Load glucose and glycerin into a suitable mixing tank.
2. Add 187 mL purified water to tank with mixing.
3. Begin bubbling N_2 protection for the balance of the process.
4. Add and dissolve saccharin sodium and sodium cyclamate, if used, with mixing.
5. Add calcium iodide to the tank with good mixing.
6. Add and dissolve ascorbic acid and sugar.
7. Dissolve the flavors in alcohol and add with mixing to the main batch.
8. Dissolve isoproterenol in 10 to 13 mL of water and add, with mixing, to the main batch.
9. Dissolve dye in 3.5 mL purified water and add solution to tank with mixing. (*Note*: Dye may be deleted.) Add caramel with mixing to main batch.
10. Move N_2 source from the bottom to the top of the tank.
11. Turn off mixer.
12. Allow to stand overnight under N_2 protection to let entrapped gases escape.
13. QS to 1 L. Mix for 1 hour.
14. Filter and circulate product through a suitable filter press until sparkling clear.

Carbamazepine Oral Suspension 2%

Formulation

Carbamazepine (Flavine), 2 g; 1,2-propylene glycol, 20 g; Kollidon 90F, 3 g; saccharine sodium, 0.1 g; sodium citrate, 1 g; sorbitol, crystalline, 25 g; Kollidon CL-M, 7 g; water, 41.9 g;

Manufacturing Directions

1. Stir the mixture of carbamazepine and propylene glycol at least during 2 hours.
2. Add Kollidon 90F, saccharine, sodium citrate, and the water and stir again until these components are dissolved.
3. Dissolve sorbitol in this mixture and add Kollidon CL-M to the well-stirred suspension to obtain a homogeneous suspension.

Carbetapentane Tannate and Chlorpheniramine Suspension

Bill of Materials			
Scale (mg/5 mL)	Item	Material Name	Qty/5 L (g)
30.00	1	Carbetapentane tannate	30.00
4.00	2	Chlorpheniramine tannate	4.00
50.00	3	Pectin medium viscosity	50.00
1000.00	4	Kaolin colloidal powder	1000.00
35.00	5	Magnesium aluminum silicate	35.00
10.00	6	Benzoic acid	10.00
2.50	7	Methyl paraben	2.50
1000.00	8	Sucrose	1000.00
0.75	9	Saccharin sodium	0.75
225.00	10	Glycerin	225.00
0.91	11	Flavor black currant imitation	0.91
2.28	12	Flavor strawberry with other flavors	2.28
0.45	13	Purpose shade "R" dye	0.45
0.80	14	FD&C red No.3 dye	0.80
0.30	15	FD&C yellow No.5	0.30
3.17	16	Sodium hydroxide solution 50%	3.17
	17	Purified water, deionized	QS to 5 mL

Carnitine and Coenzyme Q Solution

Bill of Materials			
Scale (mg/mL)	Item	Material Name	Qty/L (g)
1.00	1	Coenzyme Q10	1.00
1.00	2	Lutrol E 400	1.00
4.00	3	Cremophor RH 40	4.00
QS	4	Preservative	QS
QS	5	Water	QS to 1 L
40.00	6	Carnitine	40.00

Manufacturing Directions

1. Heat the mixture of items 1 to 5 to 60°C and stir well.
2. Add and dissolve item 6 after cooling to room temperature.

Cefaclor Suspension

Bill of Materials			
Scale (mg/5 mL)	Item	Material Name	Qty/L (g)
250.00	1	Cefaclor	50.00
5.00	2	Emulsion silicone 30%	1.00
7.50	3	Xanthan gum	1.50
10.00	4	Starch modified	2.00
4.00	5	Erythrosine aluminum lake	0.80
20.00	6	Flavor	4.00
0.75	7	Sodium lauryl sulfate	0.15
3.00	8	Methylcellulose	0.60
2960.00	9	Sucrose	592.00

Note: For 125-mg dose, adjust with sucrose the final quantity.

Cefadroxil Monohydrate Oral Suspension

Duricef for oral suspension contains the following inactive ingredients: FD&C yellow No. 6, flavors (natural and artificial), polysorbate 80, sodium benzoate, sucrose, and xanthan gum.

Cefpodoxime Proxetil Oral Suspension

Each 5 mL of Vantin oral suspension contains cefpodoxime proxetil equivalent to 50 or 100 mg of cefpodoxime activity after constitution and the following inactive ingredients: artificial flavorings, butylated hydroxy anisole, carboxymethylcellulose sodium, microcrystalline cellulose, carrageenan, citric acid, colloidal silicon dioxide, croscarmellose sodium, hydroxypropylcellulose, lactose, maltodextrin, natural flavorings, propylene glycol alginate, sodium citrate, sodium benzoate, starch, sucrose, and vegetable oil.

Cefpodoxime Proxetil Oral Suspension

Bill of Materials			
Scale (mg/g)	Item	Material Name	Qty/kg (g)
100.00	1	Cefpodoxime proxetil	123.50
563.75	2	Sucrose	563.50
290.00	3	D-Mannitol	290.00
1.25	4	Saccharin sodium	1.25
20.00	5	Hydroxypropyl cellulose	20.00
0.50	6	Dye yellow No. 5	0.50
1.00	7	Ethylenediamine tetraacetate disodium	1.00
QS	8	Orange essence	QS
QS	9	Water purified	QS

Manufacturing Directions

1. Charge item 1, sucrose, D-mannitol, saccharin sodium, and disodium ethylenediamine tetraacetate in an agitating granulator.
2. Granulate the mixture by agitation while spraying it with a binder of hydroxypropylcellulose and yellow No. 5 in water.
3. Pass wet mass through a 42-mesh screen in an extrusion granulator.
4. Dry the granules in a fluidized bed granulator.
5. Spray the granules with orange essence.
6. Dry granules further in the fluid bed dryer.
7. Pass granules through 30-mesh sieve and fill.

When purified water is added to the resulting dry syrup at a concentration of item 1 of 49.4 mg/mL, the dry syrup rapidly dissolves in it to give a clear orange solution.

Cefpodoxime Proxetil for Oral Suspension

Each 5 mL of Vantin oral suspension contains cefpodoxime proxetil equivalent to 50 or 100 mg of cefpodoxime activity after constitution and the following inactive ingredients: artificial flavorings, butylated hydroxyanisole, carboxymethylcellulose sodium, microcrystalline cellulose, carrageenan, citric acid, colloidal silicon dioxide, croscarmellose sodium, hydroxypropylcellulose, lactose, maltodextrin, natural flavorings, propylene glycol alginate, sodium citrate, sodium benzoate, starch, sucrose, and vegetable oil.

Ceftin for oral suspension, when reconstituted with water, provides the equivalent of 125 or 250 mg of cefuroxime (as cefuroxime axetil) per 5 mL of suspension. Ceftin for oral suspension contains the inactive ingredients polyvinyl pyrrolidone K30, stearic acid, sucrose, and tutti-frutti flavoring.

Cefuroxime Axetil Suspension

Bill of Materials			
Scale (mg/mL)	Item	Material Name	Qty/L (g)
25.00	1	R-Cefuroxime axetil	25.00
0.40 mL	2	Sorbitol solution 70%	0.40 L
20.00	3	Saccharin	20.00
QS	4	Water purified	QS to 1 L

Manufacturing Directions

1. Charge the sorbitol solution and 20% of item 5 in a mixing vessel.
2. Add item 1 and mix vigorously to form a suspension.
3. Add items 3 and any flavors, if needed, and mix.
4. Bring to volume.
5. Fill.

Cetirizine Hydrochloride Syrup

Bill of Materials			
Scale (mg/5 mL)	Item	Material Name	Qty/L (g)
5.00	1	Cetirizine hydrochloride	1.03
1750.00	2	Lycosin 80/55	350.00
600.00	3	Sorbitol 70%	120.00
5.00	4	Sodium citrate	1.00
300.00	5	Propylene glycol	60.00
4.50	6	Methyl paraben	0.90
0.50	7	Propyl paraben	0.10
3.75	8	Saccharin sodium	0.75
10.00	9	Flavor raspberry	2.00
QS	10	Water purified	QS to 1 L

Manufacturing Directions

1. Charge 30% of item 10 in a stainless steel jacketed kettle and heat to 90°C to 95°C.
2. Add and dissolve items 6 and 7; cool to 40°C.
3. Add to step above item 4 and item 8 and mix to dissolve.
4. Add items 2, 3, and 5 and mix to dissolve.
5. In a separate vessel, charge 30% of item 10 and add to it item 1, mix to dissolve, and then add to step 4.
6. Add flavor(s) and bring to volume with item 10.

Chlophedianol, Ipecac, Ephedrine, Ammonium Chloride, Carbinoxamine, and Balsam Tolu Syrup

Bill of Materials			
Scale (mg/tablet)	Item	Material Name	Qty/L (g)
0.001 mL	1	Ipecac fluid extract	1.00 mL
5.00	2	Chlophedianol hydrochloride	5.00
1.32	3	Ephedrine hydrochloride (powder)	1.32
8.80	4	Ammonium chloride (reagent-grade granules)	8.80
0.80	5	Carbinoxamine maleate	0.80
0.90	6	Methyl paraben	0.90
0.10	7	Propyl paraben	0.10
6.25	8	Balsam of Tolu (eq. aqueous extract)	6.25
2.66	9	Saccharin sodium (dihydrate powder)	2.66
319.22	10	Sucrose (granulated sugar)	319.22
238.33	11	Glucose liquid (corn syrup)	238.33
83.93	12	Sorbitol solution (calculate as 70% sorbitol crystals)	83.93
40.00	13	Alcohol	40.00
166.67	14	FD&C red dye (Amaranth E123)	166.67 mg
0.80	15	Raspberry flavor	0.80
100.00	16	Propylene glycol	100.00
QS	17	HyFlo filter aid	0.50
QS	18	Water purified	~450.00 mL

Manufacturing Directions

1. Charge balsam of Tolu and 25 mL of water in a steam bath.
2. Raise the temperature, stirring continuously to mix water with the balsam.
3. Boil for half an hour and allow to decant while cooling.
4. Discard extracted balsam of Tolu.
5. Filter the supernatant liquid through filter paper and store apart.
6. Charge 150 mL water in a jacketed mixing tank and heat to boiling.
7. Add and dissolve parabens with mixing.
8. Add and dissolve sugar with constant mixing.
9. Heat to 70°C to 75°C.
10. Once sugar is dissolved, add glucose, sorbitol, and saccharin sodium. Mix well until dissolved.
11. Dissolve ammonium chloride in 28 mL water.
12. Add to mixing tank.
13. Add extract balsam of Tolu from first step with mixing. Mix well and cool to 25°C to 30°C.
14. Add and dissolve ephedrine and carbinoxamine in 20 mL water and add to mixing tank. Mix well.
15. Add and dissolve chlophedianol in 50 g of propylene glycol and add to mixing tank.
16. Add balance of propylene glycol to mixing tank.
17. Add and dissolve Ipecac fluid extract and raspberry flavor in alcohol.
18. Add to mixing tank.
19. Dissolve dye in 5 mL water and add to tank with continuous mixing.
20. Rinse container with 5 mL of water and add rinsing.
21. Adjust to volume with purified water.
22. Add HyFlo filter aid to syrup and mix well.
23. Recirculate through filter press or equivalent until sparkling clear.

Chlophedianol, Ipecac, Ephedrine, Ammonium Chloride, Carbinoxamine, and Balsam Tolu Syrup

Bill of Materials			
Scale (mg/tablet)	Item	Material Name	Qty/L (g)
0.001 mL	1	Ipecac fluid extract	1.000 mL
5.000	2	Chlophedianol hydrochloride	5.000
1.320	3	Ephedrine hydrochloride	1.320
8.800	4	Ammonium chloride	8.800
0.800	5	Carbinoxamine maleate	0.800
0.900	6	Methyl paraben	0.900
0.100	7	Propyl paraben	0.100
6.250	8	Balsam, tolu (aqueous extract)	6.250
2.660	9	Saccharin sodium powder dihydrate	2.660
319.220	10	Sucrose (sugar, granulated)	0.320
238.330	11	Glucose liquid (corn syrup)	0.240
83.933	12	Sorbitol solution 70%	0.084
40.000	13	Alcohol (ethanol)	40.000
166.670	14	Dye red	0.160
0.800	15	Flavor	0.800
100.000	16	Propylene glycol	100.000
QS	17	Filter aid HyFlo	0.500
QS	18	Water purified	~450.000 mL

Manufacturing Directions

1. Charge balsam tolu and 25 mL of water in a steam bath.
2. Raise the temperature, stirring continuously, to mix water with balsam. Boil for half an hour and allow decanting while cooling. Discard extracted balsam tolu. Filter the supernatant liquid through filter paper and store apart.
3. Charge 150 mL water in a jacketed mixing tank; heat to boiling.
4. Add and dissolve parabens with mixing. Add and dissolve sugar with constant mixing. Heat to 70°C to 75°C.
5. Once sugar is dissolved, add glucose, sorbitol, and saccharin sodium.
6. Mix well until dissolved.
7. Dissolve ammonium chloride in 28 mL water. Add to mixing tank.
8. Add extract balsam tolu with mixing.
9. Mix well and cool to 25°C to 30°C. Add and dissolve ephedrine, carbinoxamine in 20 mL water and add to mixing tank. Mix well.
10. Add and dissolve chlophedianol in 50 g of propylene glycol and add to mixing tank. Add balance of propylene glycol to mixing tank.
11. Add and dissolve Ipecac fluid extract and flavor raspberry in alcohol. Add to mixing tank. Dissolve dye in 5 mL water; add to tank with continuous mixing.
12. Rinse container with 5 mL of water and add rinsing.
13. Adjust to volume with purified water.
14. Add filter aid HyFlo to syrup and mix well.
15. Recirculate through filter press or equivalent until sparkling clear.

Chloramphenicol Palmitate Oral or Topical Emulsion (2.5% = 250 mg/10 mL)

Formulation

I. Chloramphenicol palmitate, 2.5 g; Lutrol E 400 [1], 4 g; Cremophor RH 40 [1], 4 g
II. Sucrose, crystalline, 40 g; water, 40 g
III. Water, add 100 mL

Manufacturing Directions

1. Mix components I at 70°C to obtain a clear solution.
2. Cool to 40°C and add this solution slowly to the well-stirred solution II.
3. Fill up with III to 100 mL.

Chloramphenicol Palmitate Oral or Topical Emulsion (5% = 500 mg/10 mL)

Formulation

I. Chloramphenicol palmitate, 5 g; Lutrol E400 [1], 6 g; Cremophor RH 40 [1], 4 g
II. Sucrose, crystalline, 40 g; preservative, QS; water, 45 g

Manufacturing Directions

1. Mix components I at 70°C to obtain a clear solution and cool to approximately 40°C.
2. Add the warm solution II slowly to the well-stirred solution I.

Chloramphenicol Opthalmic Solution

Bill of Materials			
Scale (mg/mL)	Item	Material Name	Qty/L (g)
30.00	1	Chloramphenicol	30.00
150.00	2	Kollidon 25	150.00
QS	3	Preservatives	QS
QS	4	Water purified	QS to 1 L

Manufacturing Directions

1. Charge 90% of item 4 in a stainless steel jacketed vessel and heat to 90°C to 95°C.
2. Add and dissolve preservatives.
3. Add and dissolve item 2.
4. Add and stir item 1 until a clear solution is obtained.
5. Optionally add 0.2% to 0.5% cysteine as antioxidant to prevent discoloration of item 2.

Chloramphenicol Palmitate Oral or Topical Emulsion

Bill of Materials			
Scale (mg/mL)	Item	Material Name	Qty/L (g)
25.00	1	Chloramphenicol palmitate	25.00
40.00	2	Lutrol E 400	40.00
40.00	3	Cremophor RH 40	40.00
400.00	4	Sucrose	400.00
400.00	5	Water purified	400.00
QS	6	Water purified	QS to 1 L

Bill of Materials			
Scale (mg/mL)	Item	Material Name	Qty/L (g)
50.00	1	Chloramphenicol palmitate	50.00
60.00	2	Lutrol E 400	50.00
40.00	3	Cremophor RH 40	40.00
400.00	4	Sucrose	400.00
450.00	5	Water purified	450.00
QS	6	Water purified	QS to 1 L

Manufacturing Directions

1. Charge items 1 to 3 in a suitable stainless steel jacketed vessel. Heat to 70°C to obtain a clear solution.
2. Cool to 40°C.
3. In a separate vessel, add and dissolve items 4 and 5 and then add this solution to step 2.
4. Bring to volume with item 6. Mix.

Chlorhexidine Gel

Bill of Materials			
Scale (mg/g)	Item	Material Name	Qty/kg (g)
20.00	1	Chlorhexidine diacetate	20.00
300.00	2	1,2-Propylene glycol (pharma)	300.00
220.00	3	Lutrol F 127	220.00
460.00	4	Water	460.00

Manufacturing Directions

1. Dissolve chlorhexidine diacetate in propylene glycol at >70°C.
2. Stir well and slowly add Lutrol F 127 and water.
3. Maintain the temperature until the air bubbles escape.
4. A clear, colorless gel is obtained.

Chlorpheniramine Maleate Syrup

Bill of Materials			
Scale (mg/5 mL)	Item	Material Name	Qty/L (g)
2.00	1	Chlorpheniramine maleate	0.40
3000.00	2	Sucrose	600.00
4.50	3	Methyl paraben	0.90
1.50	4	Propyl paraben	0.30
1.00	5	Citric acid (monohydrate)	0.20
2.40	6	Sodium citrate	0.48
2.00	7	Green banana flavor	0.40
–	8	Purified water	QS to 1 L

Manufacturing Directions

1. Add 500 g of purified water to the manufacturing vessel and heat to 95°C to 98°C.
2. Add items 3 and 4 while mixing to dissolve at high speed.
3. Mix for 5 minutes.
4. Add item 2 while mixing at slow speed.
5. Maintain a temperature of 95°C to 98°C.
6. Mix for 1 hour at high speed.
7. Cool down to 30°C while mixing at slow speed.
8. Dissolve items 5 and 6 in 20 g of cooled purified water (25°C).
9. Transfer the solution to the manufacturing vessel while mixing at high speed.
10. Mix for 2 minutes.
11. Add 8 g of cold purified water (25–30°C) in a separate container and dissolve item 1 by using stirrer.
12. Mix for 10 minutes and transfer to the manufacturing vessel.
13. Rinse the container with 2 g of cooled purified water (25°C) and transfer the rinsings to the manufacturing vessel while mixing at high speed.
14. Add item 7 to the manufacturing vessel while mixing.
15. Mix for 10 minutes at high speed.
16. Bring the volume up to 1 L with purified water and finally mix for 15 to 20 minutes at high speed.
17. Check and record the pH (limit: 5.0–5.2 at 25°C).
18. If required, adjust pH with 10% citric acid or 10% sodium citrate solution.
19. Filter the syrup at 1.5 bar.
20. Bubble the syrup with nitrogen gas.

Chloroxylenol Surgical Scrub

Chloroxylenol 3% and cocamidopropyl PG-dimonium chloride phosphate 3%. Inactive ingredients: water, sodium lauryl sulfate, cocamide DEA, propylene glycol, cocamidopropyl betaine, citric acid, tetrasodium EDTA, aloe vera gel, hydrolyzed animal protein, D&C yellow No. 10. In addition, chloroxylenol 5%, terpineol 10%, absolute alcohol 20%, soft potassium soap 8.5%, and caramel 25% and lemon oil QS in a water base.

Ciclopirox Topical Solution

Each gram of Penlac nail lacquer (ciclopirox) topical solution, 8%, contains 80 mg ciclopirox in a solution base consisting of ethyl acetate, isopropyl alcohol, and butyl monoester of poly(methylvinyl ether/maleic acid) in isopropyl alcohol. Ethyl acetate and isopropyl alcohol are solvents that vaporize after application.

Bill of Materials			
Scale (mg/mL)	Item	Material Name	Qty/L (g)
80.00	1	Ciclopirox	80.00
330.00	2	Ethyl acetate	330.00
300.00	3	Butyl monoester of poly(methylvinyl ether/maleic acid) in isopropyl alcohol (50%)	300.00
QS	4	Isopropyl alcohol	QS to 1 L

Manufacturing Directions

1. Charge item 4 in a suitable stainless steel vessel in an explosion-proof room.
2. Add item 2 and item 3 in a separate vessel, mix, and add to step 1.
3. Add item 1 and mix; seal immediately.

Cimetidine Syrup

Bill of Materials			
Scale (mg/5 mL)	Item	Material Name	Qty/L(g)
200.00	1	Cimetidine USE cimetidine hydrochloride	45.80
0.161 mL	2	Alcohol	32.50 mL
5.000	3	Methyl paraben	1.00
1.000	4	Propyl paraben	0.20
20.000	5	Pluronic F68	4.00
0.500 mL	6	Propylene glycol	100.00 mL
20.000	7	Saccharin sodium	4.00
15.000	8	Sodium chloride	3.00
27.000	9	Disodium hydrogen phosphate	5.40
0.500 mL	10	Sorbitol solution 70%	100.00 mL
2.070 g	11	Sucrose	414.00
0.050	11	Yellow dye	0.01
0.0014	12	Flavor	0.28 mL
0.0014	13	Flavor	0.28 mL
2.000	14	Sweetener additional	0.40
QS	15	Water purified	QS to 1 L

Manufacturing Directions

1. Charge items 3 and 4 in a stainless steel vessel and add 70% item 15; heat to 80°C to 90°C to dissolve.
2. In a separate vessel, add and mix items 5 through 11.
3. Add step 2 to step 1.
4. Add and dissolve remaining items and mix.
5. Fill.

Ciprofloxacin Hydrochloride and Hydrocortisone Otic Suspension

Ciprofloxacin hydrochloride and hydrocortisone otic suspension contains the synthetic broad-spectrum antibacterial agent, ciprofloxacin hydrochloride, combined with the anti-inflammatory corticosteroid, hydrocortisone, in a preserved, nonsterile suspension for otic use. Each milliliter contains ciprofloxacin hydrochloride (equivalent to 2 mg ciprofloxacin), 10 mg hydrocortisone, and 9 mg benzyl alcohol as a preservative. The inactive ingredients are polyvinyl alcohol, sodium chloride, sodium acetate, glacial acetic acid, phospholipon 90HB (modified lecithin), polysorbate, and purified water. Sodium hydroxide or hydrochloric acid may be added for adjustment of pH.

Bill of Materials			
Scale (mg/mL)	Item	Material Name	Qty/L (g)
2.00	1	Ciprofloxacin (use ciprofloxacin hydrochloride)	2.33
10.00	2	Hydrocortisone	10.00
1.00	3	Polysorbate 80	1.00
20.00	4	Polyvinyl alcohol	20.00
1.50	5	Phospholipon 90H (lecithin)	1.50
9.00	6	Benzyl alcohol	9.00
7.00	7	Acetic acid glacial	7.00
4.10	8	Sodium acetate trihydrate	4.10
9.00	9	Sodium chloride	9.00
QS	10	Hydrochloric acid 1 N for pH adjustment	QS
QS	11	Sodium hydroxide 1 N for pH adjustment	QS
QS	12	Water purified	QS to 1 L

Manufacturing Directions

1. Use well-passivated stainless steel vessels; use only sodium vapor lamps or yellow light in the manufacturing area. Avoid forming foam during transfer of liquids.
2. Charge approximately 1 L of item 12 in a suitable vessel and heat to 90°C to 95°C and then cool to 20°C to 25°C under a nitrogen environment and hold for later use for premixing, rinsing, and final volume makeup.
3. To 50% of volume of item 11, add item 4 at 90°C to 95°C.
4. Add and mix item 5 while maintaining nitrogen blanket cover. Cool to 40°C to 50°C.
5. Add and mix item 6 and cool to 20°C to 25°C.
6. In a separate vessel, mix acetic acid, sodium chloride, and sodium acetate trihydrate in approximately 10% of item 12 as prepared in step 1.
7. In a separate vessel, charge item 2 and item 3 and 30% of item 12, mix, and then pass through a micronizing chamber.
8. Add to step 6 and mix well.
9. Add item 1 to in a separate vessel and 20% of item 12 and portions of item 7 and then add to the main batch.
10. Bring to volume.
11. Adjust pH to 4.75 using item 10 or 11 as needed. Fill.

Cisapride Suspension

Bill of Materials			
Scale (mg/5 mL)	Item	Material Name	Qty/L (g)
5.00	1	Cisapride USE: cisapride monohydrate	1.04
9.00	2	Methyl paraben	1.80
1.00	3	Propyl paraben	0.20
1000.00	4	Sucrose	200.00
50.00	5	Microcrystalline cellulose (Avicel RC 591)	10.00
12.50	6	Methylcellulose 4000	2.50
5.00	7	Sodium chloride	1.00
2.50	8	Polysorbate 80 (Tween 80)	0.50
2.50	9	All fruit flavor	0.50
–	10	Water purified	QS to 1 L

Manufacturing Directions

Cisapride dispersion should be uniformity mixed or levigated. Avicel RC-591 and methylcellulose dispersion should be uniform and smooth.

1. Mix item 8 in 100 g of item 10 (35–40°C) in a stainless steel vessel, using stirrer. Add item 1 and mix to make smooth dispersion and keep aside. Check the smoothness of dispersion.
2. Add 185 g of item 10 to a suitable mixer and heat to 90°C to 95°C. Dissolve items 2 and 3 while mixing. Add and dissolve item 4 while mixing.
3. Cool down to approximately 50°C to 55°C.
4. Filter the syrup through T-1500 filter pads (8–10) washed with purified water. Collect the syrup in clean stainless steel tank. Avoid any loss of syrup quantity.
5. Disperse item 6 in 150 g of hot item 10 (70–80°C) in mixer while mixing.
6. Mix and homogenize at temperature 70°C to 80°C, mixer speed 18 rpm, homogenizer high speed, and vacuum 0.4 to 0.6 bar for 5 minutes.
7. Cool down to 25°C to 30°C with continuous mixing. Check the smoothness of dispersion.
8. Disperse item 5 in 250 g of item 10 (25–30°C) in stainless steel vessel, using stirrer. Keep on stirring for 30 minutes to make smooth dispersion. Check the smoothness of dispersion.
9. Transfer syrup mixer. Transfer Avicel mucilage to mixer.
10. Mix at high homogenizer speed and under vacuum for 5 minutes.
11. Dissolve item 7 in 10 g of item 10 and add to mixer while mixing. Add drug dispersion to mixer.
12. Rinse the drug container with 40 g of item 10 and add the rinsing to mixer.
13. Add item 9 to mixer while mixing.
14. Add item 10 up to final volume 1 L.
15. Finally, mix and homogenize for 5 minutes at mixer speed 18 rpm, homogenizer at high speed, vacuum 0.4 to 0.6 bar.
16. Check the suspension for homogeneity. Transfer the suspension through 630-micron sieve to the stainless steel storage tank, previously sanitized.

Citalopram Hydrobromide Oral Solution

Celexa oral solution contains citalopram HBr equivalent to 2 mg/mL citalopram base. It also contains the following inactive ingredients: sorbitol, purified water, propylene glycol, methyl paraben, natural peppermint flavor, and propyl paraben.

Clarithromycin Suspension

Bill of Materials			
Scale (mg/5 mL)	Item	Material Name	Qty/kg (g)
125.00	1	Clarithromycin	35.47
	2	Carbopol 974P	21.28
	3	Polyvinyl pyrrolidone K90	4.96
	4	Water purified	145 mL
	5	Hydroxypropyl methylcellulose phthalate HP-55	43.17
	6	Castor oil	4.56
QS	7	Acetone, approximate	172 mL
QS	8	Ethanol, approximate	164 mL
	9	Potassium sorbate	5.96
	10	Sucrose	600.80
	11	Maltodextrin	67.58
	12	Water purified	10 mL
	13	Xanthan gum	1.08
	14	Flavor dry	10.14
	15	Silicon dioxide	1.42
	16	Citric acid	1.20
	17	Titanium dioxide	10.14
	18	Maltodextrin	13.50
QS	19	Sucrose	QS to 1 kg

Manufacturing Directions

1. This product requires coated clarithromycin granules. Add polyvinyl pyrrolidone to water and mix.
2. Use water to granulate a blend of clarithromycin and Carbopol 974P.
3. Dry granules at 70°C until loss on drying is NMT 5%.
4. Collect fraction between 177 and 420 microns.
5. Regranulate smaller particles to meet the above range.
6. Blend the regranulate in step 5 to step 6.
7. Prepare coating solution by adding ethanol and acetone and hydroxypropyl methylcellulose phthate and castor oil in a mixing vessel; mix until solution is clear.
8. Coat granules in step 6 in a particle coater and dry to loss on drying of NMT 5%.
9. Sift coated granules and retain the fraction between 149 and 590 microns.
10. In a separate vessel, dissolve potassium sorbate in purified water.
11. Blend sucrose and the maltodextrin until a homogenous mix is achieved.
12. Granulate the step 11 mixture with step 10.
13. Dry the granulation until loss on drying is NMT 1%.
14. Mill dried granules and blend.
15. Mix to clarithromycin-coated granules in appropriate quantity, add silicon dioxide, and blend. Fill appropriate quantity.
16. Reconstitute 3.13 g to yield 125 mg/5 mL solution.

Clindamycin Phosphate Topical Solution

Cleocin T topical solution and Cleocin T topical lotion contain clindamycin phosphate at a concentration equivalent to 10 mg clindamycin per milliliter. Cleocin T topical gel contains clindamycin phosphate at a concentration equivalent to 10 mg clindamycin per gram. Each Cleocin T topical solution pledget applicator contains approximately 1 mL of topical solution. Clindamycin phosphate is a water-soluble ester of the semisynthetic antibiotic produced by a 7(S)-chloro-substitution of the 7(R)-hydroxyl group of the parent antibiotic lincomycin. The solution contains isopropyl alcohol 50% v/v, propylene glycol, and water.

Clotrimazole Topical Solution

Bill of Materials			
Scale (mg/mL)	Item	Material Name	Qty/L (g)
30.00	1	Clotrimazole	30.00
300.00	2	Cremophor RH 40	300.00
QS	3	Preservatives	QS
340.00	4	Alcohol	340.00
330.00	5	Water purified	QS to 1 L

Manufacturing Directions

1. Charge item 1 and 2 in a stainless steel jacketed mixing vessel. Heat to 60°C and mix well.
2. In a separate vessel, charge items 3 to 5 at 90°C and add to step 1.
3. Mix well and fill.

Clotrimazole Topical Solution (3%)

Formulation

I. Clotrimazole, 3 g; Cremophor RH 40, 30 g
II. Preservative, QS; Ethanol 96%, 34 g; Water, 33 g

Manufacturing

Dissolve clotrimazole in Cremophor RH 40 at approximately 60°C, stir strongly, and add slowly the hot solution II.

Codeine Phosphate and Acetaminophen Elixir

Each 5 mL of elixir contains codeine phosphate 12 mg, acetaminophen 120 mg, alcohol 7%, citric acid, propylene glycol, sodium benzoate, saccharin sodium, sucrose, natural and artificial flavors, and FD&C yellow No. 6.

Colistin Sulfate, Neomycin, Thonzonium Bromide, and Hydrocortisone Otic Suspension

Cortisporin-TC otic suspension with neomycin and hydrocortisone (colistin sulfate–neomycin sulfate–thonzonium bromide–hydrocortisone acetate otic suspension) is a sterile aqueous suspension containing in each milliliter: colistin base activity, 3 mg (as the sulfate); neomycin base activity, 3.3 mg (as the sulfate); hydrocortisone acetate, 10 mg (1%); thonzonium bromide, 0.5 mg (0.05%); polysorbate 80, acetic acid, and sodium acetate in a buffered aqueous vehicle. Thimerosal (mercury derivative), 0.002%, is added as a preservative. The suspension is a nonviscous liquid, buffered at pH 5, for instillation into the canal of the external ear or direct application to the affected aural skin.

Cotrimoxazole Oral Suspension

Bill of Materials			
Scale (mg/mL)	Item	Material Name	Qty/L (g)
40.00	1	Trimethoprim micronized (98% particles less than 50 microns)	8.00
200.00	2	Sulfamethoxazole powder (100% particles less than 50 microns)	40.00
20.00	3	Magnesium aluminum silicate (Veegum HV)	4.00
22.50	4	Carboxymethylcellulose sodium	4.50
350.00	5	Glycerin	70.00
400.00	6	Propylene glycol	80.00
5.00	7	Polyvinyl pyrrolidone (polyvinyl pyrrolidone K-30)	1.00
20.00	8	Polysorbate 80	4.00
12.50	9	Colloidal silicon dioxide (Aerosil 200)	2.50
375.00	10	Sorbitol (70% solution)	75.00
5.00	11	Saccharin sodium	1.00
3.00	12	Citric acid	0.60
2200.00	13	Sucrose	440.00
5.00	14	Methyl paraben	1.00
1.50	15	Propyl paraben	0.30
0.035	16	Raspberry red color	0.007
0.025	17	FD&C red No. 40	0.005
5.00	18	Banana flavor	1.00
5.00	19	Apricot flavor	1.00
–	20	Water purified	QS to 1 L

Manufacturing Directions

1. Disperse item 4 in item 5 in a stainless steel vessel, using stirrer. Check that the dispersion is even.
2. Disperse item 3 in the dispersion of items 4 and 5 (sodium CMC-glycerol) at step 1, using stirrer. Check that the final dispersion is even.
3. Add 100 g of hot item 20 (75–85°C) to the dispersion at step 2 while stirring to make the mucilage. Mix for 30 minutes using stirrer.
4. Keep aside the mucilage, for hydration, overnight in a well-closed container.
5. Add item 6 in a stainless steel container and mix items 2 and 1 while mixing using stirrer to make homogenous slurry.
6. Add 100 g of cold item 20 (25–30°C) in a stainless steel container and dissolve item 7 to make a clear solution. Add item 8 while mixing to make a clear solution, then add item 9 while mixing at slow speed.
7. Transfer the mix from step 6 to the slurry of sulpha-trimethoprim step 3 while mixing.
8. Mix for 30 minutes.
9. Add item 10 to the slurry. Mix for 10 minutes.
10. Add 250 g of item 20 in mixer and heat to 90°C to 95°C.
11. Add items 14 and 15 while mixing to dissolve, homogenize at high speed for 2 minutes.
12. Add item 13 to the parabens solution at step 6. Mix well to dissolve completely.
13. Cool down to 30°C.
14. Filter the syrup through T-1500 filters using filter press. (Wash the filters with cooled item 20 approximately 100 mL before use.) Collect the filtered syrup in stainless steel containers.
15. Wash the mixer with item 20.
16. Load items 4 and 3 (CMC-Veegum) mucilage from step 2 to the mixer. Homogenize while mixing for 2 minutes at high speed under vacuum 0.4 to 0.6 bar, mixer speed 20 rpm, temperature 25°C. Check the suspension for uniformity.
17. Load the sulpha-trimethoprim slurry from step 5 to the mixer. Homogenize while mixing for 10 minutes at high speed under vacuum 0.4 to 0.6 bar, mixer speed 20 rpm, temperature 25°C, Check the suspension for uniformity.
18. Transfer the sugar syrup from step 7 to the mixer. Homogenize while mixing for 2 minutes at high speed under vacuum 0.4 to 0.6 bar, mixer speed 20 rpm, temperature 25°C. Check the suspension for uniformity.
19. Dissolve item 12 in 4 g of cooled item 20 and transfer to the mixer while mixing.
20. Dissolve item 11 in 10 g of cooled item 20 and transfer to the mixer while mixing.
21. Dissolve items 16 and 17 and FD&C red No. 40 in 1 g of cooled item 20 and transfer to the mixer while mixing.
22. Mix items 18 and 19 and transfer to the mixer while mixing.
23. Add cold item 20 to make up the volume to 1 L.

24. Set the mixer on high speed, rpm 20, manual mode, vacuum 0.4 to 0.6 bar, temperature 25°C. Mix for 15 minutes.
25. Check and record the pH (limit: 5.5–5.8) at 25°C. If required, adjust pH with 10% citric acid or 10% sodium citrate solution.
26. Transfer the suspension through 630-micron sieve to the stainless steel storage tank, previously sanitized by 70% ethanol.

Cromolyn Sodium Nasal Spray

Each milliliter of NasalCrom nasal spray contains 40 mg of cromolyn sodium in purified water with 0.01% benzalkonium chloride to preserve and 0.01% EDTA to stabilize the solution. Each metered spray releases the same amount of medicine, 5.2 mg cromolyn sodium.

Cromolyn Sodium Oral Concentrate

Each 5-mL ampule of oral concentrate contains 100 mg cromolyn sodium in purified water. It is an unpreserved, colorless solution supplied in a low-density polyethylene plastic unit-dose ampule with 8 ampules per foil pouch.

Crospovidone Oral Suspension (2000 mg/10 mL)

Formulation

Kollidon CL-M [1], 20 g; sorbitol, crystalline [10], 10 g; Kollidon 90F [1], 2 g; Preservatives, QS; Flavor, QS; water, add 100 mL.

Manufacturing Directions

Dissolve sorbitol, Kollidon 90F, the preservatives, and the flavors in the water; add Kollidon CL-M; and homogenize by shaking.

Cyclosporin Oral Solution

Cyclosporine oral solution: Each milliliter contains cyclosporin 100 mg and alcohol 12.5% by volume dissolved in an olive oil, Labrafil M 1944CS (polyoxyethylated oleic glycerides), vehicle that must be further diluted with milk, chocolate milk, or orange juice before oral administration.

Bill of Materials			
Scale (mg/mL)	Item	Material Name	Qty/L (g)
100.00	1	Cyclosporin	100.00
125.00	2	Alcohol	125.00
532.00	3	Olive oil	532.00
242.50	4	Labrafil M 1944CS	242.50

Manufacturing Directions

1. Charge items 2 to 4 in a mixing vessel and stir well.
2. Homogenize step 1.
3. Add item 1 and homogenize again.
4. Fill.

Cyclosporine Soft Gelatin Capsules

Cyclosporine capsules are available in 25- and 100-mg strengths. Each 25- or 100-mg capsule contains cyclosporine 25 mg and alcohol 12.7% by volume. Inactive ingredients: corn oil, gelatin, glycerol, Labrafil M 2125CS (polyoxyethylated glycolysed glycerides), red iron oxide (25- and 100-mg capsule only), sorbitol, titanium dioxide, and other ingredients.

Desmopressin Acetate Nasal Spray

Desmopressin acetate is a synthetic analogue of the natural pituitary hormone 8-arginine vasopressin, an antidiuretic hormone affecting renal water conservation. It contains 1.5 mg/mL desmopressin acetate in a pH-adjusted aqueous solution with hydrochloric acid to 4; chlorobutanol (5 mg) and sodium chloride (9 mg) are the inactive ingredients. The compression pump delivers 0.1 mL (150 (μg) of solution per spray; 2.5 mL bottle.

Dexamethasone Elixir

Dexamethasone elixir contains 0.5 mg of dexamethasone in each 5 mL. Benzoic acid, 0.1%, is added as a preservative. It also contains alcohol 5%. Inactive ingredients are FD&C red No. 40, flavors, glycerin, purified water, and sodium saccharin.

Dextromethorphan and Chlorpheniramine Maleate Solution

Bill of Materials			
Scale (mg/mg)	Item	Material Name	Qty/kg (g)
14.70	1	Dextromethorphan base	14.70
2.60	2	Chlorpheniramine maleate	
QS	2	Vehicle (pluronic F 127 55.67%, ethanol 26.55%, and water 17.79%)	QS to 1 kg
3.00	3	Sodium saccharin	3.00
QS	4	Flavors and colors (menthol, eucalyptus oil, tienzoocane)	QS
0.50	5	Monoammonium glycyrrhizinate	0.50

Manufacturing Directions

1. Mill and screen the menthol and tienzoocaine to reduce the product particle size.
2. Add the menthol, benzocaine, sodium saccharin, and monoammonium glycyrrhizinate into a clean vessel.
3. Add eucalyptus oil and ethanol to the vessel.
4. Subsequently, add the poloxamer and water to the vessel. Mix until uniform.

Dextromethorphan, Pseudoephedrine, and Chlorpheniramine Maleate Syrup

Bill of Materials			
Scale (mg/mL)	Item	Material Name	Qty/L (g)
2.00	1	Dextromethorphan hydrobromide	2.00
4.00	2	D-Pseudoephedrine hydrochloride	4.00
0.40	3	Chlorpheniramine maleate	0.40
25.00	4	Sorbitol syrup	25.00
0.20	5	Saccharin sodium	0.20
3.00	6	Hydroxyethyl cellulose (Natrosol®)	3.00
2.50	7	Sodium benzoate	2.50
1.05	8	Banana flavor	1.05
1.10	9	Custard flavor	1.10
1.20	10	Trisodium citrate dihydrate (powder)	1.20
QS	11	Deionized water	QS 1 L

Manufacturing Directions

1. In a suitable stainless steel vessel, combine sorbitol syrup, hydroxyethylcellulose, and deionized water; mix well.
2. Add sodium benzoate and stir again for 5 minutes.
3. After obtaining a clear solution, stir the hydroxyethyl cellulose suspension, rinse the container with deionized water, and transfer the rinsings to the vessel.
4. Heat the vessel to 40°C to 50°C and stir the mix for 1 hour.
5. After 1 hour, a clear gel without lumps is obtained.
6. Dilute the gel with sorbitol syrup and cool to 30°C.
7. In a separate vessel, add deionized water and heat while stirring to 50°C.
8. After reaching this temperature, dissolve, in this order, dextromethorphan hydrobromide, chlorpheniramine maleate, and pseudoephedrine hydrochloride and saccharin sodium.
9. Cool the solution to 25°C.
10. In a suitable stainless steel container, add deionized water and while stirring dissolve trisodium citrate under 0.6 bar vacuum and high speed.
11. Transfer the active substance solution to the syrup vehicle.
12. Rinse the vessel twice with deionized water.
13. Add while stirring (low) the custard and banana flavors.
14. Mix for 10 minutes.
15. Then, while stirring, add the solution from step above; keep stirring for 15 minutes at moderate speed.
16. Stop stirring and check pH (5.9–6.2); adjust with 10% trisodium citrate solution; after each addition, where necessary, stir for 5 minutes before recording pH again.
17. Finally, make up the volume with deionized water and stir once more for 15 minutes under vacuum (0.6 bar) at moderate speed.
18. Stop stirring and remove vacuum; check final volume once more.
19. Filter the clear syrup under compressed air pressure, first through a filter of 330-μm and then through a 20-μm filter of propylene type.

Dextromethorphan Liquid

Bill of Materials			
Scale (mg/mL)	Item	Material Name	Qty/L (g)
22.00	1	Dextromethorphan base	22.00
QS	2	Vehicle (pluronic 33.56%, ethanol 10.51%, water 13.42%, propylene glycol 42.51%)[a]	QS to 1 L
1.00	3	Sodium metabisulfite	1.00
1.00	4	Disodium EDTA	1.00
4.00	5	Sodium saccharin	4.00
1.50	6	Monoammonium glycyrrhizinate	1.50
5.00	7	Acesulfame	5.00
14.00	8	Flavor	14.00

[a]Alternate vehicle composition: pluronic F 27 29.08%, ethanol 10.51%, water 24.61%, propylene glycol 35.80%. Second alternate vehicle: pluronic F127 40.27%, ethanol 10.51%, water 13.42%, propylene glycol 35.80%.

Manufacturing Directions

1. Add propylene glycol and poloxamer to a clean vessel (main mix).
2. While stirring, heat the mixture as appropriate to sufficiently melt the poloxamer.
3. Once a uniform solution is obtained, remove from heat source and continue mixing.
4. In a separate vessel (alcohol premix), add alcohol, dextromethorphan base, and monoammonium glycyrrhizinate and mix until uniform.
5. In another vessel (water premix), add water, EDTA, sodium saccharin, acesulfame, and sodium metabisulfite. Mix until all materials are dissolved.
6. Add the alcohol containing premix to the main mixing vessel containing the poloxamer.
7. Mix until uniform.
8. While stirring, add the water containing premix to the main vessel and continue to mix until uniform.
9. Add desired flavor component and mix until uniform.
10. The preparation has a viscosity of approximately 0.67 Pa seconds and a triggered viscosity ratio at a 50% dilution with water of 10.5. If using alternate vehicle composition (above), the preparation has a viscosity of approximately 0.97 Pa seconds and a triggered viscosity ratio at a 50% dilution with water of 4.95. If using the second alternate vehicle, the preparation has a viscosity of approximately 2.14 Pa seconds and a triggered viscosity ratio at a 50% dilution.

Dextromethorphan Liquid

Bill of Materials			
Scale (mg/mL)	Item	Material Name	Qty/L (g)
QS	1	Vehicle (pluraflo 1220 40.90%, ethanol 10.22%, propylene glycol 46.83%, anhydrous glycerin 2.05%)	QS to 1 L
22.00	2	Dextromethorphan base	22.00
QS	3	Flavors	QS

Manufacturing Directions

1. Weigh the dextomethophan into a clean vessel, add the ethanol, and begin mixing.
2. Add propylene glycol and mix until uniform and clear.
3. Add pluraflo and mix. Add glycerin and mix until uniform.
4. Add desired flavor component and mix until uniform.

Dextromethorphan, Pseudoephedrine, and Chlorpheniramine Maleate Syrup

Bill of Materials			
Scale (mg/tablet)	Item	Material Name	Qty/L (g)
20.00	1	Dextromethorphan hydrobromide	20.00
40.00	2	D-Pseudoephedrine hydrochloride	40.00
4.00	3	Chlorpheniramine maleate	4.00
250.00	4	Sorbitol syrup	250.00
2.00	5	Saccharin sodium	2.00
30.00	6	Hydroxyethyl cellulose (Natrosol HHY)	30.00
25.00	7	Sodium benzoate	25.00
10.50	8	Banana flavor	10.50
11.00	9	Custard flavor	11.00
12.00	10	Trisodium citrate dihydrate powder	12.00
QS	11	Water purified	QS

Manufacturing Directions

1. In a suitable vessel, add sorbitol syrup and hydroxyethylcellulose and purified water; mix well.
2. Add sodium benzoate and stir again for 5 minutes.
3. After obtaining clear solution, put under stirring hydroxyethyl cellulose suspension, rinse the container with purified water, and transfer the rinsing to the vessel.
4. Heat the vessel to 40°C to 50°C and keep the mix stirring for 1 hour.
5. After 1 hour, a clear gel without lumps is obtained.
6. The gel is then diluted with sorbitol syrup and cooled to 30°C.
7. In a separate vessel, add purified water and heat under stirring to 50°C.
8. After reaching this temperature, dissolve sequentially dextromethorphan hydrobromide, chlorpheniramine maleate and pseudoephedrine hydrochloride, and saccharin sodium.
9. Cool the solution to 25°C.
10. In a suitable stainless steel container, add purified water and under stirring dissolve trisodium citrate under 00.6 bar and high speed.
11. The active substance solution from step 10 is transferred to the syrup vehicle.
12. The vessel is rinsed twice with purified water.
13. In the larger vessel, add under stirring (low) the custard flavor and banana flavor and mix for 10 minutes.
14. Then, under stirring, add the solution from step 13; keep stirring for 15 minutes at moderate speed.
15. Stop stirring and check pH (5.9–6.2); adjust with 10% trisodium citrate solution; after each addition, where necessary, stir for 5 minutes before recording pH again.
16. Finally, make up the volume with purified water and stir once more for 15 minutes under vacuum (−0.6 bar) moderate speed. Stop stirring and vacuum; check final volume once more.
17. Clear syrup is filtered under compressed air pressure first through a filter of 330 microns and then through a 20-micron filter of propylene type.

Dextromethorphan Solution

Bill of Materials			
Scale mg/mg	Item	Material Name	Qty/kg (g)
14.70	1	Dextromethorphan base	14.70
QS	2	Vehicle (pluronic F 127 55.51%, ethanol 26.48%, and water 18.01%)	QS to 1 kg
3.00	3	Sodium saccharin	3.00
QS	4	Flavors and colors	QS
0.50	5	Monoammonium glycyrrhizinate	0.50

Manufacturing Directions

1. Add the dextromethorphan base, sodium saccharin, and monoammonium glycyrrhizinate into a clean vessel.
2. Add ethanol and then the poloxamer and water. Mix until clear and uniform.
3. Good pourable formula.

Dextrose, Levulose, and Phosphoric Acid Solution

Emetrol is an oral solution containing balanced amounts of dextrose (glucose) and levulose (fructose) and phosphoric acid with controlled hydrogen ion concentration. Available in original lemon-mint or cherry flavor. Each 5-mL teaspoonful contains dextrose (glucose), 1.87 g; levulose (fructose), 1.87 g; phosphoric acid, 21.5 mg; glycerin; methyl paraben; purified water; and D&C yellow No. 10 and natural lemon-mint flavor in lemon-mint Emetrol and FD&C red No. 40 and artificial cherry flavor in cherry Emetrol.

Diazepam Rectal Solution

Bill of Materials			
Scale (mg/2.5 mL)	Item	Material Name	Qty/L (g)
10.00	1	Diazepam	4.00
2.50	2	Benzoic acid	1.00
250.00	3	Alcohol	100.00
1000.00	4	Propylene glycol	400.00
122.50	5	Sodium benzoate	49.00
37.50	6	Benzyl alcohol	19.00
QS	7	Water purified	QS to 1 L

Manufacturing Directions

1. Dissolve benzoic acid in absolute alcohol previously warmed to 35°C.
2. Add diazepam to step 1, stir to dissolve.
3. Separately mix together polypropylene glycol and benzyl alcohol.
4. Separately dissolve sodium benzoate in one-fourth quantity of purified water and filter through a 0.6-μm millipore filter.
5. Under heavy stirring, mix together steps 2 and 3.
6. Bring to volume with water under stirring and filter through a 0.22-μ millipore filter.
7. Fill solution into rectal tubes; fill volume 2.9 mL.

Diclofenac Oral Solution

Bill of Materials			
Scale (mg/mL)	Item	Material Name	Qty/L (g)
15.00	1	Diclofenac sodium	15.00
25.00	2	Kollidon 30	24.00
5.00	3	Cremophor RH 40	5.00
400.00	4	Sucrose crystalline	400.00
QS	5	Water purified	QS to 1 L

Manufacturing Directions

1. Dissolve items 2 to 5 in a suitable stainless steel vessel.
2. Add item 1 and dissolve.
3. Fill.

Didanosine for Oral Solution

Videx buffered powder for oral solution is supplied for oral administration in single-dose packets containing 100, 167, or 250 mg of didanosine. Packets of each product strength also contain a citrate–phosphate buffer (composed of dibasic sodium phosphate, sodium citrate, and citric acid) and sucrose.

Digoxin Capsules

Digoxin is one of the cardiac (or digitalis) glycosides, a closely related group of drugs having in common specific effects on the myocardium. These drugs are found in a number of plants. Digoxin is extracted from the leaves of *Digitalis lanata*. The term "digitalis" is used to designate the whole group of glycosides. The glycosides are composed of two portions: a sugar and a cardenolide (hence "glycosides"). The capsule is a stable solution of digoxin enclosed within a soft gelatin capsule for oral use. Each capsule contains the labeled amount of digoxin dissolved in a solvent comprising polyethylene glycol 400, 8% ethyl alcohol, propylene glycol, and purified water. Inactive ingredients in the capsule shell include FD&C red No. 40 (0.05-mg capsule), D&C yellow No. 10 (0.1- and 0.2-mg capsules), FD&C blue No. 1 (0.2-mg capsule), gelatin, glycerin, methyl paraben and propyl paraben (added as preservatives), purified water, and sorbitol. Capsules are printed with edible ink.

Digoxin Elixir Pediatric

This is a stable solution of digoxin specially formulated for oral use in infants and children. Each milliliter contains 50 μg (0.05 mg) digoxin. The lime-flavored elixir contains the inactive ingredients alcohol 10%, methyl paraben 0.1% (added as a preservative), citric acid, D&C green No. 5, D&C yellow No. 10, flavor, propylene glycol, sodium phosphate, and sucrose. Each package is supplied with a specially calibrated dropper to facilitate the administration of accurate dosage even in premature infants. Starting at 0.2 mL, this 1-mL dropper is marked in divisions of 0.1 mL, each corresponding to 5 μg (0.005 mg) digoxin.

Dihydroergotamine Mesylate Drops

Bill of Materials			
Scale (mg/mL)	Item	Material Name	Qty/L (g)
2.00	1	Dihydroergotamine mesylate, 10% excess	2.20
153.00	2	Glycerin	153.00
48.25	3	Alcohol	48.25
QS	4	Methanesulfonic acid	QS
QS	5	Sodium hydroxide	QS
QS	6	Water purified	QS to 1 L
QS	7	Nitrogen gas	QS

Manufacturing Directions

The product is highly susceptible to oxidation and should be manufactured until continuous bubbling and cover of nitrogen; the oxygen level should be below 10 ppm at all times; nitrogen gas used should filtered through a 0.45-micron membrane filter; also, protect product from light; all tubing used for transferring product should be of stainless steel, Teflon, or silicon.

1. Heat sufficient quantity of item 6 to 95°C and hold for 1 hour. Begin bubbling nitrogen for 1 hour, cool slowly to 22°C while continuing to bubble nitrogen.
2. In another suitable glass-lined or stainless steel container, charge glycerin.
3. In another stainless steel container, charge alcohol and bubble it with nitrogen for more than 2 hours.
4. Check oxygen levels in step 1 to less than 1 ppm.
5. Flush a suitable tank with nitrogen and transfer approximately 700 mL of purified water from step above and begin bubbling nitrogen.
6. Add approximately 40 mL of purified water from step 4 to step 2 and bubble nitrogen again for 1 hour; do not discontinue bubbling throughout manufacturing process.
7. Weigh the alcohol container above, add 49 g of alcohol to water in step above, stir.
8. Dilute approximately 0.03 mL of methanesulfonic acid with purified water to make a 20% solution; measure and adjust pH to 3.25.
9. Add item 1 to batch and stir until completely dissolved.
10. Add glycerin/water mixture to the batch and adjust volume to 995 mL.
11. Dissolve 4 g of sodium hydroxide in 100 mL purified water and use this solution to adjust pH of step 10 to 3.75; stir for 1 minute and recirculate for at least 5 minutes.
12. Adjust the volume to 1 L with item 6.
13. Filter through 0.22-micron filter previously sterilized and fill in presterilized amber-colored bottle with nitrogen flushing.

Diphenhydramine and Ammonium Chloride Syrup

Bill of Materials			
Scale (mg/5 mL)	Item	Material Name	Qty/L (g)
131.50	1	Ammonium chloride	26.30
15.00	2	Caramel	5.00
11.00	3	Citric acid	2.20
13.50	4	Diphenhydramine hydrochloride	2.70
200.00	5	Alcohol	40.00
318.00	6	Glycerin	63.60
1.10	7	Menthol	0.22
5.00	8	Flavor	1.00
9.80	9	Saccharin sodium	1.96
12.00	10	Sodium benzoate	2.40
2750.00	11	Sugar	550.00
QS	12	Water purified	QS to 1 L

Manufacturing Directions

1. Charge one-half of item 12 in a suitable stainless steel mixing vessel, heat to 90°C to 95°C, and add and mix item 11. Mix for 1 hour at 90°C to 95°C.
2. Cool to room temperature.
3. In separate vessels, charge 100 mL of item 12 in each and mix items 3, 4, or 10 separately. Then mix them all together and stir well.
4. Add item 6 to step 2 and mix well.
5. In 100 mL of water, dissolve item 4 and add to step 4.
6. Dissolve item 2 in 100 mL of water and add to step 5.
7. In a separate vessel, charge item 5 and add and mix items 7 and 8.
8. Add step 7 into step 6 and make up volume.

Diphenhydramine Hydrochloride Liquid

Bill of Materials			
Scale (mg/5 mL)	Item	Material Name	Qty/L (g)
12.50	1	Diphenhydramine hydrochloride	2.50
1000.00	2	Lycasin 80/55	200.00
12.00	3	Sodium benzoate	2.40
4.40	4	Citric acid monohydrate	0.88
7.60	5	Sodium citrate	1.52
5.00	6	Saccharin sodium	1.00
250.00	7	Propylene glycol	50.00
1.25	8	Menthol	2.50
5.00	9	Flavor	1.00
QS	10	Water purified	QS to 1 L

Manufacturing Directions

1. Charge 600 mL of item 10 in a stainless steel vessel and bring to boil, cool to 40°C to 50°C.
2. Add and mix items 2 to 4 and stir to dissolve; mix for another 10 minutes.
3. In a separate vessel, charge 100 mL of item 10 and add and mix item 6.
4. In a separate vessel, charge 100 mL of item 10 and add and mix item 1. Add to step 1.
5. Add steps 2 and 3 to step 1 and mix well.
6. Add item 2 and mix again.
7. In a separate vessel, add and mix item 7 to 9. Add to step 6 and make up volume.
8. Fill.

Dornase-Alpha Inhalation Solution

Each Pulmozyme single-use ampule will deliver 2.5 mL of the solution to the nebulizer bowl. The aqueous solution contains 1.0 mg/mL dornase alfa, 0.15 mg/mL calcium chloride dihydrate, and 8.77 mg/mL sodium chloride. The solution contains no preservative. The nominal pH of the solution is 6.3.

Doxercalciferol Capsules

Doxercalciferol, the active ingredient in Hectorol, is a synthetic vitamin D analog that undergoes metabolic activation in vivo to form 1(alpha),25-dihydroxyvitamin D_2 (1(alpha),25-$(OH)_2D2$), a naturally occurring biologically active form of vitamin D_2. Hectorol is available as soft gelatin capsules containing 2.5 μg doxercalciferol. Each capsule also contains fractionated triglyceride of coconut oil, ethanol, and butylated hydroxyanisole. The capsule shells contain gelatin, glycerin, titanium dioxide, and D&C yellow No. 10.

Dyphylline, Guaifenesin Elixir

Each 15 mL (one tablespoonful) of elixir contains dyphylline 100 mg, guaifenesin 100 mg, alcohol (by volume) 17%, citric acid, FD&C yellow No. 6, flavor (artificial), purified water, saccharin sodium, sodium citrate, and sucrose.

Electrolyte Lavage Solution

Bill of Materials			
Scale (mg/mL)	Item	Material Name	Qty/L (g)
60.00	1	Polyethylene glycol 3350	60.00
1.46	2	Sodium chloride	1.46
0.75	3	Potassium chloride	0.75
1.68	4	Sodium bicarbonate	1.68
5.68	5	Sodium sulfate	5.68
0.81	6	Flavor	0.81

Manufacturing Directions

The values given above pertain to solution on reconstitution of one flavor pack. When dissolved in sufficient water to make 4 L, the final solution contains 125 mEq/L sodium, 10 mEq/L potassium, 20 mEq/L bicarbonate, 80 mEq/L sulfate, 35 mEq/L chloride, and 18 mEq/L polyethylene glycol 3350. The reconstituted solution is isoosmotic and has a mild, salty taste. Colyte flavor packs are available in citrus berry, lemon lime, cherry, and pineapple. This preparation can be used without the Colyte flavor packs and is administered orally or via a nasogastric tube. Each citrus berry flavor pack (3.22 g) contains hydroxypropyl methylcellulose 2910, citrus berry powder, saccharin sodium, and colloidal silicon dioxide. Each lemon lime flavor pack (3.22 g) contains lemon-lime NTA powder, hydroxypropyl methylcellulose 2910, Prosweet® powder natural, saccharin sodium, and colloidal silicon dioxide. Each cherry flavor pack (3.22 g) contains hydroxypropyl methylcellulose 2910, artificial cherry powder, saccharin sodium, and colloidal silicon dioxide. Each pineapple flavor pack (3.22 g) contains hydroxypropyl methylcellulose 2910, pineapple flavor powder, Magnasweet, saccharin sodium, and colloidal silicon dioxide.

Eplerenone Solution

Bill of Materials			
Scale (mg/L) or mL/L	Item	Material Name	Quantity mg or mL/L
2.50 mg	1	Eplerenone	2.50 mg/L
200 mL	2	Ethanol	200 mL
100 mL	3	Propylene glycol	100 mL
100 mL	4	Glycerol 70%	100 mL
QS	5	Water	QS

Erythromycin Drops

Bill of Materials			
Scale (mg/2.5 mL)	Item	Material Name	Qty/kg (g)
	1	Sodium carboxymethyl cellulose	0.41
	2	Dye red FD&C No. 3	0.13
	3	Sucrose	796.81
	4	Sodium citrate dihydrate	52.60
	5	Sodium carboxy methyl cellulose	13.10
	6	Magnesium aluminum silicate type IB Veegum F	7.90
	7	Water purified	66 mL
100.00	8	Erythromycin USE erythromycin ethylsuccinate citrate, washed (850 μg/mg)	123.50
	9	Flavor	3.94

Manufacturing Directions

Erythromycin ethylsuccinate (item 9) is factored in based on the potency used in the Bill of Materials. Excess of up to 5% erythromycin may be included. The weight of sugar (item 3) is adjusted to compensate for potency variation and excess of the erythromycin ethylsuccinate to maintain the standard quantity at 1000 g.

1. Dissolve the sodium carboxymethylcellulose (item 1) and the dye (if used) in 50 mL hot purified water. Stir until the sodium carboxymethylcellulose is completely in solution. Allow to cool before using.
2. Screen the sucrose through a 2-mm aperture screen into a mixer.
3. Mill the remaining ingredients, with the exception of the flavor, through a 1-B band (1.27-mm aperture or similar) or 0 band (686 micron aperture or similar) with impact forward at high speed, or screen through a 840-micron aperture screen.
4. Load the milled or screened ingredients into the mixer with the screened sucrose and dry blend for not less than 5 minutes.
5. Mass with the solution from step 1 and QS using purified water, if necessary. Mixer must not be stopped and the sides must be scraped down several times during the massing operation to minimize the presence of white particles in the final granulation. Do not allow massed granules to stand.
6. Screen the wet mass through a 16-mm aperture mesh (hammer mill) or a 4-mm aperture screen (oscillating granulator) and spread evenly onto trays.
7. Dry granules in an oven at between 49°C and 55°C to NMT 1.0% loss on drying (15 minutes Brabender, or equivalent, at 105°C), or loss on drying at 60°C at 5 mm of mercury for 3 hours.
8. Screen the cooled, dried granules through a 1.19-mm aperture screen and grind coarse through 2-AA band (1.98-mm aperture, or similar), medium speed, knives forward, or screen through a 1.4-mm aperture screen on an oscillating granulator. Protect granules from excessive exposure to moisture.
9. Screen the flavor through a 600-micron aperture screen with an equal portion of granulation.
10. Fill into suitable approved bottles at the theoretical fill weight.

Erythromycin Topical Solution

Bill of Materials			
Scale (mg/mL)	Item	Material Name	Qty/L (g)
500.00	1	Polyethylene glycol 400	100.00
20.00	2	Erythromycin, USE erythromycin base, 15% excess	25.55
0.32	3	Acetone	65.40 mL
77% (v/v)	4	Alcohol	840.00 mL
QS	5	Nitrogen gas	QS

Manufacturing Directions

Product is sensitive to moisture. Every effort should be made to avoid exposure or incorporation of moisture into the product because the stability of the final product is affected. Check mixing tank to make sure it is clean and dry. Mixing tank must be purged with nitrogen gas, as directed, at the start of and during manufacture to replace most of the air in the mixing tank and to reduce the possibility of fire or explosion if there should be a spark.

Transfer and filling hose lines must be approved for use with solvents.

1. Charge polyethylene glycol 400 to a suitable nitrogen-purged tank; keep nitrogen cover and purging on.
2. Add and mix acetone.
3. Add item 2 (quantity adjusted for potency) and mix.
4. Turn the agitator, sample, and adjust volume.

Estradiol Nasal Spray

Charge 2.6 g of estradiol into a pressure-addition vessel and dissolve with stirring in 405.6 g of ethanol in which 0.26 g of oleic acid has previously been dissolved. After sealing and evacuation thereof, 6.7 kg of HFA 134a that has previously been aerated with carbon dioxide and adjusted to a pressure of at most 6.5 bar (20°C) in another pressure-addition vessel is added with stirring. The formulation obtained is dispensed into aluminum containers sealed with metering valves by means of the pressure-filling technique.

Ethchlorvynol Gelatin Capsule (200 mg)

Bill of Materials			
Scale (mg/capsule)	Item	Material Name	Qty/1000 capsules (g)
200.00	1	Ethchlorvynol	200.00
150.00	2	Polyethylene glycol 400	150.00
211.00	3	Gelatin colored opaque	211.00
–	4	Acetone, approximate[a]	86.00

[a]Used for cleaning purposes only and not present in final product.

Manufacturing Directions

Polyethylene glycol should be weighed into clean, dry, light-resistant containers and sealed under nitrogen protection. Bulk container should be flushed with nitrogen and resealed.

1. Mix ethchlorvynol, polyethylene glycol 400, and glycerin (if used) in an open stainless steel drum until uniform.
2. Cover with loose-fitting polyethylene cover, permitting gas to escape. Fumes will discolor metal. Retest if held for more than 1 month before encapsulating.
3. Mix gelatin to uniform consistency with minimal introduction of air. Encapsulate using the drug mixture into 1000 capsules using gelatin mass red opaque and 6.6-m size die roll.
4. Dry 3 days in a drying room at 20°C to 22°C and 22% to 33% relative humidity or lower.
5. Inspect and remove culls. Optionally, wash with acetone or rinse twice with methylene chloride if used in place of acetone.
6. Finishing: Fill.

Eucalyptus and Mint Emulsion

Bill of Materials			
Scale (mg/mL)	Item	Material Name	Qty/L (g)
427.50	1	Distilled water	427.50
375.00	2	Eucalyptamint	375.00
70.00	3	Sodium stearoyl lactylate (Pationic® SSL)	70.00
35.00	4	PEG-20 hydrogenated lanolin (Supersat ANS4)	35.00
17.50	5	Ritasynt IP	17.50
80.00	6	Cetearyl alcohol, polysorbate 60, PEG-15 stearate, and steareth-20 (Ritachol 1000)	80.00

Manufacturing Directions

1. Heat item 1 to 71°C.
2. Combine rest of the ingredients in another container and heat to 71°C.
3. Slowly add water at 71°C and mix for 1 hour.
4. Cool the mixture to 35°C to 45°C and fill.

Eucalyptol Solution

Bill of Materials			
Scale (mg/mL)	Item	Material Name	Qty/L (g)
80.00	1	Eucalyptol	80.00
40.00	2	Cremophor RH 40	40.00
QS	3	Preservative	QS
QS	4	Water	QS to 1 L

Manufacturing Directions

Mix eucalyptol and Cremophor at 65°C, stir well, and slowly add the warm solution of item 3 to produce a clear or slightly opalescent, colorless liquid.

Eucalyptol Solution (8%)

Formulation

I. Eucalyptol, 8 g; Cremophor RH 40 [1], 4 g;
II. Preservative, QS; water, add 100 mL

Manufacturing Directions

Mix eucalyptol and Cremophor at 65°C, stir well, and add slowly the warm solution II.

Fentanyl Citrate Nasal Spray

1. Charge 2.6 g of fentanyl citrate into a pressure addition vessel and dissolve with stirring in 405.6 g of ethanol in which 0.26 g of oleic acid has previously been dissolved.
2. After sealing and evacuation thereof, 6.7 kg of HFA 134a, which has previously been aerated with carbon dioxide and adjusted to a pressure of at most 6.5 bar (20°C) in another pressure addition vessel, is added with stirring.
3. The formulation obtained is dispensed into aluminum containers sealed with metering valves by means of the pressure-filling technique.

Ferrous Sulfate Oral Solution

Bill of Materials			
Scale (mg/5 mL)	Item	Material Name	Qty/L (g)
75.00[a]	1	Ferrous sulfate	125.00
294.00	2	Sucrose	490.00
147.00	3	Maltitol solution (Lycasin 80/55)	245.00
0.30	4	Citric acid (monohydrate)	0.50
0.90	5	Citric acid (monohydrate)	1.50
0.060	6	FD&C yellow No. 6 (sunset yellow FCF)	1.00
3.120	7	Guarana flavor 12144-33	5.20
0.33	8	Potassium sorbate	0.55
0.30	9	Saccharin sodium	0.50
–	10	Water purified	QS to 1 L

[a] Equivalent to 15 mg iron (Fe).

Manufacturing Directions

Bubble nitrogen throughout the process. Check and record pH of item 10 (limit: 5.0–6.5).

1. Collect 166.67 g of item 10 in mixer.
2. Heat to 90°C to 95°C for 10 minutes.
3. Add item 8. Stir to dissolve to a clear solution.
4. Add item 2. Stir to dissolve to a clear solution.
5. Add item 3. Stir for 10 minutes and cool to 30°C to 35°C.
6. Dissolve item 4 in 10 g of item 10 (30–35°C) and add to first step.
7. Dissolve item 9 in 10 g of item 10 (30–35°C) and add to first step.
8. Dissolve item 5 in 273.33 g of item 10 (30–35°C). Then add item 1 to the clear solution and dissolve slowly without aeration.
9. Add to mixer at first step.
10. Dissolve item 6 in 10 g of item 10 (25–30°C) and add to first step.
11. Add item 7 to first step. Mix at low speed for 10 minutes.
12. Make volume up to 1 L with item 10.
13. Check and record pH. Target pH: 2.20 (limit: between 1.95 and 5.15).
14. Filter the drops with recirculation.
15. Transfer the filtered drops in storage vessel under nitrogen blanket.
16. Use nitrogen blanket in the tank throughout the storage and filling period.

Ferrous Sulfate Oral Syrup

Bill of Materials			
Scale (mg/5 mL)	Item	Material Name	Qty/L (g)
200.000[a]	1	Ferrous sulfate	40.000
3350.000	2	Sucrose	670.000
750.000	3	Maltitol solution (Lycasin 80/55)	150.000
4.166	4	Citric acid (monohydrate)	833.200
8.334	5	Citric acid (monohydrate)	1.667
0.500	6	Color	0.100
15.500	7	Flavor	3.100
–	8	Water purified	QS to 1 L

[a]Equivalent to 40 mg elemental iron.

Manufacturing Directions

Bubble nitrogen throughout the process.

1. Heat 300 g of item 8 to 95°C.
2. Add item 2 while stirring at low speed.
3. Dissolve to clear solution by stirring at 95°C.
4. Add item 3. Stir at low speed and cool to 25°C to 30°C.
5. Dissolve item 4 in 17 g of item 8 and add to first step.
6. Dissolve item 5 in 180 g of item 8 in a separate stainless steel container. Then add item 1 to the clear solution and dissolve slowly without aeration.
7. Add to first step.
8. Dissolve item 6 in 16 g of item 8 and add to first step.
9. Add item 7 to first step. Mix at low speed for 10 minutes.
10. Make volume up to 1 L with item 8. Check and record pH (limit: between 2 and 5). Filter the syrup at 1.5 bar.
11. Recirculate approximately 100 to 150 mL of syrup.
12. Use nitrogen blanket in the tank throughout the storage period.

Fluconazole Oral Suspension

Diflucan for oral suspension contains 350 or 1400 mg of fluconazole and the following inactive ingredients: sucrose, sodium citrate dihydrate, citric acid anhydrous, sodium benzoate, titanium dioxide, colloidal silicon dioxide, xanthan gum, and natural orange flavor. After reconstitution with 24 mL of distilled water or purified water, each milliliter of reconstituted suspension contains 10 or 40 mg of fluconazole.

Flunisolide Spray

Nasarel is a metered-dose manual-pump spray unit containing 0.025% w/w flunisolide in an aqueous medium containing benzalkonium chloride, butylated hydroxytoluene, citric acid, EDTA, polyethylene glycol 400, polysorbate 20, propylene glycol, sodium citrate dihydrate, sorbitol, and purified water. Sodium hydroxide or hydrochloric acid may be added to adjust the pH to approximately 5.2. It contains no fluorocarbons. Each 25-mL spray bottle contains 6.25 mg of flunisolide.

Fluocinonide Topical Solution

Lidex topical solution contains fluocinonide 0.5 mg/mL in a solution of alcohol (35%), citric acid, diisopropyl adipate, and propylene glycol. In this formulation, the active ingredient is totally in solution.

Fluorouracil Solution

Efudex solution consists of 2% or 5% fluorouracil on a weight/weight basis, compounded with propylene glycol, tris(hydroxymethyl)aminomethane, hydroxypropylcellulose, parabens (methyl and propyl), and disodium edetate.

Fluorouracil Topical Solution

Fluoroplex 1% topical solution contains fluorouracil 1%, propylene glycol, sodium hydroxide or hydrochloric acid to adjust the pH, and purified water.

Fluticasone Suspension Spray

Manufacturing Directions

1. 2 g of fluticasone propionate and 0.02 g delta-tocopherol are weighed into a pressure-addition vessel.
2. After sealing and evacuation of the addition vessel, 1.5 kg of HFA 134a that has previously been aerated with carbon dioxide and adjusted to a pressure of 4.5 bar (20°C) in another pressure addition vessel is added with stirring.
3. The suspension obtained is dispensed into aluminum containers sealed with metering valves by means of the pressure-filling technique.

Furosemide Syrup

Bill of Materials			
Scale (mg/5 mL)	Item	Material Name	Qty/L (g)
5.00	1	Furosemide, 5% excess	1.05
9.00	2	Methyl paraben	1.80
1.00	3	Propyl paraben	0.20
1500.00	4	Sorbitol 70%	300.00
500.00	5	Glycerin	100.00
500.00	6	Propylene glycol	100.00
0.50	7	FD&C yellow No. 6	0.10
2.50	8	Orange flavor	0.50
QS	9	Sodium hydroxide	0.44
QS	10	Water purified	QS to 1 L

Manufacturing Directions

1. Charge 20% of item 10 to a suitable stainless steel jacketed vessel.
2. Add items 2 and 3 and heat to 90°C to 95°C to dissolve. Cool to 40°C after complete dissolution.
3. In a separate vessel, charge items 4, 5, and 6 and mix well.
4. Dissolve item 9 in a portion of item 10 in a separate vessel.
5. Add item 1 to step 4 and mix well.
6. In a separate vessel, dissolve item 7 in a portion of item 10.
7. Add to step 6.
8. Add step 2 to step 7.
9. Add item 8 and mix well.
10. Fill.

Ferrous Sulfate Oral Solution

Bill of Materials			
Scale (mg/5 mL)	Item	Material Name	Qty/L (g)
75.00	1	Ferrous sulfate[a]	125.00
294.00	2X	Sucrose	490.00
147.00	3	Maltitol solution (Lycasin® 80/55)	245.00
0.30	4	Citric acid (monohydrate)	0.50
0.90	5	Citric acid (monohydrate)	1.50
0.06	6	FD&C yellow dye No. 6 (sunset yellow FCF)	1.00
3.12	7	Guarana flavor 12144-33	5.20
0.33	8	Potassium sorbate	0.55
0.30	9	Saccharin sodium	0.50
–	10	Purified water	QS to 1 L

[a]Equivalent to 15 mg iron (Fe).

Manufacturing Directions

1. Bubble nitrogen throughout the process.
2. Check and record pH of the purified water (limit: 5.0–6.5).
3. Collect 166.67 g of purified water in mixer.
4. Heat to 90°C to 95°C for 10 minutes.
5. Add item 8 and stir to dissolve to a clear solution.
6. Add item 2 and stir to dissolve to a clear solution.
7. Add item 3 and stir for 10 minutes and cool to 30°C to 35°C.
8. Dissolve item 4 in 10 g of purified water (30–35°C) and add to first step.
9. Dissolve item 9 in 10 g of purified water (30–35°C) and add to first step.
10. Dissolve item 5 in 273.33 g of purified water (30–35°C).
11. Then add item 1 to the clear solution and dissolve slowly without aeration.
12. Add to mixer.
13. Dissolve item 6 in 10 g of purified water (25–30°C) and add to first step.
14. Add item 7 to first step.
15. Mix at low speed for 10 minutes.
16. Bring volume up to 1 L with purified water.
17. Check and record pH (target: 2.2, limit: 1.95–5.15).
18. Filter the drops with recirculation.
19. Transfer the filtered drops to a storage vessel under an N_2 blanket.
20. Use the nitrogen blanket in the tank throughout the storage and filling period.

Ferrous Sulfate Oral Syrup

Bill of Materials			
Scale (mg/5 mL)	Item	Material Name	Qty/L (g)
200.00	1	Ferrous sulfate[a]	40.00
3350.00	2	Sucrose	670.00
750.00	3	Maltitol solution (Lycasin® 80/55)	150.00
4.16	4	Citric acid (monohydrate)	833.20
8.33	5	Citric acid (monohydrate)	1.66
0.50	6	Color	0.10
15.50	7	Flavor	3.10
–	8	Purified water	QS to 1 L

[a]Equivalent to 40 mg elemental iron.

Manufacturing Directions

1. Bubble nitrogen throughout the process.
2. Heat 300 g of purified water to 95°C.
3. Add item 2 while stirring at low speed.
4. Dissolve to clear solution by stirring at 95°C.
5. Add item 3.
6. Stir at low speed and cool to 25°C to 30°C.
7. Dissolve item 4 in 17 g of item 8 and add to the first step.
8. Dissolve item 5 in 180 g of purified water in a separate stainless steel container.
9. Then add item 1 to the clear solution and dissolve slowly without aeration.
10. Add to first step.
11. Dissolve item 6 in 16 g of purified water and add to the first step.
12. Add item 7 to the first step.
13. Mix at low speed for 10 minutes.
14. Bring volume up to 1 L with purified water.
15. Check and record pH (limit: 2–5).
16. Filter the syrup at 1.5 bar.
17. Recirculate approximately 100 to 150 mL of syrup.
18. Use a nitrogen blanket in the tank throughout the storage period.

Fir Needle Oil Solution

Bill of Materials			
Scale (mg/mL)	Item	Material Name	Qty/L (g)
30.00	1	Fir needle oil (Frey & Lau)	30.00
50.00	2	Camphora	50.00
60.00	3	Cremophor RH 40	60.00
403.00	4	Ethanol (96%)	403.00
457.00	5	Water	457.00

Manufacturing Directions

1. Mix the active ingredients with Cremophor RH 40 and heat to 50°C to 60°C.
2. Add the ethanol to the well-stirred solution, then slowly add the warm water to produce a clear or slightly opalescent liquid.
3. The amount of Cremophor RH 40 required depends on the type of fir needle oil.

Foot Bath

Bill of Materials			
Scale (mg/mL)	Item	Material Name	Qty/L (g)
200.00	1	Polysorbate 20	200.00
2.50	2	Menthol	2.50
10.00	3	α-Bisabolol	10.00
20.00	4	Disodium undecylenamido MEA-sulfosuccinate	20.00
20.00	5	Perfume (menthol compatible)	20.00
QS	6	Deionized water	QS to 1 L
QS	7	Preservative, color	QS

Manufacturing Directions

1. Predissolve menthol, alpha-bisabolol, and perfume in Polysorbate 20.
2. Add mixture to the water phase while stirring.
3. Stir until homogeneous and then fill.

Gabapentin Oral Solution

Gabapentin solution contains 250 mg/5 mL of gabapentin. The inactive ingredients for the oral solution are glycerin, xylitol, purified water, and artificial cool strawberry anise flavor.

Galantamine Hydrobromide Oral Solution

Reminyl is available as a 4 mg/mL galantamine hydrobromide oral solution. The inactive ingredients for this solution are methyl parahydroxybenzoate, propylparahydroxybenzoate, sodium saccharin, sodium hydroxide, and purified water.

Glucose, Fructose, and Phosphoric Acid Antiemetic Solution

Emetrol is an oral solution containing balanced amounts of dextrose (glucose) and levulose (fructose) and phosphoric acid with controlled hydrogen ion concentration. Available in original lemon-mint or cherry flavor. Each 5-mL teaspoonful contains dextrose (glucose), 1.87 g; levulose (fructose), 1.87 g; phosphoric acid, 21.5 mg; glycerin; methyl paraben; purified water; D&C yellow No. 10; and natural lemon-mint flavor in lemon-mint Emetrol and FD&C red No. 40 and artificial cherry flavor in cherry Emetrol.

Glycol Foam, Nonaqueous

Bill of Materials			
Scale (mg/g)	Item	Material Name	Qty/kg (g)
40.00	1	Polawax A31	4.00
710.00	2	Propylene glycol	71.00
150.00	3	Ethanol DEB100	15.00

Manufacturing Directions

1. Dissolve Polawax in propylene glycol/ethanol.
2. Pack into containers and pressurize.
3. Ethanol may be omitted if desired.
4. In aerosol pack, 90% concentrate and 10% propellant 12/114 may be used.
5. Propylene glycol is a suitable vehicle for glycol-soluble medicaments.
6. The above formulation provides a mousse for such a system.

Gramicidin Opthalmic Solution

Bill of Materials			
Scale (mg/mL)	Item	Material Name	Qty/L (g)
130.00	1	Gramicidin	130.00
1.00	2	Cremophor RH 40	1.00
10.00	3	Alcohol	10.00
QS	4	Preservatives	QS
QS	5	Water purified	QS to 1 L

Manufacturing Directions

1. Charge items 1 and 2 in a suitable mixing and jacketed vessel; heat to 65°C and mix.
2. Cool to room temperature.
3. In a separate vessel, add and mix items 3 to 5.
4. Add to step 2. Mix and fill.

Guaifenesin, Pseudoephedrine, Carbinoxamine, and Chlophedianol Drops

Bill of Materials			
Scale (mg/mL)	Item	Material Name	Qty/L (g)
20.00	1	Guaifenesin	20.00
400.00	2	Sucrose	400.00
240.00	3	Glucose liquid	240.00
120.00	4	Sorbitol solution	120.00
3.00	5	Saccharin sodium powder dihydrate	3.00
2.50	6	Sodium benzoate powder	2.50
30.00	7	Pseudoephedrine hydrochloride	30.00
1.00	8	Carbinoxamine maleate	1.00
6.60	9	Chlophedianol hydrochloride	6.60
105.00	10	Dye red E123 (Amaranth)	105.00 mg
3.75	11	Dye blue FD&C No. 1	3.75 mg
QS	12	Acid hydrochloric	QS
50.00	13	Menthol crystals	50.0 mg
2.75	14	Flavors	2.75
65.00	15	Oil orange terpeneless No. 54125	65.00 mg
5.66	16	Alcohol 190 proof (10% ex)	5.66
0.52 g	17	Filter aid HyFlo	0.52
420.00 g	18	Water purified, distilled approximate	420.00

Manufacturing Directions

1. Charge 260 mL purified water into a suitable tank.
2. Begin heating water to 70°C to 80°C while adding guaifenesin and sucrose with stirring.
3. Continue stirring to dissolve ingredients.
4. Remove heat and add glucose liquid and sorbitol to solution from step 3 with stirring.
5. Add saccharin sodium, sodium benzoate, pseudoephedrine hydrochloride, carbinoxamine maleate, and chlophedianol hydrochloride to solution from step 4. Stir well to dissolve all ingredients.
6. Dissolve dye red E123 and FD&C No. 1 in 10 mL warm, purified water.
7. Add dye solution to solution from step 6 with stirring. Cool solution to 30°C to 35°C.
8. QS to 975 mL using purified water and mix well.
9. Adjust to pH 4.25 (range 4.0–4.5) with hydrochloric acid (ca. 0.65 g/L of drops).
10. Stir well after each addition of acid. Dissolve menthol, flavors, and orange oil in alcohol; add mixture to solution from step above with good stirring.
11. Stir the solution slowly for 2 hours.
12. Allow to stand overnight to cool and remove entrapped air.
13. QS to 1 L with purified water and stir well.
14. Add filter aid HyFlo to solution and mix well.
15. Recirculate through filter press or equivalent until sparkling clean.

Guaifenesin Pseudoephedrine, Carbinoxamine, and Chlophedianol Drops

Bill of Materials			
Scale (mg/mL)	Item	Material Name	Qty/L (g)
20.00	1	Guaifenesin	20.000
400.00	2	Sucrose	400.000
240.00	3	Glucose liquid	240.000
120.00	4	Sorbitol solution	120.000
3.00	5	Saccharin sodium	3.000
2.50	6	Sodium benzoate (powder)	2.500
30.00	7	Pseudoephedrine hydrochloride	30.000
1.00	8	Carbinoxamine maleate	1.000
6.60	9	Chlophedianol hydrochloride	6.600
105.00	10	Dye red E123 (Amaranth)	0.105
3.75	11	Dye blue FD&C No. 1	3.750 mg
QS	12	Acid, hydrochloric	QS
50.00	13	Menthol crystals	50.000 mg
2.75	14	Flavors	2.750
65.00	15	Orange oil terpeneless	65.000 mg
5.66	16	Alcohol (190 proof)	5.664
GS	17	HyFlo filter aid	0.526
QS	18	Purified water	~420.000

Manufacturing Directions

1. Charge 260 mL purified water into a suitable tank.
2. Begin heating water to 70°C to 80°C while adding guaifenesin and sucrose with stirring.
3. Continue stirring to dissolve ingredients.
4. Remove heat, add glucose liquid and sorbitol to solution from step above with stirring.
5. Add saccharin sodium, sodium benzoate, pseudoephedrine hydrochloride, carbinoxamine maleate, and chlophedianol hydrochloride to solution from preceding step.
6. Stir well to dissolve all ingredients.
7. Dissolve dye red E123 and dye blue FD&C No. 1 in 10 mL warm purified water.
8. Add dye solution to solution from preceding step with stirring.
9. Cool solution to 30°C to 35°C.
10. QS to 975 mL using purified water, mix well.
11. Adjust to pH 4.25 (range: 4.0–4.5) with hydrochloric acid (~0.65 g/L of drops).
12. Stir well after each addition of acid.
13. Dissolve menthol, flavors, and orange oil in alcohol; add mixture to solution from previous step with good stirring.
14. Stir the solution slowly for 2 hours.
15. Allow to stand overnight to cool and remove entrapped air.
16. QS to 1 L with purified water and stir well.
17. Add HyFlo filter aid to solution and mix well.
18. Recirculate through filter press or equivalent until sparkling clean.

Haloperidol Oral Liquid

Bill of Materials			
Scale (mg/mL)	Item	Material Name	Qty/L (g)
2.00	1	Haloperidol	2.00
11.00	2	Lactic acid	11.00
0.20	3	Propyl paraben	0.20
1.90	4	Methyl paraben	1.90
QS	5	Sodium hydroxide for pH adjustment, approximate	0.24
QS	6	Water purified, approximate	990.00 mL
QS	7	Nitrogen gas	QS
QS	8	Lactic acid	QS

Manufacturing Directions

1. Charge approximately 700 mL of water into a suitable mixing tank. Add and dissolve lactic acid with stirring; while mixing, add haloperidol. Mix until complete solution (approximately 15 minutes).
2. Charge 240 mL of water into a separate container and heat to boiling. Add and dissolve methyl and propyl parabens. Mix until complete solution. Add this solution to step 1 solution.
3. Check pH. If necessary, adjust to pH 2.75 (range: 2.5–3.0) with 2% sodium hydroxide. Continue mixing for 10 minutes after addition of sodium hydroxide. Record pH and amount of sodium hydroxide added. Lactic acid (No. 8) may also be used to adjust pH.
4. QS to 1 L with water and mix well.
5. Filter solution through 8-micron membrane filter (or similar) into a suitable container, under nitrogen protection.
6. Fill under nitrogen.

Heparin Nasal Spray

Charge 5 g of heparin into a pressure-addition vessel and suspend with stirring 50 g of ethanol in which 0.25 g of lecithin have previously been dissolved. After sealing and evacuation thereof, 1.5 kg of HFA 227 that has previously been aerated with carbon dioxide and adjusted to a pressure of 4.5 bar (20°C) in another pressure addition vessel is added with stirring and homogenized. The suspension obtained is dispensed into aluminum containers sealed with metering valves by means of the pressure-filling technique.

Hydrocodone Bitartrate Elixir

Each 5 mL contains hydrocodone bitartrate 2.5 mg, acetaminophen 167 mg, and 7% alcohol. In addition, the liquid contains the following inactive ingredients: citric acid anhydrous, ethyl maltol, glycerin, methyl paraben, propylene glycol, propyl paraben, purified water, saccharin sodium, sorbitol solution, sucrose, and D&C yellow No. 10 and FD&C yellow No. 6 as coloring and natural and artificial flavoring.

Hydrocodone Polistirex Extended-Release Suspension

Each teaspoonful (5 mL) of Tussionex Pennkinetic extended-release suspension contains hydrocodone polistirex equivalent to 10 mg of hydrocodone bitartrate and chlorpheniramine polistirex equivalent to 8 mg of chlorpheniramine maleate Tussionex. Inactive ingredients: ascorbic acid, D&C yellow No. 10, ethylcellulose, FD&C yellow No. 6, flavor, high fructose corn syrup, methyl paraben, polyethylene glycol 3350, polysorbate 80, pregelatinized starch, propylene glycol, propyl paraben, purified water, sucrose, vegetable oil, and xanthan gum.

Hydromorphone Hydrochloride Oral Liquid

Hydromorphone hydrochloride, a hydrogenated ketone of morphine, is a narcotic analgesic. Each 5 mL (one teaspoon) contains 5 mg of hydromorphone hydrochloride. In addition, other ingredients include purified water, methylparaben, propyl paraben, sucrose, and glycerin. It may contain traces of sodium bisulfite.

Hydroxyzine Pamoate Oral Suspension

Hydroxyzine pamoate 25 mg/5 mL; inert ingredients for the oral suspension formulation are carboxymethylcellulose sodium, lemon flavor, propylene glycol, sorbic acid, sorbitol solution, and water.

Hyoscine Butylbromide Syrup

Bill of Materials			
Scale (mg/5 mL)	Item	Material Name	Qty/L (g)
5.00	1	Hyoscine butylbromide	1.00
3300.00	2	Sugar	660.00
5.00	3	Methyl paraben	1.00
1.50	4	Propyl paraben	0.30
962.50	5	Sorbitol 70%	19.30
10.00	6	Sodium saccharin	2.00
35.00	7	Sodium chloride	7.00
0.70	8	Citric acid monohydrate	0.14
0.75	9	Sodium citrate	0.15
10.00	10	Flavor	2.00
5.00	11	Flavor	1.00
5.00	12	Flavor	1.00
QS	13	Water purified	QS to 1 L

Manufacturing Directions

1. In a suitable stainless steel container, charge 300 mL item 13 and heat to 90° to 95°C.
2. Add and dissolve items 3 and 4.
3. Add item 2 and dissolve.
4. Add item 5 and dissolve. Cool to room temperature
5. In 10 mL item 13, add and dissolve items 6 and 7 and add to step 4.
6. In 10 mL item 13, add and dissolve item 8 and add to step 4.
7. In 10 mL item 13, add and dissolve item 7 and add to step 4.
8. In 20 mL item 13, add and dissolve item 1 and add to step 4.
9. Add flavors.
10. Make up volume and fill.

Hyoscyamine Sulfate Elixir

Levsin elixir contains 0.125 mg hyoscyamine sulfate per 5 mL with 20% alcohol for oral administration. Levsin elixir also contains, as inactive ingredients, FD&C red No. 40, FD&C yellow No. 6, flavor, glycerin, purified water, sorbitol solution, and sucrose.

Ibuprofen Topical Solution

Bill of Materials			
Scale (mg/mL)	Item	Material Name	Qty/L (g)
QS	1	Vehicle (pluronic P105 63.16%, ethanol 18.95%, water 17.89%)	QS to 1 L
50.00	2	Ibuprofen	50.00

Manufacturing Directions

1. Screen the ibuprofen to reduce the particle size.
2. Add the ibuprofen into a clean vessel.
3. Add ethanol to the vessel.
4. Subsequently add the poloxamer and water to the vessel.
5. Mix until uniform.

Ibuprofen Pediatric Suspension

Bill of Materials			
Scale (mg/5 mL)	Item	Material Name	Qty/L (g)
100.00	1	Ibuprofen, low-density[a]	20.00
3000.00	2	Sucrose	600.00
10.00	3	Sodium benzoate	2.00
5.00	4	Saccharin sodium	1.00
5.00	5	Edetate disodium (sodium EDTA)	1.00
500.00	6	Glycerin (glycerol)	100.00
500.00	7	Sorbitol (70% solution)	100.00
10.00	8	Xanthan gum (Keltrol-F)	2.00
20.00	9	Microcrystalline cellulose (Avicel™ RC591)	4.00
5.00	10	Polysorbate 80 (Tween 80)	1.00
8.50	11	Citric acid	1.70
1.35	12	FD&C red No. 40	0.27
7.50	13	Mixed fruits flavor	1.50
5.00	14	Strawberry flavor	1.00
QS	15	Purified water	QS to 1 L

[a] Meets USP criteria with the following additional requirements: 100% particle size below 50 μm and tapped density of 0.3 to 0.4 g/mL.

Manufacturing Directions

1. Heat 302 g of item 15 to 90°C and dissolve item 2 while mixing in mixer.
2. Cool to approximately 50°C.
3. Add items 3, 5, 4, 11, and 7 to mixer while mixing and dissolve.
4. Filter the syrup through Seitz Supra 2600 filters in clean stainless steel tank.
5. In a clean stainless steel vessel, dissolve item 10 in 35 g of item 15 (40°C).
6. Add item 1 slowly while mixing with stirrer.
7. Mix for 30 minutes to make uniform dispersion. *Caution*: Avoid excessive foaming.
8. Disperse items 8 and 9 in item 6 in a clean and dry stainless steel container using stirrer.
9. Add 75 g of hot item 15 (70–90°C) at once while mixing.
10. Mix for 20 minutes to make a homogeneous smooth mucilage.
11. Add approximately 500 g syrup, ibuprofen dispersion, and mucilage to the mixer.
12. Rinse the containers of ibuprofen dispersion and mucilage with 50 g of item 15 (40°C).
13. Add the rinsings to the mixer.
14. Set the mixer: temperature, 25°C; speed, 18 rpm; and manual mode vacuum at 0.5 bar.
15. Mix for 3 minutes at low homogenizer speed.
16. Mix for 2 minutes at homogenizer high speed. Check the suspension for uniformity of dispersion.
17. Homogenize for additional 3 minutes at high speed, if required.
18. Add the balance of the syrup (approximately 507.6 g) from previous step to the mixer.
19. In a separate container, dissolve item 12 in 6 g of cooled item 15 (40°C) and transfer to the mixer.
20. Add items 13 and 14 to the mixer.
21. Set the mixer: temperature, 25°C; speed, 18 rpm; manual mode vacuum at 0.5 bar.
22. Mix for 15 minutes.
23. Mix for 5 minutes at homogenizer low speed.
24. Mix for 5 minutes at homogenizer high speed.
25. Check the suspension for uniformity.
26. Adjust the final volume to 1 L by using purified water.

Iron Infant Drops

Bill of Materials			
Scale (mg/mL)	Item	Material Name	Qty/L (g)
0.18	1	Propyl paraben	0.18
0.022	2	Methyl paraben	0.02
1000.00	3	Sorbitol solution	1.00 kg
4.00	4	Citric acid (hydrous powder)	4.00
125.00	5	Iron sulfate	125.00
0.106	6	Sodium metabisulfite	0.10
0.50	7	Guarana flavor (artificial)	0.50
20.00	8	Alcohol (ethanol)	900.14
0.14	9	Dye	0.14
QS	9	Sodium hydroxide	QS
QS	10	Citric acid (powder)	1 QS
QS	11	Purified water	QS to 1 L
QS	12	HyFlo filter aid	1.00
QS	13	Liquid nitrogen	QS
QS	14	Carbon dioxide gas	QS

Manufacturing Directions

The product is susceptible to oxidation. No effort should be spared to protect it from atmospheric air. Maintain CO_2 or nitrogen atmosphere where indicated. The product must be manufactured and held in a glass-lined or stainless steel tank. Product waiting to be filled should either be in a closed tank with a CO_2 atmosphere or in an open tank covered with polyethylene sheeting taped tightly with a constant slow stream of CO_2 gas flowing into the tank headspace. Avoid vortex formation throughout processing.

1. Charge 144 mL of purified water into a mixing tank.
2. Heat to 95°C to 100°C and add parabens with strong agitation.
3. Add sorbitol solution and citric acid (item 4) while mixing.
4. Bring solution to 90°C while mixing.
5. Cool the solution while mixing to 60°C to 65°C and hold at this temperature with CO_2 or nitrogen gas bubbling into it.
6. CO_2 gas protection is continued for the remainder of the manufacturing process.
7. Add ferrous sulfate and dissolve while mixing, holding at 60°C to 65°C.
8. Cool to 25°C with mixing.
9. Add sodium metabisulfite and dissolve while mixing.
10. Avoid vortex formation.
11. Dissolve dye in 2 mL of freshly boiled purified water and add to the tank. Mix.
12. Dissolve the guarana flavor in alcohol, add to the tank, and mix.
13. Check pH (range: 1.8–2.2). Adjust if necessary, with a solution of 10% sodium hydroxide or a solution of 10% citric acid.
14. Make up to volume with freshly boiled purified water and mix.
15. Readjust to volume if necessary with freshly boiled purified water and mix.
16. Add HyFlo filter aid and mix. Filter through press until clear.
17. Bubble CO_2 or nitrogen gas into the clear filtrate for 5 minutes, then seal tank and hold product under CO_2 or nitrogen protection.

Iron Polystyrene and Vitamin C Syrup

Bill of Materials			
Scale (mg/mL)	Item	Material Name	Qty/L (g)
125.00	1	Glycerin	125.00
1.40	2	Methyl paraben	1.40
0.16	3	Propyl paraben	0.16
79.61	4	Sorbitol; use sorbitol solution	364.33
3.30	5	Xanthan gum	3.30
10.00	6	Sucrose (granulated)	100.00
0.20	7	Saccharin (insoluble)	2.00
105.00	8	Elemental iron; use iron polystyrene sulfonate	530.31
50.00	9	Ascorbic acid, USP (35% excess)	61.95
0.10	10	Flavor	1.00 mL
0.10	11	Flavor (artificial guarana)	1.00 mL
QS	12	Sodium hydroxide	12. 1.0
QS	13	Dye	2.00
9.50	14	Distilled purified water	~95.00 mL
10.00	15	Sorbitol solution	~10.00

Manufacturing Directions

1. Add glycerin (item 1) to the tank.
2. Commence heating with agitation.
3. Add and disperse parabens.
4. Continue heating to 70°C to 80°C and mix until solution is complete.
5. Force cool to 30°C, then add and disperse xanthan gum (item 5).
6. Add sorbitol solution (item 4) and 80 mL of purified water (item 14) and heat with mixing to 60°C to 70°C until the xanthan gum is fully dissolved.
7. Add and disperse saccharin and sugar (items 6 and 7).
8. Mix at 60°C to 70°C until dispersion is complete.
9. Force cool to 25°C to 30°C with continuous mixing.
10. Commence N_2 gas protection and maintain for the remainder of the manufacturing process.
11. Add and disperse ascorbic acid.
12. Continue mixing for 30 minutes at 25°C to 30°C.
13. *Note*: Use suitable SS high-powered stirrer.
14. Mix the iron polystyrene sulfonate milled slurry in the original epoxy-lined drums under N_2 gas protection until uniform.
15. Add the slurry to the main batch and mix for 30 minutes at 25°C to 30°C.
16. *Note*: Avoid scraping the epoxy lining of the steel drum while mixing and use a plastic or rubber scraper to assist in complete transfer of the mixed slurry. Add and disperse the flavors. Mix well.
17. Check and record pH. Adjust pH using a 20% sodium hydroxide solution (1 g in 5 mL water) to a value of 3 (range: 2.8–3.2).
18. Dissolve the dye in 5 to 7 mL of water at 40°C to 45°C by stirring for 10 minutes.
19. Add this solution to the main batch through a 420-μm screen with mixing.
20. Rinse container with 2 to 3 mL water at 40°C to 45°C and add to bulk through a 420-μm screen.
21. Continue to mix under vacuum until mixture is uniform.
22. Pass the suspension through the colloid mill at a gap setting of 100 to 150 μm.
23. Adjust the flow rate such that the temperature rise of the suspension does not exceed 10°C.
24. Collect the milled suspension in a stainless steel jacketed tank with vacuum.
25. Mix at 25°C to 30°C under vacuum until a uniform suspension is achieved.
26. Flush the bulk suspension with nitrogen and seal.
27. Hold at 25°C to 30°C.

Ibuprofen Pediatric Suspension

Bill of Materials			
Scale (mg/5 mL)	Item	Material Name	Qty/L (g)
100.00	1	Ibuprofen low density (100% particle size below 50 microns, tapped density is 0.3–0.4 g/mL)	20.00
3000.00	2	Sucrose	600.00
10.00	3	Sodium benzoate	2.00
5.00	4	Saccharin sodium	1.00
5.00	5	Edetate disodium (sodium EDTA)	1.00
500.00	6	Glycerin (glycerol)	100.00
500.00	7	Sorbitol (70% solution)	100.00
10.00	8	Xanthan gum (Keltrol-F)	2.00
20.00	9	Microcrystalline cellulose (Avicel RC 591)	4.00
5.00	10	Polysorbate 80 (Tween 80)	1.00
8.50	11	Citric acid	1.70
1.35	12	FD&C red No. 40	0.27
7.50	13	Mixed fruits flavor	1.50
5.00	14	Strawberry flavor	1.00
–	15	Water purified	QS to 1 L

Manufacturing Directions

1. Heat 302 g of item 15 to 90°C and dissolve item 2 while mixing in mixer.
2. Cool to approximately 50°C.
3. Add items 3, 5, 4, 7, and 11 to mixer while mixing and dissolve.
4. Filter the syrup through Seitz Supra 2600 filters in clean stainless steel tank.
5. In a clean stainless steel vessel, dissolve item 10 in 35 g of item 15 (40°C).
6. Add item 1 slowly while mixing with stirrer.
7. Mix for 30 minutes to make uniform dispersion. Avoid excessive foaming.
8. Disperse items 8 and 9 in item 6 in a clean and dry stainless steel container using stirrer. Add 75 g of hot item 15 (70–90°C) at once while mixing.
9. Mix for 20 minutes to make homogeneous smooth mucilage.
10. Add approximately 500 g syrup, ibuprofen dispersion, and mucilage to the mixer.
11. Rinse the containers of ibuprofen dispersion and mucilage with 50 g of item 15 (40°C).
12. Add the rinsings to the mixer. Set the mixer: temperature, 25°C; mixer speed, 18 rpm; manual mode vacuum, 0.5 bar.
13. Mix for 3 minutes at low homogenizer speed.
14. Mix for 2 minutes at homogenizer high speed. Check the suspension for uniformity of dispersion.
15. Homogenize for additional 3 minutes at high speed, if required.
16. Add the balance syrup approximately 507.6 g from step above to the mixer.
17. In a separate container, dissolve item 12 in 6 g of cooled item 15 (40°C) and transfer to the mixer.
18. Add the items 13 and 14 to the mixer. Set the mixer: temperature, 25°C; mixer speed, 18 rpm; manual mode vacuum, 0.5 bar. Mix for 15 minutes.
19. Mix for 5 minutes at homogenizer low speed.
20. Mix for 5 minutes at homogenizer high speed.
21. Check the suspension for uniformity.
22. Adjust the final volume to 1 L by using purified water.

Ibuprofen Solution

Bill of Materials			
Scale (mg/mL)	Item	Material Name	Qty/L (g)
20.00	1	Ibuprofen	20.00
200.00	2	Cremophor RH 40	200.00
QS	3	Preservatives	QS
QS	4	Water purified	QS to 1 L

Manufacturing Directions

1. In a suitable stainless steel jacketed vessel, add and suspend item 1 in item 2 by heating it to 60°C.
2. In a separate vessel, add items 3 and 4 and heat to 90°C to 95°C to dissolve preservatives and add to step 1.
3. Mix and fill.

Ibuprofen Suspension

Bill of Materials			
Scale (mg/mL)	Item	Material Name	Qty/L (g)
40.00	1	Ibuprofen	40.00
250.00	2	Sucrose	250.00
80.00	3	Kollidon CL-M	80.00
20.00	4	Kollidon 90F	20.00
20.00	5	Sodium citrate	20.00
QS	6	Water purified	QS to 1 L

Manufacturing Directions

1. Charge items 2 and 4 to 6 (40%) in a suitable mixer.
2. Add and suspend item 3.
3. Add and disperse item 1. Homogenize if necessary.
4. Bring to volume with item 6. Mix and fill.

Ibuprofen Suspension, Sugar Free

Bill of Materials			
Scale (mg/mL)	Item	Material Name	Qty/L (g)
40.00	1	Ibuprofen	40.00
10.00	2	Cremophor RH 40	100.00
50.00	3	Lutron F 68	50.00
QS	4	Preservatives	QS
QS	5	Water purified	QS to 1 L

Manufacturing Directions

1. Dissolve Lutrol F 68 and the preservatives in purified water.
2. In a separate vessel, add and mix items 1 and 2.
3. Add to step 1.
4. Homogenize if necessary.
5. Bring to volume with item 5. Mix and fill.

Ibuprofen and Domperidone Maleate Suspension

Bill of Materials			
Scale (mg/5 mL)	Item	Material Name	Qty/L (g)
200.00	1	Ibuprofen	40.00
20.00	2	Domperidone maleate	4.00
2.50	3	Colloidal cellulose	0.50
15.00	4	Glycerin	3.00
10.00	5	Sorbitol	2.00
1.00	6	Kaolin	0.20
1.00	7	Polysorbate 80	0.20
QS	8	Water	QS

Manufacturing Directions

1. Item 7 is added to the water followed by the addition of glycerin with stirring.
2. The domperidone and ibuprofen are then added and also the colloidal cellulose, sorbitol, and kaolin (as thickeners) with continued stirring until a satisfactory suspension is formed.

Insulin Inhalation Spray

Bill of Materials			
Scale (mg/mL)	Item	Material Name	Qty/L (g)
10.00	1	Insulin	10.00
9.00	2	Brij 98	9.00
10.00	3	Sodium lauryl sulfate	10.00
200.00	4	Alcohol, anhydrous	200.00
QS	5	HFA 134a (1,1,1,2-tetrafluoroethane)	QS to 1 L

Manufacturing Directions

1. Weigh insulin in a clean glass container and dissolve in acid buffer and titrate to a pH of 7 with Tris buffer.
2. Add Brij 98 and sodium lauryl sulfate to the insulin solution to form a homogenous solution.
3. Lyophilize and suspend dried particles in a nonaqueous suspension medium of ethanol and then charge with hydrofluoroalkane (HFA) 134a.
4. Fill the formulation in a pressure-resistant container fitted with a metering valve.

Ipratropium Bromide Inhalation Solution

Atrovent inhalation solution is administered by oral inhalation with the aid of a nebulizer. It contains ipratropium bromide 0.02% (anhydrous basis) in a sterile, isotonic saline solution, pH adjusted to 3.4 (3–4) with hydrochloric acid.

Ipratropium Bromide Nasal Spray

Atrovent (ipratropium bromide) nasal spray 0.03% is a metered-dose manual-pump spray unit that delivers 21 μg (70 μL) ipratropium bromide per spray on an anhydrous basis in an isotonic, aqueous solution with pH adjusted to 4.7. It also contains benzalkonium chloride, EDTA, sodium chloride, sodium hydroxide, hydrochloric acid, and purified water. Each bottle contains 165 or 345 sprays.

Manufacturing Directions

1. 2.25 g of micronized ipratropium bromide and 11.25 g of micronized salbutamol are weighed into a pressure-addition vessel.
2. After sealing and evacuation thereof, 10.5 kg of HFA 227 that has previously been aerated with carbon dioxide and adjusted to a pressure of 6.25 bar (20°C) in another pressure addition vessel is added.
3. After homogenization of this mixture, the suspension obtained is dispensed into aluminum containers sealed with metering valves by means of the pressure-filling technique.

Iron Polystyrene and Vitamin C Syrup

Bill of Materials			
Scale (mg/mL)	Item	Material Name	Qty/L (g)
125.00	1	Glycerin	125.000
1.40	2	Methyl paraben	1.400
0.16	3	Propyl paraben	0.160
79.61	4	Sorbitol solution	364.330
3.30	5	Xanthan gum	3.300
10.00	6	Sucrose	100.000
0.20	7	Saccharin	2.000
105.00	8	Elemental iron USE iron polystyrene sulfonate	530.310
50.00	9	Acid ascorbic, 35% excess	61.950
0.10 v/v	10	Flavor	1.000 mL
0.10 v/v	11	Flavor guarana artificial	1.000 mL
QS	12	Sodium hydroxide	12. 1.0
QS	13	Dye	2.000
9.50	14	Water purified	95.000 mL
10.00	15	Sorbitol solution, approximate	10.000

Manufacturing Directions

1. Add glycerin (item 1) to the tank. Commence heating with agitation.
2. Add and disperse parabens. Continue heating to 70°C to 80°C and mix until solution is complete.
3. Force cool to 30°C then add and disperse xanthan gum (item 5).
4. Add sorbitol solution (item 4) and 80 mL of purified water (item 14) and heat with mixing to 60°C to 70°C until the xanthan gum is fully dissolved.
5. Add and disperse saccharin and sugar (items 7 and 6).
6. Mix at 60°C to 70°C until dispersion is complete.
7. Force cool to 25°C to 30°C with continuous mixing.
8. Commence N_2 gas protection and maintain for the remainder of the manufacturing process.
9. Add and disperse ascorbic acid. Continue mixing for 30 minutes at 25°C to 30°C. Use suitable stainless steel high-powered stirrer.
10. Mix the iron polystyrene sulfonate milled slurry, in the original epoxy lined drums, under N_2 gas protection until uniform.
11. Add the slurry to the main batch and mix for 30 minutes at 25°C to 30°C. Avoid scraping the epoxy lining of the steel drum while mixing and use a plastic or rubber scraper to assist in complete transfer of the mixed slurry.
12. Add and disperse the flavors. Mix well.
13. Check and record pH. Adjust pH using a 20% sodium hydroxide solution (1 g in 5 mL water) to a pH of 3 (range: 2.8–3.2).
14. Dissolve the dye in 5 to 7 mL of water at 40°C to 45°C by stirring for 10 minutes.
15. Add this solution to the main batch through a 420-micron aperture screen with mixing.
16. Rinse container with 2 to 3 mL water at 40°C to 45°C and add to bulk through a 420-micron screen.
17. Continue to mix under vacuum until uniform.
18. Pass suspension through the colloid mill at a gap setting of 100 to 150 micrometers.
19. Adjust flow rate such that the temperature rise of the suspension does not exceed 10°C.
20. Collect the milled suspension in a stainless steel-jacketed tank with vacuum. Mix at 25°C to 30°C under vacuum until a uniform suspension is achieved.
21. Flush the bulk suspension with N_2 and seal. Hold at 25°C to 30°C.

Isoproterenol Sulfate and Calcium Iodide Syrup

Bill of Materials			
Scale (mg/5 mL)	Item	Material Name	Qty/L (g)
1.569	1	Glucose liquid	311.60
269.500	2	Glycerin	53.90
150.000	3	Calcium iodide anhydrous, USE calcium iodide solution 27%	111.11
5.000	4	Ascorbic acid	1.00
2.428	5	Sucrose	485.30
4.000	6	Saccharin sodium	0.80
5.000	7	Sodium cyclamate	1.00
6.550	8	Flavor honey	1.31
1.660	9	Flavor mint	0.33
0.260	10	Alcohol 190 proof	51.53
3.000	11	Isoproterenol sulfate	0.60
0.250	12	Dye yellow	0.05
1.250	13	Caramel	0.25
QS	14	Water purified	QS to 1 L

Manufacturing Directions

1. Charge in a stainless steel tank items 1, 2, 5, 6, 7, 10 and 90% of item 14. Mix well; heat if necessary.
2. In a separate vessel, add and dissolve items 4, 8, 9, 12, and 13 in item 14; mix well and add to step 1.
3. Add remaining items, mix, bring to volume. Fill.

Isotretinoin Capsules

Isotretinoin, a retinoid, is available in 10-, 20-, and 40-soft gelatin capsules for oral administration. Each capsule also contains beeswax, butylated hydroxyanisole, EDTA, hydrogenated soybean oil flakes, hydrogenated vegetable oil, and soybean oil. Gelatin capsules contain glycerin and parabens (methyl and propyl), with the following dye systems: 10 mg, iron oxide (red) and titanium dioxide; 20 mg, FD&C red No. 3, FD&C blue No. 1, and titanium dioxide; 40 mg, FD&C yellow No. 6, D&C yellow No. 10, and titanium dioxide. Chemically, isotretinoin is 13-cis-retinoic acid and is related to both retinoic acid and retinol (vitamin A). It is a yellow-orange to orange crystalline powder with a molecular weight of 300.44.

Itraconazole Oral Solution

Itraconazole oral solution contains 10 mg of itraconazole per milliliter, solubilized by hydroxypropyl-(beta)-cyclo-dextrin (400 mg/mL) as a molecular inclusion complex. The solution is clear and yellowish in color with a target pH of 2. Other ingredients are hydrochloric acid, propylene glycol, purified water, sodium hydroxide, sodium saccharin, sorbitol, cherry flavor 1, cherry flavor 2, and caramel flavor.

Kaolin, Pectin, and Aluminum Hydroxide Suspension

Bill of Materials			
Scale (mg/5 mL)	Item	Material Name	Qty/L (g)
147.600	1	Sodium methyl paraben	4.92
6.720	2	Sodium propyl paraben	224.00
36.000	3	Magnesium aluminum silicate type IA	1.20
5832.000	4	Kaolin (powder)	194.40
130.000	5	Pectin	4.33
120.000	6	Sodium CMC (premium, low-viscosity)	4.00
210.000	7	Cyclamate calcium	7.00
21.00	8	Saccharin calcium (powder)	0.70
15.375	9	Flavor	0.51
1.234	10	Flavor	41.13
QS	11	Distilled purified water (approx.)	QS
QS	12	Citric acid (anhydrous powder)	QS
QS	13	Water purified, distilled	QS
QS	14	Acid citric anhydrous powder	QS
63.300	15	Aluminum hydroxide	12.72

Manufacturing Directions

1. Charge 600 mL of water into a suitable jacketed mixing tank.
2. Add methyl paraben and propyl paraben to the tank and heat to 90°C to 95°C.
3. Cool to 70°C, add the magnesium aluminum silicate, and mix for 30 minutes or until evenly dispersed.
4. Hold temperature at 70°C.
5. Add kaolin with constant mixing at 70°C until evenly dispersed.
6. Add pectin and mix for 2 hours, maintaining the temperature of 70°C.
7. Add sodium CMC premium low viscosity and mix for at least 30 minutes, maintaining the temperature at 70°C. Cool to 60°C and hold at this temperature.
8. Add aluminum hydroxide gel and mix under vacuum.
9. Add in order cyclamate calcium and saccharin calcium and mix thoroughly for 20 minutes. While mixing, cool to room temperature and allow standing overnight to hydrate.
10. After overnight standing (minimum 12 hours), mix for 30 minutes.
11. Add and mix flavors. Check and record pH (range: 4.5–7.5). If pH is more than 7.5, adjust with a 60% solution of citric acid to the desired pH.
12. Add water to 1 L and mix thoroughly for 3 hours.
13. Strain product through muslin cloth into holding tanks and cover.

Kaolin–Pectin Suspension

Bill of Materials			
Scale (mg/5 mL)	Item	Material Name	Qty/L (g)
147.60	1	Sodium methyl paraben	4.92
6.72	2	Sodium propyl paraben	0.224
36.00	3	Magnesium aluminum silicate type IA (Veegum)	1.20
5.832 g	4	Kaolin powder	194.40
130.00	5	Pectin	4.33
120.00	6	Sodium CMC premium low viscosity	4.00
210.00	7	Cyclamate calcium	7.00
21.00	8	Saccharin calcium powder	0.70
15.37	9	Flavor	0.51
1.23	10	Flavor	41.13
QS	11	Water purified approximate	QS
QS	12	Acid citric anhydrous powder	QS

Manufacturing Directions

1. Charge 600 mL of water into a suitable jacketed mixing tank.
2. Add the methyl paraben and propyl paraben to the tank and heat to 90°C to 95°C.
3. Cool to 70°C, add the magnesium aluminum silicate, and mix for 30 minutes or until evenly dispersed.
4. Hold temperature at 70°C.
5. Add kaolin with constant mixing at 70°C until evenly dispersed.
6. Add pectin and mix for 2 hours, maintaining the temperature of 70°C.
7. Add the sodium CMC premium low viscosity and mix for at least 30 minutes, maintaining the temperature at 70°C.
8. Cool to 60°C and hold at this temperature. Add in order cyclamate calcium and saccharin calcium and mix thoroughly for 20 minutes.
9. While mixing, cool to room temperature and allow standing overnight to hydrate. After overnight standing (minimum 12 hours), mix for 30 minutes.
10. Mix while adding the flavors.
11. Check and record pH (range: 4.5–7.5). If pH is above 7.5, adjust with a 60% solution of citric acid to the desired pH.
12. Add water to 1 L and mix thoroughly for 3 hours. Strain product through muslin cloth into holding tanks and cover.

Kaolin–Pectin Suspension

Bill of Materials			
Scale (mg/5 mL)	Item	Material Name	Qty/L (g)
147.60	1	Sodium methyl paraben	4.920
6.72	2	Sodium propyl paraben	0.220
36.00	3	Magnesium aluminum silicate Type IA (Veegum)	1.200
486.60	4	Kaolin powder	0.190
43.40	5	Pectin	4.330
120.00	6	Sodium CMC premium low viscosity	4.000
210.00	7	Cyclamate calcium	7.000
21.00	8	Saccharin calcium	0.700
15.37	9	Flavor	0.510
1.23	10	Flavor	0.041

Manufacturing Directions

1. Charge 600 mL of water into a suitable jacketed mixing tank.
2. Add the methyl paraben and propyl paraben to the tank and heat to 90°C to 95°C.
3. Cool to 70°C, add the magnesium aluminum silicate, and mix for 30 minutes or until evenly dispersed.
4. Hold temperature at 70°C.
5. Add kaolin with constant mixing at 70°C until evenly dispersed.
6. Add pectin, and mix for 2 hours, maintaining a temperature of 70°C.
7. Add the premium low-viscosity sodium CMC and mix for at least 30 minutes, maintaining a temperature of 70°C.
8. Cool to 60°C and hold at this temperature.
9. Add, in order, cyclamate calcium and saccharin calcium and mix thoroughly for 20 minutes.
10. While mixing, cool to room temperature and allow to stand overnight to hydrate.
11. After overnight standing (minimum 12 hours), mix for 30 minutes.
12. Add flavors while mixing.
13. Check and record pH (range: 4.5–7.5). If pH is more than 7.5, adjust with a 60% solution of citric acid to the desired pH.
14. Add water to 1 L and mix thoroughly for 3 hours.
15. Strain product through muslin cloth into holding tanks and cover.

Ketoprofen Topical Solution

Bill of Materials			
Scale (mg/mL)	Item	Material Name	Qty/L (g)
QS	1	Vehicle (pluronic F 127 56.12%, ethanol 30.61, water 13.27%)	QS to 1 L
20.00	2	Ketoprofen	20.00
QS	3	Perfumes	QS

Manufacturing Directions

1. Screen the ketoprofen to reduce the particle size.
2. Add the ketoprofen into a clean vessel.
3. Add ethanol to the vessel.
4. Subsequently add poloxamer and water to the vessel.
5. Mix until uniform.

Ketotifen Syrup

Bill of Materials			
Scale (mg/mL)	Item	Material Name	Qty/L (g)
0.20	1	Ketotifen hydrogen fumarate	0.27
0.10	2	Flavor	0.10
0.17	3	Propyl paraben	0.17
0.33	4	Methyl paraben	0.33
2.10	5	Citric acid anhydrous	2.10
3.20	6	Disodium hydrogen phosphate anhydrous	3.20
20.00	7	Ethanol	20.00
300.00	8	Sucrose	300.00
350.00	9	Sorbitol	350.00
QS	10	Water purified	QS to 1 L

Manufacturing Directions

1. Take 1.5 L of purified water and heat to 90°C to 95°C, allow to cool down to 30°C, and bubble with nitrogen gas. Keep for batch preparation.
2. Dissolve the parabens in 1 L in a separate vessel and stir until the solution is completely clear. Add citric acid, disodium hydrogen phosphate anhydrous, sucrose, and sorbitol and stir slowly to dissolve until clear solution is obtained. Cool to room temperature.
3. In a separate container, dissolve ketotifen hydrogen fumarate in ethanol until clear.
4. Add the flavor to the alcoholic solution of ketotifen and dissolve.
5. Add the alcoholic mixture slowly to the syrup while stirring at room temperature avoiding entrapment of air.
6. Pass the syrup through 100-mesh screen and then through filter press until sparkling clear.

Lamivudine Oral Solution

Epivir oral solution is for oral administration. One milliliter of Epivir oral solution contains 10 mg lamivudine (10 mg/mL) in an aqueous solution and the inactive ingredients artificial strawberry and banana flavors, citric acid (anhydrous), methyl paraben, propylene glycol, propyl paraben, sodium citrate (dihydrate), and sucrose.

One milliliter of Epivir-HBV oral solution contains 5 mg of lamivudine (5 mg/mL) in an aqueous solution and the inactive ingredients artificial strawberry and banana flavors, citric acid (anhydrous), methyl paraben, propylene glycol, propyl paraben, sodium citrate (dihydrate), and sucrose.

Levalbuterol Hydrochloride Inhalation Solution

Xopenex (levalbuterol HCl) inhalation solution is supplied in unit-dose vials and requires no dilution before administration by nebulization. Each 3-mL unit-dose vial contains either 0.63 mg of levalbuterol (as 0.73 mg of levalbuterol HCl) or 1.25 mg of levalbuterol (as 1.44 mg of levalbuterol HCl), sodium chloride to adjust tonicity, and sulfuric acid to adjust the pH to 4.0 (3.3–4.5).

Levocarnitine Oral Solution

Each 118-mL container of Carnitor (levocarnitine) oral solution contains 1 g of levocarnitine/10 mL. It also contains artificial cherry flavor, D,L-malic acid, purified water, and sucrose syrup. Methyl paraben and propyl paraben are added as preservatives. The pH is approximately 5.

Linezolid for Oral Suspension

Zyvox for oral suspension is supplied as an orange-flavored granule/powder for constitution into a suspension for oral administration. Following constitution, each 5 mL contains 100 mg of linezolid. Inactive ingredients are sucrose, citric acid, sodium citrate, microcrystalline cellulose and carboxymethylcellulose sodium, aspartame, xanthan gum, mannitol, sodium benzoate, colloidal silicon dioxide, sodium chloride, and flavors.

Lithium Carbonate Solution

Each 5 mL of syrup for oral administration contains lithium ion (Li +) 8 mEq (equivalent to amount of lithium in 300 mg of lithium carbonate), alcohol 0.3% v/v.

Lithium Citrate Syrup

Each 5 mL of syrup for oral administration contains lithium ion 8 mEq (equivalent to amount of lithium in 300 mg of lithium carbonate), alcohol 0.3% v/v. Lithium citrate syrup is a palatable oral dosage form of lithium ion. Lithium citrate is prepared in solution from lithium hydroxide and citric acid in a ratio approximately dilithium citrate.

Lomustine Nasal Spray

Charge 112.5 g of micronized lomustine into a pressure-addition vessel. After sealing and evacuation thereof, 10.5 kg of HFA 227 that has been aerated with carbon dioxide and adjusted to a pressure of 4.5 bar (20°C) in another pressure addition vessel in which 312 g of ethanol has been initially introduced is added. After homogenization of this mixture, the formulation obtained is dispensed into aluminum containers sealed with metering valves by means of the pressure-filling technique.

Loracarbef for Oral Suspension

After reconstitution, each 5 mL of Lorabid for oral suspension contains loracarbef equivalent to 100 (0.286 mmol) or 200 mg (0.57 mmol) anhydrous loracarbef activity. The suspensions also contain cellulose, FD&C red No. 40, flavors, methyl paraben, propyl paraben, simethicone emulsion, sodium carboxymethylcellulose, sucrose, and xanthan gum.

Loratadine Syrup

Bill of Materials			
Scale (mg/5 mL)	Item	Material Name	Qty/L (g)
5.00	1	Loratadine	1.00
3000.00	2	Sucrose	600.00
10.00	3	Sodium benzoate	2.00
2.50	4	Saccharin sodium	0.50
12.50	5	Citric acid (monohydrate)	2.50
250.00	6	Glycerin (glycerol)	50.00
765.00	7	Propylene glycol	153.00
6.87	8	Hydrochloric acid 37% (concentrated)	1.51
6.25	9	All fruit flavor	1.25
1.50	10	Raspberry flavor	0.30
–	11	Water purified	QS to 1 L

Manufacturing Directions

Hydrochloric acid (concentrated) is very corrosive. Care should be taken during handling. Rubber gloves and protective goggles should be worn during dispensing and manufacturing.

1. Add 380 g of item 11 to a stainless steel manufacturing vessel and heat to 90°C to 95°C.
2. Add item 2 while mixing at slow speed at a temperature of 90°C to 95°C. Cool to 50°C.
3. Add items 3 to 6 in order while mixing at low speed at 50°C. Mix for 15 minutes at low speed. Cool to 30°C.
4. Take 13.53 g of item 11 in a stainless steel container. Add item 8 carefully. Add hydrochloric acid solution quantity 13.675 g to the manufacturing vessel. Adjust the pH between 2.3 and 2.4. If required, add the additional quantity and record. Discard the remaining quantity. Mix for 5 minutes.
5. Dissolve item 1 in 145 g of item 7 in a stainless steel drum while stirring. Add to the manufacturing vessel.
6. Rinse the stainless steel drum with 8 g of item 7. Transfer to manufacturing vessel.
7. Add items 9 and 10 in to manufacturing vessel. Mix for 5 minutes at low speed.
8. Make up the volume to 1 L with item 11.
9. Filter and fill.

Mafenide Acetate Topical Solution

Sulfamylon for 5% topical solution is provided in packets containing 50 g of sterile mafenide acetate to be reconstituted in 1000 mL of sterile water for irrigation or 0.9% sodium chloride irrigation. After mixing, the solution contains 5% w/v of mafenide acetate. The solution is an antimicrobial preparation suitable for topical administration.

Magaldrate Instant Powder for Dry Syrup

Bill of Materials			
Scale (mg/sachet)	Item	Material Name	Qty/1000 Sachets (g)
800.00	1	Magaldrate	800.00
640.00	2	Kollidon CL-M	640.00
200.00	3	Sorbitol, crystalline	200.00
40.00	4	Orange flavor	40.00
40.00	5	Kollidon 90F	40.00
4.00	6	Coconut flavor	4.00
4.00	7	Banana flavor	4.00
0.80	8	Saccharine sodium	0.80
QS	9	Water	~ 280 mL

Manufacturing Directions

1. Granulate mixture 1 to 4 with solution of items 5 to 9 and pass through a 0.8-mm sieve to obtain free-flowing granules.
2. Fill 2 g in sachets or 20 g in a 100-mL flask. Instant granules in sachets: Suspend 2 g (1 sachet) in a glass of water (800 mg magaldrate).

Magaldrate Suspension

Bill of Materials			
Scale (mg/mL)	Item	Material Name	Qty/L (g)
100.00	1	Magaldrate USP	100.00
80.00	2	Kollidon® CL-M	80.00
20.00	3	Kollidon® 90F	20.00
10.00	4	Orange flavor	10.00
0.50	5	Coconut flavor	0.50
0.80	6	Banana flavor	0.80
0.20	7	Saccharine sodium	0.20
QS	8	Preservatives	QS
QS	9	Water	QS to 1 L

Manufacturing Directions

1. Dissolve or suspend all the solids in water under aseptic conditions; pH should be approximately 9.

Magaldrate with Simethicone Suspension

Bill of Materials			
Scale (mg/5 mL)	Item	Material Name	Qty/L (g)
QS	1	Distilled purified water	285.00 mL
9.00	2	Methyl paraben	1.80
1.00	3	Propyl paraben	0.20
5.00	4	Benzoic acid	1.00
3.75	5	Saccharin sodium (dihydrate powder)	0.75
400.00	6	Magaldrate (wet cake; 18–20%)	400.00
1.00 g	7	Sorbitol solution (70%)	260.00
12.50	8	Silicon dioxide (colloidal) (International)	2.50
QS	9	Citric acid (hydrous powder)	QS
200.00	10	Dimethyl polysiloxane emulsion (30%)	40.00
0.005 mL	11	Flavor	1.00 mL
1.26 g	12	Glycerin	252.00
25.00 g	13	Potassium citrate monohydrate	5.00
13.30	14	Xanthan gum	2.66

Manufacturing Directions

This product is highly prone to microbial contamination. All equipment coming into contact with the product should be treated with a freshly prepared sodium hypochlorite solution (100 ppm), made with freshly boiled and cooled down water on the day of use. Bottles and caps should also be so treated. Freshly boiled and cooled deionized water should be used for rinsing.

1. Charge 285 mL purified water into a suitable jacketed tank and heat to 90°C to 95°C.
2. Add and dissolve parabens, benzoic acid, saccharin sodium, and potassium citrate.
3. While maintaining temperature at 85°C to 90°C, add, in small quantities, half the quantity of magaldrate cake or powder, if used, and disperse well.
4. Adjust speed of the agitator and homogenizer to ensure effective mixing and to maintain free mobility of the suspension. Add sorbitol solution and mix well.
5. Raise the temperature, if necessary, maintaining temperature at 85°C to 90°C.
6. Add in small quantities the remaining half of the magaldrate cake or powder and disperse well.
7. Mix for 1 hour and then remove heat. (Adjust speed of the agitator and homogenizer to maintain the mobility of suspension.) Separately blend colloidal silicon dioxide with xanthan gum and disperse the blend in glycerin, with constant mixing.
8. While maintaining temperature at 85°C to 95°C, add and disperse the suspension from the previous step to the main tank and mix well.
9. Avoid lump formation at any stage.

10. Cool to room temperature.
11. Add dimethyl polysiloxane emulsion and mix well.
12. Add flavor and mix well.
13. Dissolve citric acid in twice the quantity of purified water and adjust pH if necessary.
14. Check and record pH (range: 7.5–8.0). Add purified water to volume and mix well for a minimum of 30 minutes.
15. Filter through a 180-μm aperture nylon cloth and store in a suitable tank.

Magaldrate with Simethicone Suspension

Bill of Materials			
Scale (mg/5 mL)	Item	Material Name	Qty/L (g)
QS	1	Water purified	QS to 1 L
9.00	2	Methyl paraben	1.80
1.00	3	Propyl paraben	0.20
5.00	4	Acid benzoic	1.00
3.75	5	Saccharin sodium powder dihydrate	0.75
2.00 g	6	Magaldrate wet cake (18 to 20%)	400.00
1.00 g	7	Sorbitol solution	260.00
12.50	8	Silicon dioxide colloidal (international)	2.50
QS	9	Acid citric powder hydrous	QS
200.00	10	Dimethyl polysiloxane emulsion (30%)	40.00
0.005 mL	11	Flavor	1.000 mL
1.26 g	12	Glycerin	252.00
25.00 g	13	Potassium citrate monohydrate	5.00
13.30	14	Xanthan gum	2.66

Manufacturing Directions

This product is highly prone to microbial contamination. All equipment coming into contact with the product should be treated with a freshly prepared sodium hypochlorite solution (100 ppm) made with freshly boiled and cooled town water on the day of use. Bottles and caps should also be so treated. Freshly boiled and cooled purified water should be used for rinsing.

1. Charge 285 mL purified water into a suitable jacketed tank and heat to 90°C to 95°C.
2. Add and dissolve parabens, acid benzoic, saccharin sodium, and potassium citrate.
3. While maintaining temperature at 85°C to 90°C, add, in small quantities, half the quantity of magaldrate cake or powder, if used, and disperse well. (Adjust the speed of agitator and of the homogenizer to ensure effective mixing and to maintain free mobility of the suspension.)
4. Add sorbitol solution and mix well. Raise the temperature, if necessary, maintaining temperature at 85°C to 90°C.
5. Add, in small quantities, the remaining half of magaldrate cake or powder and disperse well. Mix for 1 hour and then remove heat. (Adjust the speed of the agitator and of the homogenizer to maintain the mobility of suspension.)
6. Separately blend silicon dioxide colloidal with xanthan gum and disperse the blend in glycerin with constant mixing.
7. While maintaining temperature at 85°C to 95°C, add and disperse the suspension from previous step to the main tank and mix well. Avoid lump formation at any stage. Cool to room temperature.
8. Add dimethyl polysiloxane emulsion and mix well.
9. Add flavor and mix well. Dissolve acid citric in twice the quantity of purified water and adjust pH if necessary. Check and record pH (range: 7.5–8.0).
10. Add purified water to volume and mix well for a minimum of 30 minutes.
11. Filter through a 180-micron aperture nylon cloth and store in a suitable tank.

Mebendazole Oral Suspension

Bill of Materials			
Scale (mg/5 mL)	Item	Material Name	Qty/L (g)
102.00	1	Mebendazole[a]	20.40
10.00	2	Methyl paraben	2.00
1.00	3	Propyl paraben	0.20
750.00	4	Propylene glycol	150.00
8.25	5	Sodium citrate	1.65
7.50	6	Saccharin sodium	1.50
0.55	7	Citric acid (monohydrate)	0.11
52.50	8	Microcrystalline cellulose	10.50
25.00	9	Carboxymethylcellulose sodium	5.00
7.50	10	Polysorbate 80	1.50
12.50	11	All fruits flavor	2.50
–	12	Water purified	QS to 1 L

[a]2 mg/5 mL mebendazole added as an extra to compensate the loss on drying and assay of the material.

Manufacturing Directions

1. Load 300 g of item 12 (25–30°C) in mixer. In it dissolve items 5, 6, and 7 while stirring at a speed of 18 rpm.
2. Dissolve items 2 and 3 in 30 g of item 4 (45°C) in a stainless steel container while stirring by stirrer.
3. Cool to 25°C to 30°C.
4. Add the paraben solution into step 1 while mixing.
5. Disperse item 8 in 200 g of item 12 (25–30°C) in a stainless steel container while stirring by stirrer. Keep aside for 1 hour for complete hydration.
6. Disperse item 9 in 100 g of item 12 (70°C) in a stainless steel container while stirring by stirrer.
7. Cool to 25°C to 30°C. Keep aside for 1 hour for complete gelation. Cooling is necessary for gelation.
8. Dissolve item 10 in 20 g of item 12 (50°C) in a stainless steel container while stirring by stirrer.
9. Cool to 30°C. Add 120 g of item 4 while mixing.
10. Disperse item 1 while mixing. Keep aside for complete levigation.
11. Add the Avicel dispersion and sodium CMC dispersion from step 3 and step 4 into mixer in step 1. Mix and homogenize at mixer speed 18 rpm, homogenizer low speed, and vacuum 0.4 to 0.6 bar for 10 minutes.
12. Add the mebendazole dispersion from step 5 into mixer in step 1. Mix and homogenize at mixer speed 18 rpm, homogenizer low speed, and vacuum 0.4 to 0.6 bar for 10 minutes.
13. Add item 11 into step 6. Make up the volume up to 1 L with item 12. Mix at a speed of 18 rpm for 5 minutes.
14. Check the suspension for homogeneity. Transfer the suspension through 630-micron sieve to stainless steel storage tank, previously sanitized by 70% ethanol.

Mebendazole Suspension

Bill of Materials			
Scale (mg/mL)	Item	Material Name	Qty/L (g)
20.00	1	Mebendazole	20.00
30.00	2	Lutrol F 127	30.00
1.80	3	Methyl paraben	1.80
0.20	4	Propyl paraben	0.20
QS	5	Water purified	QS

Manufacturing Directions

1. Charge 80% of item 5 in a stainless steel jacketed vessel. Heat to 90°C to 95°C.
2. Add items 3 and 4 and stir to dissolve.
3. Cool to 40°C and add item 2. Stir to dissolve completely.
4. Add item 1 and mix well. Homogenize if necessary.

Megestrol Acetate Oral Suspension

Megace oral suspension is supplied as an oral suspension containing 40 mg of micronized megestrol acetate per milliliter. Megace oral suspension contains the following inactive ingredients: alcohol (maximum of 0.06% v/v from flavor), citric acid, lemon-lime flavor, polyethylene glycol, polysorbate 80, purified water, sodium benzoate, sodium citrate, sucrose, and xanthan gum.

Bill of Materials			
Scale (mg/mL)	Item	Material Name	Qty/L (g)
40.00	1	Megestrol acetate	40.00
100.00	2	Glycerin	100.00
100.00	3	Sorbitol	100.00
0.30	4	Polysorbate 90	0.30
2.20	5	Xanthan gum	2.20
2.00	6	Sodium benzoate	2.00
0.60	7	Sodium citrate	0.60
50.00	8	Sucrose	50.00
0.80	9	Lemon flavor	0.80
QS	10	Water purified	QS to 1 L

Manufacturing Directions

1. Charge glycerol, sorbitol, and polysorbate in a suitable container. Mix well.
2. Charge xanthan gum in a separate vessel with item 10 and allow overnight hydration.
3. Add sodium citrates, sucrose, sodium benzoate, and flavor to step 1 and then add step 2 to step 1.
4. Pass the gum slurry through a screen.
5. Add megestrol acetate and pass then suspension through a colloid mill or homogenizer to provide a uniform oral suspension.

Menthol and Benzocaine Solution

Bill of Materials			
Scale (mg/mg)	Item	Material Name	Qty/kg (g)
QS	1	Vehicle (pluronic F 108 56.79%, ethanol 21.69%, water 21.52%)	QS to 1 kg
10.00	2	Menthol	10.00
20.00	3	Benzocaine	20.00
0.05	4	Eucalyptus oil	0.05
1.00	5	Sodium saccharin	1.00
0.50	6	Monoammonium glycyrrhizinate	0.50
QS	7	Flavors and colors	QS

Manufacturing Directions

1. Mill and screen the menthol and benzocaine to reduce the product particle size.
2. Add the menthol, benzocaine, sodium saccharin, and monoammonium glycyrrhizinate into a clean vessel.
3. Add eucalyptus oil and ethanol to the vessel.
4. Subsequently add the poloxamer and water to the vessel.
5. Mix until uniform.

Menthol Mouthwash

Bill of Materials			
Scale (mg/mL)	Item	Material Name	Qty/L (g)
10.00	1	Menthol	10.00
10.00	2	Eucalyptus oil	10.00
40.00	3	Cremophor RH 40	40.00
4.50	4	Saccharin sodium	4.50
2.00	5	Sodium citrate	2.00
5.00	6	Citric acid	5.00
50.00	7	Lutrol F 127	50.00
67.00	8	Ethanol 96%	67.00
QS	9	Sicovit colorant	QS
801.00	10	Water	801.00

Manufacturing Directions

1. Mix components 1 to 3 and heat to approximately 60°C.
2. Prepare solution of items 4 to 10, heat to approximately 60°C, and add it slowly to the well-stirred mixture of items 1 to 3.
3. Clear, colored liquids having a fresh mint taste are the desired result.

Mesalamine Rectal Suspension Enema

The active ingredient in rectal suspension enema, a disposable (60 mL) unit, is mesalamine, also known as 5-aminosalicylic acid. Each rectal suspension enema unit contains 4 g of mesalamine. In addition to mesalamine, the preparation contains the inactive ingredients carbomer 934P, EDTA, potassium acetate, potassium metabisulfite, purified water, and xanthan gum. Sodium benzoate is added as a preservative. The disposable unit consists of an applicator tip protected by a polyethylene cover and lubricated with white petrolatum. The unit has a one-way valve to prevent backflow of the dispensed product.

Mesalamine Rectal Suspension

Each rectal suspension enema unit contains 4 g of mesalamine. In addition to mesalamine, the preparation contains the inactive ingredients carbomer 934P, EDTA, potassium acetate, potassium metabisulfite, purified water, and xanthan gum. Sodium benzoate is added as a preservative.

Metformin Liquid

Bill of Materials			
Scale (mg/mL)	Item	Material Name	Qty/L (g)
100.00	1	Metformin hydrochloride	100.00
400.00	2	Xylitol	400.00
5.00	3	Potassium bicarbonate	5.00
1.20	4	Potassium sorbate	1.20
2.75	5	Sodium saccharin	2.75
0.004 mL	6	Hydrochloric acid	4.00 mL
2.75	7	Wild cherry flavor	2.75
QS	8	Water purified	QS to 1 L

Manufacturing Directions

1. Under continuous stirring, add potassium bicarbonate and metformin hydrochloride to purified water and dissolve to get a clear solution.
2. Add hydrochloric acid solution as a dilute solution (approximately one molar) to the mixture of the previous step. This results in carbon dioxide gas formation (effervescent gas).
3. Add xylitol at a temperature of NMT 31°C and stir to get a clear solution.
4. Continue stirring and add artificial cherry flavor and saccharin.
5. Adjust the pH to a range of 4.6 to 4.9 using dilute solution of hydrochloric acid (if required).
6. Make up the volume and filter through clarifying grade filter and fill in approved container.

Metoclopramide Oral Solution

Bill of Materials			
Scale (mg/mL)	Item	Material Name	Qty/L (g)
4.00	1	Metoclopramide HCl, 10% excess	4.40
0.76	2	Saccharin sodium	0.76
1.00	3	Sorbic acid	1.00
1.48	4	Sodium metabisulfite (sodium disufite)	1.48
0.10	5	Polyoxyl 35 castor oil (Cremophor EL)	0.10
5.20	6	Sodium citrate	5.20
8.52	7	Citric acid (monohydrate)	8.52
–	8	Water purified	QS to 1 L

Manufacturing Directions

1. Load 80 g of item 8 to the mixer and heat to 90°C to 95°C.
2. Dissolve items 2 and 3 while stirring. Mix for 15 minutes at high speed to get clear solution.
3. Cool the temperature to 25°C.
4. Transfer the solution to drops manufacturing vessel.
5. Add item 5 to the drops manufacturing vessel at step 4, while stirring to dissolve.
6. Add 8 g of item 8 (25°C) in a separate container and dissolve items 6 and 7 using stirrer and transfer to the drops manufacturing vessel at step 5.
7. Add item 4 to the drops manufacturing vessel at step 6 while mixing.
8. Add 5 g of item 8 (25°C) in a separate container and dissolve item 1 using stirrer.
9. Transfer this solution to the drops manufacturing vessel at step 7 while mixing.
10. Check and record the pH (limit: 3.4–3.6).
11. Adjust the pH if required using 5% aqueous solution of citric acid or sodium citrate.
12. Make up the volume up to 1 L with item 8 (25°C).
13. Assemble the membrane filter of 0.2 micron. Filter the solution and collect the filtrate in clean HDPE containers.

Metoclopramide Syrup

Bill of Materials			
Scale (mg/5 mL)	Item	Material Name	Qty/L (g)
30.00	1	Hydroxyethyl cellulose	6.00
4.00	2	Methyl paraben	0.80
1.00	3	Propyl paraben	0.20
5.00	4	Sorbic acid	1.00
14.25	5	Citric acid (monohydrate)	2.85
4.60	6	Sodium citrate	0.92
7.50	7	Saccharin sodium	1.50
5.00	8	Metoclopramide HCl (14% excess)	1.14
40.00	9	Alcohol (ethanol 95%)	8.00
25.00	10	Propylene glycol	5.00
6.50	11	Flavor	1.30
10.00	12	Caramel	2.00
0.50	13	Flavor	0.10
–	14	Water purified	QS to 1 L

Manufacturing Directions

1. Add 200 g of item 14 to the mixer and heat to 90°C.
2. Sprinkle item 1 slowly while mixing at 20 rpm in manual mode. Check that item 1 is dispersed completely without forming lumps.
3. Start the homogenizer at high speed with recirculation, vacuum 0.4 bar.
4. Homogenize for 15 minutes at high speed. Cool to approximately 60°C.
5. Add 200 g of item 14 in a storage container.
6. Transfer the homogenized mucilage to the storage container (step 5).
7. Add 500 g of item 14 to the syrup vessel and heat to 90°C.
8. Add items 2, 3, and 4 to the syrup vessel and mix at high speed for 15 minutes to dissolve. Start cooling until temperature reaches at 50°C to 60°C.
9. Withdraw a portion of the solution and check that it is clear and colorless.
10. Transfer the mucilage to the syrup vessel and mix at high speed for 15 minutes. Start cooling and cool to 30°C.
11. Add 20 g of item 4 (25°C) in a separate container, dissolve items 5 and 6 by using stirrer, and add solution to the manufacturing vessel.
12. Add 10 g of item 14 (25°C) in a separate container, dissolve item 7 by using stirrer, and add solution to the manufacturing vessel.
13. Withdraw a portion of the solution and check that it is clear and colorless.
14. Add 10 g of item 14 (25°C) in a separate container, dissolve item 8 by using stirrer, and add solution to the manufacturing vessel.
15. Rinse the container with 5 g of item 14 (25°C) cooled and transfer the rinsing to the syrup vessel. Mix at high speed for 20 minutes.
16. Withdraw a portion of the solution and check that it is clear and colorless.
17. Mix items 9 and 10 in a clean stainless steel container. Add items 11, 12, and 13 and mix well manually.
18. Transfer the solution to the manufacturing vessel and mix for 15 minutes at high speed.
19. Make up the volume to 1 L with item 14 (25°C) and, finally, mix for 20 minutes at high speed.
20. Check and record the color and pH (limit: 2.9–3.1). Color should be clear to faint yellow.
21. Suspend 1 g of the filter aid in 40 g of cooled item 14 (25°C) and stir well. Allow the filter aid to settle. Decant off the water.
22. Transfer the washed filter aid to the syrup vessel while mixing. Mix for 30 minutes at high speed.
23. Assemble the filter press.
24. Wash the filters using approximately 250 L purified water (25°C) by passing through filters at 0.2 bar.
25. Filter the syrup at 1 bar. Recirculate approximately 100 to 150 mL syrup.
26. Transfer the filtered syrup to the storage vessel.

Metronidazole Suspension

Bill of Materials			
Scale (mg/5 mL)	Item	Material Name	Qty/L (g)
125.00	1	Metronidazole (use metronidazole benzoate)	40.20
7.50	2	Methyl paraben	1.50
1.00	3	Propyl paraben	0.20
2500.00	4	Sucrose	500.00
7.50	5	Saccharin sodium	1.50
8.75	6	Sodium phosphate monobasic	1.75
8.75	7	Sodium phosphate dibasic	1.75
40.00	8	Magnesium aluminium silicate	8.00
30.00	9	Microcrystalline cellulose	6.00
650.00	10	Propylene glycol	130.00
7.50	11	Lemon flavor	1.50
7.50	12	Bergamot flavor	1.50
–	13	Water purified	QS to 1 L

Note: For 200 mg/5 mL strength use 64.400 g of metronidazole benzoate.

Manufacturing Directions

1. Disperse item 1 in item 10 in a stainless steel vessel, using stirrer. Make smooth slurry and keep aside for use later.
2. Add 186 g of item 13 to a vessel and heat to 90°C to 95°C. Dissolve items 2 and 3 while mixing.
3. Add and dissolve item 4 while mixing at a temperature of 90°C to 95°C.
4. Cool down to 50°C to 55°C.
5. In a stainless steel container, dissolve item 5 in 4 g of item 13 and add to the vessel while mixing.
6. Filter the syrup. Collect the syrup in stainless steel tank.
7. Disperse item 8 in 120 g of hot item 13 (70–75°C) in stainless steel vessel, using stirrer. Keep on stirring for 30 minutes. Transfer the dispersion into mixer by vacuum.
8. Mix and homogenize at temperature 70°C to 80°C, mixer speed 18 rpm, homogenizer at high speed, and vacuum 0.4 to 0.6 bar for 10 minutes.
9. Cool down to 25°C to 30°C.
10. Disperse item 9 in 120 g of item 13 in stainless steel vessel, using stirrer. Keep on stirring for 30 minutes to make smooth dispersion.
11. Transfer the filtered syrup from step 7 and transfer Avicel mucilage from step 4 to mixer. Set the mixer to 25°C to 30°C, 18 rpm, high speed and vacuum 0.4 to 0.6 bar.
12. Mix and homogenize for 10 minutes.
13. Dissolve items 6 and 7 in 12 g of item 13 and add to mixer while mixing.
14. Add metronidazole benzoate and propylene glycol dispersion (step 1) to mixer.
15. Rinse the drug container with 10 g of item 13 and add the rinsing to mixer to avoid loss.
16. Add items 11 and 12 to mixer. Make up the volume to 1 L with item 13.
17. Mix and homogenize for 20 minutes at high speed, vacuum 0.4 to 0.6 bar. Check the suspension for homogeneity. Transfer the suspension through 630-micron sieve to stainless steel storage tank, previously sanitized by 70% ethanol.
18. Do not store the bulk suspension more than 48 hours in the storage tank without stirring. Before filling, stir not less than 30 minutes for uniform dispersion to avoid problem of content uniformity.

Mineral and Multivitamin Syrup

Bill of Materials			
Scale (mg/mL)	Item	Material Name	Qty/L (g)
6.65	1	Hypophosphorous acid	6.655
16.47	2	Calcium hypophosphite	16.47
31.68	3	Calcium lactate (powder)	31.68
1.00	4	Methyl paraben	1.00
0.20	5	Propyl paraben	0.20
1.00	6	Benzoic acid	1.00
150.00	7	Sucrose (granular)	150.00
5.20	8	Ferrous gluconate	5.20
2.00	9	Niacinamide (5% excess)	2.10
0.328	10	Riboflavin-5-phosphate sodium	0.33
1.00	11	D-Pantothenyl alcohol (dexpanthenol; 20% excess)	1.20
0.60 μg	12	Vitamin B_{12} (cyanocobalamin) (35% excess)	0.81 mg
0.20	13	Pyridoxine hydrochloride	0.20
0.30	14	Thiamine hydrochloride (regular powder) (55% excess)	0.46
4.782	15	Flavor, raspberry blend	4.78
1.945	16	Flavor, chocolate	1.945
0.642	17	Orange oil (terpeneless, No. 54125)	0.64
0.21	18	Lime oil, distilled	0.215
4.28	19	Alcohol	4.28
2.50	20	Saccharin sodium	2.50
10.00	21	Ascorbic acid (white powder/EP) (45% excess)	14.50
3.00	22	Caramel (acid proof)	3.00
2.00	23	Anhydrous citric acid	2.00
10.0 μg	24	Butylated hydroxyanisole (BHA)	10.00 mg
3.39	25	Corn oil	3.39
0.40	26	Vitamin A palmitate (1.5 MM U/g) (40% excess)	0.56
0.08	27	Viosterol in corn oil (syn. oleovitamin D; 1000 mg/g) (40% excess)	0.112
1.5 G	28	Acacia (special grade)	1.50
0.127	29	Sodium lauryl sulfate (acetone-washed)	0.127
171.00	30	Deionized, purified water	~171
QS	31	Glucose liquid (corn syrup)	QS to 1 L

Manufacturing Directions

Do not expose this preparation during manufacturing to direct sunlight. Riboflavin is sensitive to light.

1. Add 83.7 mL purified water to a stainless steel jacketed tank.
2. Add calcium hypophosphite, calcium lactate, the parabens, and benzoic acid.
3. Heat mixture to 60°C with agitation.
4. Shut off mixer and wash tank until free of all powders with 25.9 mL purified water.
5. Heat to and maintain a maximum temperature of 100°C until solution is complete. Do not agitate. Avoid loss of water through evaporation; cover opening of tank.
6. After solution occurs, take sample from bottom of tank and examine for clarity. Solution must be clear.
7. Add hypophosphorous acid (if used) with mixing.
8. Turn off heat, add 222 g glucose, and start agitator. (*Caution*: Use CO_2 cover throughout; wherever water is used, it should be CO_2-saturated water.) Dissolve ferrous gluconate in 7.4 mL water CO_2-saturated by heating.
9. Add 278 g glucose with mixing. Add and dissolve sugar.
10. Allow solution to cool to 35°C and mix well.

11. To 29.6 mL water add and dissolve nicotinamide, riboflavin, D-pantothenyl alcohol, vitamin B_{12}, pyridoxine, and thiamine. Mix until solution is complete and add to tank. Dissolve by heat, if necessary.
12. Charge raspberry blend flavor and chocolate flavor into tank; charge saccharin into tank and mix until dissolved.
13. Charge ascorbic acid into tank. Mix well.
14. Charge caramel into tank and mix well.
15. Dissolve citric acid in 3 mL water and add.
16. Heat corn oil to 50°C to 60°C and add and dissolve BHA. Ensure the BHA is completely dissolved before continuing.
17. Cool to room temperature. While cooling oil mixture, saturate with CO_2 and maintain heavy CO_2 coverage for balance of operation.
18. Set aside a small amount of this mixture as a rinse for the vitamin A and viosterol containers in step above.
19. Add vitamin A palmitate and viosterol to the cool corn oil mixture, rinsing the containers with the oil reserved above.
20. Add the rinse to the bulk. Mix well.
21. Add the acacia to the oil mixture with good mixing.
22. Dissolve sodium lauryl sulfate in 3 mL CO_2-saturated purified water. To avoid excessive foaming, do not bubble CO_2 gas through the water/sodium lauryl sulfate solution.
23. Add the sodium lauryl sulfate solution to the oil mixture and stir to a thick creamy emulsion.
24. Add 7.56 g glucose to the emulsion with mixing.
25. Blend 13.33 mL CO_2-saturated purified water with 77.04 g glucose and add emulsion with stirring.
26. Recycle primary emulsion back into holding tank while setting mill.
27. Homogenize until all oil globules are less than 8 μm in diameter using colloid mill with a very fine setting. Do not change mill setting after removing sample unless samples are unacceptable.
28. Add primary emulsion to syrup solution with mixing; add glucose QS to 965 mL and mix well. Allow to stand overnight to vent entrapped air.
29. Adjust the volume to 1 L using glucose or glucose and CO_2-saturated water.
30. Strain through 149-μm aperture or similar screen into clean reserve tank and recheck volume.

Minoxidil Solution

Minoxidil 5% w/v; alcohol, 30% v/v; propylene glycol, 50% v/v; and purified water.

Mint–Menthol Mouthwash

Bill of Materials			
Scale (mg/mL)	Item	Material Name	Qty/L (g)
20.00	1	Mint oil	20.00
0.40	2	Menthol	0.40
0.90	3	Eucalyptus oil	0.90
10.00	4	Alpha-bisabolol (BASF)	10.00
0.60	5	Thymian oil	0.60
40.00	6	Cremophor RH 40	40.00
4.50	7	Saccharin sodium	4.50
2.00	8	Sodium citrate	2.00
5.00	9	Citric acid	5.00
0.20	10	Sodium fluoride	0.20
50.00	11	Glycerol	50.00
50.00	12	Lutrol F 127	50.00
0.60	13	Salicylic acid	0.60
1.00	14	Benzoic acid	1.00
175.00	15	Sorbitol, crystalline	175.00
216.00	16	Ethanol 96%	216.00
QS	17	Sicovit colorant	QS
QS	18	Water	48.4

Manufacturing Directions

1. Mix components 1 to 6 and heat to approximately 60°C.
2. Prepare solution of items 7 to 18, heat to approximately 60°C.
3. Add this solution slowly to the well-stirred mixture of items 1 to 6. The result is a clear, colored liquid having a fresh mint taste.

Mint–Menthol Mouthwash

Bill of Materials			
Scale (mg/mL)	Item	Material Name	Qty/L (g)
20.00	1	Mint oil	20.00
0.40	2	Menthol	0.40
0.90	3	Eucalyptus oil	0.90
10.00	4	α-Bisabolol (BASF)	10.00
0.60	5	Thymian oil	0.60
40.00	6	Cremophor RH 40	40.00
4.50	7	Saccharin sodium	4.50
2.00	8	Sodium citrate	2.00
5.00	9	Citric acid	5.00
0.20	10	Sodium fluoride	0.20
50.00	11	Glycerol	50.00
50.00	12	Lutrol F 127	50.00
0.60	13	Salicylic acid	0.60
1.00	14	Benzoic acid	1.00
175.00	15	Sorbitol, crystalline	175.00
216.00	16	Ethanol 96%	216.00
QS	17	Sicovit colorant	QS
QS	18	Water	48.40

Manufacturing Directions

1. Mix items 1 to 6 and heat to approximately 60°C.
2. Prepare solution of items 7 to 18, heat it to approximately 60°C, and add it slowly to the well-stirred mixture of items 1 to 6.
3. Clear, colored liquids have a fresh mint taste.

Mint Oil Solution

Bill of Materials			
Scale (mg/mL)	Item	Material Name	Qty/L (g)
35.00	1	Peppermint oil	35.00
138.00	2	Cremophor RH 40	138.00
520.00	3	Ethanol 96%	520.00
QS	4	Water	307.00

Manufacturing Directions

1. Mix the peppermint oil with Cremophor RH 40, stir well, and slowly add ethanol and water.
2. Clear, colorless liquid is of low viscosity.

Mint Oil Solution

Bill of Materials			
Scale (mg/mL)	Item	Material Name	Qty/L (g)
35.00	1	Peppermint oil	35.00
138.00	2	Cremophor RH 40	138.00
520.00	3	Ethanol 96%	520.00
307.00	4	Water	307.00

Manufacturing Directions

1. Mix peppermint oil with Cremophor RH 40 and stir well.
2. Slowly add ethanol and water. A clear, colorless liquid of low viscosity is the result.

Mometasone Furoate Nasal Spray

Nasonex nasal spray, 50 μg, is a metered-dose manual-pump spray unit containing an aqueous suspension of mometasone furoate monohydrate equivalent to 0.05% w/w mometasone furoate, calculated on the anhydrous basis, in an aqueous medium containing glycerin, microcrystalline cellulose and carboxymethylcellulose sodium, sodium citrate, 0.25% w/w phenylethyl alcohol, citric acid, benzalkonium chloride, and polysorbate 80. The pH is between 4.3 and 4.9.

Monosulfiram Solution

Bill of Materials			
Scale (%, w/w)	Item	Material Name	Qty/kg (g)
25.00	1	Monosulfiram	250.00
10.00	2	Dispersol	100.00
QS	3	Methylated spirit	QS to 1 kg

Manufacturing Directions

1. Liquefy item 1 by warming to 40°C.
2. Charge item 3 in a suitable dry stainless steel mixing vessel.
3. Add item 2 to step 2 and then add item 1 with constant stirring until clear solution obtained.
4. Filter through a suitable clarifying filter.

Multivitamin and Calcium Syrup

Bill of Materials			
Scale (mg/g)	Item	Material Name	Qty/100 g (mg)
0.10	1	Vitamin A palmitate	10.00
0.50 μg	2	Vitamin D 40 mio IU/g	0.05
1.00	3	Vitamin E acetate, BASF	100.00
0.02	4	Butylhydroxytoluene	2.00
45.00	5	Cremophor RH 40	4.50 g
100.00	6	Water	10.00 g
450.00	7	Saccharose	45.00 g
2.00	8	Methyl paraben	200.00
0.80	9	Citric acid	80.00
96.00	10	Glycerol	9.60 g
0.70	11	Calcium gluconate	70.00
250.00	12	Water	25.00 g
0.15	13	Thiamine hydrochloride, BASF	15.00
0.15	14	Riboflavin 5′-phosphate sodium	15.00
0.55	15	Nicotinamide	55.00
0.15	16	Pyridoxine hydrochloride	15.00
3.00	17	Ascorbic acid, crystalline	300.00
1.00	18	Sorbic acid	100.00
50.00	19	Propylene glycol (Pharma)	5.00 g

Manufacturing Directions

1. Heat items 1 to 5 and item 6 separately to approximately 60°C and mix slowly, stirring well to obtain a clear solution.
2. Dissolve items 7 to 9 in the hot solution of items 10 to 12 to obtain a clear solution.
3. Mix all the solutions upon cooling and add solutions of items 13 to 19; adjust the pH value to 4.0 to 4.1.
4. Pass during 10 minutes nitrogen through the solution and fill in bottles under nitrogen cover.

Multivitamin and Mineral Syrup

Bill of Materials			
Scale (mg/tablet)	Item	Material Name	Qty/L (g)
6.65	1	Hypophosphorous acid (50% pure)	6.655
16.47	2	Calcium hypophosphite	16.47
31.68	3	Calcium lactate (powder)	31.68
1.00	4	Methyl paraben	1.00
0.20	5	Propyl paraben	200.00 mg
1.00	6	Acid benzoic	1.00
150.00	7	Sucrose	150.00
5.20	8	Ferrous gluconate	5.20
2.00	9	Niacinamide (white powder) (5% excess)	2.10
0.32	10	Riboflavin-5-phosphate sodium	328.77 mg
1.00	11	D-Pantothenyl alcohol (dexpanthenol; 20% excess)	1.20
0.00060	12	Vitamin B_{12} (cyanocobalamin; 35% excess)	810.00 μg
0.20	13	Pyridoxine hydrochloride	200.00 mg
0.30	14	Thiamine hydrochloride (powder, regular) (55% excess)	465.00 mg
4.78	15	Flavor, raspberry blend	4.782
1.94	16	Flavor, chocolate	1.945
0.64	17	Orange oil, terpeneless No. 54125	642.00 mg
0.21	18	Lime oil (distilled)	214.975 mg
4.28	19	Alcohol (ethanol, 190 proof)	4.28
2.50	20	Saccharin sodium	2.50
10.00	21	Acid ascorbic (45% excess)	14.50
3.00	22	Caramel (acid proof)	3.00
2.00	23	Anhydrous citric acid	2.00
0.0010	24	Butylated hydroxyanisole (BHA)	10.0 mg
3.39	25	Corn oil	3.39
0.56	26	Vitamin A palmitate (1.5 MM UA/g) (40% excess)	560.00 mg
0.08	27	Viosterol in corn oil (syn. oleovitamin D; 1000 mD/g; D_3 in arachis oil) (40% excess)	112.00 mg
1.50	28	Acacia	1.50
0.12	29	Sodium lauryl sulfate (acetone washed)	127.41 mg
171.00	30	Purified water	~171
QS	31	Glucose liquid	QS to 1 L

Manufacturing Directions

Do not expose this preparation during manufacturing to direct sunlight. Riboflavin is sensitive to light.

1. Add 83.7 mL of purified water to a stainless steel jacketed tank.
2. Add calcium hypophosphite, calcium lactate, parabens, and benzoic acid.
3. Heat mixture to 60°C with agitation.
4. Shut off mixer and wash tank free of all powders with 25.9 mL purified water.
5. Heat to and maintain a maximum temperature of 100°C until solution is complete. Do not agitate. Avoid loss of water through evaporation. Cover opening of tank. After solution occurs, take sample from bottom of tank and examine for clarity. Solution must be clear.
6. Add acid hypophosphorous (if used) with mixing.
7. Turn off heat and add 222 g glucose and start agitator. (*Caution*: Use CO_2 cover throughout; wherever water is used, it should be CO_2-saturated water.) Dissolve ferrous gluconate in 7.4 mL water CO_2 saturated by heating.
8. Add 278 g glucose with mixing. Add and dissolve sugar.
9. Allow solution to cool to 35°C and mix well.
10. To 29.6 mL water, add and dissolve nicotinamide, riboflavin, D-pantothenyl alcohol, vitamin B_{12}, pyridoxine, and thiamine.
11. Mix until solution is complete and add to tank. Dissolve by heat, if necessary.

12. Charge raspberry blend flavor and chocolate flavor into tank.
13. Charge saccharin into tank and mix until dissolved.
14. Charge ascorbic acid into tank and mix well.
15. Charge caramel into tank and mix well.
16. Dissolve citric acid in 3 mL water and add this solution to above.
17. Heat corn oil to 50°C to 60°C and add and dissolve BHA. Ensure the BHA is completely dissolved before continuing.
18. Cool to room temperature. While cooling oil mixture, saturate with CO_2 and maintain heavy CO_2 coverage for balance of operation.
19. Set aside a small amount of this mixture as a rinse for the vitamin A and viosterol containers in previous step.
20. Add vitamin A palmitate and viosterol to the cool corn oil mixture, rinsing the containers with the oil reserved earlier.
21. Add the rinse to the bulk and mix well.
22. Add the acacia to the oil mixture with good mixing.
23. Dissolve sodium lauryl sulfate in 3 mL CO_2-saturated purified water. To avoid excessive foaming, do not bubble CO_2 gas through the water/sodium lauryl sulfate solution.
24. Add the sodium lauryl sulfate solution to the oil mixture and stir to a thick creamy emulsion.
25. Add 7.56 g glucose to the emulsion with mixing.
26. Blend 13.33 mL CO_2-saturated purified water with 77.04 g glucose and add emulsion with stirring.
27. Recycle primary emulsion back into the holding tank while setting mill.
28. Homogenize until all oil globules are less than 8 μm in diameter using colloid mill with a very fine setting. After setting mill, sample. Do not change mill setting after removing sample unless samples are unacceptable.
29. Add primary emulsion to syrup solution with mixing; add glucose QS to 965 mL and mix well.
30. Allow to stand overnight to vent entrapped air. Adjust the volume to 1 L using glucose or glucose and CO_2-saturated water.
31. Strain through 149-μm aperture or similar screen into clean reserve tank and recheck volume.

Multivitamin Drops

Bill of Materials			
Scale (mg/g)	Item	Material Name	Qty/kg (g)
13600 IU	1	Vitamin A palmitate (1.7 MM IU/g)	8.00
5200 IU	2	Vitamin D3 (40 MM IU/g)	0.13
5.00	3	Vitamin E acetate	5.00
150.0	4	Cremophor EL (or Cremophor RH 40)	150.00
2.00	5	Parabens (Methyl and propyl)	2.00
525.00	6	Water purified	525.00
4.00	7	Thiamine hydrochloride	4.00
2.00	8	Riboflavin 5-phosphate sodium	2.00
2.00	9	Pyridoxine hydrochloride	2.00
2.00	10	Nicotinamide	2.00
0.20	11	Sodium bisulfite	0.20
200.00	12	Propylene glycol	200.00
QS	13	Water purified	10.00
QS	14	Hydrochloric acid	QS

Manufacturing Directions

1. Heat mixture of items 1 to 4 to approximately 60°C; stir strongly and slowly add solution of items 5 and 6 (60°C).
2. To the obtained clear solution, add solution of items 7 to 13.
3. Adjust the pH with item 14 to approximately 4 and QS to volume.

Multivitamin Infant Drops

Bill of Materials			
Scale (mg/mL)	Item	Material Name	Qty/L (g)
1125 IU	1	Vitamin A palmitate (1.7 mm IU/g) (50% excess)	1.324
416 IU	2	Vitamin D (40 mm IU/g) (cholecalciferol, 25% excess)	0.013
5.00	3	Vitamin E (oily; α-tocopheryl acetate)	5.00
52.50	4	Ascorbic acid (50% excess)	52.50
0.375	5	Thiamine hydrochloride (50% excess)	0.75
0.40	6	Pyridoxine hydrochloride	0.40
8.00	7	Nicotinamide	8.00
0.00125	8	Cyanocobalamine (50% excess)	0.0025
0.82	9	Riboflavin sodium phosphate (5% excess as riboflavin)	0.865
2.50	10	Poloxyl 20 cetostearyl ether (Cetomacrogol 1000)	2.50
12.50	11	Polysorbate 80 (Tween 80)	12.50
0.50	12	Edetate disodium (sodium EDTA)	0.50
3.75	13	Sodium hydroxide	3.75
0.25	14	Saccharin sodium	0.25
300.00	15	Glycerin (glycerol)	300.00
500.00	16	Sorbitol (70% solution)	500.00
50.00	17	Propylene glycol	50.00
1.50	18	Flavor	1.50
3.00	19	Flavor	3.00
1.50	20	Flavor	1.50
–	21	Purified water	QS to 1 L

Manufacturing Directions

The product is a microemulsion and thermolabile. The temperature of solution must not exceed 25°C at the time of processing. Store bulk at temperature 15°C to 20°C under nitrogen protection to avoid discoloration and precipitation. Period of storage should not exceed 48 hours prior to filling in the bottle.

1. Check and record pH of item 21 (limit: 5.0–6.5) and collect 250 g of it in manufacturing vessel. Heat to 90°C to 95°C for 10 minutes, then cool to 20°C to 25°C.
2. Bubble nitrogen gas into cooled item 21 for 20 minutes.
3. Load 200 g of item 21 from first step to the manufacturing vessel.
4. Bubble nitrogen gas during all stages of the process.
5. Charge items 4 to 9 and 12 to 14 one by one to the manufacturing vessel while mixing.
6. Check that all materials are dissolved completely. Solution should be clear.
7. Add item 11 in a separate stainless steel container and heat to 45°C.
8. Mix items 1, 2, 3, and 10 one by one.
9. Mix for 1 hour at slow speed.
10. Add oil phase preparation to the aqueous phase at a rate of 2 mL/min while mixing; keep on bubbling nitrogen gas throughout the process.
11. Add items 15 and 16 to the manufacturing vessel one by one while mixing.
12. Keep on bubbling nitrogen gas throughout the process.
13. Add items 18 to 20 in item 17 and add to the manufacturing vessel while mixing.
14. Adjust the volume to 1 L using nitrogen-bubbled item 21.
15. Mix for 10 minutes at slow speed without aeration.
16. Check pH (limit: 3.7–4.5).
17. Filter the product at 1.5 bar.
18. Recirculate approximately 100 to 150 mL of product.
19. Transfer the filtered product to the storage vessel under a nitrogen blanket.

Multivitamin Infant Drops

Bill of Materials			
Scale (mg/0.6 mL)	Item	Material Name	Qty/L
675.00	1	Glycerin, USP (96%)	675.00 g
10.00	2	Nicotinamide niacinamide (white powder) (5% excess)	17.50 g
2.74	3	Riboflavin-5′-phosphate sodium (0% excess)	2.74 g
0.50	4	Methyl paraben (powder)	500.00 mg
1.00	5	Benzoic acid	1.00 g
2.10	6	Saccharin sodium (powder)	2.10 g
1.50	7	Thiamine HCl (45% excess)	3.625 g
0.60	8	Pyridoxine HCl	833.34 mg
50.00	9	Ascorbic acid (white powder) (20% excess)	100.00 g
0.257	10	Orange oil terpeneless No. 54125	257.789 mg
0.095	11	Alcohol (ethanol)	95.50 mg
80.00	12	Polysorbate 80	80.00 g
0.186	13	Butylated hydroxyanisole	186.92 mg
400 IU	14	Vitamin D viosterol in corn oil (oleovitamin D) (25% excess)	833.34 mg
5000 IU	15	Vitamin A; use vitamin A palmitate (1500000 AU/g) (50% excess[a])	16.66 g
QS	16	Purified water	329 g
QS	17	Carbon dioxide gas	QS

[a]Excess includes 20% manufacturing loss and 30% stability excess.

Manufacturing Directions

Use carbon dioxide cover at all time and use stainless steel 316 or higher resistant equipment.

1. Add 300 mL of purified water and the glycerin into a suitable jacketed tank. Start mixing.
2. Add, in this order, nicotinamide, riboflavin-5-phosphate sodium, Aspetoform M, benzoic acid, and saccharin sodium.
3. Continue mixing for balance of process.
4. Heat to 90°C to 100°C to dissolve ingredients.
5. In a separate tank, boil at least 15 mL of purified water for at least 15 minutes.
6. Cool while bubbling CO_2 gas into it and hold at 30°C or lower for use later for making up the volume.
7. Start cooling the main tank. When the temperature reaches 50°C to 60°C, start bubbling CO_2 gas through the solution from the bottom of the tank.
8. Continue cooling to 25°C. Continue the CO_2 gas protection for the balance of the process.
9. Add and dissolve thiamine HCl, pyridoxine HCl, and ascorbic acid.
10. Dissolve orange oil in alcohol and add.
11. Load approximately 5.25 g of polysorbate 80 into a separate stainless steel container.
12. Heat to 50°C to 60°C; add the butylated hydroxyanisole and dissolve with mixing. Remove heat.
13. Add remaining polysorbate 80 into the container, setting aside a sufficient quantity for rinsing the vitamin containers.
14. Bubble in CO_2 gas while mixing slowly. Stop mixing.
15. Add viosterol and vitamin A palmitate.
16. Rinse bottles with remaining polysorbate 80 and drain.
17. Mix slowly for at least 30 minutes or longer, if necessary, to provide a clear solution. Continue to bubble CO_2 gas for the entire mixing period.
18. Change CO_2 gas protection on main mixing tank to the top to prevent excessive foaming upon addition of polysorbate 80 solution.
19. Add polysorbate 80 solution to the main tank from the bottom of the tank to the top to prevent excessive foaming. Stop mixing.
20. If the volume is less than 1000 mL, adjust the volume with CO_2-saturated purified water made above to 1000 mL; mix for at least 1 hour.
21. In a separate tank, boil at least 115 mL of purified water for at least 15 minutes.
22. Cool while bubbling CO_2 gas into it, and hold at 30°C or lower for use later. Stop mixing.
23. Allow to stand for at least 4 hours to eliminate entrapped CO_2 gas.
24. Readjust volume to 1000 mL with CO_2-saturated purified water; mix for at least 1 hour. Stop mixing.
25. Filter through lint-free paper and do not use filter aids.
26. Recirculate product back to mixing tank until clear.
27. Flush storage tank with CO_2 gas and continue CO_2 gas protection until product has been filled.
28. Average intake dose is 0.60 mL.

Multivitamin Mineral Syrup

Bill of Materials			
Scale (mg/mL)	Item	Material Name	Qty/L (g)
6.65	1	Acid hypophosphorous (50% pure)	6.65
16.47	2	Calcium hypophosphite	16.47
31.68	3	Calcium lactate (powder)	31.68
1.00	4	Methyl paraben	1.00
0.20	5	Propyl paraben	200.00 mg
1.00	6	Benzoic acid	1.00
150.00	7	Sucrose (granular)	150.00
5.20	8	Ferrous gluconate	5.20
2.00	9	Niacinamide (5% excess)	2.10
0.32	10	Riboflavin-5-phosphate sodium	328.77 mg
1.00	11	D-Pantothenyl alcohol (dexpanthenol) (20% excess)	1.20
0.60	12	Vitamin B_{12} (cyanocobalamin) (35% excess)	810.00 μg
0.20	13	Pyridoxine hydrochloride	200.00 mg
0.30	14	Thiamine hydrochloride (regular powder) (55% excess)	465.00 mg
4.78	15	Flavor	4.78
1.94	16	Flavor	1.94
0.64	17	Orange oil, terpeneless	642.00 mg
0.21	18	Lime oil, distilled	214.97 mg
4.28	19	Alcohol (190 proof)	4.28
2.50	20	Saccharin sodium	2.50
14.50	21	Acid ascorbic (white powder/EP) (45% excess)	14.50
3.00	22	Caramel (acid proof)	3.00
2.00	23	Anhydrous citric acid (powder/EP)	2.00
0.01	24	Butylated hydroxyanisole (BHA)	10.00 mg
3.39	25	Corn oil	3.39
0.40	26	Vitamin A palmitate (TN, 1.5 MM UA/g) (40% excess)	560.00 mg
0.08	27	Viosterol in corn oil (syn. oleovitamin D; 1000 mD/g; D_3 in arachis oil) (40% excess)	112.00 mg
1.50	28	Acacia	1.50
0.12	29	Sodium lauryl sulfate (acetone washed)	127.41 mg
171.00	30	Deionized, purified water	171.00
QS	31	Glucose liquid	QS to 1 L

Manufacturing Directions

Do not expose this preparation during manufacturing to direct sunlight. Riboflavin is sensitive to light.

1. Add 83.7 mL of purified water to a stainless steel jacketed tank.
2. Add calcium hypophosphite, calcium lactate, parabens, and benzoic acid.
3. Heat mixture to 60°C with agitation.
4. Shut off mixer and wash tank free of all powders with 25.9 mL purified water.
5. Heat mixture to and maintain a maximum temperature of 100°C until solution is complete. Do not agitate. Avoid loss of water through evaporation. Cover opening of tank.
6. After solution occurs, take sample from bottom of tank and examine for clarity. Solution must be clear.
7. Add acid hypophosphorous (if used) with mixing.
8. Turn off heat and add 222 g glucose and start agitator. (*Caution*: Use CO_2 cover throughout; wherever water is used, it should be CO_2-saturated water.) Dissolve ferrous gluconate in 7.4 mL water CO_2 saturated by heating.
9. Add 278 g glucose with mixing. Add and dissolve sugar.
10. Allow solution to cool to 35°C and mix well.

11. To 29.6 mL water, add and dissolve nicotinamide, riboflavin, D-pantothenyl alcohol, vitamin B_{12}, pyridoxine, and thiamine. Mix until solution is complete and add to tank. Dissolve by heat, if necessary.
12. Charge flavors into tank.
13. Charge saccharin into tank and mix until dissolved.
14. Charge ascorbic acid into tank and mix well.
15. Charge caramel into tank and mix well, Dissolve citric acid in 3 mL water and add to above.
16. Heat corn oil to 50°C to 60°C and add and dissolve BHA. Ensure the BHA is completely dissolved before continuing.
17. Cool to room temperature. While cooling oil mixture, saturate with CO_2 and maintain heavy CO_2 coverage for balance of operation.
18. Set aside a small amount of this mixture as a rinse for the vitamin A and viosterol containers above.
19. Add vitamin A palmitate TN and viosterol to the cool corn oil mixture, rinsing the containers with the oil reserved above.
20. Add the rinse to the bulk. Mix well.
21. Add the acacia to the oil mixture with good mixing.
22. Dissolve sodium lauryl sulfate in 3 mL CO_2-saturated purified water.
23. To avoid excessive foaming, do not bubble CO_2 gas through the water/sodium lauryl sulfate solution.
24. Add the sodium lauryl sulfate solution to the oil mixture and stir to a thick creamy emulsion.
25. Add 7.56 g glucose to the emulsion with mixing.
26. Blend 13.33 mL CO_2-saturated purified water with 77.04 g glucose and add emulsion with stirring.
27. Recycle primary emulsion back into holding tank while setting mill.
28. Homogenize until all oil globules are less than 8 μm in diameter using colloid mill with a very fine setting.
29. Add primary emulsion to syrup solution with mixing; add glucose QS to 965 mL and mix well.
30. Allow to stand overnight to vent entrapped air.
31. Adjust the volume to 1 L using glucose or glucose and CO_2-saturated water.
32. Strain through 149-μm aperture or similar screen into clean reserve tank and recheck volume.
33. Seal tank under heavy CO_2 until filled.

Multivitamin Syrup

Bill of Materials			
Scale (mg/mL)	Item	Material Name	Qty/100 mL
170.00 IU	1	Vitamin A palmitate (1.7 million IU/g)	10.00
2.00 IU	2	Vitamin D (40 million IU/g)	0.05
1.00	3	Vitamin E acetate	100.00
0.02	4	Butylhydroxytoluene	2.00
45.00	5	Cremophor RH 40	4.50 g
100.00	6	Water	10.00 g
450.00	7	Saccharose	45.00 g
2.00	8	Methyl paraben	200.00
0.08	9	Citric acid	80.00
9.60	10	Glycerol	9.60 g
250.00	11	Water	25.00 g
0.15	12	Thiamine hydrochloride	15.00
0.15	13	Riboflavin 5′-phosphate sodium	15.00
0.55	14	Nicotinamide	55.00
0.15	15	Pyridoxine hydrochloride	15.00
3.00	16	Ascorbic acid (crystalline)	300.00
1.00	17	Sorbic acid	100.00
5.00	18	Propylene glycol (pharma)	5.00 g

Manufacturing Directions

1. Mix items 1 through 5 and heat to 60°C.
2. Separately heat item 2 to approximately 60°C.
3. Mix these two solutions slowly, stirring well to obtain a clear solution.
4. Dissolve items 7 to 9 in the hot solution of items 10 and 11 to obtain a clear solution.
5. Add to solution above.
6. Add items 12 to 18 and adjust the pH to 4.0 to 4.2.
7. Pass nitrogen through the solution for 10 minutes and fill under nitrogen cover. Provides 1 to 2 RDA/20 mL.

Multivitamin Syrup

Bill of Materials			
Scale (mg/mL)	Item	Material Name	Qty/100 mL (mg)
0.17	1	Vitamin A palmitate (1.7 MM IU/g)	17.00
0.001	2	Vitamin D_3 (40 MM IU/g)	0.10
0.01	3	Butylhydroxytoluene	1.00
30.00	4	Cremophor RH 40	3.00 g
1.00	5	Parabens	100.00
170.00	6	Water	17.00 g
0.50	7	Thiamine hydrochloride	50.00
0.20	8	Riboflavin phosphate sodium	20.00
0.20	9	Pyridoxine hydrochloride	20.00
2.50	10	Ascorbic acid (crystalline)	250.00
50.00	11	Water	5.00 g
–	12	Sugar syrup	Add 100 mL

Manufacturing Directions

1. Heat mixture of items 1 to 4 to approximately 65°C.
2. Stir well and very slowly add item 6 to warm solution (65°C).
3. Mix with solution of items 7 to 11 and add item 12 to make up the volume. *Note*: Parabens are generally a 1:10 ratio of methyl and propyl paraben.

Multivitamin with Fluoride Infant Drops

Bill of Materials			
Scale (mg/tablet)	Item	Material Name	Qty/1000 Tablets (g)
8.00	1	Niacin; use niacinamide (5% excess)	8.332
0.60	2	Riboflavin, USP; use riboflavin-5′-phosphate sodium (2% excess)	0.83
0.50	3	Methyl paraben	0.50
1.00	4	Benzoic acid	1.00
5000 IU	5	Vitamin E; use D-α-tocopheryl PEG-1000 succinate (20% excess)	13.826
400 IU	6	Vitamin D; use viosterol in corn oil (syn. oleovitamin D) (25% excess)	0.522
1500 IU (0.45)	7	Vitamin A palmitate (synthetic A palmitate, 1 MM U/g), USP	1.44
35.00	8	Ascorbic acid (white powder), USP (33% excess)	46.55
0.50	9	Thiamine hydrochloride (44% excess)	0.72
0.40	10	Pyridoxine; use pyridoxine hydrochloride	0.486
0.25	11	Fluoride; use sodium fluoride (powder)	0.5526
4.013	12	Caramel (acid proof)	4.013
0.257	13	Orange oil terpeneless	0.257
QS	14	Alcohol (ethanol; 190 proof)	10.00 mL
QS	15	Distilled purified water	QS
QS	16	Acid hydrochloric	QS
QS	17	Sodium hydroxide	QS
QS	18	Carbon dioxide gas	QS

Manufacturing Directions

Use only stainless steel tanks and minimize vortex formation to prevent aeration. Product attacks glass, so avoid contact with glass.

1. Charge 350 mL of purified water into the stainless steel jacketed main tank.
2. Start mixing.
3. Add, in this order, niacinamide, riboflavin, sodium fluoride, methyl paraben, and benzoic acid.
4. Rinse the interior walls of the tank with approximately 16 mL purified water.
5. Continue mixing for the balance of the process.
6. Heat the main tank to 95°C to dissolve ingredients.
7. When the solution is complete, cool below 85°C (range: 80–90°C).
8. The main tank will have to be heated to 85°C for this step.
9. Add vitamin E to another tank, if necessary, by heating vitamin E container.
10. Melt vitamin E in the tank.
11. Add viosterol and vitamin A and heat to 60°C to 65°C with mixing.
12. Start bubbling in CO_2.
13. Mix slowly for 10 minutes or longer to produce a clear solution.
14. Start CO_2 gas protection on the main mixing tank and continue for the balance of the process.
15. With the main batch at 85°C to 90°C, add the solution of vitamins E, D, and A at 60°C to 65°C with mixing.
16. The addition may cause the temperature of the main batch to drop below the specified range, so readjust to 85°C to 90°C.
17. Mix and maintain at this temperature until solution is complete, after which cool to below 30°C.
18. Add the glycerin with mixing.
19. Adjust the temperature to 25°C ± 5°C and maintain at this temperature before proceeding.
20. Add and dissolve with mixing, in this order, ascorbic acid, thiamine, pyridoxine, and caramel.
21. Rinse the caramel container with approximately 3 mL of water and add the rinsings.
22. Rinse the tank inner walls and mixer shaft with approximately 3 mL water.
23. Dissolve the orange oil with mixing in the alcohol and add to solution above.
24. Continue mixing for at least 30 minutes to ensure a homogeneous product.
25. Stop mixing and take pH (range: 3.1–3.3). If necessary, adjust with 10% sodium hydroxide or 10% hydrochloric acid, prepared by adding 1 mL hydrochloric acid (reagent-grade) with 3.3 mL purified water. Mix.
26. Stop mixing and allow to stand for at least 4 hours to eliminate entrapped CO_2 gas.
27. In a properly cleaned separate tank, boil at least 65 mL of purified water for at least 15 minutes.
28. Cool while bubbling CO_2 into it and hold at 30°C.
29. Adjust pH to the range of 3.1 to 3.3.
30. Filter using a lint-free paper; do not use filter aids.
31. Recirculate product back to main mixing tank until clear.
32. Flush a storage tank with CO_2 for at least 10 minutes with the CO_2 valve completely open.
33. Filter product into this storage tank.
34. Fill under CO_2 cover.

Multivitamin Drops

Bill of Materials			
Scale (mg/g)	Item	Material Name	Qty/kg (g)
8.00	1	Vitamin A palmitate 1.7 mm U/g (BASF)	8.00
0.130	2	Vitamin D_3 40 mm U/g	0.130
5.00	3	Vitamin E acetate (BASF)	5.00
150.0	4	Cremophor EL (or Cremophor RH 40)	150.00
2.00	5	Parabens	2.00
525.00	6	Water	525.00
4.00	7	Thiamine hydrochloride (BASF)	4.00
2.00	8	Riboflavin 5-phosphate sodium	2.00
2.00	9	Pyridoxine hydrochloride (BASF)	2.00
2.00	10	Nicotinamide	2.00
0.20	11	Sodium bisulfite	0.20
200.00	12	Propylene glycol	200.00
QS	13	Water	10.00 g
QS	14	Hydrochloric acid	QS

Manufacturing Directions

1. Heat mixture of items 1 to 4 to approximately 60°C and stir strongly.
2. Slowly add solution of items 5 and 6 at 60°C.
3. To the obtained clear solution, add solution of items 7 to 13.
4. Adjust the pH, with item 14, to approximately 4.
5. Bring to volume.

Multivitamin Syrup

Bill of Materials			
Scale (mg/mL)	Item	Material Name	Qty/100 mL (g)
0.170	1	Vitamin A palmitate 1.7 MM U/g (BASF)	17.0 mg
0.001	2	Vitamin D3 40 MM U/g	0.1 mg
0.010	3	Butylhydroxytoluene	1.0 mg
30.000	4	Cremophor RH 40	3.00
1.000	5	Parabens	0.10
170.000	6	Water	17.00
0.500	7	Thiamine hydrochloride (BASF)	0.05
0.200	8	Riboflavin phosphate sodium	0.02
0.200	9	Pyridoxine hydrochloride (BASF)	0.02
2.500	10	Ascorbic acid, crystalline (BASF)	0.25
50.000	11	Water	5
QS	12	Sugar syrup	QS to 100 mL

Manufacturing Directions

1. Heat mixture of items 1 to 4 to about 65°C and stir well.
2. Add very slowly item 6 to the warm solution (65°C).
3. Mix with solution of items 7 to 11 and add item 12 to make up the volume. Parabens are generally a 1:10 ratio of methyl and propyl paraben.

Multivitamin Syrup

Bill of Materials			
Scale (mg/mL)	Item	Material Name	Qty/100 mL (g)
170.00 U	1	Vitamin A palmitate 1.7 MMM U/g (BASF)	0.010
2.00 U	2	Vitamin D 40 MMM U/g	0.05 mg
1.00	3	Vitamin E acetate (BASF)	0.10
0.020	4	Butylhydroxytoluene	0.0020
45.0	5	Cremophor RH 40	4.50
100.00	6	Water	10.00
450.00	7	Saccharose	45.00
2.00	8	Methyl paraben	0.20
0.080	9	Citric acid	0.080
9.60	10	Glycerol	9.60
250.00	11	Water	25.00
0.150	12	Thiamine hydrochloride (BASF)	0.015
0.150	13	Riboflavin 5'-phosphate sodium	0.015
0.55	14	Nicotinamide	0.055
0.150	15	Pyridoxine hydrochloride (BASF)	0.015
3.00	16	Ascorbic acid, crystalline (BASF)	0.30
1.00	17	Sorbic acid	0.10
5.00	18	Propylene glycol	5.00

Manufacturing Directions

1. Heat items 1 to 5 and item 2 separately to approximately 60°C and mix slowly with stirring to obtain a clear solution.
2. Dissolve items 7 to 9 in the hot solution of items 10 and 11 to obtain a clear solution.
3. Mix the cool solutions and then add items 12 to 18 and adjust the pH value to 4.0 to 4.2.
4. Pass nitrogen for 10 min through the solution and fill under nitrogen cover. Provides 1 to 2 RDA/20 mL.

Multivitamin With Fluoride-Infant Drops

Bill of Materials			
Scale (mg/mL)	Item	Material Name	Qty/1000 L (g)
8.00	1	Niacin, USE niacinamide, 5% excess	8.33
0.60	3	Riboflavin, USE riboflavin-5'-phosphate sodium 2% excess	0.84
0.50 g	5	Methyl paraben	0.50
1.00	6	Acid benzoic	1.00
5000 U	7	Vitamin E, USE D-alpha tocopheryl polyethylene glycol 1000 succinate, 20% excess	13.82
400 U	9	Vitamin D, USE viosterol in corn oil (synthetic oleovitamin D, 25% excess)	0.52
1500 U (0.45 mg)	11	Vitamin A palmitate synthetic A palmitate 1 mm	
U/g	1.44		
35.00	14	Acid, ascorbic white powder, 33% exc;	46.55
0.50	15	Thiamine hydrochloride, 44% excess	0.72
0.40	16	Pyridoxine, USE pyridoxine hydrochloride	0.48
0.25	18	Fluoride, USE sodium fluoride powder	0.55
4.01	20	Caramel acid proof	4.01
0.26	21	Oil Orange Terpeneless	0.25
0.00001 mL	22	Alcohol, ethanol, 190 proof	0.101 mL
QS	23	Water purified, distilled	QS
QS	24	Acid hydrochloric	QS
QS	25	Sodium hydroxide	QS
QS	26	Carbon dioxide gas	QS

Manufacturing Directions

Use only stainless steel tanks; minimize vortex formation to prevent aeration. Product attacks glass; avoid contact with glass.

1. Charge 350 mL of purified water into the stainless steel jacketed main tank.
2. Start mixing. Add, in order, niacinamide, riboflavin, sodium fluoride, methyl paraben, and benzoic acid.
3. Rinse the interior walls of tank with approximately 16 mL purified water.
4. Continue mixing for the balance of the process.
5. Heat the main tank to 95°C to dissolve ingredients. When the solution is complete, cool below 85°C (range 80–90°C).
6. Add vitamin E to another tank, if necessary, by heating vitamin E container. Melt vitamin E in the tank.
7. Add viosterol and vitamin A and heat to 60°C to 65°C with mixing.
8. Start bubbling in CO_2. Mix slowly for 10 minutes or longer to produce a clear solution. Start CO_2 gas protection on the main mixing tank and continue for the balance of the process.
9. With the main batch at 85°C to 90°C, add the solution of vitamins E, D, and A at 60°C to 65°C, with mixing. The addition may cause the temperature of the main batch to drop below the specified range; readjust to 85°C to 90°C.
10. Mix and maintain at this temperature until solution is complete, after which cool to below 30°C. Add the glycerin with mixing. Adjust the temperature to the 25°C to 5°C range and maintain at this temperature before proceeding.
11. Add and dissolve with mixing in the following order: ascorbic acid, thiamine, pyridoxine, and caramel. Rinse the caramel container with approximately 3 mL of water and add the rinsings.
12. Rinse the tank inner walls and mixer shaft with approximately 3 mL water.
13. Dissolve the orange oil with mixing in the alcohol and add to solution.
14. Continue mixing for at least 30 minutes to ensure a homogenous product.
15. Stop mixing, take pH (range: 3.1–3.3). If necessary, adjust with 10% sodium hydroxide or 10% hydrochloric acid (prepared by adding 1 mL hydrochloric acid, reagent grade, with 3.3 mL purified water). Mix.
16. Stop mixing and allow to stand for at least 4 hours to eliminate entrapped CO_2 gas.
17. In a separate tank, properly cleaned, boil at least 65 mL of purified water for at least 15 minutes, cool while bubbling CO_2 into it, and hold at 30°C and adjust pH in the range 3.1 to 3.3.
18. Filter using a lint-free paper; do not use filter aids.
19. Recirculate product back to main mixing tank until clear. Flush a storage tank with CO_2 for at least 10 minutes with the CO_2 valve completely open.
20. Filter product into this storage tank. Fill under carbon dioxide cover.

Nafarelin Acetate Nasal Solution

Synarel nasal solution contains nafarelin acetate (2 mg/mL, content expressed as nafarelin base) in a solution of benzalkonium chloride, glacial acetic acid, sodium ride, polysorbate 80, aroma, and water. The solution is isotonic with a pH of 7. It contains no chlorofluorocarbons.

Naproxen Suspension

Naprosyn (naproxen) suspension for oral administration contains 125 mg/5 mL of naproxen in a vehicle containing sucrose, magnesium aluminum silicate, sorbitol solution, and sodium chloride (30 mg/5 mL, 1.5 mEq), methyl paraben, fumaric acid, FD&C yellow No. 6, imitation pineapple flavor, imitation orange flavor, and purified water. The pH of the suspension ranges from 2.2 to 3.7.

Nevirapine Suspension

Viramune oral suspension is for oral administration. Each 5 mL of Viramune suspension contains 50 mg nevirapine (as nevirapine hemihydrate). The suspension also contains the following excipients: carbomer 934P, methyl paraben, propyl paraben, sorbitol, sucrose, polysorbate 80, sodium hydroxide, and water.

Nicotine Spray

Each 10-mL spray bottle contains 100 mg nicotine (10 mg/mL) in an inactive vehicle containing disodium phosphate, sodium dihydrogen phosphate, citric acid, methyl paraben, propyl paraben, EDTA, sodium chlorhydroxide, or hydrochloric acid (to adjust pH), sorbitol, and purified water.

Nimesulide Suspension

Bill of Materials			
Scale (mg/mL)	Item	Material Name	Qty/L (g)
10.00	1	Nimesulide	10.00
400.00	2	Sucrose	400.00
49.00	3	Propylene glycol	49.00
1.00	4	Methyl paraben	1.00
0.20	5	Propyl paraben	0.20
2.80	6	Sodium benzoate	2.80
0.20	7	Disodium edentate	0.20
0.50	8	Sodium citrate	0.50
0.10 mL	9	Sorbitol solution 70%	100 mL
4.00	10	Carboxymethyl cellulose sodium	4.00
2.00	11	Aerosil 200	2.00
3.30	12	Citric acid	3.30
1.00	13	Hydroxypropyl methyl cellulose	1.00
0.48	14	Simethicone emulsion	0.48
QS	15	Flavor	QS
QS	16	Water purified	QS to 1 L

Manufacturing Directions

1. In a suitable stainless steel container, heat item 16 to 70°C.
2. Add and dissolve sodium benzoate, disodium edentate, and sodium citrate.
3. Filter though a filter press.
4. Add sugar till completely dissolved.
5. Filter again through a filter press.
6. In a separate container, charge propylene glycol and sorbitol solution. Add carboxymethyl cellulose and aerosol homogenizes and store for a few hours.
7. Add and mix in step 5, hydroxypropylmethylcellulose and simethicone emulsion.
8. Add item 1 and make a slurry in step 6.
9. Add step 7 into step 4 and make up the volume with item 16.

Nimodipine Capsules

Each liquid-filled capsule contains 30 mg nimodipine in a vehicle of glycerin, peppermint oil, purified water, and polyethylene glycol 400. The soft gelatin capsule shell contains gelatin, glycerin, purified water, and titanium dioxide.

Nitroglycerin Lingual Spray

Nitrolingual pumpspray (nitroglycerin lingual spray 400 μg) is a metered-dose spray containing nitroglycerin. This product delivers nitroglycerin (400 μg per spray, 75 or 200 metered sprays) in the form of spray droplets onto or under the tongue. Inactive ingredients are medium-chain triglycerides, dehydrated alcohol, medium-chain partial glycerides, and peppermint oil.

Norephedrine Syrup

Bill of Materials			
Scale (mg/mL)	Item	Material Name	Qty/L (g)
40.00	1	DL-Norephedrine hydrochloride	40.00
10.00	2	Parabens	10.00
50.00	3	Saccharin sodium	50.00
30.00	4	Kollidon 90F	30.00
500.00	5	Sorbitol solution	500.00
460.00	6	Water	460.00

Manufacturing Directions

1. Dissolve the parabens in the hot water (90–95°C).
2. Add the sorbitol, cool to room temperature, and dissolve the other components.
3. To prevent of discoloration of Kollidon in the solution during storage, 0.1% to 0.5% of cysteine could be added as antioxidant.
4. Flavors should be added to adjust the required taste.

Norephedrine Syrup

Bill of Materials			
Scale (mg/mL)	Item	Material Name	Qty/L (g)
40.00	1	DL-norephedrine hydrochloride	40.00
4.00	2	Parabens	4.00
5.00	3	Saccharin sodium	5.00
3.00	4	Kollidon® 90F	3.00
500.00	5	Sorbitol solution	500.00
460.00	6	Water	460.00

Manufacturing Directions

1. Dissolve the parabens in the hot water, add the sorbitol, cool to room temperature, and dissolve the other components.
2. To prevent discoloration of Kollidon in the solution during storage, 0.1% to 0.5% cysteine could be added as an antioxidant.
3. Flavors should be added to adjust the taste, as needed.

Nystatin Oral Suspension

Bill of Materials			
Scale (mg/mL)	Item	Material Name	Qty/L (g)
21.05	1	Nystatin microfine (particles size not less than 90% below 45 (im, 100% below 80 (im; based on potency of 5500 U/g anhydrous; adjust accordingly; 10% overage)	21.050
600.00	2	Sucrose	600.000
1.80	3	Methyl paraben	1.8000
0.20	4	Propyl paraben	0.2000
150.00	5	Sorbitol (70% solution)	150.000
5.00	6	Microcrystalline cellulose	5.000
10.00	7	Glycerin	10.000
2.00	8	Carboxymethylcellulose sodium	2.000
2.00	9	Polysorbate 80	2.000
50.00	10	Glycerin	50.000
2.50	11	Saccharin sodium	2.500
2.00	12	Flavor	2.000
30.00	13	Alcohol (ethanol 95%)	30.000
QS	14	Sodium hydroxide	0.174
QS	15	Hydrochloric acid (37%)	0.296
–	16	Water purified	QS to 1 L

Manufacturing Directions

1. Add 200 g of item 16 (90–95°C) into mixer and heat to 90°C to 95°C. Dissolve items 3 and 4 while mixing. Add and dissolve item 2 while mixing at a speed of 18 rpm.
2. Cool down to approximately 50°C to 55°C.
3. Filter the syrup. Collect the syrup in a clean stainless steel tank. Avoid any loss of syrup. Clean the mixer.
4. Transfer the sugar syrup from the stainless steel tank into the mixer.
5. Add 100 g of item 5 into mixer while mixing.
6. Disperse item 6 in the mixture of 50 g of item 16 (25–30°C) and 50 g of item 5 in a stainless steel drum while mixing with stirrer.
7. Disperse item 8 in item 7 in a stainless steel drum while mixing with stirrer. Add 30 g of item 16 (90°C) to the solution. Stir until it becomes clear. Cool to 30°C.
8. Transfer the dispersion from step 3 and 4 into mixer.
9. Mix and homogenize under vacuum 0.4 to 0.6 bar for 10 minutes.
10. Stop homogenizer and keep continuous mixing.
11. Dissolve item 9 in 50 g of item 16 (50°C) in a stainless steel container while mixing by stirrer.
12. Add item 10 into it. Disperse item 1 while stirring by stirrer. Cool to 30°C.
13. Add the drug dispersion into mixer while mixing.
14. Dissolve item 11 in 15 g of item 16 (25–30C) in a stainless steel container while stirring by stirrer. Add to mixer while mixing.
15. Add items 12 and 13 into mixer while mixing.
16. Homogenize high speed and vacuum 0.4 to 0.6 bar. Mix and homogenize for 10 minutes.
17. Dissolve item 14 in 7 g of item 16 in a stainless steel container. Add slowly into the mixer while mixing.
18. Dissolve item 15 carefully in 7 g of item 16 in a stainless steel container. Slowly add the required quantity into mixer to adjust the pH between 6.8 and 7.1.
19. Make up the volume with item 16, up to 1 L. Mix for 5 minutes.

Nystatin Suspension

Bill of Materials			
Scale (mg/mL)	Item	Material Name	Qty/L (g)
22.50	1	Nystatin	22.50
57.50	2	Kollidon CL-M	57.50
20.00	3	Kollidon 90F	20.00
248.00	4	Sorbitol	248.00
5.00	5	Citric acid	5.00
QS	6	Water purified	QS to 1 L

Manufacturing Directions

1. Charge items 1, 2, and 4 in a suitable stainless steel vessel and suspend in item 6; mix well.
2. Add item 3 slowly while stirring and in small portions and then follow up with vigorous stirring to obtain smooth suspension. Homogenize if necessary.
3. Fill.

Ofloxacin Otic Solution

Floxin otic contains 0.3% (3 mg/mL) ofloxacin with benzalkonium chloride (0.0025%), sodium chloride (0.9%), and water for injection. Hydrochloric acid and sodium hydroxide are added to adjust the pH to 6.5 ± 0.5.

Ofloxacin Otic Solution

Bill of Materials			
Scale (mg/mL)	Item	Material Name	Qty/L (g)
3.00	1	Ofloxacin	3.00
QS	2	Vehicle (pluraflo 1220 45.48%, ethanol 5.05%, propylene glycol 41.23%, anhydrous glycerin 8.24)	QS to 1 L
QS	3	Perfumes	QS

Manufacturing Directions

1. Add propylene glycol, pluraflo, glycerin, and ethanol to a clean vessel.
2. While stirring, add ofloxacin. Stir until a clear solution is obtained.
3. Add perfume and mix until uniform.

Omeprazole Solution

Bill of Materials			
Scale (mg/mL)	Item	Material Name	Qty/L (g)
20.00	1	Omeprazole free base	20.00
QS	2	Vehicle (pluronic F127 34.07%, ethanol 10.43%, propylene glycol 42.18%)	1.00 L
1.00	3	Sodium metabisulfite	1.00
1.00	4	Disodium EDTA	1.00
2.50	5	Sodium saccharin	2.50
1.10	6	Monoammonium glycerhizzinate	1.10
3.50	7	Acesulfame	3.50
QS	8	Flavor	QS

Manufacturing Directions

1. Add propylene glycol and poloxamer to a clean vessel (main mix).
2. While stirring, heat the mixture as appropriate to sufficiently melt the poloxamer.
3. Once a uniform solution is obtained, remove from heat source and continue mixing.
4. In a separate vessel (alcohol premix), add alcohol, omeprazole base, and monoammonium glycerizzinate and mix until uniform. In another vessel (water premix), add water, EDTA, sodium saccharin, acesulfame, and sodium metabisulfite.
5. Mix until all materials are dissolved.
6. Add the alcohol containing premix to the main mixing vessel containing the poloxamer.
7. Mix until uniform.
8. While stirring, add the water containing premix to the main vessel and continue to mix until uniform.
9. Subsequently, add desired flavor component and mix until uniform.

Ondansetron Hydrochloride Dihydrate Oral Solution

Each 5 mL of Zofran oral solution contains 5 mg of ondansetron HCl dihydrate equivalent to 4 mg of ondansetron. Zofran oral solution contains the inactive ingredients citric acid anhydrous, purified water, sodium benzoate, sodium citrate, sorbitol, and strawberry flavor.

Orciprenaline Sulfate and Clobutinol Hydrochloride Syrup

Bill of Materials			
Scale (mg/5 mL)	Item	Material Name	Qty/L (g)
10.00	1	Natrosol 250 M	2.00
5.00	2	Sodium benzoate	1.00
10.00	3	Saccharin sodium	2.00
35.00	4	Ammonium chloride	7.00
26.24	5	Citric acid	5.25
4.00	6	Sodium citrate	0.80
2500.00	7	Sorbitol 70%	500.00
500.00	8	Glycerin	100.00
5.00	9	Orciprenaline sulfate, 5% excess	1.05
20.00	10	Clobutinol hydrochloride	4.20
40.40	11	Alcohol	8.00
0.20	12	Anise oil	0.04
QS	13	Water purified	QS to 1 L

Manufacturing Directions

1. In a suitable stainless steel mixing vessel, charge 250 mL of item 13 and heat to 70°C to 75°C. Add item 1 and mix well; cool to room temperature.
2. In 10 mL of item 13, add and dissolve item 2 and 3 and add to step 2.
3. In 20 mL of item 13, add and dissolve item 4 and add to step above.
4. In a separate vessel, add items 50 mL of item 13 and item 8 and mix well; add to step 4.
5. In 50 mL of item 13, add item 10, mix well, and add to step 5.
6. In 50 mL of item 13, add item 9, mix well, and add to step 6.
7. Adjust pH to 3.1 to 3.2 using item 5.
8. Filter through 100-micron filter and then through filter pads.
9. Make up volume and fill.

Oxitropium and Formoterol Nasal Spray

1. Charge 4.5 g of micronized oxitropium bromide and 0.675 g of micronized formoterol fumarate into a pressure-addition vessel.
2. After sealing and evacuation thereof, 10.5 kg of HFA 227, which has previously been aerated with carbon dioxide and adjusted to a pressure of 6.25 bar (20°C) in another pressure addition vessel, is added.
3. After homogenization of this mixture, the suspension obtained is dispensed into aluminum containers sealed with metering valves by means of the pressure-filling technique.

Oxycodone Hydrochloride Oral Concentrate Solution

Each 1 mL of Oxyfast concentrate solution contains oxycodone hydrochloride, 20 mg citric acid, FD&C yellow No. 10, sodium benzoate, sodium citrate, sodium saccharine, and water.

Oxymetazoline Hydrochloride Congestion Nasal Spray

Each milliliter of Afrin severe congestion nasal spray contains oxymetazoline hydrochloride 0.05%. It also contains benzalkonium chloride, benzyl alcohol, camphor, EDTA, eucalyptol, menthol, polysorbate 80, propylene glycol, sodium phosphate dibasic, sodium phosphate monobasic, and water.

Oxymetazoline Hydrochloride Nasal Solution

Bill of Materials			
Scale (g/100 mL)	Item	Material Name	Qty/L (g)
0.025	1	Oxymetazoline hydrochloride	0.25
0.03	2	Benzalkonium chloride (50% Solution)	0.30
0.05	3	Disodium edetate (sodium EDTA)	0.50
0.025	4	Sodium hydroxide (1N solution)	0.25
1.02	5	Monobasic sodium phosphate	10.20
2.80	6	Dibasic sodium phosphate	28.00
–	7	Water purified	QS to 1 L

Manufacturing Directions

Oxymetazoline hydrochloride is toxic. There is a risk of serious intoxication if inhaled or swallowed. This product is a colorless, odorless membrane-filtered solution. Thus, make sure that the receiving tank for the filtered solution is cleaned and free of any contamination.

1. Heat 1 kg of item 7 up to 85°C to 90°C in the manufacturing vessel. Hold the temperature at 85°C to 90°C for 30 minutes.
2. Cool item 7 to 30°C and transfer into mobile tank.
3. Add 900 g of cold item 7 (from step 2) into manufacturing vessel.
4. Dissolve items 1 to 6 one by one while mixing in manufacturing vessel containing cold item 7.
5. After completion of addition mix for 20 more minutes.
6. Make up the volume to 1 L with cold item 7 and, finally, mix for 20 minutes.
7. Check and record the pH (limit: 6.8 ± 0.1).
8. Filter the solution through Sartorius prefilter and membrane filter 0.2 μm into receiving tanks.

Oxymetazoline Moisturizing Nasal Spray

Each milliliter of Afrin extra moisturizing nasal spray contains oxymetazoline hydrochloride, 0.05%. It also contains benzalkonium chloride, EDTA, glycerin, polyethylene glycol, polyvinyl pyrrolidone, propylene glycol, sodium phosphate dibasic, sodium phosphate monobasic, and water.

Oxymetazoline Nasal Spray

Each milliliter of Afrin original nasal spray and pump mist contains oxymetazoline hydrochloride 0.05%. It also contains benzalkonium chloride, EDTA, polyethylene glycol, polyvinyl pyrrolidone, propylene glycol, sodium phosphate dibasic, sodium phosphate monobasic, and water.

Oxymetazoline Sinus Nasal Spray

Each milliliter of Afrin sinus nasal spray contains oxymetazoline hydrochloride 0.05%. It also contains benzalkonium chloride, benzyl alcohol, camphor, EDTA, eucalyptol, menthol, polysorbate 80, propylene glycol, sodium phosphate dibasic, sodium phosphate monobasic, and water.

Oxymetazoline Nasal Solution

Bill of Materials			
Scale (mg/mL)	Item	Material Name	Qty/L (g)
QS	1	Vehicle (pluronic F127 40.27%, ethanol 26.18%, water 33.55%)	QS to 1 L
0.50	2	Oxymetazoline	0.50
1.50	3	Tyloxapol	1.50
0.40	4	Dibasic sodium phosphate	0.40
1.30	5	Monobasic potassium phosphate	1.30
0.40	6	Benzalkonium chloride	0.40
2.60	7	Chlorhexidine gluconate	2.60
0.10	8	Disodium EDTA	0.10

Manufacturing Directions

1. Add the dibasic sodium phosphate, monobasic potassium phosphate, disodium EDTA, benzalkonium chloride, and oxymetazoline HCl to a clean vessel.
2. Add tyloxapol, chlorhexidine gluconate, and ethanol to the vessel.
3. Subsequently, add the poloxamer and water to the vessel.
4. Mix until uniform.

Peptide Topical Liquid

Formulation

Peptide such as thymic fraction 5, glycerin 44.5, propylene glycol 44.9, methyl nicotinate 0.1, water 50, polysorbate 80, 0.5% by weight.

Pheniramine Maleate Syrup

Bill of Materials			
Scale (mg/5 mL)	Item	Material Name	Qty/L (g)
15.00	1	Pheniramine maleate	3.00
2980.00	2	Sugar	596.00
5.40	3	Methyl paraben	1.08
0.60	4	Propyl paraben	0.11
0.60	5	Citric acid monohydrate	0.11
1.50	6	Sodium citrate	0.30
3.50	7	Flavor	0.70
QS	8	Water purified	QS to 1 L

Manufacturing Directions

1. Charge 700 mL item 8 in a suitable mixing vessel and heat to 90°C to 95°C.
2. Add and mix item 2.
3. Add items 3 and 4 and mix to dissolve.
4. In separate vessels in approximately 100 mL item 8, add and dissolve items 5 to 7 and item 1 separately.
5. Add the two mixtures in step 3 to step 2 at room temperature.
6. Make up the volume.

Phenobarbital, Hyoscyamine Sulfate, Atropine Sulfate, and Scopolamine Hydrobromide Elixir

Each 5 mL (teaspoonful) of elixir (23% alcohol) contains phenobarbital 16.2 mg, hyoscyamine sulfate 0.1037 mg, atropine sulfate 0.0194 mg, and scopolamine hydrobromide 0.0065 mg; D&C yellow No. 10, FD&C blue No. 1, FD&C yellow No. 6, flavors, glucose, saccharin sodium, water.

Phenylephrine Tannate and Chlorpheniramine Tannate Pediatric Suspension

Rynatan® pediatric suspension is an antihistamine/nasal decongestant combination available for oral administration as a suspension. Each 5 mL (one teaspoonful) of the slate purple-colored, natural strawberry, artificial currant-flavored suspension contains phenylephrine tannate 5 mg, chlorpheniramine tannate 4.5 mg, benzoic acid, FD&C blue No. 1, FD&C red No. 3, FD&C red No. 40, FD&C yellow No. 5, flavors (natural and artificial), glycerin, kaolin, magnesium aluminum silicate, methylparaben, pectin, purified water, saccharin sodium, and sucrose.

Phenylephrine Tannate and Pyrilamine Tannate Suspension

RYNA-12 S suspension is an antihistamine/nasal decongestant combination available for oral administration as a suspension. Each 5 mL (one teaspoonful) of the pink-colored, natural strawberry, artificial currant-flavored suspension contains phenylephrine tannate 5 mg, pyrilamine tannate 30 mg, benzoic acid, FD&C red No. 3, flavors (natural and artificial), glycerin, kaolin, magnesium aluminum silicate, methyl paraben, pectin, purified water, saccharin sodium, and sucrose.

Phenylpropanolamine, Chlorpheniramine, Dextromethorphan, Vitamin C Syrup

Bill of Materials			
Scale (mg/mL)	Item	Material Name	Qty/L (g)
150.00	1	Polyethylene glycol 400	150.00
21.66	2	Acetaminophen	21.66
0.075 mL	3	Glycerin	75.000 mL
0.35 mL	4	Sorbitol solution	350.000 mL
1.00	6	Acid, benzoic	1.00
1.75	7	Saccharin sodium, powder, dihydrate	1.75
0.91	8	Phenylpropanolamine hydrochloride	0.92
0.065	9	Chlorpheniramine maleate (10% excess)	0.073
0.66	10	Dextromethorphan hydrobromide	0.67
20.00	11	Sodium CMC premium low viscosity	0.02
70.00	12	Dye	0.070
6.00	13	Dye	0.006
5.00	14	Ascorbic acid, USE sodium ascorbate fine powder	5.62
0.50	15	Flavor orange	0.50
0.25	16	Flavor orange	0.25
QS	17	Carbon dioxide gas	QS
QS	18	Water purified	QS to 1 L

Manufacturing Directions

1. In a covered stainless steel container, heat 500 mL water to boiling. Boil for 30 minutes.
2. Turn off the heat and, while keeping the container covered, cool the water to 30°C while purging it with carbon dioxide.
3. Keep this water in a covered container blanketed with carbon dioxide gas and use where indicated.
4. Transfer to the main stainless steel mixing tank the polyethylene glycol 400, cover, start bubbling CO_2 gas, and then, while mixing, slowly heat to 60°C to 65°C. Maintain at this temperature.
5. While mixing, add and dissolve the acetaminophen. Maintain the temperature and CO_2 protection.
6. When all the acetaminophen has dissolved, add, while mixing, the glycerin and sorbitol.
7. Continue mixing while maintaining the temperature and CO_2 gas protection until used later. Do not allow the temperature to go above 65°C. During this mixing period, remove samples through the bottom valve of the mixing tank and inspect for clarity. Return samples to the mixing tank.
8. Continue mixing and sampling until absolutely clear.
9. In a separate stainless steel mixing tank, add 300 mL water, cover, and then heat to 90°C.
10. While maintaining at this temperature, start bubbling CO_2 gas and then, while mixing, add and dissolve successively the benzoic acid, saccharin sodium, and phenylpropanolamine hydrobromide.
11. Continue mixing until all have dissolved. Reduce the temperature to 60°C to 65°C while mixing. Do not force cool.
12. To the solution in the main mixing tank add, while mixing and bubbling CO_2 gas, the solution from step above. Rinse the container with two lots of 5 mL carbon dioxide-saturated water and add the rinsings to the batch while mixing.
13. Continue mixing for 15 minutes while maintaining the temperature at 60°C to 65°C and CO_2 gas protection.
14. While mixing the batch, sprinkle on the sodium CMC.
15. Continue mixing until all the sodium CMC has been dispersed. Check to be sure there are no undissolved lumps.
16. Add CO_2-saturated water from step above and mix while cooling the batch to 30°C. Dissolve the dyes in 10 mL carbon dioxide-saturated water then add to the batch with mixing.
17. Rinse the container with two lots of 5 mL the same water and add the rinsings to the batch. Mix until a homogenously colored batch is formed.
18. Stop bubbling in CO_2 gas but maintain CO_2 protection of the tank headspace. In a stainless steel container, dissolve the sodium ascorbate in 25 mL carbon dioxide-saturated water, taking care to minimize exposure of the solution to air or light.
19. Mix all solutions, add rinsings where necessary, and continue mixing for 15 minutes.
20. Add the flavors, complete the batch to 1 L with carbon dioxide-saturated water, and mix well for 1 hour.
21. Stop mixing, saturate the head space with CO_2, and leave overnight to release any entrapped air.

Phenylpropanolamine, Chlorpheniramine, Dextromethorphan, Vitamin C Syrup

Bill of Materials			
Scale (mg/mL)	Item	Material Name	Qty/L (g)
150.00	1	PEG-400 (low color), NF	150.00
21.66	2	Acetaminophen, USP	21.66
0.075 mL	3	Glycerin, USP (96%)	75.00 mL
0.35 mL	4	Sorbitol; use sorbitol solution, USP	350.00 mL
1.00	5	Benzoic acid, USP	1.00
1.75	6	Saccharin sodium (dihydrate powder), USP	1.75
0.91	7	Phenylpropanolamine hydrochloride, USP	916.70 mg
0.06	8	Chlorpheniramine maleate, USP (plus 10% manufacturing)	73.30 mg
0.66	9	Dextromethorphan hydrobromide, USP	667.00 mg
20.00	10	Sodium CMC (premium low viscosity)	20.00
70.00	11	Dye	70.00 mg
6.00	12	Dye	6.00 mg
5.00	13	Ascorbic acid; use sodium ascorbate (fine powder)	5.62
0.50	14	Flavor, orange	500.00 mg
0.25	15	Flavor, orange	250.00 mg
QS	16	Carbon dioxide gas	QS
QS	17	Purified water, USP	QS to 1 L

Manufacturing Directions

Manufacture under complete CO_2 protection. Bubble the CO_2 gas through the solution from the bottom of the tank.

If excessive foaming occurs, change CO_2 gas protection from the bottom to the top of the tank. Minimize vortex formation while mixing to prevent aeration of the product.

1. In a covered stainless steel container, heat 500 mL of water to boiling. Boil for 30 minutes.
2. Turn off the heat; while keeping the container covered, cool the water to 30°C while purging the water with CO_2.
3. Keep this water in a covered container blanketed with CO_2 gas and use where indicated.
4. Transfer the PEG-400 to the main stainless steel mixing tank and cover.
5. Start bubbling CO_2 gas; while mixing, slowly heat to 60°C to 65°C. Maintain at this temperature.
6. While mixing, add and dissolve the acetaminophen. Maintain the temperature and CO_2 protection.
7. When all the acetaminophen has dissolved, add, while mixing, the glycerin and sorbitol.
8. Continue mixing while maintaining the temperature and CO_2 gas protection until mixture is used later.
9. Do not allow the temperature to go above 65°C.
10. During this mixing period, remove samples through the bottom valve of the mixing tank and inspect for clarity; return samples to the mixing tank. Continue mixing and sampling until absolutely clear.
11. In a separate stainless steel mixing tank, heat 300 mL of water, covered, to 90°C.
12. While maintaining at this temperature, start bubbling CO_2 gas.
13. While mixing, add and dissolve successively the benzoic acid, saccharin sodium, and phenylpropanolamine hydrobromide. Continue mixing until all have dissolved.
14. Reduce the temperature to 60°C to 65°C while mixing. Do not force-cool.
15. Add the solution from step above to the solution in the main mixing tank, while mixing and bubbling CO_2 gas.
16. Rinse the container with two lots of 5 mL of CO_2-saturated water and add the rinsings to the batch while mixing.
17. Continue mixing for 15 minutes while maintaining the temperature at 60°C to 65°C and under CO_2 gas protection.
18. While mixing the batch, sprinkle on the sodium CMC.
19. Continue mixing until all the sodium CMC has been dispersed.
20. Check on the absence of any undissolved lumps.
21. Add CO_2-saturated water from step 3 to 900 mL and mix while cooling the batch to 30°C.
22. Dissolve the dyes in 10 mL of CO_2-saturated water, then add to the batch with mixing.
23. Rinse the container with two lots of 5 mL of the same water and add the rinsings to the batch.
24. Mix until a homogenously colored batch is formed.
25. Stop bubbling in CO_2 gas but maintain CO_2 protection of the tank headspace.
26. In a stainless steel container, dissolve the sodium ascorbate in 25 mL of CO_2-saturated water, taking care to minimize exposure of the solution to air or light.
27. Mix all solutions, add rinsings where necessary, and continue mixing for 15 minutes.
28. Add the flavors, complete the batch to 1 L with CO_2-saturated water, and mix well for 1 hour.
29. Stop mixing, saturate the headspace with CO_2, and leave overnight to release any entrapped air.

Phenylpropanolamine Controlled-Release Capsules

Bill of Materials			
Scale (mg/mL)	Item	Material Name	Qty/L (g)
33.00	1	Phenylpropanolamine	33.00
QS	2	Vehicle (pluraflo 1220 70.12%, ethanol 2.26%, anhydrous glycerin 16.35%)	QS to 1 L
1.00	3	Sodium metabisulfite	1.00
1.00	4	Disodium EDTA	1.00

Manufacturing Directions

1. Add alcohol, propylene glycol, EDTA, sodium metabisulfite, and phenylpropanolamine to a clean vessel and begin mixing.
2. Subsequently, add pluraflo and glycerin to the vessel.
3. Mix until uniform.
4. This liquid may be filled into hard gelatin capsules that are then banded to prevent leakage or it may be used as the fill for a soft elastic gelatin capsule. One capsule is made to contain 0.75 mL of the liquid and, taken 3 times daily, provides controlled release of the phenylpropanolamine active. After swallowing, the gelatin shell dissolves in the gastrointestinal tract and the liquid fill immediately transforms into a slow-dissolving gel that provides controlled release of the phenylpropanolamine.

Phenytoin Suspension

Each teaspoonful of suspension contains 125 mg phenytoin, with maximum alcohol content not greater than 0.6%. It also contains carboxymethylcellulose sodium; citric acid, anhydrous; flavors; glycerin; magnesium aluminum silicate; polysorbate 40; purified water; sodium benzoate; sucrose; vanillin; and FD&C yellow No. 6.

Phenytoin Suspension

Bill of Materials			
Scale (mg/mL)	Item	Material Name	Qty/L (g)
50.00	1	Phenytoin	50.00
80.00	2	Kollidon CL-M	80.00
10.00	3	Kollidon 90F	10.00
QS	4	Preservative	QS
QS	5	Water purified	QS to 1 L

Manufacturing Directions

1. Charge in a suitable stainless steel-jacketed vessel item 5 and heat to 90°C to 95°C.
2. Add and dissolve preservatives (e.g., parabens). Stir to complete solution.
3. Cool to 40°C.
4. Add item 3 and dissolve.
5. Add item 2 and suspend.
6. Add item 1 and suspend. Homogenize if necessary.
7. Fill.

Pipenzolate Methyl Bromide and Phenobarbital Drops

Bill of Materials			
Scale (mg/5 mL)	Item	Material Name	Qty/L (g)
20.00	1	Pipenzolate methyl bromide	4.00
30.00	2	Phenobarbital	6.00
350.00	3	Alcohol	70.00
1000.00	4	Propylene glycol	200.00
450.00	5	Propylene glycol	90.00
33.00	6	Sodium saccharin	6.66
2500.00	7	Glycerin	500.00
5.00	8	Peppermint oil	1.00
1.65	9	Flavor	0.33
1.65	10	Flavor	0.33
0.20	11	Dye	0.04
10.00	12	Sodium citrate	2.00
17.70	13	Citric acid monohydrate	3.54
QS	14	Water purified	QS to 1 L

Manufacturing Directions

1. Charge 150 mL item 14 in a suitable stainless steel vessel and heat to 90°C for 1 hour and then cool to room temperature.
2. Add items 1, 6, 11, 12, and 13 and mix well.
3. In a separate vessel, charge items 4 and 7 and mix well for 10 minutes.
4. In a separate vessel, charge items 2, 3, 5, flavors, and item 7 and mix well.
5. Add step 4 to step 3 and mix well.
6. Add step 5 to step 1 and make up volume and mix well.
7. Fill.

Podofilox Solution

Condylox is the brand name of podofilox, an antimitotic drug that can be chemically synthesized or purified from the plant families *Coniferae* and *Berberidaceae* (e.g., species of Juniperus and Podophyllum). Condylox 0.5% solution is formulated for topical administration. Each milliliter of solution contains 5 mg of podofilox in a vehicle containing lactic acid and sodium lactate in alcohol 95%.

Polidocanol Wound Spray

Bill of Materials			
Scale (mg/g)	Item	Material Name	Qty/kg (g)
5.00	1	I. Polidocanol	5.00
50.00	2	Kollidon VA 64	50.00
50.00	3	Ethocel® 20	50.00
20.00	4	Lutrol E 400	20.00
675.00	5	Ethyl acetate	675.00
200.00	6	Isopropanol	200.00

Manufacturing Directions

1. Dissolve the items 1 to 4 in the solvent mixture of items 5 and 6.
2. Fill the solution into spray cans with the necessary quantity of propellant (e. g., propane/butane) or in a mechanical pump bottle.

Polidocanol Wound Spray

Bill of Materials			
Scale (mg/g)	Item	Material Name	Qty/kg (g)
5.00	1	Polidocanol	5.00
50.00	2	Kollidon® VA 64	50.00
50.00	3	Ethocel® 20	50.00
20.00	4	Lutrol E 400	20.00
675.00	5	Ethyl acetate	675.00
200.00	6	Isopropanol	200.00

Manufacturing Directions

1. Dissolve items 1 to 4 in the solvent mixture of items 5 and 6.
2. Fill the solution into spray cans with the necessary quantity of propellant (e.g., propane/butane) or in a mechanical pump bottle.

Polyvinyl Pyrrolidone–Iodine Gargle Solution

Bill of Materials			
Scale (mg/mL)	Item	Material Name	Qty/L (g)
10.00	1	Polyvinyl pyrrolidone-iodine, powder, 35% excess	13.500
10.00	2	Glycerin (96%)	10.000
QS	3	Water purified	QS to 1 L

Manufacturing Directions

Wear gloves and mask during all phases of manufacturing and filling. Do not keep the lid of the manufacturing or storage tank open unless necessary, as iodine may be liberated.

1. Add 600 mL purified water to a suitable stainless steel manufacturing tank.
2. Add polyvinyl pyrrolidone–iodine powder, slowly to first step (with continuous stirring).
3. Stir for 30 minutes or until a clear brown solution is obtained.
4. Add glycerin to the manufacturing tank. Stir until uniform solution is obtained.
5. Make up volume to 1 L with purified water and mix well for 5 minutes.
6. Check pH (range: 2–4). Filter the solution through a 100-mesh nylon cloth and transfer to a stainless steel storage tank.
7. Keep the storage tank tightly closed.

Polyvinyl Pyrrolidone–Iodine Gargle Solution Concentrate

Bill of Materials			
Scale (mg/mL)	Item	Material Name	Qty/L (g)
100.00	1	Polyvinyl pyrrolidone-Iodine 30/06	100.00
10.00	2	Propylene glycol (pharma)	10.00
90.00	3	Ethanol 96%	90.00
800.00	4	Water	800.00

Manufacturing Directions

1. Dissolve the polyvinyl pyrrolidone–iodine in the solvent mixture.
2. Brown transparent liquid: Dilute 10 mL the concentrate with approximately 100 mL water before use.

Polyvinyl Pyrrolidone–Iodine Liquid Spray

Bill of Materials			
Scale (mg/g)	Item	Material Name	Qty/kg (g)
100.00	1	Polyvinyl pyrrolidone-Iodine 30/06	100.00
150.00	2	Kollidon VA 64	150.00
750.00	3	*N*-Propanol	750.00
750.00	4	Ethanol	750.00

Manufacturing Directions

1. Dissolve Kollidon VA 64 in the mixture of solvents.
2. Slowly add polyvinyl pyrrolidone–iodine to the well-stirred solution.
3. Fill in aerosol cans with propellants such as propane and butane or with manual valves.

Polyvinyl Pyrrolidone–Iodine Mouthwash

Bill of Materials			
Scale (mg/g)	Item	Material Name	Qty/kg (g)
100.0	1	Polyvinyl pyrrolidone-Iodine	100.0
5.0	2	Sodium saccharin	5.0
2.0	3	Menthol	2.0
0.5	4	Oil aniseed	0.5
0.5	5	Eucalyptus oil	0.5
160.0	6	Polyethylene glycol 400	160.0
300.0	7	Ethanol	300.0
440.0	8	Water purified	440.0

Manufacturing Directions

1. Dissolve polyvinyl pyrrolidone–iodine powder and sodium saccharin in 440 g water to obtain a clear solution.
2. In a separate container, add alcohol and mix and dissolve aniseed oil, eucalyptus oil, menthol, and polyethylene glycol 400 to obtain a clear solution.
3. Add solution from step above and mix with stirring. Package in HDPE plastic bottles.

Polyvinyl Pyrrolidone–Iodine Mouthwash and Gargle Solution Concentrate

Bill of Materials			
Scale (mg/g)	**Item**	**Material Name**	**Qty/kg (g)**
75.00	1	Polyvinyl pyrrolidone-Iodine 30/06	75.00
5.00	2	Saccharin sodium	5.00
150.00	3	Water	150.00
2.00	4	Menthol	2.00
1.00	5	Anise oil + eucalyptus oil, 1+1	1.00
150.00	6	Lutrol E 400	150.00
500.00	7	Ethanol 96%	500.00

Manufacturing Directions

1. Dissolve polyvinyl pyrrolidone–iodine and saccharin in water and mix with solution of items 4 to 7.
2. A brown, transparent liquid having a fresh odor is formed.
3. Dilute 10 to 20 mL with a glass of water. A brown liquid is obtained having a fresh taste.

Polyvinyl Pyrrolidone–Iodine Scrub

Bill of Materials			
Scale (mg/mL)	Item	Material Name	Qty/L (g)
75.00	1	Polyvinyl pyrrolidone-iodine, powder,	
40% excess	105.000		
250.00	2	Sodium lauryl sulfate	250.000
35.00	3	Lauric diethanolamide	35.000
QS	4	Water purified, distilled	QS to 1 L

Manufacturing Directions

1. Add 600 mL purified water to a suitable stainless steel manufacturing tank.
2. Add, by sprinkling, sodium lauryl sulfate in the manufacturing tank.
3. Continue to mix slowly under vacuum and begin to heat until product temperature is 70°C.
4. Continue to mix vigorously under vacuum at 65°C to 70°C for 15 minutes or until completely dissolved. Do not add detergent quickly, as a gel may form that is difficult to dissolve. Stop mixer, release vacuum, and open tank.
5. Add and disperse the previously broken lauric diethanolamide in the warmed solution in step above.
6. Maintain vacuum and then mix vigorously for 30 minutes at 65°C to 70°C or until completely dissolved.
7. Slowly cool under vacuum to room temperature with slow mixing. Do not force cool with cold water, otherwise the mixture will adhere to the walls of the manufacturing tank.
8. When temperature reaches 30°C, release vacuum and open tank.
9. While mixing slowly, add polyvinyl pyrrolidone–iodine in small portions.
10. Rinse the container of polyvinyl pyrrolidone–iodine with 150 mL purified water and add to the main tank. Do not keep the lid of the manufacturing or storage tank open unless necessary, as iodine may liberate.
11. Mix under vacuum until a clear, reddish-brown solution is obtained.
12. Make volume to 1 L with purified water and mix well under vacuum for at least 15 minutes to ensure product uniformity and to deaerate the product.
13. Stop mixing, release the vacuum, and open the tank.
14. Check and record pH (range: 3–6).
15. Filter the solution through 100-mesh nylon cloth.

Polyvinyl Pyrrolidone–Iodine Solution

Bill of Materials			
Scale (mg/g)	Item	Material Name	Qty/kg (g)
100.00	1	Polyvinyl pyrrolidone-iodine 30/06	100.00
0.230	2	Texapon K 12	0.230
1.40	3	Sodium biphosphate	1.40
0.30	4	Sodium citrate	0.30
20.80	5	Sodium hydroxide solution, 1 molar	20.80
10.00	6	Glycerol	10.00
864.20	7	Water	864.20

Manufacturing Directions

1. Dissolve Texapon K 12 in solution of items 3 to 7.
2. Slowly add polyvinyl pyrrolidone–iodine to the well-stirred solution. This creates a brown, transparent liquid having a pH of 4.5.

Polyvinyl Pyrrolidone–Iodine Solution

Bill of Materials			
Scale (mg/g)	Item	Material Name	Qty/kg (g)
100.00	1	Polyvinyl pyrrolidone-iodine 30/06	100.00
10.00	2	Natrosol® HR 250	10.00
2.00	3	Lutrol F 127	2.00
32.00	4	Sodium hydroxide, 1 molar solution	32.00
856.00	5	Water	856.00

Manufacturing Directions

1. Dissolve Lutrol F 127 and then Natrosol in the water.
2. As soon as both are dissolved, slowly add the polyvinyl pyrrolidone–iodine to the well-stirred solution.
3. Adjust the pH with the sodium hydroxide solution to about 3.5.

Polyvinyl Pyrrolidone–Iodine Solution

Bill of Materials			
Scale (mg/g)	Item	Material Name	Qty/kg (g)
20.00	1	Tylose M 300	20.00
2.00	2	Texapon K 12	2.00
595.00	3	Citric acid solution 0.1 molar	595.00
283.00	4	Sodium biphosphate solution 0.2 molar	283.00

Manufacturing Directions

1. Dissolve Tylose M 300 in the mixture of the citric acid and sodium biphosphate solutions.
2. Add Texapon and slowly dissolve the polyvinyl pyrrolidone–iodine. This creates a brown, clear solution having a certain viscosity and a pH of 3 to 4.

Polyvinyl Pyrrolidone–Iodine Solution

Bill of Materials			
Scale (mg/g)	Item	Material Name	Qty/kg (g)
100.00	1	Polyvinyl pyrrolidone-iodine 30/06	100.00
3.00	2	Lutrol F 127	3.00
5.00	3	Lutrol E 400	5.00
432.00	4	Citric acid 0.1 molar solution	432.00
460.00	5	$Na2HPO_4 \cdot 12H_2O$ 0.2 molar solution	460.00

Manufacturing Directions

1. Dissolve the polyvinyl pyrrolidone–iodine (and Lutrol F 127) in the mixture of the buffer solutions (and Lutrol E 400).
2. A brown, clear solution is formed that has a low viscosity and a pH of about 4.5.
3. Items 2 and 3 can be deleted and compensated with item 5.

Polyvinyl Pyrrolidone–Iodine Solution

Bill of Materials			
Scale (mg/mL)	Item	Material Name	Qty/1000 Tabs. (g)
100.00	1	Polyvinyl pyrrolidone-iodine powder, 35% excess	135.00
9.318	2	Acid, citric, anhydrous, powder	9.318
14.62	3	Sodium phosphate, dibasic, anhydrous	14.62
QS	4	Water purified, distilled	QS to 1 L

Manufacturing Directions

1. Add 600 mL purified water to a suitable stainless steel manufacturing tank. With gentle stirring, add citric acid into the purified water in the manufacturing tank.
2. Stir for 10 minutes or until completely dissolved. During this mixing period, remove samples from the bottom valve of the manufacturing tank and inspect for clarity.
3. Return samples to the manufacturing tank.
4. Continue mixing and sampling until the solution is completely clear.
5. With gentle stirring, add sodium phosphate, dibasic, into the solution. Stir for 10 minutes or until completely dissolved. During this mixing period, remove samples from the bottom valve of the manufacturing tank and inspect for clarity. Return samples to the manufacturing tank.
6. Continue mixing and sampling until the solution is completely clear. Make up volume to 1 L with purified water and mix well for 5 minutes.
7. Check and record pH (range: 4.8–5.2). Filter the solution through a 100-mesh nylon cloth.
8. Transfer into a suitable stainless steel storage tank and keep tightly closed. This solution should be freshly prepared and should not be stored for more than 24 hours.
9. Dissolve polyvinyl pyrrolidone–iodine in about 600 mL citric acid–phosphate buffer (pH 5) solution (made above) in a suitable stainless steel mixing tank.
10. Stir evenly for 10 minutes or until a clear, brown solution is obtained. Make up volume to 1 L with citric acid–phosphate buffer solution.
11. Mix well for 10 minutes.
12. Check and record pH (range: 3.0–4.5).
13. Filter the solution through a 100-mesh nylon cloth.
14. Transfer into a suitable stainless steel storage tank and keep tightly closed

Polyvinyl Pyrrolidone–Iodine Surgical Scrub

Bill of Materials			
Scale (mg/g)	Item	Material Name	Qty/kg (g)
75.00	1	Polyvinyl pyrrolidone-Iodine 30/06	75.00
250.00	3	Lutensit AES	250.00
40.00	4	Monoamide 150 MAW	40.00
QS	6	Floral bouquet	QS
635.00	7	Water	635.00

Manufacturing Directions

1. Dissolve monoamide in hot water, cool to room temperature.
2. Dissolve polyvinyl pyrrolidone–iodine.
3. Add Lutensit to form a brown, clear viscous solution.

Polyvinyl Pyrrolidone–Iodine Surgical Scrub

Bill of Materials			
Scale (mg/g)	Item	Material Name	Qty/kg (g)
75.00	1	Polyvinyl pyrrolidone-Iodine 30/06	75.00
250.00	2	Neutronyx S 60	250.00
40.00	3	Super amide L 9	40.00
QS	4	Floral bouquet	QS
635.00	5	Water	635.00

Manufacturing Directions

1. Dissolve Super Amide in hot water and then cool.
2. Dissolve polyvinyl pyrrolidone–iodine and add Neutronyx.
3. A brown, clear viscous solution is formed, with pH of about 3.4.

Polyvinyl Pyrrolidone–Iodine Vaginal Douche Concentrate

Bill of Materials			
Scale (mg/g)	Item	Material Name	Qty/kg (g)
100.00	1	Polyvinyl pyrrolidone-iodine 30/06	100.00
5.00	2	Lutrol E 400	5.00
3.00	3	Lutrol F 127	3.00
432.00	4	Citric acid, 0.1 molar solution	432.00
460.00	5	$Na_2HPO_4 \cdot 12H_2O$, 0.2 molar solution	460.00

Manufacturing Directions

1. Dissolve polyvinyl pyrrolidone–iodine and Lutrol F 127 in the mixture of the buffer solutions with Lutrol E 400.
2. A brown, clear solution is created having a low viscosity and a pH of about 4.3.

Polyvinyl Pyrrolidone–Iodine Viscous Solution

Bill of Materials			
Scale (mg/g)	Item	Material Name	Qty/kg (g)
10.00	1	Polyvinyl pyrrolidone-Iodine 30/06	10.00
15.00	2	Natrosol HR 250	15.00
QS	3	Buffer	QS
QS	4	Water	975.00

Manufacturing Directions

1. Clear brown viscous liquid viscosity (Brookfield) of 7500 mPas is obtained.
2. Dissolve polyvinyl pyrrolidone–iodine and natrosol in the well-stirred water.

Polyvinylpyrrolidone–Iodine Mouthwash

Bill of Materials			
Scale (mg/g)	Item	Material Name	Qty/kg (g)
100.00	1	Polyvinylpyrrolidone (PVP)-Iodine	100.00
5.00	2	Saccharin sodium	5.00
2.00	3	Menthol	2.00
0.50	4	Aniseed oil	0.50
0.50	5	Eucalyptus oil	0.50
160.00	6	PEG-400	160.00
300.00	7	Ethanol	300.00
QS	8	Purified water	QS to 1 kg

Manufacturing Directions

1. Dissolve PVP–iodine powder and saccharin sodium in 440 g of water to obtain a clear solution.
2. In a separate container, add alcohol.
3. Mix and dissolve aniseed oil, eucalyptus oil, menthol, and PEG-400 to obtain a clear solution.
4. QS with water.
5. Add solution from step above and mix with stirring.
6. Package in HDPE plastic bottles.

Povidone–Iodine Concentrates for Broilers and Cattle

Bill of Materials			
Scale (mg/g)	Item	Material Name	Qty/kg (g)
200.00	1	Polyvinylpyrrolidone (PVP)-Iodine 30/06	200.00
50.00	2	Texapon® K 12	50.00
50.00	3	Cremophor NP 14	50.00
73.00	4	Tartaric acid	73.00
43.00	5	Sulfuric acid, diluted	43.00
100.00	6	Ethanol 96%	100.00
QS	7	Water	QS to 1 kg

Manufacturing Directions

1. Dissolve surfactant items 2 and 3 in solution of items 4 to 7 and slowly add PVP–iodine.
2. Brown, transparent liquids having a pH of about 1.
3. Dilute about 3 mL of the concentrate with 1 L of water prior to use.

Povidone–Iodine Foam Spray

Bill of Materials			
Scale (mg/g)	Item	Material Name	Qty/kg (g)
100.00	1	Polyvinylpyrrolidone (PVP)-Iodine 30/06	100.00
0.10	2	Cremophor A 25	0.10
QS	3	Water	QS to 1 kg

Manufacturing Directions

1. Dissolve PVP–iodine in the solution of Cremophor A 25 in water.
2. Fill the aerosol cans with 90 parts of this solution and 10 parts of propane plus 1 part butane.

Povidone–Iodine Gargle

Bill of Materials			
Scale (mg/mL)	Item	Material Name	Qty/L (g)
10.00	1	Polyvinylpyrrolide-Iodine (powder) (35% excess)	13.50
10.00	2	Glycerin, USP (96%)	10.00
–	3	Purified water, USP	QS to1 L

Manufacturing Directions

Wear gloves and mask during all phases of manufacturing and filling. Do not keep the lid of the manufacturing or storage tank open, unless necessary, as iodine may be liberated.

1. Add 600 mL purified water to a suitable stainless steel manufacturing tank.
2. Slowly add povidone–iodine powder to the water (with continuous stirring).
3. Stir for 30 minutes or until a clear, brown solution is obtained.
4. Add glycerin to the manufacturing tank.
5. Stir until uniform solution is obtained.
6. Make up volume to 1 L with purified water and mix well for 5 minutes.
7. Check pH (range: 2.0–4.0).
8. Filter the solution through a 100-mesh nylon cloth and transfer to a stainless steel storage tank.
9. Keep the storage tank tightly closed.

Povidone–Iodine Gargle Solution Concentrate

Bill of Materials			
Scale (mg/mL)	Item	Material Name	Qty/L (g)
100.00	1	Polyvinylpyrrolidone (PVP)–Iodine 30/06	100.00
10.00	2	Propylene glycol	10.00
90.00	3	Ethanol (96%)	90.00
800.00	4	Water	800.00

Manufacturing Directions

1. Dissolve the PVP–iodine in the solvent mixture to produce a brown transparent liquid.
2. Dilute 10 mL of the concentrate with approximately 100 mL of water prior to use.

Povidone–Iodine Liquid Spray

Bill of Materials			
Scale (mg/g)	Item	Material Name	Qty/kg (g)
100.00	1	Polyvinylpyrrolidone (PVP)–Iodine 30/06	100.00
150.00	2	Kollidon® VA 64	150.00
750.00	3	*N*-Propanol	750.00
750.00	4	Ethanol	750.00

Manufacturing Directions

1. Dissolve Kollidon VA 64 in the mixture of solvents and slowly add PVP–iodine to the well-stirred solution.
2. Fill in aerosol cans with propellants such as propane and butane or with manual valves.

Povidone–Iodine Mouthwash and Gargle Solution Concentrate

Bill of Materials			
Scale (mg/g)	Item	Material Name	Qty/kg (g)
75.00	1	Polyvinylpyrrolidone (PVP)–Iodine 30/06	75.00
5.00	2	Saccharin sodium	5.00
150.00	3	Water	150.00
2.00	4	Menthol	2.00
1.00	5	Anise oil + eucalyptus oil (1+1)	1.00
150.00	6	Lutrol E 400	150.00
500.00	7	Ethanol (96%)	500.00

Manufacturing Directions

1. Dissolve PVP–iodine and saccharin in water and mix with solution of items 4 to 7.
2. Brown transparent liquid has a fresh odor.
3. Dilute 10 to 20 mL with a glass of water.
4. A brown liquid with a fresh taste is obtained.

Povidone–Iodine Powder Spray

Bill of Materials			
Scale (mg/g)	Item	Material Name	Qty/kg (g)
250.00	1	Polyvinylpyrrolidone (PVP)-Iodine 30/06	250.00
250.00	2	Maize PO_4 aerosol	250.00
15.00	3	Isopropyl myristate	15.00
100.00	4	Dow Corning® 344 fluid	100.00
500.00	5	Pentane	500.00
220.00	6	Propane + butane (1+3)	220.00

Manufacturing Directions

1. Suspend PVP–iodine and maize PO_4 aerosol in the liquid mixture of items 3 to 5.
2. Fill in aerosol cans with the propellants.

Povidone–Iodine Pump Spray

Bill of Materials			
Scale (mg/g)	Item	Material Name	Qty/kg (g)
10.00	1	Polyvinylpyrrolidone (PVP)-Iodine 30/06	10.00
100.00	2	Water	100.00
1.00	3	Potassium iodide	1.00
100.00	4	Xylitol	100.00
787.50	5	Propylene glycol	787.50
1.00	6	Menthol (crystalline)	1.00
0.50	7	Peppermint oil (double rectified)	0.50

Manufacturing Directions

1. Dissolve potassium iodide in water, warm up to 40°C, and dissolve xylitol.
2. At room temperature, dilute with propylene glycol, dissolve PVP–iodine, and add flavors to produce a clear, brown liquid with a sweet, refreshing taste.

Povidone–Iodine Shampoo

Bill of Materials			
Scale (mg/g)	Item	Material Name	Qty/kg (g)
75.00	1	Polyvinylpyrrolidone (PVP)-Iodine 30/06	75.00
250.00	2	Neutronyx® S 60	250.00
40.00	3	Super Amide® L 9	40.00
5.0-7.0	4	Natrosol® 250 HR	5.0-7.0
–	5	Water	QS to 1 kg

Manufacturing Directions

1. Dissolve Super Amide and Natrosol in hot water (about 60°C), then dissolve PVP–iodine.
2. After cooling, incorporate Neutronyx.
3. A brown, clear solution is obtained.
4. The viscosity can be changed by modification of the amount of Natrosol 250 HR.

Povidone–Iodine Solution

Bill of Materials			
Scale (mg/mL)	Item	Material Name	Qty/L (g)
100.00	1	Povidone-Iodine powder (35% excess)	135.00
9.318	2	Anhydrous citric acid (powder)	9.318
14.62	3	Anhydrous sodium phosphate (dibasic)	14.62
QS	4	Purified water	QS to 1 L

Manufacturing Directions

Wear gloves and mask during all phases of manufacturing and filling. Do not keep the lid of the manufacturing or storage tank open, unless necessary, as iodine may be liberated.

1. Citric acid–phosphate buffer solution (pH 5): Add 600 mL purified water to a suitable stainless steel manufacturing tank.
2. With gentle stirring add citric acid to the purified water in the manufacturing tank.
3. Stir for 10 minutes or until completely dissolved.
4. During this mixing period, remove samples from the bottom valve of the manufacturing tank and inspect for clarity.
5. Return samples to the manufacturing tank.
6. Continue mixing and sampling until the solution is completely clear.
7. With gentle stirring add dibasic sodium phosphate to the solution.
8. Stir for 10 minutes or until completely dissolved.
9. During this mixing period, remove samples from the bottom valve of the manufacturing tank and inspect for clarity.
10. Return samples to the manufacturing tank.
11. Continue mixing and sampling until the solution is completely clear.
12. Make up volume to 1 L with purified water and mix well for 5 minutes.
13. Check and record pH (range: 4.8–5.2).
14. Filter the solution through a 100-mesh nylon cloth.
15. Transfer into a suitable stainless steel storage tank and keep tightly closed.
16. This solution should be freshly prepared and should not be stored for more than 24 hours.
17. Preparation of solution: Dissolve povidone–iodine in approximately 600 mL of citric acid/phosphate buffer (pH 5) solution in a suitable stainless steel mixing tank.
18. Stir evenly for 10 minutes or until a clear brown solution is obtained.
19. Make up volume to 1 L with citric acid/phosphate buffer solution.
20. Mix well for 10 minutes.
21. Check and record pH (range: 3.0–4.5).
22. Filter the solution through a 100-mesh nylon cloth.
23. Transfer into a suitable stainless steel storage tank and keep it tightly closed.

Povidone–Iodine Solution

Bill of Materials			
Scale (mg/g)	Item	Material Name	Qty/kg (g)
100.00	1	Polyvinylpyrrolidone (PVP)-Iodine 30/06	100.00
3.00	2	Lutrol F 127	3.00
5.00	3	Lutrol E 400	5.00
432.00	4	Citric acid (0.1-M solution)	432.00
460.00	5	$Na_2HPO_4 \cdot 12H_2O$ (0.2-M solution)	460.00

Manufacturing Directions

1. Dissolve the PVP–iodine (and Lutrol F 127) in the mixture of buffer solutions (and Lutrol E 400).
2. Brown clear solutions having a low viscosity and pH of approximately 4.5.
3. Items 2 and 3 can be deleted and compensated with item 5.

Povidone–Iodine Solution

Bill of Materials			
Scale (mg/g)	Item	Material Name	Qty/kg (g)
100.00	1	Polyvinylpyrrolidone (PVP)–Iodine 30/06	100.00
0.23	2	Texapon® K 12	0.23
1.40	3	Sodium biphosphate	1.40
0.30	4	Sodium citrate	0.30
20.80	5	Sodium hydroxide (1-M solution)	20.80
10.00	6	Glycerol	10.00
QS	7	Water	QS to 1 kg

Manufacturing Directions

1. Dissolve Texapon K 12 in solution of items 3 to 7 and slowly add PVP–iodine to the well-stirred solution.
2. The brown, transparent liquid has a pH of 4.5.

Povidone–Iodine Solution

Bill of Materials			
Scale (mg/g)	Item	Material Name	Qty/kg (g)
100.00	1	Polyvinylpyrrolidone (PVP)–Iodine 30/06	100.00
10.00	2	Natrosol® HR 250	10.00
2.00	3	Lutrol F 127	2.00
32.00	4	Sodium hydroxide (1-M solution)	32.00
QS	5	Water	QS to 1 kg

Manufacturing Directions

1. Dissolve Lutrol F 127 and then Natrosol in the water.
2. As soon as both are dissolved, slowly add the PVP–iodine to the well-stirred solution.
3. Adjust the pH with the sodium hydroxide solution to approximately 3.5.

Povidone–Iodine Solution

Bill of Materials			
Scale (mg/g)	Item	Material Name	Qty/kg (g)
20.00	1	Tylose® M 300	20.00
2.00	2	Texapon® K 12	2.00
595.00	3	Citric acid (0.1-M solution)	595.00
283.00	4	Sodium biphosphate (0.2-M solution)	283.00

Manufacturing Directions

1. Dissolve Tylose M 300 in the mixture of the citric acid and sodium biphosphate solutions.
2. Add Texapon and slowly dissolve the PVP–iodine.
3. The brown, clear solution has a pH of 3 to 4.

Povidone–Iodine Scrub

Bill of Materials			
Scale (mg/mL)	Item	Material Name	Qty/L (g)
75.00	1	Polyvinylpyrrolidone-Iodine (powder) (40% excess)	105.00
250.00	2	Sodium lauryl sulfate	250.00
35.00	3	Lauric diethanolamide	35.00
–	4	Distilled purified water, USP	QS to 1 L

Manufacturing Directions

1. Add 600 mL purified water to a suitable stainless steel manufacturing tank.
2. Add, by sprinkling, the sodium lauryl sulfate to the manufacturing tank.
3. Continue to mix slowly under vacuum and begin to heat until product temperature is 70°C.
4. Continue to mix vigorously under vacuum at 65°C to 70°C for 15 minutes or until completely dissolved.
5. (*Note*: Do not add detergent quickly, as a gel may form that is difficult to dissolve.) Stop mixer, release vacuum, and open tank.
6. Add and disperse the previously broken lauric diethanolamide in the warmed solution from the step above.
7. Maintain vacuum and mix vigorously for 30 minutes at 65°C to 70°C or until completely dissolved.
8. Slowly cool under vacuum to room temperature with slow mixing. (*Note*: Do not force cool with cold water; otherwise, the mixture will adhere to the walls of the manufacturing tank.) When temperature reaches 30°C, release vacuum and open tank.
9. While mixing slowly, add povidone–iodine in small portions.
10. Rinse the container of povidone–iodine with 150 mL purified water and add to the main tank. (*Note*: Do not keep the lid of the manufacturing or storage tank open, unless necessary, as iodine may liberate.) Mix under vacuum until a clear reddish brown solution is obtained.
11. Make volume up to 1 L with purified water and mix well under vacuum for at least 15 minutes to ensure product uniformity and to deaerate the product.
12. Stop mixing, release the vacuum, then open the tank.
13. Check and record pH (range: 3–6).
14. Filter the solution through 100-mesh nylon cloth.

Povidone–Iodine Surgical Scrub

Bill of Materials			
Scale (mg/g)	Item	Material Name	Qty/kg (g)
75.00	1	Polyvinylpyrrolidone (PVP)-Iodine 30/06	75.00
250.00	2	Neutronyx® S 60	250.00
40.00	3	Super Amide® L 9	40.00
QS	4	Floral bouquet	QS
QS	5	Water	QS to 1 kg

Manufacturing Directions

1. Dissolve Super Amide in hot water, cool, dissolve PVP–iodine, and add Neutronyx to produce a brown, clear viscous solution with pH of approximately 3.4.

Povidone–Iodine Surgical Scrub

Bill of Materials			
Scale (mg/g)	Item	Material Name	Qty/kg (g)
75.00	1	Polyvinylpyrrolidone (PVP)-Iodine 30/06	75.00
250.00	2	Lutensit® AES	250.00
40.00	3	Monoamide® 150 MAW	40.00
QS	4	Floral bouquet	QS
QS	5	Water	QS to 1 kg

Manufacturing Directions

1. Dissolve Monoamide in hot water, cool, dissolve PVP–iodine, and add Lutensit to produce a brown, clear viscous solution.

Povidone–Iodine Vaginal Douche Concentrate

Bill of Materials			
Scale (mg/g)	Item	Material Name	Qty/kg (g)
100.00	1	Polyvinylpyrrolidone (PVP)-Iodine 30/06	100.00
5.00	2	Lutrol E 400	5.00
3.00	3	Lutrol F 127	3.00
432.00	4	Citric acid (0.1-M solution)	432.00
460.00	5	$Na_2HPO_4 \cdot 12H_2O$ (0.2-M solution)	460.00

Manufacturing Directions

1. Dissolve PVP–iodine and Lutrol F 127 in the mixture of buffer solutions with Lutrol E 400.
2. The brown, clear solution has a low viscosity and pH of approximately 4.3.

Povidone–Iodine Viscous Solution

Bill of Materials			
Scale (mg/g)	Item	Material Name	Qty/kg (g)
10.00	1	Polyvinylpyrrolidone (PVP)-Iodine 30/06	10.00
15.00	2	Natrosol® HR 250	15.00
QS	3	Buffer	QS
QS	4	Water	975.00

Manufacturing Directions

1. Dissolve PVP–iodine and Natrosol in the well-stirred buffered solution in water to produce a clear brown viscous liquid.
2. Viscosity (Brookfield) is 7500 mPa.

Prednisone Oral Solution

Each 5 mL oral solution contains prednisolone 5 mg and alcohol 5% or 30%. Inactive ingredients include alcohol, citric acid, disodium edetate, fructose, hydrochloric acid, maltol, peppermint oil, polysorbate 80, propylene glycol, saccharin sodium, sodium benzoate, vanilla flavor, and water. Prednisone 30% alcohol solution contains citric acid, poloxamer 188, propylene glycol, and water.

Prednisolone Sodium Phosphate Oral Solution

Pediapred (prednisolone sodium phosphate) oral solution is a dye-free, colorless to light-straw-colored, raspberry-flavored solution. Each 5 mL (teaspoonful) of Pediapred contains 6.7 mg prednisolone sodium phosphate (5 mg prednisolone base) in a palatable, aqueous vehicle.

Prednisolone Syrup

The syrup contains 15 or 5 mg prednisolone in each 5 mL. Benzoic acid 0.1% is added as a preservative. The syrup also contains alcohol 5%, citric acid, edetate disodium, glycerin, propylene glycol, purified water, sodium saccharin, sucrose, artificial wild cherry flavor, and FD&C blue No. 1 and red No. 40.

Progesterone Capsules

Progesterone capsules contain micronized progesterone for oral administration. Capsules are available in multiple strengths to afford dosage flexibility for optimum management. Capsules contain 100 or 200 mg micronized progesterone. The inactive ingredients for 100-mg capsules include peanut oil, gelatin, glycerin, lecithin, titanium dioxide, D&C yellow No. 10, and FD&C red No. 40. The inactive ingredients for capsules 200 mg include peanut oil, gelatin, glycerin, lecithin, titanium dioxide, D&C yellow No. 10, and FD&C yellow No. 6.

Promethazine and Codeine Syrup

Each teaspoon (5 mL) of Phenergan VC with codeine contains 10 mg codeine phosphate (*Warning*:—this may be habit forming), 6.25 mg promethazine hydrochloride, and 5 mg phenylephrine hydrochloride in a flavored syrup base with a pH between 4.8 and 5.4; alcohol, 7%. The inactive ingredients present are artificial and natural flavors, citric acid, D&C red No. 33, FD&C yellow No. 6, glycerin, saccharin sodium, sodium benzoate, sodium citrate, sodium propionate, water, and other ingredients.

Promethazine and Dextromethorphan Syrup

Each teaspoon (5 mL) of Phenergan with dextromethorphan contains 6.25 mg promethazine hydrochloride and 15 mg dextromethorphan hydrobromide in a flavored syrup base with a pH between 4.7 and 5.2; alcohol, 7%. The inactive ingredients present are artificial and natural flavors, citric acid, D&C yellow 10, FD&C yellow 6, glycerin, saccharin sodium, sodium benzoate, sodium citrate, sodium propionate, water, and other ingredients.

Promethazine Hydrochloride Syrup

Each teaspoon (5 mL) of Phenergan syrup plain contains 6.25 mg promethazine hydrochloride in a flavored syrup base with a pH between 4.7 and 5.2; alcohol, 7%. The inactive ingredients present are artificial and natural flavors, citric acid, D&C red No. 33, D&C yellow No. 10, FD&C blue No. 1, FD&C yellow No. 6, glycerin, saccharin sodium, sodium benzoate, sodium citrate, sodium propionate, water, and other ingredients. Each teaspoon (5 mL) of Phenergan syrup fortis contains 25 mg promethazine hydrochloride in a flavored syrup base with a pH between 5.0 and 5.5; alcohol, 1.5%. The inactive ingredients present are artificial and natural flavors, citric acid, saccharin sodium, sodium benzoate, sodium propionate, water, and other ingredients.

Promethazine Hydrochloride Syrup

Bill of Materials			
Scale (mg/mL)	Item	Material Name	Qty/L (g)
1.00	1	Promethazine HCl (5% excess)	1.05
675.00	2	Sucrose	675.00
1.00	3	Citric acid (monohydrate)	1.00
2.40	4	Sodium citrate	2.40
0.50	5	Ascorbic acid	0.50
0.25	6	Sodium metabisulfite (sodium disulfite)	0.25
0.25	7	Anhydrous sodium sulfite	0.25
50.00	8	Alcohol (ethanol, 95%)	50.00
0.15	9	Flavor	0.15
0.30	10	Flavor	0.30
0.50	11	Polysorbate 80 (Tween 80)	0.50
0.15	12	Caramel color	0.15
QS	13	Purified water	QS to 1 L

Manufacturing Directions

Promethazine HCl undergoes thermal and photochemical oxidation. Protect from light, heat, and oxygen as practicable. Avoid vortex or overmixing to avoid air entrapment. Use nitrogen gas whenever necessary to expel air.

1. Add 400 g of item 13 to the manufacturing vessel and heat to 90°C to 95°C.
2. Add item 2 while mixing at slow speed.
3. After addition of item 2, mix for 30 minutes at high speed and a temperature of 90°C to 95°C.
4. Cool down to 30°C to 35°C while mixing at low speed.
5. Add items 3 and 4 to the manufacturing vessel while mixing and mix until dissolved.
6. Add items 6 and 7 to the manufacturing vessel while mixing and mix until dissolved.
7. Add item 5 to the manufacturing vessel while mixing and mix until dissolved.
8. Mix items 9 and 10 with items 8 and 11 in a separate container by using stirrer.
9. Mix for 10 minutes and add to the manufacturing vessel while mixing.
10. Add 8 g of cold purified water (25–30°C) to a separate container and dissolve item 12 by using stirrer.
11. Mix for 10 minutes and add to the manufacturing vessel while mixing.
12. Start flushing the syrup with nitrogen gas pressure at 20 to 40 psi.
13. Add 10 g of cold purified water (cooled and flushed with N_2 gas) in a separate container with lid.
14. Pass nitrogen gas at 20 to 40 psi pressure for 15 minutes.
15. Dissolve item 1 in nitrogen-flushed cold purified water (25–30°C) by using stirrer.
16. Mix for 10 minutes and add to the manufacturing vessel while mixing. Do not produce vortex.
17. Bring volume up to 1 L with nitrogen-flushed purified water.
18. Continue flushing nitrogen gas at 20 to 40 psi pressure for 30 minutes while mixing at slow speed.
19. Check and record the pH (limit: 4.5–5.5). If required, adjust pH with 10% citric acid or 10% sodium citrate solution.
20. Filter the syrup at 1.5 bar.
21. Recirculate approximately 20 to 30 mL syrup.
22. Transfer the filtered syrup to the storage vessel.
23. Flush with nitrogen gas and seal the tank.

Promethazine Rectal Solution

Bill of Materials			
Scale (mg/mL)	Item	Material Name	Qty/L (g)
QS	1	Pluronic L62	QS to 1 L
2.50	2	Promethazine hydrochloride	2.50

Manufacturing Directions

1. Mill and screen the promethazine HCl to reduce particle size.
2. Add the poloxamer and the promethazine HCl into a clean vessel.
3. Mix until uniform.

Promethazine Rectal Solution

Bill of Materials			
Scale (mg/mL)	Item	Material Name	Qty/L (g)
QS	1	Pluronic L62	QS to 1 L
10.00	2	Carbopol 974	10.00
2.50	3	Promethazine hydrochloride	2.50

Manufacturing Directions

1. Mill the promethazine HCl to reduce particle size.
2. Sieve the carbomer and promethazine HCl and add to a clean vessel.
3. Add the poloxamer. Mix until uniform.

Pseudoephedrine Hydrochloride Syrup

Bill of Materials			
Scale (mg/mL)	Item	Material Name	Qty/L (g)
6.00	1	Pseudoephedrine HCl (3.0% excess)	6.18
600.00	2	Sucrose	600.00
100.00	3	Glycerin (glycerol)	100.00
100.00	4	Sorbitol (70% solution)	100.00
15.00	5	Propylene glycol	15.00
1.00	6	Methyl paraben	1.00
0.30	7	Propyl paraben	0.30
0.50	8	Saccharin sodium	0.50
0.02	9	Dye (if needed)	0.02
0.05	10	Menthol	0.05
0.13	11	Citric acid	0.13
1.15	12	Sodium citrate	1.15
QS	13	Purified water	QS to 1 L

Manufacturing Directions

1. Add 390 g of purified water to the manufacturing vessel and heat to 90°C to 95°C.
2. Add items 6 and 7 while mixing to dissolve at high speed.
3. Add item 2 while mixing at slow speed at a temperature of 90°C to 95°C.
4. Mix for 1 hour at high speed.
5. Cool down to 50°C while mixing at slow speed.
6. Dissolve items 8 and 12 in 10 g of item 13 and add to the manufacturing vessel while mixing at high speed.
7. Dissolve item 11 in 10 g of purified water and add to the manufacturing vessel while mixing at high speed.
8. Load items 4 and 3 into the manufacturing vessel using a transfer pump while mixing at high speed.
9. Mix for 5 minutes.
10. Cool down to 30°C while mixing at slow speed.
11. Add 20 g of item 13 (30°C) in a separate container and dissolve item 1 by using stirrer.
12. Mix for 10 minutes and add to the manufacturing vessel while mixing at high speed.
13. Add 6 g of item 13 in a separate container and dissolve item 9 manually.
14. Add color to the manufacturing vessel while mixing at high speed.
15. Dissolve item 10 in item 5.
16. Add this flavor mixture to the manufacturing vessel while mixing at high speed.
17. Bring the volume up to 1 L with item 13 and finally mix for 15 to 20 minutes at high speed.
18. Check and record the pH (limit: 5.5–6.5 at 25°C).
19. If required, adjust pH with 20% citric acid or 20% sodium citrate solution.
20. Filter the syrup at 1.5 bar.
21. Recirculate approximately 100 to 150 mL syrup.

Pseudoephedrine Hydrochloride, Carbinoxamine Maleate Oral Drops

Bill of Materials			
Scale (mg/mL)	Item	Material Name	Qty/L (g)
500.00	1	Sucrose	500.00
300.00	2	Glucose liquid	300.00
150.00	3	Glycerin (96%)	150.00
30.00	4	D-Pseudoephedrine hydrochloride	30.00
1.00	5	Carbinoxamine maleate	1.00
4.00	6	Saccharin sodium (powder)	4.00
2.50	7	Sodium benzoate (powder)	2.50
1.25	8	Flavor	1.25
0.03	9	Dye	0.03
0.03	10	Dye	0.03
QS	11	Hydrochloric acid reagent-grade bottles	QS
QS	12	HyFlo filter aid	1.32
QS	13	Purified water	455.00
QS	14	Sodium hydroxide for pH adjustment	QS

Manufacturing Directions

1. Charge 315 mL of deionized water into a suitable tank.
2. Begin heating water to 60°C to 70°C while adding sucrose with stirring.
3. Stir until sugar is dissolved.
4. Remove heat.
5. Add glucose liquid and 125 g of glycerin in this step.
6. Add and dissolve D-pseudoephedrine HCl, carbinoxamine maleate, saccharin sodium, and sodium benzoate with mixing.
7. Cool solution to 30°C to 35°C.
8. Mix flavor with 25 g of glycerin.
9. (*Note*: Temperature of syrup must not be higher than 35°C.) Dissolve dyes, if used, in 5 mL of deionized water and add to syrup with mixing.
10. Adjust to pH 4.25 (range: 4.0–4.5), if necessary, with hydrochloric acid or sodium hydroxide.
11. QS to 1 L with deionized water and mix well.
12. Allow product to stand overnight to let entrapped air escape.
13. Readjust volume to 1 L with deionized water.
14. Add and mix 1.320 g of HyFlo filter aid to the product.
15. Circulate through a press.
16. Filter into tank for filling.

Pseudoephedrine Hydrochloride, Carbinoxamine Maleate Oral Drops

Bill of Materials			
Scale (mg/mL)	Item	Material Name	Qty/L (g)
500.00	1	Sucrose	500.000
300.00	2	Glucose, liquid	300.000
150.00	3	Glycerin (96%)	150.000
30.00	4	D-Pseudoephedrine hydrochloride	30.000
1.00	5	Carbinoxamine maleate	1.000
4.00	6	Saccharin sodium powder	4.000
2.50	7	Sodium benzoate powder	2.500
1.25	8	Flavor	1.250
0.032	9	Dye	0.032
0.036	10	Dye	0.036
–	11	Acid hydrochloric reagent-grade bottles	QS
1.320	12	Filter aid HyFlo	1.320
455.00	13	Water purified	455
QS	14	Sodium hydroxide for pH adjustment	QS

Manufacturing Directions

1. Charge 315 mL purified water into a suitable tank. Begin heating water to 60°C to 70°C while adding sugar with stirring.
2. Stir until sugar is dissolved. Remove heat. Add glucose liquid and 125 g glycerin in this step.
3. Add and dissolve D-pseudoephedrine HCl, carbinoxamine maleate, saccharin sodium, and sodium benzoate with mixing. Cool solution to 30°C to 35°C.
4. Mix flavor with 25 g of glycerin. Temperature of syrup must not be higher than 35°C.
5. Dissolve dyes, if used, in 5 mL purified water and add to syrup with mixing. Adjust to pH 4.25 (range: 4.0–4.5), if necessary, with hydrochloric acid or sodium hydroxide.
6. QS to 1 L with purified water and mix well. Allow product to stand overnight to let entrapped air escape.
7. Readjust volume to 1 L with purified water.
8. Add and mix 1.320 g of filter aid HyFlo to the product.
9. Circulate through a press. Filter into tank for filling.

Pseudoephedrine and Carbinoxamine Drops

Bill of Materials			
Scale (mg/mL)	Item	Material Name	Qty/L (g)
500.00	1	Sucrose	500.00
300.00	2	Glucose liquid	300.00
150.00	3	Glycerin	150.00
30.00	4	Pseudoephedrine hydrochloride	30.00
1.00	5	Carbinoxamine maleate	1.00
4.00	6	Saccharine sodium	4.00
2.50	7	Sodium benzoate	2.50
1.25	8	Flavor black currant	1.25
0.032	9	Dye red	0.032
0.036	10	Dye yellow	0.036
QS	11	Hydrochloric acid, to adjust pH	QS
1.32	12	Filter aid HyFlo	1.32
QS	13	Water purified	QS to 1 L
QS	14	Sodium hydroxide, to adjust pH	QS

Manufacturing Directions

1. Charge 315 mL purified water into a suitable tank.
2. Begin heating water to 60°C to 70°C while adding sugar with stirring. Stir until sugar is dissolved.
3. Remove heat. Add glucose liquid and 40 g sorbitol solution with mixing. Hold balance of sorbitol for step 6.
4. Add and dissolve D-pseudoephedrine HCl, carbinoxamine maleate, saccharin sodium, and sodium benzoate with mixing.
5. Cool solution to 30°C to 35°C.
6. Mix flavors with balance of sorbitol and add to syrup.
7. Add glycerin. Temperature of syrup must not be higher than 35°C.
8. Dissolve dyes, if used, in 5 mL purified water and add to syrup with mixing. Adjust to pH 4.25 (range: 4.0–4.5), if necessary, with hydrochloric acid or sodium hydroxide.
9. QS to 1 L with purified water and mix well.
10. Allow product to stand overnight to let entrapped air escape. Readjust volume to 1 L.
11. Add and mix 1.32 g of filter aid HyFlo to the product. Circulate through a press until sparkling clear.
12. Filter into tank for filling. Fill into suitable approved containers.

Pseudoephedrine Hydrochloride Syrup

Bill of Materials			
Scale (mg/mL)	Item	Material Name	Qty/L (g)
6.00	1	Pseudoephedrine HCl, 3% excess	6.18
600.00	2	Sucrose	600.00
100.00	3	Glycerin (glycerol)	100.00
100.00	4	Sorbitol (70% solution)	100.00
15.00	5	Propylene glycol	15.00
1.00	6	Methyl paraben	1.00
0.30	7	Propyl paraben	0.30
0.50	8	Saccharin sodium	0.50
0.02	9	Dye (if needed)	0.02
0.05	10	Menthol	0.05
0.132	11	Citric acid	0.13
1.150	12	Sodium citrate	1.15
–	13	Water purified	QS to 1 L

Manufacturing Directions

1. Add 390 g of item 13 to the manufacturing vessel and heat to 90°C to 95°C.
2. Add items 6 and 7 while mixing to dissolve at high speed.
3. Add item 2 while mixing at slow speed. Temperature 90°C to 95°C.
4. Mix for 1 hour at high speed. Cool down to 50°C while mixing at slow speed.
5. Dissolve items 8 and 12 in 10 g of item 13 and add to the manufacturing vessel while mixing at high speed.
6. Dissolve item 11 in 10 g of item 13 and add to the manufacturing vessel while mixing at high speed. Load items 4 and 3 into the manufacturing vessel using transfer pump while mixing at high speed.
7. Mix for 5 minutes. Cool down to 30°C while mixing at slow speed.
8. Add 20 g of item 13 (30°C) in a separate container and dissolve item 1 by using stirrer.
9. Mix for 10 minutes and add to the manufacturing vessel while mixing at high speed. Add 6 g of item 13 in a separate container and dissolve item 9 manually.
10. Add color to the manufacturing vessel while mixing at high speed.
11. Dissolve item 10 in item 5. Add this flavor mixture to the manufacturing vessel while mixing at high speed. Make up the volume to 1 L with item 13 and finally mix for 15 to 20 minutes at high speed.
12. Check and record the pH (limit: 5.5–6.5 at 25°C).
13. If required, adjust pH with 20% citric acid or 20% sodium citrate solution.
14. Filter the syrup at 1.5 bar. Recirculate about 100 to 150 mL syrup.

Ribavirin Inhalation Solution

Virazole is a brand name for ribavirin, a synthetic nucleoside with antiviral activity. Virazole for inhalation solution is a sterile, lyophilized powder to be reconstituted for aerosol administration. Each 100-mL glass vial contains 6 g ribavirin, and when reconstituted to the recommended volume of 300 mL with sterile water for injection or sterile water for inhalation (no preservatives added) contains 20 mg of ribavirin per milliliter, with a pH of approximately 5.5. Aerosolization is to be carried out in a small particle aerosol generator (SPAG-2) nebulizer only.

Risperidone Oral Solution

Risperdal is available as a 1 mg/mL oral solution. The inactive ingredients for this solution are tartaric acid, benzoic acid, sodium hydroxide, and purified water.

Ritonavir Capsules

Norvir soft gelatin capsules are available for oral administration in a strength of 100 mg ritonavir with the following inactive ingredients: butylated hydroxytoluene, ethanol, gelatin, iron oxide, oleic acid, polyoxyl 35 castor oil, and titanium dioxide.

Ritonavir Oral Solution

Norvir oral solution is available for oral administration as 80 mg/mL ritonavir in a peppermint- and caramel-flavored vehicle. Each 8-oz bottle contains 19.2 g ritonavir. Norvir oral solution also contains ethanol, water, polyoxyl 35 castor oil, propylene glycol, anhydrous citric acid to adjust pH, saccharin sodium, peppermint oil, creamy caramel flavoring, and FD&C yellow No. 6.

Ritonavir and Lopinavir Oral Solution

Kaletra oral solution is available for oral administration as 80 mg lopinavir and 20 mg ritonavir per milliliter with the following inactive ingredients: acesulfame potassium, alcohol, artificial cotton candy flavor, citric acid, glycerin, high fructose corn syrup, Magnasweet-110 flavor, menthol, natural and artificial vanilla flavor, peppermint oil, polyoxyl 40 hydrogenated castor oil, polyvinyl pyrrolidone, propylene glycol, saccharin sodium, sodium chloride, sodium citrate, and water.

Rivastigmine Tartarate Oral Solution

Exelon oral solution is supplied as a solution containing rivastigmine tartrate, equivalent to 2 mg/mL rivastigmine base for oral administration. Inactive ingredients are citric acid, D&C yellow No. 10, purified water, sodium benzoate, and sodium citrate.

Salbutamol Aerosol

Bill of Materials			
Scale (mg/g)	Item	Material Name	Qty/1000 units (g)
1.17	1	Salbutamol, 10% excess	26.40
0.11	2	Oleic acid, 10% excess	2.64
277.61	3	Trichloromonofluoromethane	5664.00
721.09	4	Dichlorodifluoromethane	14700.00

Manufacturing Directions

1. Filter approximately 5 kg of the trichloromonofluoromethane and the oleic acid through a suitable 0.2-micron filter into a stainless steel concentrate container.
2. Slowly add the salbutamol to the solution in step 1 and mix for about 15 minutes.
3. Filter most of the remaining trichloromonofluoromethane through a suitable 0.2-micron filter into the suspension holding tank.
4. Add the slurry from step 2 to the holding tank.
5. Rinse the concentrate container with filtered trichloromonofluoromethane and add the rinses to the holding tank.
6. Make up the final mass of 5.693 kg with filtered trichloromonofluoromethane.
7. Mix for 5 minutes. Sample (to determine nonvolatile matter, range: 0.49–0.53 w/w).
8. Fill 5.7 g of suspension into a clean aluminum vial and immediately crimp on the metering valve. Pressure fill, through metering valve, sufficient dichlorodifluoromethane to produce a final fill weight of 20.4 g. Check-weigh each aerosol to ensure that the fill weight is in the range of 20 to 20.8 g. At the start of manufacture, fill the vials and apply nonmetering valves. Pressure-test these vials using a special gauge adaptor to ensure the correct propellant mix is being used. The internal pressure measured at 22°C should be 50 to 60 psi.
9. Store the filled aerosols for a period of 2 weeks and check the weight again.
10. Test each aerosol by actuation to ensure correct operation.

Salbutamol Syrup Sugar Free

Bill of Materials			
Scale (mg/5 mL)	Item	Material Name	Qty/L (g)
20.75	1	Citric acid (monohydrate)	4.15
10.00	2	Sodium benzoate	2.00
6.25	3	Sodium citrate	1.25
3.75	4	Saccharin sodium	0.75
2.00	5	Salbutamol sulfate, 20% excess	0.48
5.00	6	Sodium chloride	1.00
5.00	7	Strawberry flavor	1.00
10.00	8	Tangerine flavor	2.00
15.00	9	Hydroxypropyl methylcellulose (Methocel E4M)	3.00
–	10	Water purified	QS to 1 L

Manufacturing Directions

1. Add 700 g of item 10 to the manufacturing vessel and heat to 70°C.
2. Add item 9 slowly while mixing at low speed. Mix for 30 minutes.
3. Cool down to 25°C with continuous mixing at low speed.
4. Add 20 g of item 10 (25°C) in a separate stainless steel container and dissolve items 3, 4, and 6 and add to the manufacturing vessel.
5. Add 20 g of item 10 (25°C) in a separate container and dissolve item 1 by and add to the manufacturing vessel.
6. Add 20 g of item 10 (25°C) in a separate container and dissolve item 2 and add to the manufacturing vessel.
7. Add 20 g of item 10 (25°C) in a separate container and dissolve item 5 by and add to the manufacturing vessel.
8. Add items 7 and 8 to the manufacturing vessel while mixing.
9. Make up the volume up to 1 L with item 10 (25°C) and finally mix for 20 minutes at high speed.
10. Assemble the Seitz filter press and wash the filters using about 250 L purified water (25°C) by passing through filters at 0.2 bar.
11. Filter the syrup at 1.5 bar. Recirculate about 30 to 40 mL syrup.
12. Transfer the filtered syrup to the storage vessel.

Salbutamol Syrup

Bill of Materials			
Scale (mg/5 mL)	Item	Material Name	Qty/L (g)
2.00	1	Salbutamol sulphate (20%)	0.480
2500.00	2	Sucrose	500.000
5.00	3	Methyl paraben	1.000
1.00	4	Propyl paraben	0.20
5.00	5	Citric acid (monohydrate)	1.00
2.80	6	Sodium citrate	0.57
1000.00	7	Sorbitol (70% solution)	200.00
1.10	8	Flavor	0.22
1.10	9	Flavor	0.22
50.00	10	Propylene glycol	10.00
–	11	Water purified	QS to 1 L

Manufacturing Directions

See above.

Salicylic Acid Collodion

Salicylic acid 17% w/w, alcohol, 26.3% w/w, t-butyl alcohol, denatonium benzoate, flexible collodion, and propylene glycol dipelargonate.

Salmeterol Xinafoate Inhalation Aerosol

Salmeterol xinafoate inhalation aerosol contains salmeterol xinafoate as the racemic form of the 1-hydroxy-2-naphthoic acid salt of salmeterol. It is a pressurized, metered-dose aerosol unit for oral inhalation. It contains a microcrystalline suspension of salmeterol xinafoate in a mixture of two chlorofluorocarbon propellants (trichlorofluoromethane and dichlorodifluoromethane) with lecithin. 36.25 μg of salmeterol xinafoate is equivalent to 25 μg of salmeterol base. Each actuation delivers 25 μg of salmeterol base (as salmeterol xinafoate) from the valve and 21 μg of salmeterol base (as salmeterol xinafoate) from the actuator. Each 6.5-g canister provides 60 inhalations and each 13-g canister provides 120 inhalations.

Salmeterol Xinafoate Inhalation Aerosol

Bill of Materials			
Scale (mg/application)	Item	Material Name	Qty/1000 application (g)
0.25	1	Salmeterol (used as salmeterol xinafoate)	0.250
7.28	2	Miglyol 829 (caprylic/capric diglycerol succinate)	7.280
0.15	3	Peppermint oil	0.150
0.18	4	Menthol	0.180
113.00	5	*N*-Butane	QS to 113.000

Manufacturing Directions

1. Transfer Miglyol 829 by pumping from the released and tared container into mixing vessel.
2. After pumping Miglyol 829, set the propeller with optimum circulation and revolution to ensure no air entrapment.
3. Weigh out required amount of salmeterol xinafoate transfer directly into mixing vessel while mixing slowly.
4. Keep the preparation under stirring without interruption or change in rpm.
5. Dissolve menthol in peppermint oil at 25°C by slow stirring in another mixing vessel. Continue stirring until the solution becomes clear.
6. Transfer the clean menthol solution (step 5) into step 4 while stirring at the set speed. Continue stirring for 1 hour.
7. Store the base solution in aluminum can with polyethylene stopper and screw cap.

Scopolamine Nasal Spray

Charge 2.6 g of scopolamine into a pressure-addition vessel and dissolve with stirring in 405.6 g of ethanol in which 0.26 g of oleic acid has previously been dissolved. After sealing and evacuation thereof, 6.7 kg of HFA 134a that has previously been aerated with carbon dioxide and adjusted to a pressure of 8 bar (20) in another pressure addition vessel is added by stirring. The solution obtained is dispensed into aluminum containers sealed with metering valves by means of the pressure-filling technique.

Selenium Sulfide Shampoo with Conditioner

Bill of Materials			
Scale (mg/mL)	Item	Material Name	Qty/L (g)
10.00	1	Selenium sulfide	10.00
2.00	2	Methyl paraben	2.00
10.00	3	Magnesium aluminum silicate type IIA	10.00
20.00	4	Titanium	20.00
0.17	5	Dye	0.17
230.00	6	Sodium alkyl ether sulfate/sulfonate	230.00
30.00	7	Cocamide DEA surfactant	30.00
40.00	8	Cocoamphocarboxyglycinate	40.00
10.00	9	Hydrolyzed protein	10.00
4.00	10	Perfume	4.00
QS	11	Citric acid	QS
QS	12	Sodium chloride	QS
QS	13	Deionized purified water	QS to 1 L

Note: Item 11 is used for pH adjustment, if necessary and item 12 is used for viscosity adjustment, if necessary.

Manufacturing Directions

1. Selenium sulfide is toxic; handle carefully and use approved respiratory protection.
2. Add 7 mL of purified water to an appropriate mill containing full-charge alumina grinding cylinder media.
3. Add selenium sulfide.
4. Seal the mill and agitate for approximately 10 minutes to wet down the powdered material.
5. Recycle for approximately 5 minutes with the pump set at 1040 mm Hg.
6. Stop agitation.
7. If necessary, add purified water (25–30°C) to nearly cover the grinding media.
8. Seal the mill and recirculate the slurry for 1 to 2 hours with the pump set to obtain the required particle size specifications for the selenium sulfide.
9. Load 250 mL of purified water into a suitable jacketed mixing tank and heat to 60°C to 70°C.
10. With good stirring, add and dissolve methyl paraben.
11. Slowly add and disperse the magnesium aluminum silicate. Continue mixing until fairly smooth.
12. Stop mixing and allow to hydrate for 1 hour.
13. Add and disperse titanium dioxide.
14. Mix for 30 minutes.
15. With good stirring, add the selenium sulfide slurry and rinse the mill with purified water.
16. Mix for 30 minutes.
17. Stop mixing and add sodium lauryl ether sulfate/sulfonate.
18. Mix slowly for 5 minutes.
19. Add cocamide DEA.
20. Mix slowly for approximately 3 minutes.
21. Add coco-amphocarboxyglycinate.
22. Mix slowly for 30 minutes.
23. Separately dissolve hydrolyzed protein (hydrogel) in 4 mL of purified water and mix until uniform.
24. Add solution from above to the tank and mix until uniform.
25. Add perfume and mix for 1 minute.
26. Dissolve dye in 2 mL of warm purified water (50–60°C) and add to mixing tank.
27. Mix until uniform.
28. Check and record pH; adjust to 4.5 to 5.0, if necessary, using citric acid. Record amount of citric acid used and the adjusted pH.
29. Add purified water QS to 980 mL and mix for 30 minutes.
30. Check and record viscosity.
31. If necessary, adjust by adding sodium chloride.
32. Deaerate by slow stirring under vacuum or use of a suitable deaerator.
33. Mix for 1 hour.

Sertraline Hydrochloride Oral Concentrate

Sertraline hydrochloride is a selective serotonin reuptake inhibitor for oral administration. It is chemically unrelated to other selective serotonin reuptake inhibitors or tricyclic, tetracyclic, or other available antidepressant agents. It is supplied in a multidose 60-mL bottle. Each milliliter of solution contains sertraline hydrochloride equivalent to 20 mg of sertraline. The solution contains the following inactive ingredients: glycerin, alcohol (12%), menthol, butylated hydroxytoluene. The oral concentrate must be diluted before administration.

Sertraline Hydrochloride Solution

Zoloft oral concentrate is available in a multidose 60-mL bottle. Each milliliter of solution contains sertraline hydrochloride equivalent to 20 mg of sertraline. The solution contains the following inactive ingredients: glycerin, alcohol (12%), menthol, butylated hydroxytoluene.

Simethicone Drops

Bill of Materials			
Scale (mg/mL)	Item	Material Name	Qty/L (g)
144.00	1	Simethicone emulsion 30% (Simethicone Antifoam M30)[a]	144.00
60.00	2	Polyethylene glycol (PEG 6000)	60.00
1.50	3	Xanthan gum (Keltrol F)	1.50
1.50	4	Methylcellulose 4000 (Methocel A4M)	1.50
1.50	5	Potassium sorbate	1.50
1.20	6	Methyl paraben	1.20
0.20	7	Propyl paraben	0.20
1.500	8	Saccharin sodium	1.50
0.80	9	Banana green flavor	0.80
1.02	10	Citric acid (monohydrate)	1.02
0.24	11	Sodium citrate powder	0.24
–	12	Water purified	QS to 1 L

[a]Equivalent to 43.2 mg of simethicone.

Manufacturing Directions

1. Load 240 g of item 12 in mixer. Heat to 90° to 95°C. Dissolve items 6 and 7 by mixing with recirculation for 5 minutes.
2. Load item 2 in mixer. Mix to clear solution at 90°C to 95°C for 5 minutes, under vacuum 0.4 to 0.6 bar.
3. Cool down to 25°C to 30°C. Take the PEG paraben solution out of the mixer and keep in a stainless steel container.
4. Load 512 g of item 12 in mixer. Heat to 90°C to 95°C and then cool to 65°C to 70°C.
5. Take out 208 g of item 12 (65–70°C) from the mixer in a stainless steel container. Disperse item 3 by continuous stirring by mixer.
6. Disperse item 4 in mixer containing item 12 at 65°C to 70°C (step 4) while mixing and homogenizing at high speed for 5 minutes under vacuum 0.4 to 0.6 bar.
7. Cool to 20°C to 25°C with continuous mixing and recirculation.
8. Add PEG paraben solution from step 3 to mixer while mixing at speed 18 rpm.
9. Add item 3 mucilage from step 5 to mixer while mixing at speed 18 rpm.
10. Homogenize at high speed under vacuum 0.4 to 0.6 bar for 5 minutes while mixing.
11. Dissolve items 5 and 8 in 12 g of item 12 in a stainless steel container and add to mixer while mixing.
12. Add item 1 to the mixer while mixing.
13. Rinse the container of item 1 (step 12) with 12 g of item 12 and add the rinsing to the mixer.
14. Add item 9 to the mixer while mixing.
15. Mix and homogenize at low speed under vacuum 0.4 to 0.6 bar for 5 minutes.
16. pH is a critical factor for Simethicone emulsion. Limit is between 4.4 and 4.6. Carefully adjust the pH.
17. Add item 12 (25–30°C) to make up the volume up to 1 L.
18. Mix at slow speed under vacuum 0.4 to 0.6 bar for 5 minutes.
19. Filter the bulk through 630-micron sieve in a clean stainless steel storage tank.

Sirolimus Solution

Sirolimus is an immunosuppressive agent. Sirolimus is a macrocyclic lactone produced by *Streptomyces hygroscopicus*. It is available for administration as an oral solution containing 1 mg/mL sirolimus; the inactive ingredients include phosphatidylcholine, propylene glycol, mono- and diglycerides, ethanol, soy fatty acids, and ascorbyl palmitate, and polysorbate 80. The oral solution contains 1.5% to 2.5% ethanol.

Sodium Chloride Nasal Drops

Bill of Materials			
Scale (mg/mL)	Item	Material Name	Qty/L (g)
90.00	1	Sodium chloride	90.00
3.00	2	Benzalkonium chloride solution 5%	3.00
QS	3	Water purified	QS to 1 L

Manufacturing Directions

1. Charge 50% item 1 in a suitable stainless steel container and heat to 85°C to 90°C.
2. Add and dissolve item 2 at room temperature.
3. Add item 1 and make up volume.

Stavudine for Oral Suspension

Zerit (stavudine) for oral solution is supplied as a dye-free, fruit-flavored powder in bottles with child-resistant closures providing 200 mL, 1 mg/mL, stavudine solution on constitution with water per label instructions. The powder for oral solution contains the following inactive ingredients: methyl paraben, propyl paraben, sodium carboxymethylcellulose, sucrose, and antifoaming and flavoring agents.

Sucralfate Suspension

Carafate suspension for oral administration contains 1 g sucralfate per 10 mL. Carafate suspension also contains colloidal silicon dioxide, FD&C red No. 40, flavor, glycerin, methylcellulose, methyl paraben, microcrystalline cellulose, purified water, simethicone, and sorbitol solution.

Bill of Materials			
Scale (mg/5 mL)	Item	Material Name	Qty/L (g)
1000.00	1	Sucralfate	200.00
5.00	2	Methyl paraben	1.00
1.50	3	Propyl paraben	0.30
1500.00	4	Sorbitol 70%	300.00
2.50	5	Saccharin sodium	0.50
20.00	6	Natrosol 250M	4.00
30.00	7	Avicel HC 591	6.00
20.00	8	Sodium phosphate dibasic	4.00
7.50	9	Sodium phosphate monobasic	1.50
1.00	10	Lemon flavor	0.20
QS	11	Water purified	QS to 1 L

Manufacturing Directions

1. Charge 40% of item 11 in a stainless steel jacketed vessel and heat to 90°C to 95°C.
2. Add items 2 and 3 and mix to dissolve. Cool to 40°C.
3. Charge item 11 and item 6 in a separate vessel at 70°C to 80°C and stir for 30 minutes.
4. Add and disperse item 7 in step 3.
5. Transfer to step 1 and mix to disperse.
6. In a separate vessel, add and mix item 4 with items 1 and 11.
7. Add to step 6.
8. Add flavor and bring to volume.

Sulfacetamide Sodium and Sulfur Cleanser and Suspension

Each gram of Plexion (sodium sulfacetamide 10% and sulfur 5%) cleanser contains 100 mg sodium sulfacetamide and 50 mg sulfur in a cleanser base containing water, sodium methyl oleyltaurate, sodium cocoyl isethionate, disodium oleamido MEA sulfosuccinate, cetyl alcohol, glyceryl stearate and PEG-100 stearate, stearyl alcohol, PEG-55 propylene glycol oleate, magnesium aluminum silicate, methyl paraben, disodium EDTA, butylated hydroxytoluene, sodium thiosulfate, fragrance, xanthan gum, and propyl paraben. Each gram of Plexion (sodium sulfacetamide 10% and sulfur 5%) topical suspension contains 100 mg sodium sulfacetamide and 50 mg sulfur in a topical suspension containing water, propylene glycol, isopropyl myristate, light mineral oil, polysorbate 60, sorbitan monostearate, cetyl alcohol, hydrogenated cocoglycerides, stearyl alcohol, fragrances, benzyl alcohol, glyceryl stearate and PEG-100 stearate, dimethicone, zinc ricinoleate, xanthan gum, disodium EDTA, and sodium thiosulfate.

Sulfadiazine and Trimethoprim Veterinary Oral Suspension

Bill of Materials			
Scale (mg/mL)	Item	Material Name	Qty/L (g)
400.00	1	Sulfadiazine	400.00
80.00	2	Trimethoprim	80.00
50.00	3	Sodium hydroxide	50.00
20.00	4	Kollidon CL-M	20.00
QS	5	Water purified	QS to 1 L

Manufacturing Directions

1. Charge item 3 into a stainless steel vessel along with item 5. Mix and dissolve.
2. Add and suspend item 4. Mix well.
3. Add and suspend items 1 and 2. Homogenize if necessary.
4. Fill.

Sulfamethoxazole and Trimethoprim Suspension

Bill of Materials			
Scale (mg/5 mL)	Item	Material Name	Qty/L (g)
200.00	1	Sulfamethoxazole	40.00
40.00	2	Trimethoprim	8.00
2.50	3	Carrageenan (Hydrogel 843T)	0.50
18.75	4	Tragacanth	3.75
2.50	5	Saccharin sodium dihydrate	0.50
0.625	6	Anise oil	0.125
3.125	7	Methyl paraben	0.625
2.70	8	Propyl paraben	0.54
2.17	9	Alcohol dehydrated	0.435
2914.00	10	Sorbitol solution	582.80
403.75	11	Glycerin	80.75
QS	12	Water purified	QS to 1 L

Manufacturing Directions

1. Add and disperse Hydrogel 843T in approximately 8 mL purified water.
2. Heat 30 mL purified water to 100°C and add to dispersion from step 1 with mixing.
3. Let stand overnight.
4. Load trimethoprim and 7 g sulfamethoxazole into a suitable mixer. Blend.
5. Moisten blend with approximately 25 mL water.
6. Spread mass as small pancakes onto oven trays and dry at 50°C for approximately 14 hours.
7. Retain balance of sulfamethoxazole for later use.
8. While mixing, add 75 mL water. Mix until homogenous.
9. Charge approximately 350 mL water into a suitable stainless steel mixing tank. Add and dissolve saccharin with mixing.
10. Add tragacanth and continue mixing for 4 hours.
11. Separately add and dissolve the following ingredients in alcohol: methyl paraben, propyl paraben, and anise oil.
12. Add solution from step above and sorbitol to the preparation from step 1. Mix for 3 hours and let stand overnight.
13. Add gel from step above with mixing. Mix for approximately 15 minutes.
14. Pass trimethoprim/sulfamethoxazole mass from step 4 and balance of sulfamethoxazole through a 595-micron aperture screen in Fitz mill knives forward, medium speed, and slowly add to main tank with continuous agitation.
15. Add glycerin to main tank with mixing.
16. Pass the whole batch through a colloid mill until particle size and homogeneity meet specifications. Rinse mill and other equipment with purified water. Add the rinsings to the batch and mix.
17. If necessary, deaerate the product mixing under vacuum (ca. 20–25 in of mercury). Release vacuum and check volume.
18. Bring to volume with water and mix.
19. Stir the suspension until homogeneous. Fill while stirring.

Sulfamethoxazole and Trimethoprim Suspension

Bill of Materials			
Scale (mg/mL)	Item	Material Name	Qty/L (g)
80.00	1	Sulfamethoxazole	80.00
16.00	2	Trimethoprim	16.00
30.00	3	Kollidon CL-M	30.00
100.00	4	Sucrose	100.00
QS	5	Water purified	QS to 1 L
2.00	6	Vanillin	2.00
2.00	7	Flavor chocolate	2.00

Manufacturing Directions

1. Charge in a suitable stainless steel jacketed vessel items 4 and 5. Heat to dissolve.
2. Cool to 40°C.
3. Add, after passing through 200-mesh sieve, items 1 to 3 into step 2. Mix to dissolve.
4. Add flavors. Mix and fill.

Sulfamethoxazole and Trimethoprim Suspension

Bill of Materials			
Scale (mg/mL)	Item	Material Name	Qty/L (g)
80.00	1	Sulfamethoxazole	80.00
16.00	2	Trimethoprim	16.00
50.00	3	Sucrose	5.00
30.00	4	Lutrol F 127 or Lutrol F 68	30.00
QS	5	Water purified	QS to 1 L
QS	6	Vanillin	QS
QS	7	Flavor chocolate	QS

Manufacturing Directions

1. Charge in a suitable stainless steel jacketed vessel items 3 and 4. Heat to dissolve.
2. Cool to 40°C.
3. Add, after passing through 200-mesh sieve, items 1, 2, and 4 into step 2. Mix to dissolve.
4. Add flavors, if used. Mix and fill.

Sulfathiazole Veterinary Oral Solution

Bill of Materials			
Scale (mg/mL)	Item	Material Name	Qty/L (g)
8.00	1	Sulfathiazole	8.00
225.00	2	Kollidon 25	225.00
QS	3	Preservative	QS
QS	4	Water purified	QS to 1 L

Manufacturing Directions

1. Charge item 4 in a suitable stainless steel jacketed vessel. Heat to 70°C.
2. Add and disperse item 2.
3. Add and dissolve item 1 to a clear solution
4. Filter, if necessary, and fill.
5. Optionally, an antioxidant such as 0.02% sodium bisulfite or 0.5% cysteine may be added if necessary.

Sulfidoxine Solution

Bill of Materials			
Scale (mg/mL)	Item	Material Name	Qty/L (g)
20.00	1	Sulfidoxine	20.00
680.00	2	Lutrol E 400	680.00
QS	3	Preservatives	QS
QS	4	Water purified	QS to 1 L

Manufacturing Directions

1. Charge items 1 and 2 in a suitable stainless steel jacketed vessel. Heat to 60°C and mix.
2. In a separate vessel, charge item 4 and heat to 90°C to 95°C and then add item 3 (e. g., parabens) and dissolve. Cool to 40°C.
3. Add step 2 into step 1. Mix to clear solution.

Sulfidoxine and Pyrimethamine Suspension

Bill of Materials			
Scale (mg/mL)	Item	Material Name	Qty/L (g)
2.70	1	Tylose	2.70
1.00	2	Methyl paraben	1.00
0.20	3	Propyl paraben	0.20
600.00	4	Sugar	600.00
0.15	5	Sodium hydroxide	0.15
6.00	6	Trisodium citrate dehydrate	6.00
2.00	7	Benzoic acid	2.00
100.00	8	Sorbitol syrup	100.00
4.00	9	Tween 80	4.00
100.00	10	Sulfadoxine micronized	100.00
5.00	11	Pyrimethamine	5.00
0.20	12	Flavor	0.20
0.20	13	Flavor	0.20
0.20	14	Flavor	0.20
QS	15	Water purified	QS to 1 L

Manufacturing Directions

1. Boil a suitable quantity of item 15, cool down to 70°C, and add and dissolve items 2 and 3.
2. Add item 1 and dissolve in item 15 in a separate container and then add to step 1.
3. In a separate container add and dissolve sodium hydroxide, sodium citrate, and benzoic acid in item 15 and add to step 1.
4. Add and mix sorbitol with Tween 60 and item 10, stir for 15 minutes, and add to step above.
5. Add item 11 to step above and mix to dissolve.
6. Add flavors and bring to volume.

Sumatriptan Nasal Spray

Each Imitrex nasal spray contains 5 or 20 mg of sumatriptan in a 100-μL unit-dose aqueous buffered solution containing monobasic potassium phosphate, anhydrous dibasic sodium phosphate, sulfuric acid, sodium hydroxide, and purified water. The pH of the solution is approximately 5.5. The osmolality of the solution is 372 or 742 mOsmol for the 5- and 20-mg Imitrex nasal spray respectively.

Sumatriptan Nasal Spray

Manufacturing Directions

1. Charge 2.6 g of sumatriptan into a pressure-addition vessel and dissolve with stirring in 405.6 g of ethanol in which 0.26 g of oleic acid has previously been dissolved.
2. After closing and evacuation thereof, 6.7 kg of HFA 134a that has previously been aerated with carbon dioxide and adjusted to a pressure of 7 bar (20°C) in another pressure-addition vessel is added with stirring.
3. The preparation obtained is dispensed into aluminum containers sealed with metering valves by means of the pressure-filling technique.

Terfenadine Oral Suspension

Bill of Materials			
Scale (mg/5 mL)	Item	Material Name	Qty/L (g)
30.00	1	Terfenadine, 8% excess	6.48
2250.00	2	Sucrose	450.00
7.50	3	Sodium methyl paraben	1.50
2.500	4	Sodium propyl paraben	0.50
300.00	5	Propylene glycol	60.00
15.00	6	Polysorbate 80 (Tween 80)	3.00
50.00	7	Benzyl alcohol	10.00
0.24	8	Anise oil	0.048
15.00	9	Magnesium aluminium silicate (Veegum HV)	3.00
125.00	10	Glycerin	25.00
18.74	11	Carboxymethylcellulose sodium	3.74
0.76	12	Citric acid (monohydrate)	0.15
–	13	Water purified	QS to 1 L

Manufacturing Directions

1. Add 240 g of item 13 to the mixer and heat to 90°C. Add and dissolve item 2 while mixing.
2. Add and dissolve items 3 and 4 in the mixer at step 1 while mixing at speed 18 to 20 rpm for 15 minutes.
3. Cool down to about 50°C to 55°C.
4. Filter the syrup.
5. Collect the syrup in clean stainless steel tank.
6. Clean mixer with item 13 and transfer the filtered syrup from step 4. Maintain temperature at 35°C.
7. Add 80 g of item 13 (70°C) in a separate stainless steel container and disperse item 9 by using stirrer. Keep aside for 1 hour for hydration.
8. Add item 10 in a separate stainless steel container and disperse item 11 while mixing with stirrer.
9. Add 80 g of item 13 (70°C) while mixing. Make a gel and keep aside.
10. Add 160 g of item 13 (60°C) in a separate stainless steel container.
11. Dissolve item 6. Avoid foam formation. Add item 1 slowly while mixing at slow speed. Add item 5 while mixing at slow speed. Keep the solution aside.
12. Transfer items 1, 9, and 11 dispersions from steps 3, 4, and 5, respectively to the mixer.
13. Mix at speed 18 rpm for 10 minutes.
14. Mix item 8 in item 7 and add to the mixer. Mix for 2 minutes.
15. Dissolve item 12 in 3.2 g of item 13 and add to the mixer. Mix for 2 minutes.
16. Add cold item 13 (25°C) to make up the volume to 1 L.
17. Homogenize for 10 minutes at high speed under vacuum 0.5 bar, 18 to 20 rpm, temperature 25°C.
18. Check the dispersion for uniformity.
19. Check the pH (limit: 8–9 at 25°C). If required, adjust the pH with 20% solution of citric acid or sodium citrate.
20. Filter the suspension through a 500-micron sieve to storage tank.

Terfenadine Suspension

Bill of Materials			
Scale (mg/mL)	Item	Material Name	Qty/L (g)
12.00	1	Terfenadine	12.00
30.00	2	Lutrol F 127	30.00
36.00	3	Cremophor RH 40	36.00
QS	4	Preservatives	QS
QS	5	Water purified	QS to 1 L

Manufacturing Directions

1. Charge item 5 in a suitable stainless steel jacketed vessel and heat to 40°C.
2. Add and dissolve item 2 and 3 in step 1.
3. While stirring, add item 1 and suspend.
4. Homogenize if necessary and fill.

Theophylline Sodium Glycinate Elixir

Bill of Materials			
Scale (mg/5 mL)	Item	Material Name	Qty/L (g)
125.00	1	Theophylline sodium glycinate[a]	25.00
4000.00	2	Sucrose	800.00
7.50	3	Sodium benzoate	1.50
0.75	4	Saccharin sodium	0.15
0.025	5	FD&C red No. 40	0.005
1.00	6	Flavor	0.20
QS	7	Water purified	QS to 1 L

[a]125 mg theophylline sodium glycinate is equivalent to 60 mg theophylline hydrate.

Manufacturing Directions

1. Add 400 g of item 7 to the manufacturing vessel and heat to 95°C to 98°C. Add items 3 and 4 to dissolve. Mix for 10 minutes at low speed.
2. Add item 2 while mixing at low speed, temperature 95°C to 98°C. When addition is over, mix for 30 minutes at high speed.
3. Cool to 30°C while mixing at low speed.
4. Add 50 g of item 7 (25–30°C) in a separate container and dissolve item 1 by using stirrer. Mix for 10 minutes and transfer to the manufacturing vessel at step 3.
5. Rinse the container (step 3) with 1 g of item 7 (25–30°C) and transfer the rinsings to the manufacturing vessel while mixing at low speed.
6. Dissolve item 5 in 1 g of item 7 in a stainless steel container with slow stirring by stirrer. Transfer to the manufacturing vessel while mixing at low speed.
7. Add item 6 to the manufacturing vessel step 4 while mixing. Mix for 10 minutes at low speed.
8. Make up the volume to 1 L with item 7 and, finally, mix for 5 to 10 minutes at high speed.
9. Check and record the pH (limit: 8.5–9.0 at 25°C).
10. Filtration: Assemble the filter press. Wash the filters using about 1 L of purified water (25°) by passing through filters at 0.2 bar. Filter the syrup at 1.5 bar. Recirculate about 20 to 30 mL syrup.
11. Transfer the filtered syrup to the storage vessel.

Thiabendazole Suspension

Mintezol (Thiabendazole) is an anthelmintic provided as a suspension, containing 500 mg thiabendazole per 5 mL. The suspension also contains sorbic acid 0.1% added as a preservative. Inactive ingredients in the tablets are acacia, calcium phosphate, flavors, lactose, magnesium stearate, mannitol, methylcellulose, and sodium saccharin. Inactive ingredients in the suspension are an antifoam agent, flavors, polysorbate, purified water, sorbitol solution, and tragacanth.

Thiothixene Oral Concentrate

Ingredients are thiothixene (2–30 mg/30 mL), alcohol, cherry flavor, dextrose, passion fruit flavor, sorbitol solution, and water.

Timolol Maleate Opthalmic Drops

Bill of Materials			
Scale (mg/mL)	Item	Material Name	Qty/L (g)
2.50	1	Timolol maleate	2.50
QS	2	Vehicle (pluraflo 1220 92.37%, ethanol 2.11%, anhydrous glycerin 5.16%)	QS to 1 L

Manufacturing Directions

1. Add timolol. Cover tightly and stir until a clear solution is obtained.
2. Add glycerin, ethanol, and pluraflo to a clean vessel.

Tolnaftate Foot Care Microemulsion

Bill of Materials			
Scale (mg/g)	Item	Material Name	Qty/kg (g)
155.00	1	Ethoxydiglycol	155.00
130.00	2	Polyglyceryl-6 dioleate	130.00
450.00	3	PEG-8 caprylic/capric glycerides	450.00
10.00	4	Tolnaftate	10.00
100.00	5	Water purified	100.00
50.00	6	Apricot kernel oil PEG-6 esters	50.00
100.00	7	Caprylic/Capric triglycerides	100.00
5.00	8	Chlorocresol	5.00

Manufacturing Directions

1. Mix items 1 to 3 and dissolve item 4 in this mixture.
2. Add items 5 to 8 and mix until uniform.

Tolu Balsam Cough Syrup

Bill of Materials			
Scale (mg/mL)	Item	Material Name	Qty/L (g)
11.03	1	Tolu balsam tincture	11.03
2.50	2	Magnesium carbonate	2.50
15.00	3	Sucrose	15.00
QS	4	Water purified	90.000 mL
0.77	5	Methyl paraben	0.77
0.086	6	Propyl paraben	0.086
514.36	7	Sucrose	0.51
129.24	8	Glycerin (96%)	0.13
2.00	9	Dextromethorphan hydrobromide	2.00
1.00	10	Ephedrine HCl[a]	1.00
8.00	11	Ammonium chloride	8.00
0.40	12	Chlorpheniramine maleate	0.40
1.00	13	Phenylephrine hydrochloride	1.00
333.32	14	Glucose liquid	0.33
0.35	15	Flavor	0.35
0.15	16	Flavor	0.15
1.02	17	Ipecac fluid extract	1.01
8.57	18	Alcohol[b]	8.57
0.0375	19	Dye	0.037
QS	20	Acid hydrochloric	QS
QS	21	Water purified	QS to 1 L

[a] May be deleted.
[b] Tolu balsam tincture contains 80% alcohol. Use this item optionally to dissolve flavors.

Manufacturing Directions

1. Charge tolu balsam tincture into mixing tank and add magnesium carbonate.
2. Mix well to suspend.
3. Add sugar (item 3) with mixing. Add 90 mL purified water (item 4) and mix thoroughly.
4. Allow to set for 1 hour.
5. Mix periodically while circulating through filter.
6. Solution must be brilliantly clear. Filter and save for next part.
7. Charge 210.5 mL purified water (item 21) into suitable tank.

8. Add and dissolve aseptoforms M and P with heat 90°C to 95°C and mixing.
9. Add and dissolve sugar (item 7) with mixing.
10. Heat if necessary. Add glycerin, continue agitation, and cool to room temperature. Add filtrate from step above to cooled syrup.
11. Add and dissolve the following ingredients with mixing: dextromethorphan HBr, ephedrine HCl (if used), ammonium chloride, chlorpheniramine maleate, and phenylephrine HCl.
12. Add glucose. Mix well. Add and dissolve in alcohol: flavors and ipecac fluid extract.
13. Add to tank, or in a separate container add flavors and ipecac extract to 10 mL glucose liquid, and mix. Add this to the main mixture.
14. Rinse the container with a further 5 mL glucose liquid and add the rinsing to the mixture.
15. Add the remaining glucose liquid. Mix well.
16. Dissolve in 1.75 mL purified water and add.
17. Check pH (range: 4–5). Adjust to pH 4 to 5 with hydrochloric acid.
18. Make the volume to 1 L with purified water.
19. Filter until sparkling clear. Add 0.5 g Hyflo® to mixing tank, mixing until uniform.
20. Filter into tank for filling.

Tolu Balsam Cough Syrup

Bill of Materials			
Scale (mg/mL)	Item	Material Name	Qty/L (g)
11.03	1	Tolu balsam tincture	11.03
2.50	2	Magnesium carbonate (powder)	2.50
15.00	3	Sucrose (granulated sugar)	15.00
QS	4	Purified water	90.00 mL
0.77	5	Methyl paraben	0.77
0.086	6	Propyl paraben	0.86
514.36	7	Sucrose (granulated sugar)	514.36
129.24	8	Glycerin (96%)	129.24
2.00	9	Dextromethorphan hydrobromide	2.00
1.00	10	Ephedrine HCl (powder)	1.00
8.00	11	Ammonium chloride	8.00
0.40	12	Chlorpheniramine maleate	0.40
1.00	13	Phenylephrine HCl	1.00
333.32	14	Glucose (liquid)	333.32
0.35	15	Flavor	0.35
0.15	16	Flavor	0.15
1.01	17	Ipecac (fluid extract)	1.01
8.57	18	Alcohol (ethanol, 190 proof)	8.57
0.037	19	Dye	0.037
QS	20	Hydrochloric acid (reagent-grade bottles)	QS
QS	21	Purified water	212.00 mL

Manufacturing Directions

1. Charge tolu balsam tincture into mixing tank and add magnesium carbonate.
2. Mix well to suspend.
3. Add sugar (item 3) with mixing.
4. Add 90 mL purified water (item 4) and mix thoroughly.
5. Allow to set for 1 hour.
6. Mix periodically while circulating through Shriver filter (or equivalent).
7. Solution must be brilliantly clear.
8. Filter and save for next part.
9. Charge 210.5 mL purified water (item 21) into suitable tank.
10. Add and dissolve parabens with heat (90–95°C) and mixing.
11. Add and dissolve sugar (item 7) with mixing. Heat if necessary.
12. Add glycerin, continue agitation, and cool to room temperature.
13. To cooled syrup, add filtrate from step above.
14. Add and dissolve the following ingredients with mixing: dextromethorphan hydrobromide, ephedrine HCl, ammonium chloride, chlorpheniramine maleate, and phenylephrine HCl.
15. Add glucose. Mix well.
16. Add and dissolve flavors and Ipecac fluid extract in 190-proof alcohol.
17. To the tank or in a separate container add flavors and Ipecac extract to 10 mL of glucose liquid and mix.
18. Add this mixture to the main mixture.

19. Rinse the container with a further 5 mL of liquid glucose and add the rinsing to the mixture.
20. Add the remaining liquid glucose. Mix well.
21. Dissolve in 1.75 mL purified water and add.
22. Check pH (range: 4–5).
23. Use hydrochloric acid to adjust pH to 4 to 5, with 4.5 being optimum (~0.3 mL HCl per liter of syrup).
24. QS to 1 L with purified water.
25. Filter until sparkling clear.
26. Add a suitable filter aid and mix until uniform.
27. Filter into tank for filling.

Tretinoin Solution (50 mg/100 g)

Formulation

I. Tretinoin (BASF), 0.05 g; Cremophor RH 40 [1], 14.0 g; propylene glycol [1], 15.0 g; butylhydroxytoluene, 0.05 g; alpha-bisabolol nat. (BASF), 0.1 g
II. Water, 70.0 g; parabens/sorbic acid, QS

Manufacturing

Heat mixture I to 40°C to 50°C to obtain a clear solution. Introduce this warm solution slowly in solution II. It forms a clear yellow solution.

Tretinoin Solution

Bill of Materials			
Scale (mg/mL)	Item	Material Name	Qty/L (g)
0.50	1	Tretinoin (BASF)	0.50
140.00	2	Cremophor RH 40	140.00
150.00	3	Propylene glycol	150.00
0.50	4	Butylated hydroxytoluene	0.50
1.00	5	Alpha bisabolol natural (BASF)	1.00
QS	6	Water purified	QS to 1 L
QS	7	Parabens	QS
QS	8	Sorbic acid	QS

Manufacturing Directions

1. Charge items 1 to 5 in a suitable stainless steel jacketed vessel. Heat to 40°C to 50°C to obtain a clear solution.
2. In a separate jacketed vessel, charge item 6 and heat to 90°C to 95°C.
3. Add and dissolve items 7 and 8. Cool to 40°C.
4. Add step 3 into step 1.
5. Mix to clear solution.
6. Filter if necessary and fill.

Triamcinolone Acetonide Nasal Spray

Tri-Nasal spray is a metered-dose manual-spray pump in an amber polyethylene terephthalate bottle with 0.05% w/v triamcinolone acetonide in a solution containing citric acid, EDTA, polyethylene glycol 3350, propylene glycol, purified water, sodium citrate, and 0.01% benzalkonium chloride as a preservative. Tri-Nasal Spray pH is 5.3.

Manufacturing Directions

Dissolve 20 g triamcinolone acetonide in 1.5 kg ethanol. The solution is dispensed into open aluminum containers and these are sealed with suitable metering valves. The containers are filled by means of the pressure-filling technique with a total of 4 kg of HFA 227 that has been aerated with carbon dioxide and adjusted to a pressure of 5 bar (20°C).

Triclosan Oral Solution

Bill of Materials			
Scale (mg/mL)	Item	Material Name	Qty/L (g)
QS	1	Vehicle (pluronic F108 55.80%, ethanol 21.30%, water 22.90%)	QS to 1 L
2.80	2	Triclosan monophosphate	2.80
10.00	3	Menthol	10.00
1.00	4	Sodium saccharin	1.00
0.50	5	Monosodium glycyrhizzinate	0.50
QS	6	Flavors and colors	QS

Manufacturing Directions

1. Mill and screen the menthol and triclosan monophosphate to reduce particle size.
2. Add the menthol, triclosan monophosphate, sodium saccharin, and monoammonium glycyrizzinate into a clean vessel.
3. Add propylene glycol to the vessel.
4. Subsequently add the poloxamer and water to the vessel.
5. Mix until uniform.

Triprolidine and Pseudoephedrine Hydrochloride Syrup

Bill of Materials			
Scale (mg/mL)	Item	Material Name	Qty/L (g)
0.25	1	Triprolidine HCl, 4.8% excess	0.26
6.00	2	Pseudoephedrine HCl, 3.0% excess	6.18
600.00	3	Sucrose	600.00
100.00	4	Glycerin (glycerol)	100.00
100.00	5	Sorbitol (70% solution)	100.00
15.00	6	Propylene glycol	15.00
1.00	7	Methyl paraben	1.00
0.30	8	Propyl paraben	0.30
0.50	9	Saccharin sodium	0.50
0.04	10	Quinoline yellow	0.04
0.05	11	Menthol	0.05
0.25	12	Raspberry flavor	0.25
1.15	13	Sodium citrate	1.15
QS	14	Water purified	QS to 1 L

Manufacturing Directions

1. Add 400 g of item 14 to the manufacturing vessel and heat to 90°C to 95°C.
2. Add items 7 and 8 while mixing to dissolve at high speed.
3. Add item 3 while mixing at slow speed. Temperature 90°C to 95°C.
4. Mix for 1 hour at high speed. Cool down to 50°C while mixing at slow speed.
5. Add items 9 and 13 to the manufacturing vessel while mixing at high speed.
6. Load items 5 and 4 into the manufacturing vessel using transfer pump while mixing at high speed.
7. Add 20 g of cold item 14 (30°C) in a separate container and dissolve items 1 and 2 by using stirrer.
8. Mix for 10 minutes and add to the manufacturing vessel while mixing at high speed.
9. Add 1 g of item 14 in a separate container and dissolve item 10 manually.
10. Add color to the manufacturing vessel while mixing at high speed. Dissolve item 11 in item 12. Then add item 6 to it. Add this flavor mixture to the manufacturing vessel while mixing at high speed.
11. Make up the volume 1 L with item 14 and, finally, mix for 15 to 20 minutes at high speed.
12. Check and record the pH (limit: 5.8–6.8 at 25°C).
13. If required, adjust pH with 20% citric acid or 20% sodium citrate solution.
14. Filter the syrup at 1.5 bar. Recirculate about 20 to 30 mL syrup.

Tulobuterol Syrup

Bill of Materials			
Scale (mg/5 mL)	Item	Material Name	Qty/L (g)
1.00	1	Tulobuterol hydrochloride	0.20
5.00	2	Water purified	100.00 mL
3.75	3	Glycerin	75.00 mL
0.03	4	Methyl paraben	0.60
0.0075	5	Propyl paraben	0.15
QS	6	Red dye	25.00 mg
QS	7	Flavor	5.00
QS	8	Sorbitol (70%)	QS to 1 L

Manufacturing Directions

1. Heat 50 mL water to approximately 80°C and 95°C in a suitable vessel.
2. Add the methyl paraben and propyl paraben. Rinse the containers with some of the remaining water if necessary. Stir until dissolved, maintaining temperature at about 80°C.
3. Warm about 340 mL sorbitol solution to 40°C and 55°C in a suitable vessel.
4. Transfer the warm sorbitol to the final mixing vessel and add the hot paraben solution from step 2, stirring continuously. Rinse paraben solution container with 5 mL hot water and add to the bulk.
5. Dissolve tulobuterol and the dye in about 25 mL remaining water, rinsing the containers with some of the remaining water if necessary.
6. Add the solution from step above to the final vessel, mixing continuously. It is important to ensure all of the colored solution is transferred. Rinse the container with a portion of the remaining water.
7. Add the glycerol and flavor to the bulk solution. Rinse the glycerol container with the remaining water and add to the bulk. Make up to volume with the sorbitol solution.
8. Mix gently until a uniform syrup is obtained, avoiding incorporation of air bubbles.
9. If necessary, circulate through a filter press until sparkling clear.
10. Pass filtered clear syrup into a suitable holding tank.

Tolnaftate Foot Care Microemulsion

Bill of Materials			
Scale (mg/g)	Item	Material Name	Qty/kg (g)
155.00	1	Ethoxydiglycol	155.00
130.00	2	Polyglyceryl-6 dioleate	130.00
450.00	3	PEG-8 caprylic/capric glycerides	450.00
10.00	4	Tolnaftate	10.00
100.00	5	Deionized water	100.00
50.00	6	Apricot kernel oil PEG-6 esters	50.00
100.00	7	Caprylic/Capric triglycerides	100.00
5.00	8	Chlorocresol	5.00

Manufacturing Directions

1. Mix items 1 to 3 and dissolve item 4 in this mixture.
2. Add items 5 to 8 and mix until uniform.

Triprolidine and Pseudoephedrine Hydrochloride Syrup

Bill of Materials			
Scale (mg/mL)	Item	Material Name	Qty/L (g)
0.25	1	Triprolidine HCl (4.8% excess)	0.26
6.00	2	Pseudoephedrine HCl (3.0% excess)	6.18
600.00	3	Sucrose	600.00
100.00	4	Glycerin (glycerol)	100.00
100.00	5	Sorbitol (70% solution)	100.00
15.00	6	Propylene glycol	15.00
1.00	7	Methyl paraben	1.00
0.30	8	Propyl paraben	0.30
0.50	9	Saccharin sodium	0.50
0.04	10	Quinoline yellow	0.04
0.05	11	Menthol	0.05
0.25	12	Raspberry flavor	0.25
1.15	13	Sodium citrate	1.15
QS	14	Purified water	QS to 1 L

Manufacturing Directions

1. Add 400 g of purified water to the manufacturing vessel and heat to 90°C to 95°C.
2. Add items 7 and 8 while mixing to dissolve at high speed.
3. Add item 3 while mixing at slow speed (temperature: 90–95°C).
4. Mix for 1 hour at high speed.
5. Cool down to 50°C while mixing at slow speed.
6. Add items 9 and 13 to the manufacturing vessel while mixing at high speed.
7. Load items 5 and 4 into the manufacturing vessel using a transfer pump while mixing at high speed.
8. Add 20 g of cold purified water (30°C) in a separate container and dissolve items 1 and 2 by using stirrer.
9. Mix for 10 minutes and add to the manufacturing vessel while mixing at high speed.
10. Add 1 g of purified water in a separate container and manually dissolve item 10.
11. Add color to the manufacturing vessel while mixing at high speed.
12. Dissolve item 11 in item 12, then add item 6.
13. Add this flavor mixture to the manufacturing vessel while mixing at high speed.
14. Bring the volume up to 1 L with item 14 and finally mix for 15 to 20 minutes at high speed.
15. Check and record the pH (limit: 5.8–6.8 at 25°C).
16. If required, adjust pH with 20% citric acid or 20% sodium citrate solution.
17. Filter the syrup at 1.5 bar.
18. Recirculate about 20 to 30 mL syrup.

Undecylenic Acid and Chloroxylenol Solution

This is an antifungal solution for topical use containing 25% undecylenic acid and 3% chloroxylenol as its active ingredients in a penetrating oil base. Available in 1-oz bottles with special brush applicator.

Urea Peroxide Ear Drops

Bill of Materials			
Scale (mg/g)	Item	Material Name	Qty/kg (g)
65.00	1	Urea peroxide (40% excess)	91.00
15.00	2	Sodium citrate (dihydrate, powder)	15.00
5.00	3	Polysorbate 20 (Tween 20)	5.00
2.50	4	Tartaric acid (12663)	2.50
QS	5	Anhydrous glycerin	QS
QS	6	Nitrogen	QS

Manufacturing Directions

1. Add 500 mL of glycerin into a suitable tank.
2. Start mixing at slow speed, and heat the contents to 70°C to 75°C.
3. Flood tank with nitrogen, increase mixing speed, and slowly add sodium citrate.
4. Add tartaric acid.
5. Mix for at least 30 minutes or until dissolved.
6. Maintain the temperature at 70°C to 75°C.
7. When sodium citrate is completely dissolved, cool to 25°C to 30°C with constant mixing.
8. Prepare urea peroxide by breaking up lumps and screening to remove large particles.
9. Wear gloves.
10. Add an additional 250 to 300 mL of glycerin into tank.
11. Add urea peroxide slowly to prevent lumping, while mixing constantly.
12. Mix at high speed after addition.
13. Add polysorbate 20 with constant mixing and QS to final volume with glycerin.
14. Mix for at least 30 minutes and until solution is clear.
15. Pass solution through an approximately No. 100 mesh (150-μm or similar) screen and collect in clean, dry carboys. (The filter support screen in a millipore holder may be used for filtering; the solution is too viscous to flow through a membrane or any cellulosic filter.)

Valproic Acid Capsules

Valproic acid is a carboxylic acid designated as 2-propylpentanoic acid. It is also known as dipropylacetic acid. Capsules and syrup are antiepileptics for oral administration. Each soft elastic capsule contains 250 mg valproic acid. Ingredients for the 250-mg capsules are corn oil, FD&C yellow No. 6, gelatin, glycerin, iron oxide, methyl paraben, propyl paraben, and titanium dioxide.

Valproic Acid Syrup

Valproic acid is a carboxylic acid designated as 2-propylpentanoic acid. It is also known as dipropylacetic acid. Capsules and syrup are antiepileptics for oral administration. The syrup contains the equivalent of 250 mg valproic acid per 5 mL as the sodium salt. Inactive ingredients are FD&C red No. 40, glycerin, methyl paraben, propyl paraben, sorbitol, sucrose, water, and natural and artificial flavors.

Vancomycin Hydrochloride Oral Solution

Vancocin HCl for oral solution contains vancomycin hydrochloride equivalent to 10 g (6.7 mmol) or 1 g (0.67 mmol) vancomycin. Calcium disodium edetate, equivalent to 0.2 mg edetate per gram of vancomycin, is added at the time of manufacture. The 10-g bottle may contain up to 40 mg of ethanol per gram of vancomycin.

Vitamin A and Vitamin D Infant Drops

Bill of Materials			
Scale (mg/mL)	Item	Material Name	Qty/L (g)
1500 IU	1	Vitamin A palmitate (1.7 MM IU/g) (50% excess)	1.323
400 IU	2	Vitamin D (40 MM IU/g) (Cholecalciferol) (25% excess)	0.012
10.00	3	Polysorbate 80 (Tween 80)	10.00
0.88	4	Vitamin E (oily; α-tocopheryl acetate)	0.88
0.50	5	Edetate disodium (sodium EDTA)	0.50
1.00	6	Ascorbic acid	1.00
0.10	7	Saccharin sodium	0.10
600.00	8	Glycerin (glycerol)	600.00
100.00	9	Sorbitol (70% solution)	100.00
50.00	10	Propylene glycol	50.00
1.00	11	Flavor	1.00
1.50	12	Flavor	1.50
QS	13	Dye	QS
QS	14	Dye	QS
–	15	Purified water	QS to 1 L

Manufacturing Directions

1. This product is a microemulsion and thermolabile preparation. The temperature of solution must not exceed 25°C at the time of processing. Store bulk at a temperature of 15°C to 20°C under nitrogen protection. Period of storage should not exceed 48 hours prior to filling in the bottle.
2. Collect 200 g of purified water in a melting vessel.
3. Heat to 90°C to 95°C for 10 minutes and then cool to 20°C to 25°C.
4. Bubble nitrogen gas into purified water for 20 minutes.
5. Load 100 g of purified water into the manufacturing vessel.
6. Bubble nitrogen gas during all stages of the processing.
7. Add items 5, 6, and 7 one by one to the manufacturing vessel while mixing.
8. Check that all materials are dissolved completely.
9. Add items 8 and 9 and 20 g of item 10 one by one to the manufacturing vessel while mixing at slow speed.
10. Mix for 5 minutes.
11. Avoid aeration.
12. Add item 3 in a stainless steel container.
13. Mix items 1, 2, and 4 one by one using a stirrer.
14. Mix for 1 hour at slow speed.
15. Avoid aeration.
16. Add the oil phase to the aqueous phase in the manufacturing vessel at a rate of 4 mL/min while mixing; keep on bubbling nitrogen gas throughout the process.
17. Dissolve items 11 and 12 in 30 g of item 10 in a stainless steel container by slow stirring.
18. Add to manufacturing vessel while mixing.
19. Dissolve items 14 and 13 in 40 g of purified water (25–30°C) in a stainless steel container with slow stirring.
20. Add to manufacturing vessel while mixing.
21. Adjust the volume to 1.0 L with cooled purified water.
22. Check and record the volume and pH (limit: 2.5–4.8).
23. Filter the solution through a prefilter and 0.2-μm membrane filter into the receiving tank.
24. Bubble with nitrogen gas for 15 minutes.
25. Store the solution with a nitrogen blanket.

Vitamins A and D Infant Drops

Bill of Materials			
Scale (mg/mL)	Item	Material Name	Qty/L (g)
1500 U	1	Vitamin A palmitate 1.7 million U/g, 50% excess	1.32
400 U	2	Vitamin D 40 MU/g (Cholecalciferol), 25% excess	0.0125
10.00	3	Polysorbate 80 (Tween 80)	10.00
0.88	4	Vitamin E oil (alpha-tocopheryl acetate)	0.88
0.50	5	Edetate disodium (sodium EDTA)	0.50
1.00	6	Ascorbic acid	1.00
0.100	7	Saccharin sodium	0.10
600.00	8	Glycerin (glycerol)	600.00
100.00	9	Sorbitol (70% solution)	10000
50.00	10	Propylene glycol	50.00
1.00	11	Flavor	1.00
1.50	12	Flavor	1.50
0.02	13	Dye	0.02
0.003	14	Dye	0.003
–	15	Water purified	QS to 1 L

Manufacturing Directions.

1. Collect 200 g of item 15 in melting vessel.
2. Heat to 90°C to 95°C for 10 minutes and then cool to 20°C to 25°C.
3. Bubble nitrogen gas into item 15 for 20 minutes.
4. Load 100 g of item 15 to the manufacturing vessel.
5. Bubble nitrogen gas during all stages of the processing.
6. Add items 5, 6, and 7 one by one to the manufacturing vessel while mixing.
7. Check that all materials are dissolved completely.
8. Add items 8 and 9 and 20 g of item 10 one by one to the manufacturing vessel while mixing at slow speed. Mix for 5 minutes. Avoid aeration.
9. Add item 3 in a stainless steel container.
10. Mix items 1, 2, and 4 one by one using stirrer. Mix for 1 hour at slow speed. Avoid aeration.
11. Add oil phase to the aqueous phase in the manufacturing vessel at a rate of 4 mL/min while mixing, continuing to bubble nitrogen gas, throughout the process.
12. Dissolve items 11 and 12 in 30 g of item 10 in a stainless steel container by slow stirring. Add into manufacturing vessel while mixing.
13. Dissolve items 14 and 13 in 40 g of item 15 (25–30°C) in a stainless steel container by slow stirring.
14. Add into manufacturing vessel while mixing.
15. Adjust the volume to 1 L with cooled item 15.
16. Check and record the volume and pH (limit: between 2.5 and 4.8).
17. Filter the solution through a prefilter and a membrane filter of 0.2 micron into the receiving tank.
18. Bubble with nitrogen gas for 15 minutes. Store the solution with nitrogen blanket.

Vitamin A and Vitamin D_3 Drops

Bill of Materials			
Scale (mg/g)	Item	Material Name	Qty/L (g)
30000 IU	1	Vitamin A palmitate (1.7 MM IU/g)	1.90
3000 IU	2	Vitamin D_3 (40 MM IU/g)	7.50 mg
12.00	3	Cremophor (relative humidity, 40%)	12.00
0.30	4	Butylhydroxytoluene	0.30
10.00	5	Lutrol E 400	10.00
0.80	6	Paraben	0.80
0.20	7	Sorbic acid	0.20
QS	8	Water	QS to 1 L

Manufacturing Directions

1. Heat mixture of items 1 to 5 and solution of items 6 to 8 to about 65°C and add this slowly to the well-stirred mixture of items 1 to 5.
2. Clear or slightly opalescent yellow liquid is obtained.

Vitamin A and Vitamin D_3 Drops

Bill of Materials			
Scale (mg/g)	Item	Material Name	Qty/L (g)
30000 U	1	Vitamin A palmitate 1.7 million U/g	1.90
3000 U	2	Vitamin D_3 40 million U/g	7.5 mg
12.0	3	Cremophor RH 40	12.00
0.3	4	Butylhydroxytoluene	0.30
10.0	5	Lutrol E 400	10.00
0.8	6	Parabens (propyl and methyl)	0.80
0.2	7	Sorbic acid	0.20
74.8	8	Water purified	74.80

Manufacturing Directions

1. Heat mixture of items 1 to 5 and solution of items 6 to 8 to about 65°C.
2. Add this slowly to the well-stirred mixture of items 1 to 5. Yellow clear or slightly opalescent liquid is obtained.

Vitamin A and Vitamin D_3 Oral Solution

Bill of Materials			
Scale (mg/mL)	Item	Material Name	Qty/L (mg)
1000 IU	1	Vitamin A palmitate (1.7 MM IU/g)	60.00
100 IU	2	Vitamin D_3 (40 MM IU/g)	0.30
0.002	3	Butylhydroxytoluene	0.20
3.00	4	Cremophor EL or Cremophor (relative humidity, 40%)	3.00 g
QS	5	Preservative	QS
QS	6	Flavor	QS
QS	7	Water	QS to 1 L

Manufacturing Directions

1. Heat mixture of items 1 to 4 to about 65°C, stir well, and slowly add the hot solution of item 5 (65°C).
2. Cool to room temperature and add item 6 to obtain a clear, yellow liquid.

Vitamin A and Vitamin D_3 Oral Solution

Bill of Materials			
Scale (mg/mL)	Item	Material Name	Qty/L (mg)
1000 U	1	Vitamin A palmitate 1.7 million U/g	60.00
100 U	2	Vitamin D_3 40 million U/g	0.30
0.002	3	Butylhydroxytoluene	0.20
3.00	4	Cremophor EL or Cremophor RH 40	3000.00
QS	5	Preservative	QS
QS	6	Flavor	QS
QS	7	Water purified	QS to 1 L

Manufacturing Directions

1. Heat mixture of items 1 to 4 to about 65°C. Stir well.
2. Add slowly the hot solution of item 5 (65°C).
3. Cool to room temperature and add item 6. A clear, yellow liquid is formed.

Vitamin A and Vitamin D_3 Syrup

Bill of Materials			
Scale (mg/mL)	Item	Material Name	Qty/L (g)
30000 IU	1	Vitamin A palmitate (1.7 MM IU/g)	19.00
10000 IU	2	Vitamin D_3 (40 MM IU/g)	0.25
70.00 mg	3	Cremophor (relative humidity, 40%)	7.00
QS	4	II. Sugar syrup (50%)	QS to 1 L

Manufacturing Directions

1. Heat mixture of items 1 to 3 to approximately 45°C, stir well, and slowly add item 4 to obtain a clear, yellow liquid (pH 6.2).

Vitamin A and Vitamin D_3 Syrup

Bill of Materials			
Scale (mg/mL)	Item	Material Name	Qty/L (g)
30000 U	1	Vitamin A palmitate 1.7 million U/g	19.00
10000 U	2	Vitamin D_3 40 million U/g	0.25
70.00	3	Cremophor RH 40	7.0
QS	4	Sugar syrup 50%	QS to 1 L

Manufacturing Directions

1. Heat mixture of items 1 to 3 to about 45°C. Stir well.
2. Add slowly the item 4. A clear, yellow liquid with pH 6.2 is formed.

Vitamin A and Vitamin E Drops

Bill of Materials			
Scale (mg/mL)	Item	Material Name	Qty/L (g)
25000 U	1	Vitamin A palmitate 1.7 million U/g	15.00
50.00	2	Vitamin E acetate	50.00
210.00	3	Cremophor RH 40[a]	210.00
QS	4	Preservative	QS
QS	5	Water purified	QS to 1 L

[a]The quantity is reduced by 1.0 g if DL-alpha-tocopherol is also added at 1.0-g level in the formulation.

Manufacturing Directions

1. Mix the vitamins with Cremophor RH 40 (and DL-alpha-tocopherol, if used) at 60°C.
2. Add solution of preservatives (at 37°C) slowly, with stirring. Clear, yellow viscous liquids are formed.

Vitamin A and Vitamin E Drops

Bill of Materials			
Scale (mg/mL)	Item	Material Name	Qty/L (g)
5000 U	1	Vitamin A palmitate 1.7 million U/g	3.33
50.00	2	Vitamin E acetate	60.00
150.00	3	Cremophor RH 40	150.00
150.00	4	Alcohol	150.00
QS	5	Water purified	QS to 1 L

Manufacturing Directions

1. Heat mixture items 1 to 3 to about 65°C. Stir well.
2. Slowly add the mixture of items 4 and 5. Color is yellow and clarity should be clear (turbity units: 25 FTU). It must be tested to see whether the ethanol concentration has a sufficient preservative efficiency. The addition of butylhydroxytoluene as antioxidant is recommended.

Vitamin A and Vitamin E Drops

Bill of Materials			
Scale (mg/mL)	Item	Material Name	Qty/L (g)
5000 IU	1	Vitamin A palmitate (1.7 MM IU/g)	3.33
50.00	2	Vitamin E acetate	60.00
150.00	3	Cremophor (relative humidity, 40%)	150.00
150.00	4	Ethanol (96%)	150.00
QS	5	Water	QS to 1 L

Manufacturing Directions

1. Heat mixture of items 1 to 3 to about 65°C, stir well, and slowly add the mixture of items 4 and 5.
2. Color is yellow; clarity is clear (turbity units 25 FTU).
3. It must be determined whether or not the ethanol concentration has a sufficient preservative efficiency.
4. The addition of butylhydroxytoluene as an antioxidant is recommended.

Vitamin A and Vitamin E Drops

Bill of Materials			
Scale (mg/mL)	Item	Material Name	Qty/L
25000 IU	1	Vitamin A palmitate (1.7 Mio IU/g)	1.50
50.00	2	Vitamin E acetate	5.00
210.00	3	Cremophor (relative humidity, 40%)[a]	21.00
QS	5	Preservative	QS
QS	6	Water	71.50

[a] The quantity is reduced by 1.0 g if 1.0 g of d,l-α-tocopherol is also added in the formulation.

Manufacturing Directions

1. Mix the vitamins with Cremophor (and d,l-α-tocopherol, if used) at 60°C.
2. Add solution of preservatives (at 37°C) slowly, with stirring to produce clear, yellow viscous liquids.

Vitamin A Concentrate, Water-Miscible

Bill of Materials			
Scale (mg/mL)	Item	Material Name	Qty/L (g)
100000 U	1	Vitamin A palmitate 1.7 million U/g	65.00
2.00	2	Butylhydroxytoluene	2.00
210.00	3	Cremophor RH 40	210.00
QS	4	Preservative	QS
QS	5	Water purified	QS to 1 L

Manufacturing Directions

1. Heat the mixture of items 1 to 3 to about 65°C. Stir well.
2. Add very slowly the warm solution of items 4 and 5 (65°C). Clear, yellow liquid, miscible with water, is formed.

Vitamin A Concentrate, Water-Miscible

Bill of Materials			
Scale (mg/mL)	Item	Material Name	Qty/L (g)
100000 IU	1	Vitamin A palmitate (1.7 MM IU/g)	6.50
2.00	2	Butylhydroxytoluene	0.20
210.00	3	Cremophor (relative humidity, 40%)	21.00
QS	4	Preservative	QS
QS	5	Water	QS to 1 L

Manufacturing Directions

1. Heat the mixture of items 1 to 3 to approximately 65°C. Stir well.
2. Add slowly the warm solution of items 4 and 5 (65°C) to obtain a clear, yellow liquid that is miscible with water.

Vitamin A Drops

Bill of Materials			
Scale (mg/mL)	Item	Material Name	Qty/1000 Tablets (g)
50000 IU	1	Vitamin A palmitate (1.7 Mio IU/g)	3.00
110.00	2	Cremophor (relative humidity, 40%)	11.00
1.00	3	Butylhydroxytoluene	0.10
QS	4	Water	85.90

Manufacturing Directions

1. Heat the mixture of items 1 to 3 to about 65°C. Stir well.
2. Add slowly the hot water (65°C) to obtain a clear or slightly opalescent yellow solution of low viscosity.
3. Lutrol E 400 can be added at a level of 5% (compensated for by item 4).

Vitamin A Drops

Bill of Materials			
Scale (mg/mL)	Item	Material Name	Qty/L (g)
50000 U	1	Vitamin A palmitate 1.7 million U/g	30.00
110.00	2	Cremophor RH 40	110.00
1.00	3	Butylhydroxytoluene	1.00
QS	4	Water purified	QS to 1 L

Manufacturing Directions

1. Heat the mixture of items 1 to 3 to approximately 65°C. Stir well.
2. Add slowly the hot water (65°C). The solution should be yellow and clear or slightly opalescent and of low viscosity. Lutrol E 400 can be added at a level of 5%, compensated by item 4.

Vitamin B Complex Syrup

Bill of Materials			
Scale (mg/g)	Item	Material Name	Qty/kg (g)
0.600	1	Thiamine hydrochloride	0.600
0.550	2	Riboflavin 5-phosphate sodium	0.550
2.50	3	Nicotinamide	2.50
1.20	4	Dexpanthenol	1.20
0.550	5	Pyridoxine hydrochloride	0.550
2.00	6	Sorbic acid	2.00
0.05	7	EDTA sodium	0.05
2.25	8	Vanillin	2.25
465.00	9	Sucrose	465.00
25.00	10	Kollidon 25	25.00
90.00	11	Glycerol	90.00
100.00	12	Propylene glycol (pharma)	100.00
310.00	13	Water purified	310.00

Manufacturing Directions

1. Dissolve the sucrose in the heat mixture of glycerol, propylene glycol and water. Cool to room temperature.
2. Dissolve the other components to obtain a clear solution.

Vitamin B Complex Syrup

Bill of Materials			
Scale (mg/mL)	Item	Material Name	Qty/L (g)
0.66	1	Dexpanthenol	0.66
4.40	2	Nicotinamide	4.44
0.22	3	Pyridoxine HCl	0.22
0.60	4	Riboflavin-5-phosphate sodium	0.60
1.50	5	Thiamine HCl	1.50
350.00	6	Sorbitol (70% solution)	350.00
11.20	7	Propylene glycol	11.20
0.84	8	Methyl paraben	0.84
0.16	9	Propyl paraben	0.16
550.00	10	Maltitol solution (Lycasin 80/55)	550.00
0.15	11	Edetate disodium (sodium EDTA)	0.15
3.72	12	Citric acid (monohydrate)	3.72
3.72	13	Sodium citrate	3.72
2.50	14	Sodium benzoate	2.50
0.50	15	Saccharin sodium	0.50
150.00	16	Glycerin (glycerol)	150.00
1.50	17	Flavor	1.50
1.00	18	Flavor	1.00
–	19	Water purified	QS to 1 L

Manufacturing Directions

1. Load items 6, 10, and 16 in a suitable manufacturing vessel and mix for 5 minutes.
2. Dissolve items 8 and 9 in item 7 in a stainless steel container.
3. Put the whole container in hot water (60–70°C) and stir to dissolve.
4. Add the clear solution to mixer.
5. Dissolve items 11 and 12 in 40 g of item 19 in a stainless steel container.
6. Add the clear solution to mixer.
7. Dissolve items 13, 14, and 15 in 50 g of item 19 in a stainless steel container. Add the clear solution to mixer and mix for 5 minutes.
8. Dissolve item 1 in 10 g of item 19 in a stainless steel container.
9. Add the clear solution to mixer. Dissolve items 3 and 5 in 10 g of item 19 in a stainless steel container. Add the clear solution to mixer.
10. Dissolve items 2 and 4 in 30 g of item 19 in a stainless steel container.
11. Add the clear yellow solution to mixer and mix for 5 minutes.
12. Add items 17 and 18 to mixer. Make up the volume up to 1 L with item 19 and finally mix for 15 to 20 minutes.
13. Check and record the pH (limit: 4.4–4.8 at 25°C). If required, adjust pH with 20% citric acid or 20% sodium citrate solution.
14. Filter the syrup at 1.5 bar. Recirculate about 200 to 300 mL syrup.
15. Transfer the filtered syrup to the storage vessel, flushing with nitrogen gas. Store the syrup under nitrogen blanket NMT 2 days before filling.

Vitamin B Complex Syrup

Bill of Materials			
Scale (mg/mL)	Item	Material Name	Qty/L (g)
0.60	1	Thiamine hydrochloride (BASF)	0.60
0.55	2	Riboflavin 5-phosphate sodium	0.55
2.50	3	Nicotinamide	2.50
12.00	4	Dexpanthenol (BASF)	12.00
0.55	5	Pyridoxine hydrochloride	5.50
2.00	6	Sorbic acid	20.00
0.050	7	EDTA sodium	0.50
2.25	8	Vanillin	22.50
465.00	9	Sucrose	465.00
25.00	10	Kollidon 25	25.00
90.00	11	Glycerin	90.00
100.00	12	Propylene glycol	100.00
QS	13	Water purified	QS to 1 L

Manufacturing Directions

1. Charge glycerin, propylene glycol, and purified water in a suitable stainless steel jacketed vessel. Heat to 65°C.
2. Add and dissolve sucrose in step 1.
3. Cool to room temperature.
4. Add and dissolve all other items.
5. Filter if necessary. Fill.

Vitamin B Complex and Vitamin C Syrup

Bill of Materials			
Scale (mg/mL)	Item	Material Name	Qty/L (g)
0.150	1	Thiamine hydrochloride	0.15
0.15	2	Riboflavin phosphate sodium	0.15
0.70	3	Nicotinamide	0.70
0.035	4	Dexpanthenol	0.035
0.15	5	Pyridoxine hydrochloride	0.15
2.25	6	Ascorbic acid, crystalline	2.25
0.28	7	Orange aroma	0.28
0.56	8	EDTA sodium	0.56
186.50	9	Propylene glycol (pharma) + water (2:1)	186.50
0.15	10	Parabens	0.155
84.30	11	Sorbitol, crystalline	84.30
562.50	12	Sucrose, crystalline	562.50
QS	13	Water purified	QS to 1 L

Manufacturing Directions

1. Dissolve items 1 to 8 in item 2.
2. Prepare solution of items 10 to 13 by heating, cool, and mix with solution balance of formulation.
3. Adjust to pH 4.2 to 4.5. Adjust volume with item 13; use more if necessary. Use nitrogen as inert gas during packaging.

Vitamin B Complex (without B_{12}) Syrup

Bill of Materials			
Scale (mg/mL)	Item	Material Name	Qty/L (g)
570.00	1	Sucrose	570.00
70.00	2	Glycerin	70.00
3.72	3	Citric acid (monohydrate)	3.72
1.00	4	Edetate disodium (sodium EDTA)	1.00
0.90	5	Calcium pantothenate, 10% excess	1.00
5.70	6	Sodium citrate	5.70
0.84	7	Methyl paraben	0.84
0.18	8	Propyl paraben	0.16
1.90	9	Benzoic acid	1.90
1.14	10	Strawberry flavor manefils	1.14
9.60	11	Alcohol	9.60
1.50	12	Thiamine HCl, 50% excess	1.50
0.20	13	Pyridoxine hydrochloride, 10% excess	0.22
4.00	14	Nicotinamide, 10% excess	4.40
0.30	15	Riboflavin sodium phosphate, 50% excess	0.60
–	16	Water purified	QS to 1 L

Manufacturing Directions

1. Flush with nitrogen gas (purity 99.95%).
2. Add 400 g of item 16 to the manufacturing vessel and heat to 90°C to 95°C.
3. Add item 1 while mixing at low speed. After addition of item 1 mix for 30 to 35 minutes at high speed and temperature 90°C to 95°C.
4. Cool to 40°C while mixing at low speed.
5. Disperse 1 g filter aid in 10 g cooled item 16 (25–30°C) in a stainless steel container to prepare a slurry.
6. Add the slurry to syrup in syrup vessel. Mix for 15 minutes at high speed.
7. Filter the syrup at 1.5 bar.
8. Recirculate about 40 to 60 mL syrup.
9. Transfer the filtered syrup to the storage vessel. Recharge the filtered syrup to the manufacturing vessel. Start mixing.
10. Add item 2 to the syrup vessel while mixing at high speed.
11. Add item 3 to the syrup vessel while mixing to dissolve at high speed.
12. Dissolve item 4 in 6 g of cooled item 16 (25–30°C) and add to the syrup vessel while mixing at high speed.
13. Dissolve item 5 in 6 g of cooled item 16 and add to the syrup vessel while mixing at high speed for 30 minutes.
14. Dissolve item 6 in 10 g of cooled item 16 (25 –30°C) and add to the syrup vessel while mixing at high speed.
15. Dissolve items 7, 8, 9, and 10 in item 11 in a stainless steel container and add to the syrup vessel while mixing at high speed for 15 minutes.
16. Dissolve items 12 and 13 in 6 g of cooled item 16 (25–30°C) in a separate stainless steel container and add to the syrup vessel while mixing at high speed.
17. Rinse the container with 1 g of cooled item 16 (25–30°C) and add the rinsing to the syrup vessel while mixing at high speed.
18. Flush the vessel with nitrogen gas purity 99.95% for 15 minutes.
19. Dissolve item 14 in 9 g of cooled item 16 in a separate stainless steel container and add to the syrup vessel while mixing at high speed.
20. Rinse the container with 1 g of cooled item 16 (25–30°C) and add the rinsing to the syrup vessel while mixing at high speed.
21. Dissolve item 15 in 4 g of cooled item 16 (25–30°C) in a separate stainless steel container and add to the syrup vessel while mixing at high speed.
22. Rinse the container with 1 g of cooled item 16 and add the rinsing to the syrup vessel while mixing at high speed.
23. Make up the volume to 1 L with cooled item 16 (25–30°C) and finally mix for 15 minutes at high speed.
24. Check and record the pH (limit: 4.3–4.7 at 25°C).
25. If required, adjust pH with 10% solution of citric acid or sodium citrate.
26. Flush the syrup with nitrogen gas purity 99.95% for 15 minutes.
27. Close the tank. Hold the syrup for 12 hours. Filter the syrup at 1.5 bar. Recirculate about 40 to 60 mL syrup.
28. Transfer the filtered syrup to the storage vessel.

Vitamin B Complex, A, C, D, and Calcium Drops

Bill of Materials			
Scale (mg/mL)	Item	Material Name	Qty/L (g)
675.00	1	Glycerin	675.00
16.66	2	Niacinamide powder white	16.66
2.739	3	Riboflavin-5′-phosphate sodium, 3% excess	2.822
0.500	4	Methyl paraben	0.500
1.0	5	Acid benzoic	1.00
105.0	6	Saccharin sodium powder	105.00
73.360	7	Calcium chloride granules (dihydrate)	73.36
28.785	8	Ferrous gluconate	28.78
2.25	9	Thiamine HCl powder regular, 35% excess	3.37
1.000	10	Pyridoxine hydrochloride	1.00
83.33	11	Acid ascorbic white powder, 35% excess	112.50
0.258	12	Oil orange terpeneless	0.25
0.081	13	Alcohol	0.081
80.00	14	Polysorbate 80	80.00
0.167	15	Butylated hydroxyanisole	0.16
0.666	16	Viosterol in corn oil (synthetic oleovitamin D USP 1000 mD/g), 25% excess	0.83
0.056	17	Vitamin A palmitate 1500000 U/g	0.056
10.000	18	Carmel acid proof	10.00
QS	19	Water purified	QS to 1 L

Manufacturing Directions

Product must not stand more than 1 week before filling. Avoid unnecessary exposure of product to light, air, and heat. Manufacture and store product under complete CO_2 protection. Avoid vigorous mixing.

1. Charge glycerin and 210 mL purified water into a stainless steel jacketed tank.
2. Add with mixing in the following order: niacinamide, riboflavin-5′-phosphate sodium, methylparaben, benzoic acid, and saccharin sodium.
3. Continue mixing and heat to 95°C to 100°C and hold to completely dissolve the ingredients.
4. Add, in portions, calcium chloride and stir until complete solution.
5. Continue mixing and cool to 70°C to 75°C. Add with mixing and dissolve ferrous gluconate at 70°C to 75°C. Check for absence of nondissolved material.
6. Check volume if necessary replace the purified water lost by heating with additional purified water, previously boiled, QS to 750 mL.
7. Cool with mixing to room temperature 25°C to 30°C while bubbling CO_2 gas through. Continue the CO_2 gas bubbling for balance of process.
8. Add and dissolve each ingredient in the order named: thiamine HCl, pyridoxine HCl, and ascorbic acid. Dissolve oil orange in ethyl alcohol and add with stirring.
9. Heat polysorbate 80 to 50°C to 60°C and hold for approximately 10 minutes with slow mixing.
10. Add and dissolve butylated hydroxyanisole.
11. Mix slowly and saturate with CO_2 while cooling to 25°C to 30°C.
12. Add and dissolve viosterol in corn oil and vitamin A palmitate, mixing well with CO_2 gas blowing.
13. Add polysorbate solution to main batch and mix thoroughly. Rinse container with a portion of main batch.
14. Heat 50 mL purified water to 35°C to 40°C while bubbling CO_2 gas through.
15. Add caramel color. Mix well until uniform.
16. Add to main batch. Rinse container with a small quantity of purified water that has been previously saturated with CO_2 gas.
17. Add to main batch. Add purified water that has been previously saturated with CO_2 gas.
18. Bring to volume.
19. Filter, without using filter aid. Cycle to achieve clarity. Keep carbon dioxide cover.

Vitamin B Complex and Iron Syrup

Bill of Materials			
Scale (mg/mL)	Item	Material Name	Qty/L (g)
910.00	1	Sorbitol solution	910.00
0.019	2	Propyl paraben	0.019
0.170	3	Methyl paraben	0.170
1.500	4	Niacinamide powder white	1.500
0.300	5	Riboflavin	0.300
103.600	6	Propylene glycol	103.60
126.400	7	Glycerin	126.40
26.132	8	Iron sulfate granular	26.13
0.0375	9	Dye	0.037
0.250	10	Pyridoxine hydrochloride	0.25
1.200	11	Saccharin sodium powder dihydrate	1.20
22.000	12	Sodium cyclamate powder	22.00
30.000	13	Acid ascorbic white powder	30.00
0.800 g	14	Sodium bicarbonate	0.80
0.360	15	Thiamine hydrochloride powder regular	0.36
0.625	16	D-Pantothenyl alcohol (dexpanthenol FCC)	0.62
0.0020	17	Vitamin B_{12} μg (cyanocobalamin)	2.00 mg
0.007	18	Flavor	0.700 mL
QS	19	Water purified	QS to 1 L
QS	20	Filter aid HyFlo	QS
QS	21	Acid hydrochloric	QS
QS	22	Sodium hydroxide	QS

Manufacturing Directions

1. Manufacture under complete CO_2 protection.
2. Load 780 g (portion of item 2) of sorbitol solution into a stainless steel jacketed tank. Remaining sorbitol to be used later.
3. Add parabens (unless added previously), niacinamide, and riboflavin to the sorbitol or glucose solution.
4. Heat solution to 85°C to 90°C and mix until the ingredients are dissolved.
5. Remove heat. While mixing, cool the main solution to 50°C to 60°C.
6. Hold at this temperature while bubbling CO_2 into it. CO_2 protection is continued for the remainder of the manufacturing procedure.
7. Heat 50 mL purified water to boiling and bubble CO_2 into it while cooling to 55°C.
8. Add and dissolve, with mixing, iron sulfate with 30 mL purified water at 55°C. Use CO_2 protection.
9. Warm the solution to 50°C to 55°C while mixing to dissolve. Then add the solution slowly, with good mixing, to the solution.
10. The above addition should be made as soon as possible to prevent oxidation. Add the pyridoxine, saccharin sodium, and sodium cyclamate and mix until dissolved.
11. Cool the solution to 30°C. Add the ascorbic acid with good stirring to 78 g of reserved sorbitol; make a slurry. Use a container that has plenty of headspace.
12. Add the sodium bicarbonate slowly in small portions to the ascorbic acid slurry with stirring until all of the powder has been added and most of the foaming has stopped.
13. Add this slurry slowly to the solution from the step above with vigorous mixing until a uniform solution results.
14. Rinse the mixing container with 22 g of the reserved sorbitol and add to the product with stirring.
15. Add and dissolve thiamine hydrochloride with mixing. If necessary, warm the D-pantothenyl alcohol until liquefied and add it to the 0.5 mL CO_2-saturated purified water.
16. Use an additional 0.5 mL CO_2-saturated purified water to thoroughly rinse the container of D-pantothenyl alcohol and add this to the D-pantothenyl alcohol solution.
17. Mix the D-pantothenyl alcohol solution thoroughly until homogeneously dispersed.
18. Add the D-pantothenyl alcohol solution to the main solution with mixing. Use an additional 0.5 mL CO_2-saturated purified water to rinse out the container in which the D-pantothenyl alcohol solution is made and add to the product with mixing.
19. Dissolve vitamin B_{12} in 0.5 mL purified water to make a clear solution and add this solution to the product with good mixing.
20. Dissolve the flavor in 10 g of propylene glycol, reserved from step above, with good stirring. Add this solution to the product with good mixing. Check pH (range: 3.0–3.3).

Adjust, if necessary, with a solution of 10% sodium hydroxide or 10% hydrochloric acid depending on the test results.

21. Adjust the volume of the product with the remaining 30 g of the sorbitol solution or, if necessary, purified water to 1 L.
22. Mix for 1 hour. Allow to stand overnight to eliminate entrapped CO_2 gas. Readjust volume to 1 L with purified water. Mix for 1 hour. Filter by adding HyFlo filter aid and mixing it, followed by passing through filter press. Do not allow temperature to exceed 30°C. Bubble CO_2 gas into clear filtrate for 5 minutes. Then seal tank and hold product under CO_2 protection.

Vitamin B Complex and Iron Syrup

Bill of Materials			
Scale (mg/mL)	Item	Material Name	Qty/L (g)
910.00	1	Sorbitol solution	910.00
0.019	2	Propyl paraben	0.019
0.17	3	Methyl paraben	0.17
1.50	4	Niacinamide (white powder)	1.50
0.30	5	Riboflavin	0.30
103.60	6	Propylene glycol	103.60
126.40	7	Glycerin	126.40
26.13	8	Iron sulfate (granular)	26.132
0.037	9	Dye	37.50 mg
0.25	10	Pyridoxine hydrochloride	0.25
1.20	11	Saccharin sodium (dihydrate powder)	1.20
22.00	12	Sodium cyclamate (powder)	22.00
30.00	13	Ascorbic acid (white powder)	30.00
0.80	14	Sodium bicarbonate (powder)	0.80
0.36	15	Thiamine hydrochloride (powder, regular)	0.36
0.625	16	D-Pantothenyl alcohol (dexpanthenol)	0.62
0.002	17	Vitamin B_{12} (cyanocobalamin)	2.00 mg
0.007	18	Flavor	0.70 mL
QS	19	Deionized purified water	QS to 1 L
QS	20	HyFlo filter aid	QS
QS	21	Hydrochloric acid	QS
QS	22	Sodium hydroxide	QS

Manufacturing Directions

1. Manufacture under complete carbon dioxide (CO_2) protection.
2. Load 780 g (portion of item 2) of sorbitol solution into a jacketed stainless steel tank; the remaining sorbitol will be used later.
3. Add parabens (unless added previously), niacinamide, and riboflavin to the sorbitol or glucose solution.
4. Heat solution to 85°C to 90°C and mix until the ingredients are dissolved.
5. Remove heat.
6. While mixing, cool the main solution to 50°C to 60°C.
7. Hold at this temperature while bubbling CO_2 into it.
8. CO_2 protection must be continued for the remainder of the manufacturing procedure.
9. Heat 50 mL of purified water to boiling and bubble CO_2 into it while cooling to 55°C.
10. Add and dissolve, with mixing, iron sulfate with 30 mL of purified water at 55°C.
11. Use CO_2 protection.
12. Warm the solution to 50°C to 55°C while mixing to dissolve, then slowly add the solution, with good mixing, to the solution above.
13. The above addition should be made as soon as possible to prevent oxidation.
14. Add the pyridoxine, saccharin sodium, and sodium cyclamate and mix until dissolved.
15. Cool the solution to 30°C.
16. Add the ascorbic acid, with good stirring, to 78 g of reserved sorbitol. Make a slurry.
17. Use a container that has plenty of headspace.
18. Then add the sodium bicarbonate slowly in small portions to the ascorbic acid slurry, with stirring, until all of the powder has been added and most of the foaming has stopped.
19. Add this slurry slowly to the solution from the step above with vigorous mixing until a uniform solution results.

20. Rinse the mixing container with 22 g of the reserved sorbitol and add to the product with stirring.
21. Add and dissolve thiamine hydrochloride with mixing.
22. If necessary, warm the D-pantothenyl alcohol until liquefied and add it to the 0.5-mL CO_2-saturated purified water.
23. Use an additional 0.5 mL of CO_2-saturated purified water to thoroughly rinse the container of D-pantothenyl alcohol and add this to the D-pantothenyl alcohol solution.
24. Mix the D-pantothenyl alcohol solution thoroughly until it is homogeneously dispersed.
25. Add the D-pantothenyl alcohol solution to the main solution with mixing.
26. Use an additional 0.5 mL of CO_2-saturated purified water to rinse out the container in which the D-pantothenyl alcohol solution is made and add to the product with mixing.
27. Dissolve the vitamin B_{12} in 0.5 mL of purified water to make a clear solution and add this to the product with good mixing.
28. Dissolve the guarana flavor in 10 g of propylene glycol, reserved from earlier step, with good stirring.
29. Add this solution to the product with good mixing.
30. Check pH (range: 3.0–3.3).
31. Adjust, if necessary, with a solution of 10% sodium hydroxide or 10% hydrochloric acid depending on the test results.
32. Adjust the volume of the product with the remaining 30 g of the sorbitol solution and, if necessary, purified water to 1 L.
33. Mix for 1 hour.
34. Allow to stand overnight to eliminate entrapped CO_2 gas.
35. Readjust volume to 1 L with purified water.
36. Mix for 1 hour.
37. Filter by adding HyFlo filter aid and mixing it, followed by passing through a filter press.
38. Do not allow temperature to exceed 30°C.
39. Bubble CO_2 gas into clear filtrate for 5 minutes, then seal tank, and hold product under CO_2 protection.

Vitamin B Complex and Vitamin C Syrup

Bill of Materials			
Scale (mg/g)	Item	Material Name	Qty/kg (g)
0.60	1	Thiamine hydrochloride	0.60
0.55	2	Riboflavin phosphate sodium	0.55
2.50	3	Nicotinamide	2.50
1.20	4	Dexpanthenol	1.20
0.55	5	Pyridoxine hydrochloride	0.55
9.00	6	Ascorbic acid, crystalline	9.00
0.25	7	Orange flavor	0.25
0.05	8	EDTA sodium	0.05
0.50	9	Propyl gallate	0.50
2.00	10	Sorbic acid	2.00
5.00	11	Kollidon 25	5.00
10.00	12	Sorbitol, crystalline	10.00
9.00	13	Glycerol	9.00
10.00	14	1,2-Propylenglycol Pharma	10.00
5.00	15	Water purified	5.00
60.00	16	Sugar syrup (64% sucrose in water)	60.00

Manufacturing Directions

1. Mix solution of items 1 to 5 with sugar syrup.
2. Adjust the clear solution to about pH 4.2.
3. Use nitrogen as an inert gas in the final packaging. 10 g provides 2 to 3 times the recommended daily allowance.

Vitamin B Complex and Vitamin C Syrup

Bill of Materials			
Scale (mg/g)	Item	Material Name	Qty/kg (g)
0.60	1	Thiamine hydrochloride	0.60
0.55	2	Riboflavin phosphate sodium	0.55
2.50	3	Nicotinamide	2.50
1.20	4	Dexpanthenol	1.20
0.55	5	Pyridoxine hydrochloride	0.55
9.00	6	Ascorbic acid (crystalline)	9.00
0.25	7	Orange flavor	0.25
0.05	8	EDTA sodium	0.05
0.50	9	Propyl gallate	0.50
2.00	10	Sorbic acid	2.00
5.00	11	Kollidon® 25	5.00
10.00	12	Sorbitol (crystalline)	10.00
9.00	13	Glycerol	9.00
10.00	14	1,2-Propylenglycol (Pharma)	10.00
5.00	15	Water	5.00
QS	16	Sugar syrup (64% sucrose in water)	QS to 1 kg

Manufacturing Directions

1. Mix solution of items 1 to 5 with sugar syrup, adjust the clear solution to about pH 4.2, and use nitrogen as an inert gas in the final packaging; 10 g provides two to three RDA.

Vitamin B Complex and Vitamin C Syrup

Bill of Materials			
Scale (mg/mL)	Item	Material Name	Qty/L (g)
0.15	1	Thiamine hydrochloride	0.15
0.15	2	Riboflavin phosphate sodium	0.15
0.70	3	Nicotinamide	0.70
0.035	4	Dexpanthenol	0.035
0.150	5	Pyridoxine hydrochloride	0.15
2.25	6	Ascorbic acid (crystalline)	2.25
0.28	7	Orange aroma	0.28
0.56	8	EDTA sodium	0.56
186.50	9	Propylene glycol (Pharma) + water (2:1)	186.50
0.15	10	Paraben	0.15
84.30	11	Sorbitol (crystalline)	84.30
562.50	12	Sucrose (crystalline)	562.50
42.00	13	Water	42.00

Manufacturing Directions

1. Dissolve items 1 to 8 in item 2.
2. Prepare a solution of items 10 to 13 by heating.
3. Cool and mix with solution of the balance of the formulation.
4. Adjust to a pH of 4.2 to 4.5.
5. Adjust volume with water; use more, if necessary.
6. Use nitrogen as an inert gas during packaging.

Vitamin B Complex, A, C, and D Syrup

Bill of Materials			
Scale (mg/mL)	Item	Material Name	Qty/L (g)
60.00	1	Sucrose	600.00
51.00	2	Methyl paraben	1.00
0.20	3	Propyl paraben	0.20
1.00	4	Edetate disodium	1.00
10.00	5	Ascorbic acid, 50% excess	15.00
0.80	6	Sodium hydroxide	0.80
4.00	7	Nicotinamide, 5% excess	4.20
0.40	8	Riboflavin sodium phosphate, 8% excess	0.43
1.00	9	Thiamine hydrochloride, 50% excess	1.50
1.20	10	Pyridoxine hydrochloride, 10% excess	1.32
0.50	11	Monosodium glutamate	0.50
1.26 μg	12	Cyanocobalamin, 50% excess	0.0018
150.00	13	Propylene glycol	150.00
1000.0 U	14	Vitamin A palmitate 1.75 million/g, 54% excess	0.88
100.0 U	15	Cholecalciferol 40 million/g, 52% excess	0.0038
13.20	16	Polysorbate 80	13.20
2.50	17	Polyoxyl 20 cetostearyl ether	2.50
0.30	18	Lemon oil terpenless	0.30
0.84	19	Strawberry oil composed	0.84
–	20	Purified water	QS to 1 L

Manufacturing Directions

This product is an aqueous solution of water-soluble vitamins with oily vitamin A palmitate and cholecalciferol solubilized in water using the surfactant system of Tween 80 and cetomacrogol. This syrup is a solubilized oil surfactant system and is liable to heat and rate of mixing. The temperature of solution must not exceed 30°C at the time of final mixing. The final mixing must be in continuous manner without any interruption. For the preparation of oily phase, the container must be dry.

1. Before start of batch, cool approximately 80 mL purified water and flush with nitrogen gas (purity 99.95%). Use this water for making solutions and for adjusting the volume.
2. Add 420 g of item 20 to the manufacturing vessel and heat to 90°C to 95°C.
3. Add items 2 and 3 while mixing to dissolve.
4. Add item 1 while mixing at slow speed. After addition of item 1, mix for 30 to 35 minutes at high speed, temperature 90°C to 95°C. Cool to 25°C to 30°C while mixing at low speed.
5. Bubble nitrogen gas for 10 minutes. Add item 4 to the syrup while mixing at high speed to dissolve.
6. Add item 5 to the syrup while mixing at high speed to dissolve.
7. Add 4 g of item 20 (25°C) in a separate container and dissolve item 6 by using stirrer.
8. Transfer the cooled item 6 solution to the syrup tank while mixing at high speed. Mix for 15 minutes.
9. Check pH of the syrup (limit: 3.75–3.85). Add items 7 to 11 one by one to the syrup in manufacturing vessel while mixing at high speed to dissolve.
10. Mix for 10 minutes. Add 6 g of cold item 20 (25°C) in a separate container and dissolve item 12.
11. Add to the manufacturing vessel while mixing at high speed. Rinse the container with cooled item 20, about 2 mL, and transfer the rinsing to the syrup-manufacturing vessel and mix well at high speed.
12. Add item 13 to the manufacturing vessel while mixing at high speed.
13. Warm item 14 to 70°C in a separate stainless steel container in water bath.
14. Warm item 16 to 70°C and mix well with item 14 under nitrogen atmosphere.
15. Add item 15 while mixing. Melt item 17 in stainless steel container and add with stirring to mix well.
16. Cool to 30°C while mixing under nitrogen atmosphere.
17. Add items 18 and 19 to the oily phase solution and mix for 15 minutes at high speed.
18. Check and record the volume of oily phase. Start mixing and continue mixing. Mixing must be continuous.
19. Start the addition of oily phase solution in a thin stream. Do not stop mixing during addition of oily phase. After the addition is over, mix for a further 15 minutes at high speed.
20. Rinse the oily phase vessel with a sufficient quantity of syrup from the syrup vessel. Transfer the rinsing to the syrup vessel.
21. Makeup the volume to 1 L with cooled item 20 (25°C) and, finally, mix for 20 minutes at high speed.
22. Check and record the pH (limit: 3.75–3.85 at 25°C). Filter the syrup at 1.5 bar. Recirculate about 40 to 60 mL syrup.

Vitamin B Complex Syrup

Bill of Materials			
Scale (mg/g)	Item	Material Name	Qty/kg (g)
0.60	1	Thiamine hydrochloride	0.60
0.55	2	Riboflavin 5-phosphate sodium	0.55
2.50	3	Nicotinamide	2.50
1.20	4	Dexpanthenol	1.20
0.55	5	Pyridoxine hydrochloride	0.55
2.00	6	Sorbic acid	2.00
0.05	7	EDTA sodium	0.05
2.25	8	Vanillin	2.25
465.00	9	Sucrose	465.00
25.00	10	Kollidon® 25	25.00
90.00	11	Glycerol	90.00
100.00	12	Propylene glycol (pharma)	100.00
310.00	13	Water	310.00

Manufacturing Directions

1. Dissolve the sucrose in the heat mixture of glycerol, propylene glycol, and water.
2. Cool to room temperature and dissolve the other components to obtain a clear solution.

Vitamin B Complex Syrup

Bill of Materials			
Scale (mg/mL)	Item	Material Name	Qty/L (g)
0.66	1	Dexpanthenol	0.66
4.40	2	Nicotinamide	4.40
0.22	3	Pyridoxine hydrochloride	0.22
0.60	4	Riboflavin-5-phosphate sodium	0.60
1.50	5	Thiamine hydrochloride	1.50
350.00	6	Sorbitol (70% solution)	350.00
11.20	7	Propylene glycol	11.20
0.84	8	Methyl paraben	0.84
0.168	9	Propyl paraben	0.168
550.00	10	Maltitol solution (Lycasin 80/55)	550.00
0.15	11	Edetate disodium (sodium EDTA)	0.15
3.72	12	Citric acid (monohydrate)	3.72
3.72	13	Sodium citrate	3.72
2.50	14	Sodium benzoate	2.50
0.50	15	Saccharin sodium	0.50
150.00	16	Glycerin (glycerol)	150.00
1.50	17	Flavor	1.50
1.00	18	Flavor	1.00
–	19	Purified water	QS to 1 L

Manufacturing Directions

1. Load items 6, 10, and 16 in a manufacturing vessel and mix for 5 minutes.
2. Dissolve items 8 and 9 in item 7 in a stainless steel container.
3. Put the entire container in hot water (60–70°C) and stir to dissolve.
4. Add the clear solution to the mixer.
5. Dissolve items 11 and 12 in 40 g of purified water in a stainless steel container.
6. Add the clear solution to the mixer.
7. Dissolve items 13, 14, and 15 in 50 g of purified water in a stainless steel container.
8. Add the clear solution to mixer and mix for 5 minutes.
9. Dissolve item 1 in 10 g of purified water in a stainless steel container.
10. Add the clear solution to mixer.
11. Dissolve items 5 and 3 in 10 g of purified water in a stainless steel container.
12. Add the clear solution to mixer.
13. Dissolve items 2 and 4 in 30 g of purified water in a stainless steel container.
14. Add the clear yellow solution to mixer and mix for 5 minutes.
15. Add items 17 and 18 to mixer.
16. Bring the volume up to 1 L with purified water and finally mix for 15 to 20 minutes.
17. Check and record the pH (limit: 4.4–4.8 at 25°C).
18. If required, adjust pH with 20% citric acid or 20% sodium citrate solution.
19. Filter the syrup at 1.5 bar.
20. Recirculate about 200 to 300 mL syrup.
21. Transfer the filtered syrup to the storage vessel, flushing with nitrogen gas.
22. Store the syrup under a nitrogen blanket for NMT 2 days prior to filling.

Vitamin B Complex Syrup (without B_{12})

Bill of Materials			
Scale (mg/mL)	Item	Material Name	Qty/L (g)
570.00	1	Sucrose[a]	570.00
70.00	2	Glycerin (glycerol)	70.00
3.72	3	Citric acid (monohydrate)	3.72
1.00	4	Edetate disodium (sodium EDTA)	1.00
0.90	5	Calcium pantothenate (10% excess)	1.00
5.70	6	Sodium citrate	5.70
0.84	7	Methyl paraben	0.84
0.168	8	Propyl paraben	0.168
1.90	9	Benzoic acid	1.90
1.14	10	Strawberry flavor manefils	1.14
9.60	11	Alcohol (ethanol, 95%)	9.60
1.50	12	Thiamine hydrochloride (50% excess)	1.50
0.20	13	Pyridoxine hydrochloride (10% excess)	0.22
4.00	14	Nicotinamide (10% excess)	4.40
0.30	15	Riboflavin sodium phosphate (50% excess)	0.60
QS	16	Purified water	QS to 1 L

[a] 513 mg for thiamine mononitrate and 504 mg for thiamine hydrochloride

Manufacturing Directions

1. Flush with nitrogen gas (purity 99.95%).
2. Add 400 g of purified water to the manufacturing vessel and heat to 90°C to 95°C.
3. Add item 1 while mixing at low speed.
4. After addition of item 1, mix for 30 to 35 minutes at high speed (temperature: 90–95°C).
5. Cool to 40°C while mixing at low speed.
6. Disperse 1 g of filter aid in 10 g of cooled purified water (25–30°C) in a stainless steel container to prepare a slurry.
7. Add the slurry to the syrup in syrup vessel.
8. Mix for 15 minutes at high speed.
9. Filter the syrup at 1.5 bar.
10. Recirculate about 40 to 60 mL syrup.
11. Transfer the filtered syrup to the storage vessel.
12. Recharge the filtered syrup to the manufacturing vessel.
13. Start mixing.
14. Add item 2 to the syrup vessel while mixing at high speed.
15. Add item 3 to the syrup vessel while mixing to dissolve at high speed.
16. Dissolve item 4 in 6 g of cooled purified water (25–30°C) and add to the syrup vessel while mixing at high speed.
17. Dissolve item 5 in 6 g of cooled purified water and add to the syrup vessel while mixing at high speed for 30 minutes.
18. Dissolve item 6 in 10 g of cooled purified water (25–30°C) and add to the syrup vessel while mixing at high speed.
19. Dissolve items 7 to 10 in item 11 in a stainless steel container and add to the syrup vessel while mixing at high speed for 15 minutes.
20. Dissolve items 12 and 13 in 6 g of cooled purified water (25–30°C) in a separate stainless steel container and add to the syrup vessel while mixing at high speed.
21. Rinse the container with 1 g of cooled, purified water (25–30°C) and add the rinsing to the syrup vessel while mixing at high speed.
22. Flush the vessel with nitrogen gas (purity 99.95%) for 15 minutes.
23. Dissolve item 14 in 9 g of cooled purified water in a separate stainless steel container and add to the syrup vessel while mixing at high speed.
24. Rinse the container with 1 g of cooled purified water (25–30°C) and add the rinsing to the syrup vessel while mixing at high speed.
25. Dissolve item 15 in 4 g of cooled, purified water (25–30°C) in a separate stainless steel container and add to the syrup vessel while mixing at high speed.
26. Rinse the container with 1 g of cooled, purified water and add the rinsing to the syrup vessel while mixing at high speed.
27. Bring the volume up to 1 L with cooled, purified water (25–30°C) and finally mix for 15 minutes at high speed.
28. Check and record the pH (limit: 4.3–4.7 at 25°C).
29. If required, adjust pH with 10% solution of citric acid or sodium citrate.
30. Flush the syrup with nitrogen gas (purity 99.95%) for 15 minutes.
31. Close the tank.
32. Hold the syrup for 12 hours.
33. Filter the syrup at 1.5 bar.
34. Recirculate about 40 to 60 mL syrup.
35. Transfer the filtered syrup to the storage vessel.

Vitamin B Complex, Vitamin A, Vitamin C, and Vitamin D Syrup

Bill of Materials			
Scale (mg/mL)	Item	Material Name	Qty/L (g)
60.00	1	Sucrose	600.00
51.00	2	Methyl paraben	1.00
0.20	3	Propyl paraben	0.20
1.00	4	Edetate disodium (sodium EDTA)	1.00
10.00	5	Ascorbic acid (50% excess)	15.00
0.80	6	Sodium hydroxide	0.80
4.00	7	Nicotinamide (5% excess)	4.20
0.40	8	Riboflavin sodium phosphate (8% excess)	0.43
1.00	9	Thiamine hydrochloride (50% excess)	1.50
1.20	10	Pyridoxine hydrochloride (10% excess)	1.32
0.50	11	Monosodium glutamate (sodium glutamate)	0.50
1.26 μg	12	Cyanocobalamin (50% excess)	0.0018
150.00	13	Propylene glycol	150.00
1000.00 IU	14	Vitamin A palmitate (1.75 MM IU/g) (54% excess)	0.88
100.00 IU	15	Cholecalciferol (40 MM IU/g) (52% excess)	0.0038
13.20	16	Polysorbate 80 (Tween 80)	13.20
2.50	17	Polyoxyl 20 cetostearyl ether (Cetomacrogol 1000)	2.50
0.30	18	Lemon oil terpeneless	0.30
0.84	19	Strawberry oil (composed)	0.84
QS	20	Purified water	QS to 1 L

Manufacturing Directions

1. This product is an aqueous solution of water-soluble vitamins with oily vitamin A palmitate and cholecalciferol solubilized in water using the surfactant system of Tween 80 and cetomacrogol.
2. This syrup is a solubilized oil surfactant system and is affected by heat and rate of mixing.
3. The temperature of the solution must not exceed 30°C at the time of final mixing.
4. The final mixing must be continuous, without any interruption.
5. For the preparation of oily phase, the container must be dry.
6. Before start of batch, cool about 80 mL of purified water and flush with nitrogen gas (purity 99.95%).
7. Use this water for making solutions and for adjusting the volume.
8. Add 420 g of purified water to the manufacturing vessel and heat to 90 to 95°C.
9. Add items 2 and 3 while mixing to dissolve.
10. Add item 1 while mixing at slow speed.
11. After addition of item 1, mix for 30 to 35 minutes at high speed and a temperature of 90°C to 95°C.
12. Cool to 25°C to 30°C while mixing at low speed.
13. Bubble nitrogen gas for 10 minutes.
14. Add item 4 to the syrup while mixing at high speed to dissolve.
15. Add item 5 to the syrup while mixing at high speed to dissolve.
16. Add 4 g of purified water (25°C) in a separate container and dissolve item 6 by using a stirrer.
17. Transfer the cooled item 6 solution to the syrup tank while mixing at high speed.
18. Mix for 15 minutes.
19. Check the pH of the syrup (limit: 3.75–3.85).
20. Add items 7 to 11 one by one to the syrup in the manufacturing vessel while mixing at high speed to dissolve.
21. Mix for 10 minutes.
22. Add 6 g of cold purified water (25°C) in a separate container and dissolve item 12.
23. Add to the manufacturing vessel while mixing at high speed.
24. Rinse the container with cooled purified water (approximately 2 mL) and transfer the rinsing to the syrup-manufacturing vessel; mix well at high speed.
25. Add item 13 to the manufacturing vessel while mixing at high speed.
26. Warm item 14 to 70°C in a separate stainless steel container in a water bath.
27. Warm item 16 to 70°C and mix well with item 14 under nitrogen atmosphere.
28. Add item 15 while mixing.
29. Melt item 17 in a stainless steel container and add with stirring to mix well.
30. Cool to 30°C while mixing under nitrogen atmosphere.
31. Add items 18 and 19 to the oily phase solution and mix for 15 minutes at high speed.
32. Check and record the volume of the oily phase.

33. Start mixing and continue mixing (mixing must be continuous).
34. Start the addition of the oily phase solution in a thin stream (do not stop mixing during addition of oily phase).
35. After the addition is complete, mix for an additional 15 minutes at high speed.
36. Rinse the oily phase vessel with a sufficient quantity of syrup from the syrup vessel.
37. Transfer the rinsing to the syrup vessel.
38. Bring the volume up to 1 L with cooled purified water (25°C) and finally mix for 20 minutes at high speed.
39. Check and record the pH (limit: 3.75–3.85 at 25°C).
40. Filter the syrup at 1.5 bar.
41. Recirculate about 40 to 60 mL syrup.

Vitamin B Complex, Vitamin A, Vitamin C, Vitamin D, and Calcium Drops

Bill of Materials			
Scale (mg/mL)	Item	Material Name	Qty/L (g)
675.00	1	Glycerin (96%)	675.00
16.66	2	Niacinamide (white powder)	16.66
2.73	3	Riboflavin-5′-phosphate sodium (3% excess)	2.82
0.50	4	Methyl paraben	0.50
1.00	5	Acid benzoic	1.00
105.00	6	Saccharin sodium (powder)	105.00
73.36	7	Calcium chloride (granules, dihydrate)	73.36
28.78	8	Ferrous gluconate	28.78
2.25	9	Thiamine hydrochloride (powder, regular) (35% excess)	3.375
1.00	10	Pyridoxine hydrochloride	1.00
83.33	11	Ascorbic acid (white powder) (35% excess)	112.50
0.25	12	Oil orange terpeneless	0.25
0.081	13	Alcohol (ethanol; 190 proof, Nonbeverage)	0.081
80.00	14	Polysorbate 80	80.00
0.16	15	Butylated hydroxyanisole (BHA)	0.16
0.66	16	Viosterol in corn oil (syn., oleovitamin D; 1000 mD/g) (25% excess)	0.83
0.056	17	Vitamin A palmitate (1500000 Units/g)	0.056
10.00	18	Caramel (acid proof)	10.00
QS	19	Deionized purified water	QS to 1 L

Manufacturing Directions

1. Product must not stand more than 1 week before filling.
2. Avoid unnecessary exposure of product to light, air, and heat.
3. Manufacture and store product under complete CO_2 protection.
4. Avoid vigorous mixing.
5. Charge glycerin and 210 mL purified water into a stainless steel jacketed tank.
6. Add, with mixing, in the following order: niacinamide, riboflavin-5′-phosphate sodium, methyl paraben, USP, benzoic acid, and saccharin sodium.
7. Continue mixing, heat to 95°C to 100°C, and hold to completely dissolve the ingredients.
8. Add in calcium chloride portions and stir until complete solution is obtained.
9. Continue mixing and cool to 70°C to 75°C.
10. Add ferrous gluconate with mixing and dissolve at 70°C to 75°C.
11. Check for the absence of undissolved material.
12. Check volume; if necessary, replace lost purified water by heating with additional previously boiled purified water; QS to 750 mL.
13. Cool with mixing to room temperature (25–30°C) while bubbling CO_2 gas through.
14. Continue the CO_2 gas bubbling for balance of the process.
15. Add and dissolve each ingredient in this order: thiamine hydrochloride, pyridoxine hydrochloride, and ascorbic acid.
16. Dissolve oil orange in ethyl alcohol and add to mixture with stirring.
17. Heat polysorbate 80 to 50°C to 60°C and hold for approximately 10 minutes with slow mixing.
18. Add and dissolve butylated hydroxyanisole.
19. Mix slowly and saturate with CO_2 while cooling to 25°C to 30°C.
20. Add and dissolve viosterol in corn oil and vitamin A palmitate, mixing well, and continuing CO_2 gas bubbling.
21. Add polysorbate solution to main batch and mix thoroughly.
22. Rinse container with a portion of the main batch and add.
23. Heat 50 mL purified water to 35°C to 40°C while bubbling CO_2 gas through.
24. Add the caramel color.
25. Mix well until uniform consistency is obtained.

26. Add to main batch.
27. Rinse container with a small quantity of purified water that has been previously saturated with CO_2 gas.
28. Add to the main batch.
29. Add purified water that has been previously saturated with CO_2 gas; QS to 1 L.
30. Filter, without using a filter aid; cycle to achieve clarity.
31. Maintain carbon dioxide cover.

Vitamin B Complex, Vitamin A, Vitamin C, Vitamin D, and Vitamin E Pediatric Drops

Bill of Materials			
Scale (mg/mL)	Item	Material Name	Qty/L (g)
8333 IU	1	Vitamin A palmitate (1.7 M IU/g) (50% excess)	7.35
666 IU	2	Vitamin D (40 M IU/g) (cholecalciferol)	0.021
75.00	3	Polysorbate 80 (Tween 80)	75.00
0.005	4	Lemon oil terpeneless	0.50
0.88	5	Vitamin E (oily) (α-tocopheryl acetate)	0.88
0.50	6	Edetate disodium (sodium EDTA)	0.50
83.33	7	Ascorbic acid (30% excess)	108.33
1.00	8	Saccharin sodium	1.00
2.50	9	Thiamine hydrochloride (50% excess)	3.75
16.66	10	Nicotinamide (5% excess)	17.50
0.833	11	Pyridoxine hydrochloride (5.6% excess)	0.88
2.00	12	Riboflavin sodium phosphate (7.9% excess as riboflavin)	2.16
700.00	13	Glycerin (glycerol)	700.00
250.00	14	Purified water	250.00

Manufacturing Directions

1. This product is a microemulsion and is a thermolabile preparation.
2. The temperature of the solution must not exceed 25°C at the time of processing.
3. Add 200 g of purified water to the manufacturing vessel.
4. Bubble nitrogen gas during all stages of the process.
5. Charge items 6 to 12 one by one into the manufacturing vessel while mixing.
6. Check that all materials are dissolved completely.
7. Load item 13 into the manufacturing vessel while mixing at slow speed.
8. Mix for 5 minutes.
9. Add item 3 in a separate stainless steel container.
10. Mix items 1, 2, 4, and 5 one by one using stirrer.
11. Mix for 1 hour at slow speed.
12. Add oil phase preparation to the aqueous phase at a rate of 4 mL/min while mixing at slow speed and continue nitrogen gas bubbling throughout the process.
13. Rinse the oil phase container with 50 g of nitrogen-bubbled and cooled purified water and transfer the rinsing to the manufacturing vessel.
14. Adjust the volume to 1 L using nitrogen-bubbled purified water.
15. Mix for 15 minutes at slow speed.
16. Check and record the volume and pH (limit: pH 2.8–4.2).
17. Filter the solution through a Sartorius prefilter and 0.2-μm membrane filter into receiving tank.
18. Bubble with nitrogen gas for 15 minutes.

Vitamin B Complex, Vitamin C, and Iron Syrup

Bill of Materials			
Scale (mg/mL)	Item	Material Name	Qty/L (g)
QS	1	Glucose (liquid), NF	QS to 1 L
225.00	2	Purified water, USP	225.00
0.30	3	Methyl paraben	0.30
1.00	4	Acid benzoic, USP	1.00
5.00	5	Alcohol (ethanol; 190 proof, nonbeverage), USP	5.00
10.00	6	Nicotinamide niacinamide (white powder), USP	10.00
10.00	7	Riboflavin; use riboflavin 5 phosphate sodium	1.64
2.00	8	Pyridoxine hydrochloride, USP	2.00
20.00	9	Ascorbic acid (white powder), USP	28.00
0.03	10	Dye	0.03
0.02	11	Dye	0.02
2.00	12	Thiamine hydrochloride (powder, regular), USP	2.40
2.00	13	D-pantothenyl alcohol	2.50
2.00 μg	14	Vitamin B_{12} (cyanocobalamin, USP)	3.40 mg
200.00	15	Sucrose, NF	200.00
0.028 mL	16	Flavor	2.80 mL
QS	17	Hydrochloric acid	2.00 mL
QS	18	Carbon dioxide gas	QS

Manufacturing Directions

1. This preparation is susceptible to oxidation and must be protected from air and sunlight at all times.
2. Carbon dioxide must be used extensively to prevent oxygen from reacting with the materials.
3. All purified water must be boiled prior to use for 10 minutes and cooled under CO_2 protection.
4. Charge 100 mL of purified water into a suitably sized stainless steel tank.
5. Add the riboflavin, nicotinamide, benzoic acid, and paraben.
6. Rinse the tank down with 10 mL purified water, seal, and heat with mixing to 95°C.
7. Continue mixing and heating for 15 minutes, until solution is complete.
8. Commence cooling with continuous mixing.
9. When the solution has cooled to 50 to 70°C, add and dissolve the sugar.
10. Commence CO_2 protection when the temperature reaches 40°C.
11. Slurry the ascorbic acid in 75 or 110 mL of CO_2-saturated purified water (use the smaller quantity only if using a total of 225 mL water) and add to bulk solution when temperature has reached 25°C to 35°C.
12. Rinse the ascorbic acid vessel with 10 mL purified water and add rinsing to bulk.
13. Mix for at least 30 minutes.
14. Dissolve thiamine and pyridoxine in 20 mL CO_2-saturated purified water and add to bulk solution at 25 to 35°C.
15. Add 10 mL CO_2-saturated purified water to the D-pantothenyl alcohol and warm on a water bath until solution is complete.
16. Add vitamin B_{12} and mix until dissolved.
17. Add and dissolve dyes.
18. Add this solution to the bulk solution and mix thoroughly.
19. Mix flavor with 95% of alcohol and add to the bulk solution.
20. Rinse the container with the remaining alcohol and add to the bulk with vigorous agitation.
21. Check pH (range: 3.0–3.3).
22. Use hydrochloric acid to adjust, if necessary.
23. Adjust the final volume with liquid glucose.
24. Filter through suitable medium until clear and bright.

Vitamin B Complex, Vitamin C, and Iron Syrup

Bill of Materials			
Scale (mg/tablet)	Item	Material Name	Qty/L (g)
QS	1	Sorbitol solution, USP	QS to 1 L
QS	2	Purified water, USP	225.00
0.20	3	Methyl paraben	0.20
0.20	4	Propyl paraben, NF	0.02
2.00	5	Nicotinamide niacinamide (white powder), USP	10.00
10.00	6	Riboflavin; use riboflavin 5 phosphate sodium	1.64
10.00	7	Iron sulfate (ferrous sulfate; granular), USP	10.00
3.60	8	Saccharin sodium (powder), USP	3.60
2.00	9	Pyridoxine hydrochloride, USP	2.00
25.00	10	Ascorbic acid (white powder), USP	28.00
0.03	11	Dye	0.030
0.02	12	Dye	0.020
2.00	13	Thiamine hydrochloride (powder, regular), USP	2.40
2.00	14	D-Pantothenyl alcohol	2.50
2.0 μg	15	Vitamin B_{12} cyanocobalamin, USP	3.40 mg
1.00	16	Flavor	1.00
10.00	17	Propylene glycol, USP	10.00
QS	18	Hydrochloric acid	2.00 mL
–	19	HyFlo filter aid	1 g
QS	20	Carbon dioxide gas	QS

Manufacturing Directions

1. This preparation is susceptible to oxidation and must be protected from air and sunlight at all times.
2. Carbon dioxide must be used extensively to prevent oxygen from reacting with the materials.
3. All purified water must be boiled prior to use for 10 minutes and cooled under CO_2 protection.
4. Charge 950 g of sorbitol solution into a jacketed stainless steel tank and heat to 95°C to 100°C.
5. Heat 250 mL of purified water to boiling for 10 minutes and bubble CO_2 into it while cooling to room temperature.
6. Add, with stirring, the parabens, niacinamide, and riboflavin 5-phosphate sodium.
7. Rinse the container with 5 mL of water.
8. Stir well.
9. Mix until solution is obtained and check the clarity.
10. Remove the source of heat from the vessel.
11. Thoroughly deoxygenate the liquid by bubbling CO_2 through the liquid and allow to cool to 50°C to 60°C.
12. Heat 15 mL of water to 70°C, saturate with CO_2, and dissolve saccharin sodium (item 8) and pyridoxine hydrochloride in 5 mL of water; add to the main bulk.
13. Rinse the container with 2.5 mL of water.
14. Cool the solution to 30°C with CO_2 protection.
15. Dissolve ascorbic acid in 120 mL of water.
16. Rinse the container with 5 mL of water.
17. Dissolve dyes in 3 mL of water.
18. Rinse the container with 2 mL of water.
19. Mix dye solution with ascorbic acid solution.
20. Add this to the main bulk with stirring.
21. Dissolve thiamine in 30 mL of water and add to the main bulk.
22. Rinse the container with 2.5 mL of water.
23. Add 10 mL of water to the D-pantothenyl and warm up on a water bath until in solution.
24. Add this mixture to the main bulk.
25. Rinse the container with 2.5 mL of water.
26. Dissolve vitamin B_{12} in 12.5 mL of water and add to the main bulk.
27. Rinse the container with 2.5 mL of water.
28. Mix flavor with 7.5 g of propylene glycol until mixture is homogeneous and add to the main bulk.
29. Rinse the container with 2.5 g of propylene glycol and add to the main bulk with vigorous agitation.
30. Check pH (range: 3.0–3.3).
31. Use hydrochloric acid to adjust, if necessary.
32. Adjust the volume of the product with sorbitol solution and mix for 30 minutes to ensure homogeneity.
33. Add the HyFlo filter aid and mix.
34. Filter the liquid through a filter press previously washed in purified water.
35. Transfer the clear filtrate into a clean closed vessel.
36. Mix for 15 minutes while bubbling CO_2 gas.

Vitamin C Drops

Bill of Materials			
Scale (mg/mL)	Item	Material Name	Qty/L (g)
100.00	1	Ascorbic acid (white powder), USP	100.00
979.00	2	Propylene glycol, USP	979.00

Manufacturing Directions

1. Keep under CO_2 protection at all times. Avoid contact with iron. Use stainless steel or glass-lined equipment only.
2. Load 868 g propylene glycol into a glass-lined or suitable stainless steel jacketed tank.
3. While mixing, heat to 70 to 80°C.
4. Bubble CO_2 gas into the propylene glycol from the bottom of the tank.
5. Add and dissolve the ascorbic acid into the propylene glycol with a minimum of stirring under CO_2 protection.
6. When the ascorbic acid is in solution, immediately cool to approximately 25°C while continuing to mix.
7. Also, while cooling, change adding CO_2 from the bottom of the tank to adding it at the top of the tank.
8. QS to 1 L, using propylene glycol and mix for at least 10 minutes.
9. Use a prefilter pad and a lint-free filter paper; recirculate the product through the filter press until sparkling clear.

Vitamin E and Benzocaine Solution

Bill of Materials			
Scale (mg/mL)	Item	Material Name	Qty/L (g)
50.00	1	Vitamin E acetate	50.00
20.00	2	Benzocaine	20.00
50.00	3	Lutrol F 127	50.00
250.00	4	Cremophor (relative humidity, 40%)	250.00
2.00	5	Sorbic acid	2.00
628.00	6	Water	628.00

Manufacturing Directions

1. Dissolve sorbic acid and benzocaine in water at 60°C. Slowly add the heated mixture of vitamin E acetate and Cremophor at a relative humidity of 40% and temperature of 60°C to 65°C.
2. Cool the clear solution to about 5°C and dissolve Lutrol F 127 to obtain a clear, colorless viscous liquid.

Vitamin E Concentrate, Water-Miscible

Bill of Materials			
Scale (mg/mL)	Item	Material Name	Qty/L (g)
105.00	1	Vitamin E acetate	105.00
250.00	2	Cremophor (relative humidity, 40%)	250.00
QS	3	Preservative	QS
QS	4	Water	QS to 1 L

Manufacturing Directions

1. Heat the mixture of items 1 and 2 and solution of item 3 in item 4 separately to about 65°C.
2. Slowly add to the well-stirred solution to obtain a clear, colorless liquid that is miscible with water.

Vitamin E Drops

Bill of Materials			
Scale (mg/mL)	Item	Material Name	Qty/L (g)
50.00	1	Vitamin E acetate	50.00
160.00	2	Cremophor (relative humidity, 40%)	160.00
QS	3	Preservative	QS
QS	4	Water	QS to 1 L

Manufacturing Directions

1. Heat mixture of items 1 and 2 and solution of item 3 in 4 to about 65°C.
2. Add them slowly to obtain a clear or lightly opalescent, colorless liquid.

Vitamin E Soft Gel Capsules

Bill of Materials			
Scale (mg/capsule)	Item	Material Name	Qty/1000 Capsules (g)
400.00	1	Vitamin E preparation, USP	400.00
25.00	2	Soybean oil, USP	25.00
QS	3	Gelatin mass (clear)	QS

Manufacturing Directions

1. Weigh items 1 and 2 and transfer into a suitable stainless steel container, mix for a minimum of 1 hour, screen transfer to tanks through a No. 80 to No. 100 mesh stainless sieve.
2. Encapsulate 425 mg of mixture into size 7.5 oval capsules using clear gelatin mass.

Vitamin E Solution with Ethanol

Bill of Materials			
Scale (mg/tablet)	Item	Material Name	Qty/L (g)
0.10	1	Vitamin E acetate	0.10
4.00–5.00	2	Cremophor, EL	4.00–5.00
570.00	3	Water	570.00
380.00	4	Ethanol (96%)	380.00

Manufacturing Directions

1. Heat mixture of item 1 and 2 to about 60°C. Stir well.
2. Add slowly add the warm solvent mixture of items 3 and 4 to obtain a clear, colorless liquid of low viscosity.

Vitamin E and Benzocaine Solution

Bill of Materials			
Scale (mg/mL)	Item	Material Name	Qty/L. (g)
50.00	1	Vitamin E acetate	50.00
20.00	2	Benzocaine	20.00
50.00	3	Lutrol F 127	50.00
250.00	4	Cremophor RH 40	250.00
2.00	5	Sorbic acid	2.00
628.00	6	Water	628.00

Manufacturing Directions

1. Dissolve sorbic acid and benzocaine in water at 60°C.
2. Add slowly the heated mixture of Vitamin E acetate and Cremophor RH 40 (60–65°C).
3. Cool the clear solution to about 5°C and dissolve Lutrol F 127. A clear, colorless viscous liquid is formed.

Vitamin E and Benzocaine Solution

Bill of Materials			
Scale (mg/mL)	Item	Material Name	Qty/L (g)
50.00	1	Vitamin E acetate	50.00
20.00	2	Benzocaine	20.00
50.00	3	Lutrol F 127	50.00
250.00	4	Cremophor RH 40	250.00
2.00	5	Sorbic acid	2.00
QS	6	Water purified	QS to 1 L

Manufacturing Directions

1. Charge item 6 in suitable stainless steel jacketed vessel. Heat to 60°C.
2. Add and dissolve items 2 and 5.
3. In a separate vessel, charge items 1 and 4 (preheated to 60–65°C) and heat the mixture to 60°C to 65°C.
4. Add step 3 to step 2 and mix until clear solution is obtained.
5. Add and dissolve item 3 and mix.

Vitamin E Capsules

Bill of Materials			
Scale (mg/capsule)	Item	Material Name	Qty/1000 caps (g)
400.00	1	Vitamin E (D-alpha tocopherol 1000 units E/g)	400.00
25.00	2	Soybean oil	25.00
QS	3	Gelatin mass clear	QS

Manufacturing Directions

1. Weigh and transfer into a suitable stainless steel container soybean oil and preparation of D-alpha tocopherol.
   - Mix for a minimum for 1 hour.
   - Transfer into a suitable tank through an 80- to 100-mesh stainless steel screen.
   - Encapsulate 425 mg of mixture of step 3 into size 7.5 oval capsules using gelatin mass clear.

Vitamin E Drops

Bill of Materials			
Scale (mg/mL)	Item	Material Name	Qty/L (g)
50.00	1	Vitamin E acetate	50.00
160.00	2	Cremophor RH 40	160.00
QS	3	Preservative	QS
QS	4	Water	QS to 1 L

Manufacturing Directions

1. Separately heat mixture of items 1 and 2 and solution of item 3 in 4 to about 65°C.
2. Add the two solutions slowly. A clear or lightly opalescent, colorless liquid should be formed.

Vitamin E Drops

Bill of Materials			
Scale (mg/mL)	Item	Material Name	Qty/L (g)
50.00	1	Vitamin E acetate	50.00
150.00	2	Cremophor RH 40	150.00
QS	3	Preservatives	QS
QS	4	Water purified	QS to 1 L

Manufacturing Directions

1. Charge items 1 and 2 in a stainless steel jacketed vessel and heat to 65°C.
2. In a separate vessel, charge item 4 and heat to 90°C to 95°C and add and dissolve preservatives. Cool to 40°C.
3. Add step 2 into step 1.
4. Fill.

Vitamin E Solution with Ethanol

Bill of Materials			
Scale (mg/tablet)	Item	Material Name	Qty/L (g)
0.10	1	Vitamin E acetate	0.100
4.50	2	Cremophor EL	4.50
570.00	3	Water	570.00
380.00	4	Ethanol	380.00

Manufacturing Directions

1. Heat mixture of item 1 and 2 to about 60°C. Stir well.
2. Slowly add the warm solvent mixture of items 3 and 4. A clear, colorless liquid of low viscosity should be formed.

Vitamin E Solution with Ethanol

Bill of Materials			
Scale (mg/mL)	Item	Material Name	Qty/L (g)
0.10	1	Vitamin E acetate (BASF)	0.10
45.00	2	Cremophor EL	45.00
QS	3	Water purified	QS to 1 L
380.00	4	Ethanol	380.00

Manufacturing Directions

1. Charge items 1 and 2 in a suitable stainless steel jacketed vessel. Heat to 60°C.
2. In a separate vessel (jacketed and explosion proof), charge item 3 and 4 and heat to 40°C.
3. Add step 2 to step 1 and stir well.
4. Fill.

Xylometazoline Hydrochloride Nasal Solution

Xylometazoline hydrochloride 0.05%, purified water, sorbitol, and mono and dibasic sodium phosphates.

Xylometazoline Hydrochloride Nasal Solution

Bill of Materials			
Scale (g/100 mL)	Item	Material Name	Qty/L (g)
0.100	1	Xylometazoline HCl	1.00
0.100	2	Disodium edetate (sodium EDTA)	1.00
0.700	3	Sodium chloride	7.00
0.030	4	Benzalkonium chloride (50% solution)	0.30
0.285	5	Monobasic sodium phosphate	2.85
0.306	6	Dibasic sodium phosphate	3.06
–	7	Water purified	QS to 1 L

Manufacturing Directions

This product is a colorless membrane filtered solution; therefore, ensure that the storage tanks for solution are cleaned and free of any contamination. Use freshly boiled and cooled purified water for the manufacturing. Prepare approximately 2 L of freshly boiled and cooled purified water and store in a clean stainless steel storage vessel.

1. Add 800 g of item 7 (20–25°C) to the manufacturing vessel.
2. Dissolve items 2 to 6 one by one in step 1 while mixing for 10 minutes. Check the clarity of the solution.
3. Dissolve item 1 in 100 g of item 7 (25–30°C) in a stainless steel container and add to the manufacturing vessel.
4. Rinse the drug container with 20 g of item 7 and add the rinsing to manufacturing vessel.
5. Make the volume up to 1 L with item 7 (20–25°C) and finally mix for 5 minutes.
6. Check and record the pH at 25°C (limit: 6.3 ± 0.2).
7. Check the cleanliness of the storage tank. Filter the solution through a prefilter and membrane filter, 0.2 micron, into the storage tank. Recirculate first 200 to 300 mL solution.
8. Store the filtered solution in tightly closed stainless steel storage tank. Do not store more than 24 hours in stainless steel storage tank after manufacturing.

Xylometazoline Hydrochloride Children's Nasal Solution

Bill of Materials			
Scale (g/100 mL)	Item	Material Name	Qty/L (g)
0.05	1	Xylometazoline hydrochloride	0.50
0.10	2	Disodium edetate (Sodium EDTA)	1.00
0.70	3	Sodium chloride	7.00
0.30	4	Benzalkonium chloride (50% solution)	0.30
0.28	5	Monobasic sodium phosphate	2.85
0.30	6	Dibasic sodium phosphate	3.06
–	7	Water purified	QS to 1 L

Manufacturing Directions

See above.

Zinc Pyrithione Shampoo

Bill of Materials			
Scale (mg/g)	Item	Material Name	Qty/1000 Tablets (g)
547.50	1	Deionized water	547.50
7.50	2	Hydroxyethylcellulose	7.50
347.00	3	TEA-lauryl sulfate	347.00
43.00	4	PEG-20 lanolin alcohol ether	43.00
20.00	5	Glycol stearate	20.00
15.00	6	Cocamide MEA	15.00
10.00	7	Zinc pyrithione (48%)	20.00
QS	8	Fragrance, preservative	QS

Manufacturing Directions

1. Add item 2 to the water and mix.
2. In a separate vessel, combine items 3 to 5, heat to 80°C, and mix.
3. Cool to 50°C.
4. Add items 6 and 7 and mix.
5. Add this mixture to mixture of item 2.
6. Cool to 40°C and add item 8.

COMMERCIAL PHARMACEUTICAL PRODUCTS

- Alupent® (metaproterenol sulfate USP) inhalation aerosol containing 75 mg of metaproterenol sulfate as micronized powder is sufficient medication for 100 inhalations. The Alupent inhalation aerosol containing 150 mg of metaproterenol sulfate as micronized powder is sufficient medication for 200 inhalations. Each metered dose delivers through the mouthpiece 0.65 mg of metaproterenol sulfate (each milliliter contains 15 mg). The inert ingredients are dichlorodifluoromethane, dichlorotetrafluoroethane, and trichloromonofluoromethane as propellants and sorbitan trioleate.
- Custodiol® contains 0.8766 g sodium chloride; 0.6710 g potassium chloride; 0.1842 g potassium hydrogen 2-ketoglutarate; 0.8132 g magnesium chloride • 6 H_2O; 3.7733 g histidine • HCl • H_2O; 27.9289 g histidine; 0.4085 g tryptophan; 5.4651 g mannitol; 0.0022 g calcium chloride – 2 H_2O in sterile water for injection. Anion: Cl – 50 mval. Physical properties: pH 7.02 to 7.20 at 25°C [77° F, pH 7.4–7.45 at 4°C (39.2° F)]. Osmolality: 310 mOsmol/kg.
- Depakene syrup (valproic acid) contains FD&C red No. 40, glycerin, methyl paraben, propyl paraben, sorbitol, sucrose, water, and natural and artificial flavors.
- Dilaudid oral liquid (hydromorphone hydrochloride), each 5 mL (one teaspoon) contains 5 mg of hydromorphone hydrochloride. In addition, other ingredients include purified water, methyl paraben, propyl paraben, sucrose, and glycerin. Dilaudid oral liquid may contain traces of sodium metabisulfite.
- Erythromycin ethylsuccinate (EES) is an ester of erythromycin suitable for oral administration. EES 200 liquid: Each 5-mL teaspoonful of fruit-flavored suspension contains erythromycin ethylsuccinate equivalent to 200 mg of erythromycin. EES 400 liquid: Each 5-mL teaspoonful of orange-flavored suspension contains erythromycin ethylsuccinate equivalent to 400 mg of erythromycin. Inactive: EES 200 liquid: FD&C red No. 40, methyl paraben, polysorbate 60, propyl paraben, sodium citrate, sucrose, water, xanthan gum and natural and artificial flavors. EES 400 liquid: D&C yellow No. 10, FD&C yellow No. 6, methyl paraben, polysorbate 60, propyl paraben, sodium citrate, sucrose, water, xanthan gum, and natural and artificial flavors.
- Gengraf® [cyclosporine capsules, USP (modified)] is a modified oral formulation of cyclosporine that forms an aqueous dispersion in an aqueous environment. Gengraf® capsules [cyclosporine capsules, USP (modified)] are available in 25- and 100-mg strengths. Each 25-mg capsule contains cyclosporine, 25 mg; alcohol, USP, absolute, 12.8% v/v (10.1% wt/vol.). Each 100-mg capsule contains cyclosporine, 100 mg; alcohol, USP, absolute, 12.8% v/v (10.1% wt/vol.). Inactive ingredients: FD&C blue No. 2, gelatin NF, polyethylene glycol NF, polyoxyl 35 castor oil NF, polysorbate 80 NF, propylene glycol USP, sorbitan monooleate NF, titanium dioxide.
- Indocin suspension for oral use contains 25 mg of indomethacin per 5 mL, alcohol 1%, and sorbic acid 0.1% added as a preservative, and the following inactive ingredients: antifoam AF emulsion, flavors, purified water, sodium hydroxide or hydrochloric acid to adjust pH, sorbitol solution, and tragacanth.
- Kaletra (lopinavir/ritonavir) oral solution is available for oral administration as 80 mg lopinavir and 20 mg ritonavir per milliliter with the following inactive ingredients: acesulfame potassium, alcohol, artificial cotton candy flavor, citric acid, glycerin, high fructose corn syrup, magnasweet-110 flavor, menthol, natural & artificial vanilla flavor, peppermint oil, polyoxyl 40 hydrogenated castor oil, povidone, propylene glycol, saccharin sodium, sodium chloride, sodium citrate, and water.
- Miacalcin® (calcitonin-salmon) nasal spray is provided in a 3.7-mL fill glass bottle as a solution for nasal administration. This is sufficient medication for at least 30 doses. Active ingredient: calcitonin-salmon, 2200 IU/mL (corresponding to 200 IU/0.09 mL actuation). Inactive

ingredients: sodium chloride, benzalkonium chloride, hydrochloric acid (added as necessary to adjust pH), and purified water.

- Norvir (ritonavir) oral solution also contains ethanol, water, polyoxyl 35 castor oil, propylene glycol, anhydrous citric acid to adjust pH, saccharin sodium, peppermint oil, creamy caramel flavoring, and FD&C yellow No. 6.
- Omnicef® (cefdinir) for oral suspension after reconstitution contains 125 mg cefdinir per 5 mL or 250 mg cefdinir per 5 mL and the following inactive ingredients: sucrose, NF; citric acid, USP; sodium citrate, USP; sodium benzoate, NF; xanthan gum, NF; guar gum, NF; artificial strawberry and cream flavors; silicon dioxide, NF; and magnesium stearate, NF.
- Rhinocort aqua nasal spray (budesonide) is an unscented, metered-dose manual-pump spray formulation containing a micronized suspension of budesonide in an aqueous medium. Microcrystalline cellulose and carboxymethyl cellulose sodium, dextrose anhydrous, polysorbate 80, disodium edetate, potassium sorbate, and purified water are contained in this medium; hydrochloric acid is added to adjust the pH to a target of 4.5. Rhinocort aqua nasal spray delivers 32 μg of budesonide per spray. Each bottle of Rhinocort aqua nasal spray 32 μg contains 120 metered sprays after initial priming.
- Suprane® (desflurane, USP) is a nonflammable liquid administered via vaporizer and is a general inhalation anesthetic. Desflurane is a colorless, volatile liquid below 22.8°C. Desflurane does not corrode stainless steel, brass, aluminum, anodized aluminum, nickel-plated brass, copper, or beryllium.
- Witch hazel, 50%, inactive ingredients: aloe barbadensis gel, capryl/capramidopropyl betaine, citric acid, diazolidinyl urea, glycerin, methyl paraben, propylene glycol, propyl paraben, sodium citrate, water.
- Abilify (aripiprazole) 1 mg/mL oral solution: Inactive ingredients for this solution include fructose, glycerin, DL-lactic acid, methyl paraben, propylene glycol, propyl paraben, sodium hydroxide, sucrose, and purified water. The oral solution is flavored with natural orange cream and other natural flavors.
- Accuzyme spray contains papain, USP (6.5 × 10.5 USP units of activity based on Lot I0C389 per gram of spray) and urea, USP 10% in a base composed of anhydrous lactose, cetearyl alcohol & ceteth-20 phosphate & dicetyl phosphate, fragrance, glycerin, methyl paraben, mineral oil, potassium phosphate monobasic, propyl paraben, purified water, and sodium hydroxide.
- Aerobid (flunisolide) inhaler is delivered in a metered-dose aerosol system containing a microcrystalline suspension of flunisolide as the hemihydrate in propellants (trichloromonofluoromethane, dichlorodifluoromethane, and dichlorotetrafluoroethane) with sorbitan trioleate as a dispersing agent. Aerobid-M also contains menthol as a flavoring agent. Each activation delivers approximately 250 μg of flunisolide to the patient. One Aerobid inhaler system is designed to deliver at least 100 metered inhalations.
- Astelin® (azelastine hydrochloride) nasal spray, 137 μg, contains 0.1% azelastine hydrochloride in an aqueous solution at pH 6.8 ± 0.3. It also contains benzalkonium chloride (125 μg/mL), EDTA, hypromellose, citric acid, dibasic sodium phosphate, sodium chloride, and purified water.
- Avar™ cleanser (sodium sulfacetamide 10% and sulfur 5%) in each gram contains 100 mg of sodium sulfacetamide and 50 mg of colloidal sulfur in a mild aqueous based cleansing vehicle containing purified water USP, sodium magnesium silicate, sodium thiosulfate, propylene glycol, sodium lauryl sulfate, cetyl alcohol, stearyl alcohol, phenoxyethanol, fragrance.
- Beconase AQ nasal spray, beclomethasone dipropionate, monohydrate, the active component of Beconase AQ nasal spray is a metered-dose manual pump spray unit containing a microcrystalline suspension of beclomethasone dipropionate, monohydrate equivalent to 42 μg of beclomethasone dipropionate, calculated on the dried basis, in an aqueous medium containing microcrystalline cellulose, carboxymethylcellulose sodium, dextrose, benzalkonium chloride, polysorbate 80, and 0.25% v/w phenylethyl alcohol. The pH through expiry is 5.0 to 6.8.
- Celexa® (citalopram HBr) oral solution contains citalopram HBr equivalent to 2 mg/mL citalopram base. It also contains the following inactive ingredients: sorbitol, purified water, propylene glycol, methyl paraben, natural peppermint flavor, and propyl paraben.
- Clarinex syrup is a clear orange-colored liquid containing 0.5 mg/1 mL desloratadine. The syrup contains the following inactive ingredients: propylene glycol USP, sorbitol solution USP, citric acid (anhydrous) USP, sodium citrate dihydrate USP, sodium benzoate NF, disodium edetate USP, purified water USP. It also contains granulated sugar, natural and artificial flavor for bubble gum and FDC yellow No. 6 dye.
- Clindets® (clindamycin phosphate pledgets) contain clindamycin phosphate, USP, at a concentration equivalent to 10 mg clindamycin per milliliter in a vehicle of isopropyl alcohol 52% v/v, propylene glycol, and water. Each Clindets® pledget applicator contains approximately 1 mL of clindamycin phosphate topical solution. Clindamycin phosphate topical solution has a pH range between 4 and 7.
- Clobex® (clobetasol propionate) spray, 0.05%, contains clobetasol propionate, a synthetic fluorinated corticosteroid, for topical use. Each gram of Clobex (clobetasol propionate) spray, 0.05%, contains 0.5 mg of clobetasol propionate, in a vehicle base composed of alcohol, isopropyl myristate, sodium lauryl sulfate, and undecylenic acid.
- Clobex (clobetasol propionate) shampoo, 0.05%, contains clobetasol propionate, a synthetic fluorinated corticosteroid, for topical dermatologic use. Each milliliter of Clobex (clobetasol propionate) shampoo, 0.05%, contains clobetasol propionate, 0.05%, in a shampoo base consisting of alcohol, citric acid, cocobetaine, polyquaternium-10, purified water, sodium citrate, and sodium laureth sulfate. Each gram of Clobex (clobetasol propionate) lotion, 0.05%, contains 0.5 mg of clobetasol propionate, in a vehicle base composed of hypromellose, propylene glycol, mineral oil, polyoxyethylene glycol 300 isostearate, carbomer 1342, sodium hydroxide, and purified water.
- Colace® syrup [docusate sodium, in each tablespoonful (15 mL)] contains docusate sodium 60 mg. Inactive ingredients: citric acid, D&C red No. 33, FD&C red No. 40, flavors, glycerin, propylene glycol, purified water, sodium citrate, sodium saccharin, sorbitol. Colace® liquid 1% solution: each mL contains 10 mg of docusate sodium.
- Depacon solution, valproate sodium, is the sodium salt of valproic acid designated as sodium 2-propylpentanoate. It is available in 5-mL single-dose vials for intravenous injection. Each milliliter contains valproate sodium equivalent to 100 mg valproic acid, EDTA 0.40 mg, and water for injection to volume. The pH is adjusted to 7.6 with sodium

hydroxide and/or hydrochloric acid. The solution is clear and colorless.

- Dextromethorphan–Pseudoephedrine active ingredients: Each 0.8 mL contains 2.5 mg dextromethorphan hydrobromide, USP; 7.5 mg pseudoephedrine hydrochloride, USP. Inactive ingredients: citric acid, flavors, glycerin, high fructose corn syrup, maltol, menthol, polyethylene glycol, propylene glycol, sodium benzoate, sorbitol, sucrose, water.
- Diuril (chlorothiazide) oral suspension contains 250 mg of chlorothiazide per 5 mL, alcohol 0.5%, with methyl paraben 0.12%, propyl paraben 0.02%, and benzoic acid 0.1% added as preservatives. The inactive ingredients are D&C yellow No. 10, flavors, glycerin, purified water, sodium saccharin, sucrose, and tragacanth.
- Dovonex® (calcipotriene solution) scalp solution 0.005% is a colorless topical solution containing 0.005% calcipotriene in a vehicle of isopropanol (51% v/v) propylene glycol, hydroxypropyl cellulose, sodium citrate, menthol, and water.
- Ferrochel® (elemental iron) 70 mg, ferrous fumerate (elemental iron) 81 mg, vitamin C as Ester-C®, ascorbic acid (as calcium ascorbate) 60 mg, threonic acid (as calcium threonate) 0.8 mg, folic acid, USP 1 mg, vitamin B_{12} (cyanocobalamin) 10 μg, Ferrochel® (ferrous bisglycinate chelate) is a registered trademark of Albion International, Inc., Clearfield, Utah, and is protected under U.S. Patent Nos. 4,599,152 and 4,830,716. Ester-C® is a patented pharmaceutical grade material consisting of calcium ascorbate and calcium threonate. Ester-C® is a licensed trademark of Zila Nutraceuticals, Inc. Inactive ingredients: soybean oil, gelatin, glycerin, lecithin (unbleached), yellow beeswax, titanium dioxide, methyl paraben, ethyl vanillin, FD& yellow No. 6, FD& red No. 40, propyl paraben, FD& blue No. 1.
- Efudex solutions and cream are topical preparations containing the fluorinated pyrimidine 5-fluorouracil. Efudex solution consists of 2% or 5% fluorouracil on a weight/weight basis, compounded with propylene glycol, tris (hydroxymethyl) aminomethane, hydroxypropyl cellulose, parabens (methyl and propyl), and disodium edetate.
- Epinephrine inhalation active ingredient (in each inhalation), epinephrine 0.22 mg. Inactive ingredients: ascorbic acid, dehydrated alcohol (34%), dichlorodifluoromethane (CFC 12), dichlorotetrafluoroethane (CFC 114), hydrochloric acid, nitric acid, purified water.
- Epivir (also known as 3TC) is lamivudine, a white to off-white crystalline solid with a solubility of approximately 70 mg/mL in water at 20°C. Epivir oral solution is for oral administration. One milliliter of Epivir oral solution contains 10 mg of lamivudine (10 mg/mL) in an aqueous solution and the inactive ingredients artificial strawberry and banana flavors, citric acid (anhydrous), methyl paraben, propylene glycol, propyl paraben, sodium citrate (dihydrate), and sucrose (200 mg).
- Epivir-HBV is lamivudine, a white to off-white crystalline solid with a solubility of approximately 70 mg/mL in water at 20°C. Epivir-HBV oral solution is for oral administration. One milliliter of Epivir-HBV oral solution contains 5 mg of lamivudine (5 mg/mL) in an aqueous solution and the inactive ingredients artificial strawberry and banana flavors, citric acid (anhydrous), methyl paraben, propylene glycol, propyl paraben, sodium citrate (dihydrate), and sucrose (200 mg).
- Exelon® (rivastigmine tartrate) oral solution is supplied as a solution containing rivastigmine tartrate, equivalent to 2 mg/mL of rivastigmine base for oral administration. Inactive ingredients are citric acid, D&C yellow No. 10, purified water, sodium benzoate, and sodium citrate.
- Fleet® Phospho-soda® EZ-Prep™ contains active ingredients (each 15 mL) monobasic sodium phosphate monohydrate 7.2 g and dibasic sodium phosphate heptahydrate 2.7 g.
- Flovent HFA 44 μg inhalation aerosol, Flovent HFA 110 μg inhalation aerosol, and Flovent HFA 220 μg inhalation aerosol contain fluticasone propionate. Flovent HFA 44 μg inhalation aerosol, Flovent HFA 110 μg inhalation aerosol, and Flovent HFA 220 μg inhalation aerosol are pressurized, metered-dose aerosol units intended for oral inhalation only. Each unit contains a microcrystalline suspension of fluticasone propionate (micronized) in propellant HFA-134a (1, 1, 1, 2-tetrafluoroethane). It contains no other excipients. Each 10.6-g canister (44 μg) and each 12-g canister (110 and 220 μg) provides 120 inhalations. Flovent HFA should be primed before using for the first time by releasing four test sprays into the air away from the face, shaking well before each spray. In cases where the inhaler has not been used for more than 7 days or when it has been dropped, prime the inhaler again by shaking well and releasing one test spray into the air away from the face. This product does not contain any chlorofluorocarbon (CFC) as the propellant. Under standardized in vitro test conditions, Flovent DISKUS 50 μg delivers 46 μg of fluticasone propionate when tested at a flow rate of 60 L/min for 2 seconds. In adult patients with obstructive lung disease and severely compromised lung function (mean forced expiratory volume in 1 second [FEV 1] 20–30% of predicted), mean peak inspiratory flow (PIF) through a Diskus® is 82.4 L/min (range: 46.1–115.3 L/min). In children with asthma 4 and 8 years old, mean PIF through Flovent Diskus is 70 and 104 L/min, respectively (range: 48–123 L/min).
- Flumadine® (rimantadine hydrochloride, 5 mL) of the syrup contains 50 mg of rimantadine hydrochloride in a dye-free, aqueous solution containing citric acid, parabens (methyl and propyl), saccharin sodium, sorbitol, and flavors.
- Fluticasone propionate, Flonase nasal spray, 50 μg, is an aqueous suspension of microfine fluticasone propionate for topical administration to the nasal mucosa by means of a metering, atomizing spray pump. Flonase nasal spray also contains microcrystalline cellulose and carboxymethylcellulose sodium, dextrose, 0.02% w/w benzalkonium chloride, polysorbate 80, and 0.25% w/w phenylethyl alcohol and has a pH between 5 and 7. It is necessary to prime the pump before first use or after a period of nonuse (1 week or more). After initial priming (6 actuations), each actuation delivers 50 μg of fluticasone propionate in 100 mg of formulation through the nasal adapter. Each 16-g bottle of Flonase nasal spray provides 120 metered sprays. After 120 metered sprays, the amount of fluticasone propionate delivered per actuation may not be consistent and the unit should be discarded.
- Fosamax (alendronate sodium) oral solution contains 91.35 mg of alendronate monosodium salt trihydrate, which is the molar equivalent to 70 mg of free acid. Each bottle also contains the following inactive ingredients: sodium citrate dihydrate and citric acid anhydrous as buffering agents, sodium saccharin, artificial raspberry flavor, and purified water. Added as preservatives are sodium propyl paraben 0.0225% and sodium butylparaben 0.0075%.
- Frotical (calcitonin) calcitonin-salmon (rDNA origin) nasal spray is provided in a 3.7-mL fill glass bottle as a

solution for intranasal administration with sufficient medication for at least 30 doses. Each spray delivers 200 IU calcitonin-salmon in a volume of 0.09 mL. Active ingredient: Calcitonin-salmon 2200 IU/mL, corresponding to 200 IU per actuation (0.09 mL). Inactive ingredients: Sodium chloride USP, citric acid USP, phenylethyl alcohol USP, benzyl alcohol NF, polysorbate 80 NF, hydrochloric acid NF or sodium hydroxide NF (added as necessary to adjust pH), and purified water USP.

- Gets The Dry Out® and Visine® pure tears portables preservative free lubricant eye. Glycerin 0.2%, hypromellose 0.2%, polyethylene glycol 400 1%.
- Gordochom containing 25% undecylenic acid and 3% chloroxylenol as its active ingredients in a penetrating oil base.
- Guaifenesin, active ingredient (in each 5 mL tsp): guaifenesin, USP 100 mg, Inactive ingredients: caramel, citric acid, FD&C red No. 40, flavors, glucose, glycerin, high fructose corn syrup, menthol, saccharin sodium, sodium benzoate, water.
- Hydroquinone USP 4% also contains avobenzone, ceteareth-20, cetostearyl alcohol, citric acid, diethylaminoethyl stearate, dimethicone, EDTA, glyceryl dilaurate, glyceryl monostearate, glyceryl stearate, PEG-100 stearate, hydroxyethylcellulose, methyl paraben, octyldodecyl stearoyl stearate, octinoxate, oxybenzone, polysorbate 80, propylene glycol, propyl gallate, propyl paraben, purified water, quaternium-26, sodium metabisulfite, sodium PCA, squalane, ubiquinone, stearyl alcohol, water, glycerin, *Rumex occidentalis* extract.
- Ibuprofen, active ingredient (in each 5 mL), Ibuprofen 100 mg, inactive ingredients (fruit flavor): artifical flavors, carboxymethylcellulose sodium, citric acid, EDTA, FD&C red No. 40, glycerin, microcrystalline cellulose, polysorbate 80, purified water, sodium benzoate, sorbitol solution, sucrose, xanthan gum. Inactive ingredients (grape flavor): acetic acid, artifical flavor, butylated hydroxytoluene, carboxymethylcellulose sodium, citric acid, EDTA, FD&C blue No. 1, FD&C red No. 40, glycerin, microcrystalline cellulose, polysorbate 80, propylene glycol, purified water, sodium benzoate, sorbitol solution, sucrose, xanthan gum. Inactive ingredients (blue raspberry flavor): carboxymethylcellulose sodium, citric acid, edetate disodium, FD&C blue No. 1, glycerin, microcrystalline cellulose, natural and artificial flavors, polysorbate 80, propylene glycol, purified water, sodium benzoate, sodium citrate, sorbitol solution, sucrose, xanthan gum.
- Ibuprofen 200 mg, inactives: FD&C green No. 3, gelatin, light mineral oil, pharmaceutical ink, polyethylene glycol, potassium hydroxide, purified water, sorbitan, sorbitol.
- Ibuprofen liquid gel, active ingredients (in each LiquiGel): solubilized ibuprofen equal to 200 mg ibuprofen (present as the free acid and potassium salt) pseudoephedrine HCl 30 mg. Inactive ingredients (LiquiGel): D&C yellow No. 10, FD&C red No. 40, fractionated coconut oil, gelatin, pharmaceutical ink, polyethylene glycol, potassium hydroxide, purified water, sorbitan, sorbitol.
- Imitrex (sumatriptan) nasal spray contains sumatriptan. Each Imitrex nasal spray contains 5 or 20 mg of sumatriptan in a 100-μL unit dose aqueous buffered solution containing monobasic potassium phosphate NF, anhydrous dibasic sodium phosphate USP, sulfuric acid NF, sodium hydroxide NF, and purified water USP. The pH of the solution is approximately 5.5. The osmolality of the solution is 372 or 742 mOsmol for the 5- and 20-mg Imitrex nasal spray, respectively.
- Iron protein succinylate is a proprietary stabilized iron compound. The iron is wrapped in a casein protective layer, which allows the iron to pass through the stomach to the intestinal tract for immediate safe and efficacious absorption. Ferretts IPS liquid is for use as a dietary supplement. Each 1 mL contains 2.67 mg iron. Serving size: 15 mL, amount per 15 mL, iron 40 mg (from iron protein succinylate). Other ingredients: purified water, sorbitol solution, propylene glycol, casein (milk protein) strawberry flavor, sodium hydroxide, methyl paraben sodium, propyl paraben sodium, saccharin sodium.
- Kaopectate®: Each 15 mL of Kaopectate antidiarrheal contains bismuth subsalicylate 262 mg, contributing 130 mg total salicylates. Kaopectate antidiarrheal is low sodium, with each 15 mL tablespoonful containing 10 mg sodium. Extra-strength Kaopectate: Each 15 mL of extra-strength Kaopectate antidiarrheal contains bismuth subsalicylate 525 mg, contributing 236 mg total salicylates. Extra-strength Kaopectate is low sodium. Each 15 mL tablespoonful contains sodium 11 mg.
- Keppra® oral solution contains 100 mg of levetiracetam per milliliter. Inactive ingredients: ammonium glycyrrhizinate, citric acid monohydrate, glycerin, maltitol solution, methyl paraben, potassium acesulfame, propyl paraben, purified water, sodium citrate dihydrate, and natural and artificial flavor.
- Lexapro® (escitalopram oxalate) oral solution contains escitalopram oxalate equivalent to 1 mg/mL escitalopram base. It also contains the following inactive ingredients: sorbitol, purified water, citric acid, sodium citrate, malic acid, glycerin, propylene glycol, methyl paraben, propyl paraben, and natural peppermint flavor.
- Loprox® (ciclopirox) shampoo 1% contains the synthetic antifungal agent, ciclopirox. Each gram (equivalent to 0.96 mL) of Loprox shampoo contains 10 mg ciclopirox in a shampoo base consisting of purified water USP, sodium laureth sulfate, disodium laureth sulfosuccinate, sodium chloride USP, and laureth-2. Loprox shampoo is a colorless, translucent solution.
- Loratadine, active ingredient (in each 5-mL teaspoon): loratadine 5 mg. Inactive ingredients: artificial flavor, citric acid, glycerin, propylene glycol, purified water, sodium benzoate, sucrose.
- Lortab elixir, hydrocodone bitartrate and acetaminophen are supplied in liquid form for oral administration. It is affected by light. Lortab elixir contains per 5 mL hydrocodone bitartrate 2.5 mg, acetaminophen 167 mg, alcohol 7%. In addition, the liquid contains the following inactive ingredients: citric acid anhydrous, ethyl maltol, glycerin, methyl paraben, propylene glycol, propyl paraben, purified water, saccharin sodium, sorbitol solution, sucrose, with D&C yellow No. 10 and FD&C yellow No. 6 as coloring and natural and artificial flavoring.
- Lotrimin topical solution contains 10 mg clotrimazole, USP, in a nonaqueous vehicle of PEG-400 NF.
- Marinol® Dronabinol capsules for oral administration: Marinol capsules are supplied as round, soft gelatin capsules containing either 2.5, 5, or 10 mg dronabinol. Each Marinol capsule is formulated with the following inactive ingredients: FD&C blue No. 1 (5 mg), FD&C red No. 40 (5 mg), FD&C yellow No. 6 (5 and 10 mg), gelatin, glycerin, methyl paraben, propyl paraben, sesame oil, and titanium dioxide.
- Megace® ES (megestrol acetate) oral suspension contains megestrol acetate. Megace ES (megestrol acetate) is a concentrated formula supplied as an oral suspension

containing 125 mg of megestrol acetate per mL. Megace ES (megestrol acetate) oral suspension contains the following inactive ingredients: alcohol (max 0.06% v/v from flavor), artificial lime flavor, citric acid monohydrate, docusate sodium, hydroxypropylmethylcellulose (hypromellose), natural and artificial lemon flavor, purified water, sodium benzoate, sodium citrate dihydrate, and sucrose.

- Mepron (atovaquone) suspension is a formulation of microfine particles of atovaquone. The atovaquone particles, reduced in size to facilitate absorption, are significantly smaller than those in the previously marketed tablet formulation. Mepron suspension is for oral administration and is bright yellow with a citrus flavor. Each teaspoonful (5 mL) contains 750 mg of atovaquone and the inactive ingredients benzyl alcohol, flavor, poloxamer 188, purified water, saccharin sodium, and xanthan gum.
- Migranal® is ergotamine hydrogenated in the 9, 10 position as the mesylate salt. Migranal (dihydroergotamine mesylate, USP) nasal spray is provided for intranasal administration as a clear, colorless to faintly yellow solution in an amber glass vial containing dihydroergotamine mesylate, USP 4 mg; caffeine, anhydrous, USP 10 mg; dextrose, anhydrous, USP 50 mg; carbon dioxide, USP QS; purified, USP QS 1 mL.
- Namenda® (memantine hydrochloride) oral solution contains memantine hydrochloride in a strength equivalent to 2 mg of memantine hydrochloride in each milliliter. The oral solution also contains the following inactive ingredients: sorbitol solution (70%), methyl paraben, propyl paraben, propylene glycol, glycerin, natural peppermint flavor No. 104, citric acid, sodium citrate, and purified water.
- Nasacort® HFA nasal aerosol contains triamcinolone acetonide. Nasacort HFA nasal aerosol is a metered-dose aerosol unit containing a microcrystalline suspension of triamcinolone acetonide in tetrafluoroethane (HFA-134a) and dehydrated alcohol USP 0.7% w/w. Each canister contains 15 mg of triamcinolone acetonide.
- Nasonex nasal spray 50 µg mometasone furoate monohydrate is a metered-dose manual pump spray unit containing an aqueous suspension of mometasone furoate monohydrate equivalent to 0.05% w/w mometasone furoate calculated on the anhydrous basis; in an aqueous medium containing glycerin, microcrystalline cellulose and carboxymethylcellulose sodium, sodium citrate, citric acid, benzalkonium chloride, and polysorbate 80. The pH is between 4.3 and 4.9. After initial priming (10 actuations), each actuation of the pump delivers a metered spray containing 100 mg of suspension containing mometasone furoate monohydrate equivalent to 50 µg of mometasone furoate calculated on the anhydrous basis. Each bottle of Nasonex nasal spray 50 µg provides 120 sprays.
- Neoral® is an oral formulation of cyclosporine that immediately forms a microemulsion in an aqueous environment. Neoral soft gelatin capsules (cyclosporine capsules, USP) modified are available in 25- and 100-mg strengths. Each 25-mg capsule contains cyclosporine 25 mg; alcohol, USP dehydrated 11.9% v/v (9.5% wt/vol.). Each 100-mg capsule contains cyclosporine 100 mg alcohol, USP dehydrated 11.9% v/v (9.5% wt/vol.). Inactive ingredients: Corn oil-mono-di-triglycerides, polyoxyl 40 hydrogenated castor oil NF, DL-(alpha)-tocopherol USP, gelatin NF, glycerol, iron oxide black, propylene glycol USP, titanium dioxide USP, carmine, and other ingredients.
- Neoral oral solution (cyclosporine oral solution, USP) modified is available in 50 mL bottles. Each milliliter contains cyclosporine 100 mg/mL; alcohol, USP dehydrated 11.9% v/v (9.5% wt/vol.). Inactive ingredients: Corn oil-mono-di-triglycerides, polyoxyl 40 hydrogenated castor oil NF, DL-(alpha)-tocopherol USP, propylene glycol USP.
- Neurontin® (gabapentin) oral solution contains 250 mg/5 mL of gabapentin. The inactive ingredients for the oral solution are glycerin, xylitol, purified water, and artificial cool strawberry anise flavor.
- Nicotrol® inhaler (nicotine inhalation system) consists of a mouthpiece and a plastic cartridge delivering 4 mg of nicotine from a porous plug containing 10 mg nicotine. The cartridge is inserted into the mouthpiece prior to use. Nicotine is the active ingredient; inactive components of the product are menthol and a porous plug which are pharmacologically inactive. Nicotine is released when air is inhaled through the inhaler.
- Nicotrol NS (nicotine nasal spray) is an aqueous solution of nicotine intended for administration as a metered spray to the nasal mucosa. Each 10 mL spray bottle contains 100 mg nicotine (10 mg/mL) in an inactive vehicle containing disodium phosphate, sodium dihydrogen phosphate, citric acid, methyl paraben, propyl paraben, edetate disodium, sodium chloride, polysorbate 80, aroma, and water. The solution is isotonic with a pH of 7. It contains no chlorofluorocarbons. After priming the delivery system for Nicotrol NS, each actuation of the unit delivers a metered dose spray containing approximately 0.5 mg of nicotine. The size of the droplets produced by the unit is in excess of 8 microns. One Nicotrol NS unit delivers approximately 200 applications.
- Nitrolingual® pumpspray (nitroglycerin lingual spray 400 µg) is a metered dose spray containing nitroglycerin. This product delivers nitroglycerin (400 µg per spray, 60 or 200 metered sprays) in the form of spray droplets onto or under the tongue. Inactive ingredients: medium-chain triglycerides, dehydrated alcohol, medium-chain partial glycerides, peppermint oil.
- Oxsoralen ultra lotion: Each milliliter of Oxsoralen lotion contains 10 mg methoxsalen in an inert vehicle containing alcohol (71% v/v), propylene glycol, acetone, and purified water.
- Oxyfast® oral concentrate solution: Each 1 mL of Oxyfast concentrate solution contains oxycodone hydrochloride 20 mg. Inactive ingredients: citric acid, D&C yellow No. 10, sodium benzoate, sodium citrate, sodium saccharine, and water.
- Panafil spray contains papain, USP (not less than 405, 900 units of activity based on Lot IOC389 per gram of spray); urea, USP 10%; and chlorophyllin copper complex sodium, USP 0.5% in a base composed of anhydrous lactose, cetearyl alcohol & ceteth-20 phosphate & dicetyl phosphate, glycerin, methyl paraben, mineral oil, propyl paraben, purified water, and sodium hydroxide.
- Paxil CR (paroxetine hydrochloride) suspension for oral administration: Each 5 mL of orange-colored, orange-flavored liquid contains paroxetine hydrochloride equivalent to paroxetine 10 mg. Inactive ingredients consist of polacrilin potassium, microcrystalline cellulose, propylene glycol, glycerin, sorbitol, methyl paraben, propyl paraben, sodium citrate dihydrate, citric acid anhydrate, sodium saccharin, flavorings, FD&C yellow No. 6, and simethicone emulsion, USP.
- Pediapred (prednisolone sodium phosphate, USP) oral solution is a dye-free, colorless to light straw-colored, raspberry-flavored solution. Each 5 mL (teaspoonful) of Pediapred contains 6.7 mg prednisolone sodium phosphate

(5 mg prednisolone base) in a palatable, aqueous vehicle. Pediapred also contains dibasic sodium phosphate, edetate disodium, methyl paraben, purified water, sodium biphosphate, sorbitol, natural and artificial raspberry flavor.

- Penlac® nail lacquer (ciclopirox) topical solution, 8%, contains a synthetic antifungal agent ciclopirox. It is intended for topical use on fingernails and toenails and immediately adjacent skin. Each gram of Penlac nail lacquer (ciclopirox) topical solution, 8%, contains 80 mg ciclopirox in a solution base consisting of ethyl acetate, NF; isopropyl alcohol, USP; and butyl monoester of poly(methylvinyl ether/maleic acid) in isopropyl alcohol. Ethyl acetate and isopropyl alcohol are solvents that vaporize after application. Penlac nail lacquer (ciclopirox) topical solution, 8%, is a clear, colorless to slightly yellowish solution.
- Plexion®, sodium sulfacetamide, each gram of Plexion (sodium sulfacetamide USP 10% and sulfur USP 5%) cleanser contains 100 mg of sodium sulfacetamide USP and 50 mg of sulfur USP in a cleanser base containing purified water USP, sodium methyl oleyltaurate, sodium cocoyl isethionate, disodium oleamido MEA sulfosuccinate, cetyl alcohol NF, glyceryl stearate (and) PEG-100 stearate, stearyl alcohol NF, PEG-55 propylene glycol oleate, magnesium aluminum silicate, methyl paraben NF, edetate disodium USP, butylated hydroxytoluene, sodium thiosulfate USP, fragrance, xanthan gum NF, and propyl paraben NF. Each cloth of Plexion (sodium sulfacetamide USP 10% and sulfur USP 5%) Cleansing cloths are coated with a cleanser-based formulation. Each gram of this cleanser-based formulation contains 100 mg of sodium sulfacetamide USP and 50 mg of sulfur USP. The cleanser base consists of purified water USP, sodium methyl oleyltaurate, sodium cocoyl isethionate, disodium laureth sulfosuccinate (and) sodium lauryl sulfoacetate, disodium oleamido MEA sulfosuccinate, glycerin USP, sorbitan monooleate NF, glyceryl stearate (and) PEG-100 stearate, stearyl alcohol NF, propylene glycol (and) PEG-55 propylene glycol oleate, cetyl alcohol NF, edetate disodium USP, methyl paraben NF, PEG-150 pentaerythrityl tetrastearate, butylated hydroxytoluene NF, sodium thiosulfate USP, aloe vera gel decolorized, allantoin, alpha bisabolol natural, fragrance, propyl paraben NF. Each gram of Plexion SCT® (sodium sulfacetamide USP 10% and sulfur USP 5%) contains 100 mg of sodium sulfacetamide USP and 50 mg of sulfur USP in a cream containing purified water USP, kaolin USP, glyceryl stearate (and) PEG-100 stearate, witch hazel USP, silicon dioxide, magnesium aluminum silicate, benzyl alcohol NF, water (and) propylene glycol (and) quillaia saponaria extract, xanthan gum NF, sodium thiosulfate USP, fragrance.
- Prevacid for delayed-release oral suspension is composed of the active ingredient lansoprazole, in the form of enteric-coated granules and also contains inactive granules. The packets contain lansoprazole granules which are identical to those contained in Prevacid delayed-release capsules and are available in 15- and 30-mg strengths. Inactive granules are composed of the following ingredients: confectioner's sugar, mannitol, docusate sodium, ferric oxide, colloidal silicon dioxide, xanthan gum, crospovidone, citric acid, sodium citrate, magnesium stearate, and artificial strawberry flavor. The lansoprazole granules and inactive granules, present in unit dose packets, are constituted with water to form a suspension and consumed orally.
- Proventil HFA (albuterol sulfate) inhalation aerosol contains a microcrystalline suspension of albuterol sulfate in propellant HFA-134a (1, 1, 1, 2-tetrafluoroethane), ethanol, and oleic acid. Each actuation delivers 120 μg albuterol sulfate, USP, from the valve and 108 μg albuterol sulfate, USP, from the mouthpiece (equivalent to 90 μg of albuterol base from the mouthpiece). Each canister provides 200 inhalations.
- Proventil inhalation solution contains albuterol sulfate. Proventil inhalation solution is a clear, colorless to light yellow solution and requires no dilution before administration by nebulization. Each milliliter of Proventil inhalation solution 0.083% contains 0.83 mg of albuterol (as 1 mg of albuterol sulfate) in an isotonic aqueous solution containing sodium chloride. Sulfuric acid may be added to adjust pH (3–5). Proventil inhalation solution contains no sulfiting agents or preservatives.
- Prozac® (fluoxetine hydrochloride) oral solution contains fluoxetine hydrochloride equivalent to 20 mg/5 mL (64.7 μmol) of fluoxetine. It also contains alcohol 0.23%, benzoic acid, flavoring agent, glycerin, purified water, and sucrose.
- Rapamune® (sirolimus) is available for administration as an oral solution containing 1 mg/mL sirolimus. The inactive ingredients in Rapamune oral solution are Phosal 50 PG ® (phosphatidylcholine, propylene glycol, mono- and diglycerides, ethanol, soy fatty acids. Oral solution contains 1.5%–2.5% ethanol.
- Retrovir (zidovudine) syrup is for oral administration. Each teaspoonful (5 mL) of Retrovir syrup contains 50 mg of zidovudine and the inactive ingredients sodium benzoate 0.2% (added as a preservative), citric acid, flavors, glycerin, and liquid sucrose. Sodium hydroxide may be added to adjust pH.
- Robitussin CF, active ingredients (in each 5 mL tsp Robitussin CF): dextromethorphan HBr, USP 10 mg, guaifenesin, USP 100 mg, pseudoephedrine HCl, USP 30 mg (in each 2.5 mL Robitussin cough & cold infant drops), dextromethorphan HBr, USP 5 mg, guaifenesin, USP 100 mg, pseudoephedrine HCl, USP 15 mg. Active ingredients (in each 5 mL tsp: Robitussin DM, Robitussin sugar free cough): dextromethorphan HBr, USP 10 mg guaifenesin, USP 100 mg. Active ingredients (in each 2.5 mL Robitussin DM infant drops): dextromethorphan HBr, USP 5 mg, guaifenesin, USP 100 mg, pseudoephedrine HCl, USP 30 mg. Inactive ingredients (Robitussin DM): citric acid, FD&C red No. 40, flavors, glucose, glycerin, high fructose corn syrup, menthol, saccharin sodium, sodium benzoate, water. Inactive ingredients (Robitussin sugar free cough): acesulfame potassium, citric acid, flavors, glycerin, methyl paraben, polyethylene glycol, povidone, propylene glycol, saccharin sodium, sodium benzoate, water. Inactive ingredients (Robitussin DM infant drops): citric acid, FD&C red No. 40, flavors, glycerin, high fructose corn syrup, maltitol, maltol, polyethylene glycol, povidone, propylene glycol, saccharin sodium, sodium benzoate, sodium chloride, sodium citrate, water. Robitussin DM infant drops in 1fl oz bottle: Active ingredients (in each 5 mL tsp): guaifenesin, USP 100 mg, Inactive ingredients: citric acid, FD&C red No. 40, flavors, glucose, glycerin, high fructose corn syrup, maltol, menthol, propylene glycol, saccharin sodium, sodium benzoate, water. Active ingredients (in each 5 mL tsp): chlorpheniramine maleate, USP 1 mg, dextromethorphan HBr, USP 7.5 mg, pseudoephedrine HCl, USP 15 mg. Inactive ingredients: citric acid, FD&C red No. 40, glycerin, high fructose corn syrup, natural and artificial flavors, propylene glycol, purified water, saccharin sodium, sodium benzoate, sodium chloride, sodium citrate. Active ingredient (in each drop): natural honey center

and honey lemon tea: menthol, USP 5 mg, honey citrus and almond with natural honey center: menthol, USP 2.5 mg, inactive ingredients: natural honey center: caramel, corn syrup, glycerin, high fructose corn syrup, honey, natural herbal flavor, sorbitol, sucrose. Honey lemon tea: caramel, citric acid, corn syrup, honey, natural flavor, sucrose, tea extract. Honey citrus: citric acid, corn syrup, flavors, honey, sucrose. almond with natural honey center: caramel, corn syrup, glycerin, honey, natural almond flavor, natural anise flavor, natural coriander flavor, natural fennel flavor, natural honey flavor and other natural flavors, sorbitol, sucrose. Inactive ingredients: citric acid, D&C red No. 33, FD&C yellow No. 6, flavor, glycerin, high fructose corn syrup, polyethylene glycol, purified water, sodium benzoate, sodium citrate, sorbitol solution, sucralose. Active ingredient (in each drop) menthol eucalyptus: menthol, USP 10 mg, cherry and honey-lemon: menthol, USP 5 mg. Active ingredients (in each 5 mL tsp), acetaminophen, USP 160 mg, chlorpheniramine maleate, USP 1 mg, dextromethorphan HBr, USP 5 mg, pseudoephedrine HCl, USP 15 mg. Inactive ingredients: menthol eucalyptus: corn syrup, eucalyptus oil, flavor, sucrose. Cherry: corn syrup, FD&C red No. 40, flavor, methyl paraben, propyl paraben, sodium benzoate, sucrose. Honey-Lemon: citric acid, corn syrup, D&C yellow No. 10, FD&C yellow No. 6, honey, lemon oil, methyl paraben, povidone, propyl paraben, sodium benzoate, sucrose.

- Sandimmune® oral solution (cyclosporine oral solution, USP) is available in 50-mL bottles. Each milliliter contains cyclosporine, USP 100 mg, alcohol, Ph. Helv. 12.5% by volume dissolved in an olive oil, Ph. Helv./Labrafil M 1944 CS (polyoxyethylated oleic glycerides) vehicle which must be further diluted with milk, chocolate milk, or orange juice before oral administration.
- Sandimmune soft gelatin capsules (cyclosporine capsules, USP) are available in 25- and 100-mg strengths. Each 25-mg capsule contains cyclosporine, USP 25 mg, alcohol, USP dehydrated max 12.7% by volume. Each 100-mg capsule contains cyclosporine, USP 100 mg, alcohol, USP dehydrated max 12.7% by volume. Inactive ingredients: corn oil, gelatin, glycerol, Labrafil M 2125 CS (polyoxyethylated glycolysed glycerides), red iron oxide (25- and 100-mg capsule only), sorbitol, titanium dioxide, and other ingredients.
- Sulfamylon® for 5% topical solution is provided in packets containing 50 g of sterile mafenide acetate to be reconstituted in 1000 mL of sterile water for irrigation, USP or 0.9% sodium chloride irrigation, USP. After mixing, the solution contains 5% w/v of mafenide acetate. The solution is an antimicrobial preparation suitable for topical administration. The solution is not for injection. The reconstituted solution may be held up to 28 days after preparation if stored in unopened containers.
- Tahitian Noni® juice is reconstituted *Morinda citrifolia* fruit juice from pure juice puree from French Polynesia, natural grape juice concentrate, natural blueberry juice concentrate, and natural flavors. Not made from dried or powdered *M. citrifolia*.
- Triaz® (benzoyl peroxide) 3%, 6%, and 9% gels, cleansers, and pads are topical, gel-based benzoyl peroxide–containing preparations for use in the treatment of acne vulgaris. Triaz 3% gel contains benzoyl peroxide USP 3% as the active ingredient in a gel-based formulation consisting of purified water USP, C12–15 alkyl benzoate, glycerin USP, cetearyl alcohol, polyacrylamide (and) C13–14 isoparaffin (and) laureth-7, glyceryl stearate (and) PEG-100 stearate, steareth-2, steareth-20, dimethicone, glycolic acid, zinc lactate, lactic acid USP, edetate disodium USP, sodium hydroxide NF.
- Trileptal® (oxcarbazepine) is available as a 300 mg/5 mL (60 mg/mL) oral suspension contains the following inactive ingredients: ascorbic acid, dispersible cellulose, ethanol, macrogol stearate, methyl parahydroxybenzoate, propylene glycol, propyl parahydroxybenzoate, purified water, sodium saccharin, sorbic acid, sorbitol, yellow-plum-lemon aroma.
- Tussionex, each teaspoonful (5 mL) of Tussionex Pennkinetic extended-release suspension contains hydrocodone polistirex equivalent to 10 mg of hydrocodone bitartrate and chlorpheniramine polistirex equivalent to 8 mg of chlorpheniramine maleate. Hydrocodone polistirex: sulfonated styrene-divinylbenzene copolymer complex with 4, 5(alpha)-epoxy-3-methoxy-17-methylmorphinan-6-one. Chlorpheniramine polistirex: sulfonated styrene-divinylbenzene copolymer complex with 2-[p-chloro-(alpha)-[2-(dimethylamino)ethyl]-benzyl]pyridine. Inactive ingredients: ascorbic acid, D&C yellow No. 10, ethylcellulose, FD&C yellow No. 6, flavor, high fructose corn syrup, methyl paraben, polyethylene glycol 3350, polysorbate 80, pregelatinized starch, propylene glycol, propyl paraben, purified water, sucrose, vegetable oil, xanthan gum.
- Zmax (azithromycin extended release) for oral suspension contains the active ingredient azithromycin (as azithromycin dihydrate). Zmax is a single-dose, extended release formulation of microspheres for oral suspension containing azithromycin (as azithromycin dihydrate) and the following excipients: glyceryl behenate, poloxamer 407, sucrose, sodium phosphate tribasic anhydrous, magnesium hydroxide, hydroxypropyl cellulose, xanthan gum, colloidal silicon dioxide, titanium dioxide, artificial cherry flavor, and artificial banana flavor. Each bottle contains azithromycin dihydrate equivalent to 2 g of azithromycin. It is constituted with 60 mL of water and the entire contents are administered orally as a single dose.
- Zoloft oral concentrate is available in a multidose 60 mL bottle. Each milliliter of solution contains sertraline hydrochloride equivalent to 20 mg of sertraline. The solution contains the following inactive ingredients: glycerin, alcohol (12%), menthol, butylated hydroxytoluene (BHT).
- Zomig® (zolmitriptan) nasal spray contains zolmitriptan is supplied as a clear to pale yellow solution of zolmitriptan, buffered to a pH 5. Each Zomig nasal spray contains 5 mg of zolmitriptan in a 100-μL unit dose aqueous buffered solution containing citric acid, anhydrous USP, disodium phosphate dodecahydrate USP, and purified water USP. Zomig nasal spray is hypertonic. The osmolarity of Zomig nasal spray 5 mg is 420 to 470 mOsmol.
- Zyrtec syrup is a colorless to slightly yellow syrup containing cetirizine hydrochloride at a concentration of 1 mg/mL (5 mg/5 mL) for oral administration. The pH is between 4 and 5. The inactive ingredients of the syrup are banana flavor, glacial acetic acid, glycerin, grape flavor, methyl paraben, propylene glycol, propyl paraben, sodium acetate, sugar syrup, and water.

Index